GREEN'S CHILD AND ADOLESCENT CLINICAL PSYCHOPHARMACOLOGY

GREEN'S CHILD AND ADOLESCENT CLINICAL PSYCHOPHARMACOLOGY

5TH EDITION

WILLIAM M. KLYKYLO, AM, MD
Professor and Director
Division of Child and Adolescent Psychiatry
Wright State University Boonshoft
    School of Medicine
Dayton, Ohio

CHRISTINA WESTON, MD
Associate Professor
Division of Child and Adolescent Psychiatry
Wright State University Boonshoft
    School of Medicine
Dayton, Ohio

RICK BOWERS, MD
Clinical Associate Professor
Division of Child and Adolescent Psychiatry
Wright State University Boonshoft
    School of Medicine
Dayton, Ohio

JULIA JACKSON, MD
Assistant Professor
Division of Child and Adolescent Psychiatry
Wright State University Boonshoft
    School of Medicine
Dayton, Ohio

Wolters Kluwer | Lippincott Williams & Wilkins
Health

Philadelphia • Baltimore • New York • London
Buenos Aires • Hong Kong • Sydney • Tokyo

Acquisitions Editor: Julie Goolsby
Product Manager: Tom Gibbons
Vendor Manager: Alicia Jackson
Senior Manufacturing Manager: Beth Welsh
Marketing Manager: Alexander Burns
Design Coordinator: Steve Druding
Production Service: S4Carlisle Publishing Services

Printed in China

Library of Congress Cataloging-in-Publication Data

Klykylo, William M., author.
  Green's child and adolescent clinical psychopharmacology / William M. Klykylo.—Fifth edition.
    p. ; cm.
  Child and adolescent clinical psychopharmacology
  Preceded by Child and adolescent clinical psychopharmacology / Wayne Hugo Green. 4th ed. c2007.
  Includes bibliographical references and index.
  ISBN 978-1-4511-0714-2—ISBN 1-4511-0714-5
  I. Green, Wayne H. Child and adolescent clinical psychopharmacology. Preceded by (work):
II. Title.   III. Title: Child and adolescent clinical psychopharmacology.
  [DNLM: 1. Mental Disorders—drug therapy.   2. Adolescent.   3. Child.   4. Psychopharmacology—methods.   5. Psychotropic Drugs—therapeutic use. WS 350.2]
  RC483
  616.89'18—dc23
                                                                            2013018393

Care has been taken to confirm the accuracy of the information presented and to describe generally accepted practices. However, the authors, editors, and publisher are not responsible for errors or omissions or for any consequences from application of the information in this book and make no warranty, expressed or implied, with respect to the currency, completeness, or accuracy of the contents of the publication. Application of the information in a particular situation remains the professional responsibility of the practitioner.

The authors, editors, and publisher have exerted every effort to ensure that drug selection and dosage set forth in this text are in accordance with current recommendations and practice at the time of publication. However, in view of ongoing research, changes in government regulations, and the constant flow of information relating to drug therapy and drug reactions, the reader is urged to check the package insert for each drug for any change in indications and dosage and for added warnings and precautions. This is particularly important when the recommended agent is a new or infrequently employed drug.

Some drugs and medical devices presented in the publication have Food and Drug Administration (FDA) clearance for limited use in restricted research settings. It is the responsibility of the health care provider to ascertain the FDA status of each drug or device planned for use in their clinical practice.

To purchase additional copies of this book, call our customer service department at (800) 638-3030 or fax orders to (301) 223-2320. International customers should call (301) 223-2300.

Visit Lippincott Williams & Wilkins on the Internet: at LWW.com. Lippincott Williams & Wilkins customer service representatives are available from 8:30 am to 6:00 pm, EST.

10 9 8 7 6 5 4 3 2 1

*To our teachers, our students, our patients,
and our families, and to Wayne Hugo Green*

Contributor

Ryan Mast, MBA, DO
Assistant Professor
Division of Child and Adolescent Psychiatry
Wright State University Boonshoft
    School of Medicine
Dayton, Ohio

Preface

It has been both a great honor and a daunting challenge to prepare a fifth edition of Wayne Hugo Green's seminal *Child and Adolescent Clinical Psychopharmacology*. Words cannot express our respect for Dr. Green's magnum opus; perhaps it is best demonstrated by our efforts as four editors to revisit what Dr. Green has done by himself through four editions. This book has exerted a major beneficial influence on the conduct of our specialty and the care of our patients, and we have endeavored to be worthy of this tradition.

We have maintained Dr. Green's attention to FDA Black Box and Bold Print warnings, as increasing evidence appears that modern psychopharmacology, despite its great benefits, is no more exempt from adversity than other medical interventions. Modern agents are not without undesirable effects in some cases, and they are never panaceas or replacements for psychosocial and educational interventions. The possibility of misadventure becomes increasingly apparent as more of these agents are administered to more children. At the same time, however, the increasing use of these medications is also an indication of their utility and promise to children. We have approached this book as we approach our clinical work, with optimism balanced by realistic expectations and clinical caution.

The general format of this book has been carried on from previous editions, but with some modifications. Notably, drugs used to enhance attentional function are now grouped together. A number of older drugs that are less commonly used today are covered in an appendix. We have done this in the interest of utility and not as a disparagement of the continued value and frequent cost-effectiveness of these agents for some patients. We have included mention of thioridazine not as endorsement but in recognition of the use of that agent by a few practitioners. Since the last edition, there has been an increase in the number of extended-release psychostimulant preparations and of new second-generation antipsychotic drugs, and these are noted herein. Child and adolescent psychopharmacology has largely been conducted on an "off-label" basis, but with evolving research, an increasing number of indications for specific drugs have been approved by the FDA, and we have recognized these. Inevitably, indications (and possible contraindications) will continue to appear after any book goes to print, and the reader is strongly encouraged to maintain currency with www.fda.gov and related sources. Finally, in view of the growing recognition of the moral as well as legal challenges related to the use of psychotropic medication in minors, we have added a section on the ethics of psychopharmacology.

We hope that this edition will continue the book's tradition of authority and utility. Whatever its merits, preparing it required the help of many others. Dr. Green has been personally supportive, and we would not have undertaken this project without his kind encouragement. The staff of Lippincott Williams & Wilkins, most notably Tom Gibbons, have made our work pleasurable through their encouragement, advice, and patience. Here at Wright State University, Megan Schwartz assisted with research and Elizabeth Huber employed her very considerable editorial abilities in organizing our texts and references. No such work as this could ever come about without the assistance of our colleagues and the tolerance of our families, to whom we are forever in debt.

WMK, RB, CGW, JJ

Preface to the First Edition

This book is written with the conviction that proper psychiatric treatment of children and adolescents will, on some occasions, necessitate the use of psychopharmacotherapy. It is not intended to suggest that psychopharmacotherapy is warranted for most patients in this age group.

Most children and adolescents seen in private practices and in mental hygiene clinics do not require medication. Indeed, medication is not appropriate for many patients of this age group seen on inpatient psychiatric services.

Clinicians who administer psychoactive medication to children and adolescents will almost certainly encounter individuals with strong viewpoints on this treatment. Some are convinced that drugs are the answer to a child's or adolescent's problem. Others are equally certain that drugs are an anathema and ought to be avoided at all costs.

In this second, antidrug group, two lines of reasoning seem to appear with regularity in a significant minority of cases.

Some health and educational professionals working with children and adolescents maintain that in the face of compelling psychological explanations for a mental disorder, or for significant contributions to it, drugs should not be used. This group argues that drugs may have inimical effects and, further, that psychotherapy alone should be able to do the job.

A few professionals, but more often parents and relatives, offer a variation on this theme. They believe drugs should be avoided because the drugs will make their children "zombies" or "dope them up" or "make them become drug addicts later on."

The author's point of view is that the etiology of virtually all psychiatric disorders is multiply determined. Each individual case must be fully assessed and evaluated for the potential benefits and risks of administering a specific medication. In those cases where potential benefits appear to significantly outweigh risks, usually a trial of medication is indicated.

Still, extreme caution is required in employing psychoactive medications. The long-term effects of psychoactive medications on the maturation and development of children and adolescents are at best only partially known, and many of their known untoward effects are potentially harmful.

But when a mental illness is delaying or disrupting the maturation and development of a patient, effective medication may aid considerably in bringing about more normal development and socialization. The medication often will augment the patient's ability to respond to other treatment modalities as well.

The clinician must successfully negotiate among these conflicting viewpoints and objectives in order to undertake a clinical trial of a psychoactive drug in a reasonably favorable or at least dispassionately neutral atmosphere.

Time and reality are two extremely important factors often overlooked by critics of psychopharmacotherapy. In deciding about medication, it is essential to employ a realizable goal, not some unattainable ideal.

For example, a latency-age child is diagnosed with a conduct disorder and attention-deficit hyperactivity disorder. School officials threaten to suspend the child, with eventual placement in a special education class for children with behavioral problems.

In many such cases, an argument can be made that the child's problems are primarily psychological, that they could be helped by tutoring and individual and family therapies, and that medication should be withheld.

However, the realities of the case and the time frame for behavior change may call for trying medication. It may be exceedingly difficult to engage and work with the parents and the child. The child's symptoms may not have responded to the initial evaluation and intervention. The attitude of the school officials may be that the child's behavior must improve quickly.

In a situation such as this, if psychopharmacotherapy is likely to significantly hasten the therapeutic response to other treatments, or to prevent the patient from being removed from the regular classroom, the author recommends a trial of medication, unless other compelling factors are involved.

This book provides a framework for making an informed decision to undertake a clinical trial of a psychoactive medication and guides the clinician through the myriad issues involved in that decision.

Wayne Hugo Green, MD

Contents

SECTION ONE

General Principles

Introduction

WILLIAM KLYKYLO

The fifth edition of *Child and Adolescent Clinical Psychopharmacology* is an update of Wayne H. Green's seminal work and bears his strong influence. As in the previous editions, this book will review selected topics and most drugs used in child and adolescent psychopharmacology from a practical, clinically oriented perspective. It is intended primarily for clinicians actively engaged in treating children and adolescents with psychoactive medications. These include child psychiatrists, pediatricians, family physicians, residents in child and adolescent psychiatry, residents in general psychiatry, pediatric residents, and other health care professionals who may prescribe drugs to patients in this age group. In addition, other clinicians and mental health personnel who work with children receiving psychoactive medication may wish to review the medications their patients are receiving, as may some parents/caregivers of such children.

The first part of the book focuses rather intensively on the general principles of psychopharmacotherapy for children and adolescents. This section, although updated by the current editors, is unabashedly derivative of Dr. Green's work, restating his enduring standards. The reader is presented with a clinically useful way of thinking about psychopharmacotherapy, beginning with the initial clinical contact and continuing through the psychiatric evaluation, psychodynamic formulation, diagnosis, and development of the treatment plan. For those cases in which psychoactive medication is recommended as a part of the treatment plan, the necessary medicolegal responsibilities of the clinician in introducing and explaining the purpose of medication to the relevant caretakers and the patient, steps to obtain informed consent and assent to administer medication, ways of maximizing the chances of the legal guardian's and patient's acceptance of a trial of the medication and cooperation with its administration, and the necessary documentation of these facts in the clinical record are reviewed. Following this, the entire process of administering medication is discussed. This begins with a consideration of which drug to choose for the initial trial of medication and subsequent medications, should the first choice(s) not result in adequate clinical improvement. Examples of algorithms, which are often helpful in medicating complicated clinical cases, are also included. The necessary documentation of target symptoms and any baseline behavioral ratings that will be useful in assessing clinical response or the development of untoward effects and the baseline physical and laboratory assessments to be selected are then discussed. This part of the book ends with a detailed presentation of the principles of administering psychoactive medication from the initial dose, through titration and determining the optimal dose, to maintenance therapy, duration of treatment, and issues in terminating medication. These principles are generalizable and provide clinical guidelines for selecting and administering any psychoactive medication to children and adolescents.

The second portion of the book begins with a short chapter discussing the history of child psychopharmacology and some issues concerning psychopharmacological research in children and adolescents. The purpose of this review is to remind the reader where the information that follows is placed in the history of child psychopharmacology and of the importance of research and a critical assessment of the presented data for informed clinical practice.

After these brief introductory comments, the remainder of Section II focuses on specific psychopharmacological agents that are presently the most important in the clinical practice of child and adolescent psychiatry. This section necessarily is more extensively modified than is the first. The drugs are presented by their class. Many specific psychoactive medications are presently used to treat diverse psychiatric disorders or symptoms across psychiatric diagnoses (e.g., lithium for its antiaggressive effects), and this method of organization avoids repeating similar information under several diagnoses. In exception to this rule, one agent, topiramate, is treated twice, because of the two particularly divergent uses for it.

As we learn more about the etiopathogenesis of psychiatric disorders, it becomes increasingly useful and important, both scientifically and clinically, to think about how drugs affect basic neurotransmitter and psychoneuroendocrine functioning across diagnoses. Drugs may affect one or more neurotransmitter systems. For example, the atypical or second-generation antipsychotics have a very complex mixture of pharmacologic properties. They primarily influence not only the dopamine and serotonin systems as antagonists but also the noradrenergic and cholinergic systems and have antihistaminic and other properties (Stahl, 2000). Likewise, a specific neurotransmitter system may be important in one or more diagnostic categories. For example, there appears to be a relationship between the serotonergic system's functioning and aggressive or violent behavior and self-destructive behavior among various diagnostic groups (Linnoila et al., 1989; Mann et al., 1989). Several books devoted solely to the behavioral pharmacology of serotonin have been published (e.g., Bevan et al., 1989; Brown and van Praag, 1991; Coccaro and Murphy, 1990).

As might be expected in a clinically oriented book, the standard, often older, psychopharmacological treatments established by investigational and clinical studies as both efficacious and safe for use in children and adolescents and approved by the U.S. Food and Drug Administration (FDA) for advertising as such are still included. The literature reviews determining the efficacy of these treatments, however, are kept to a minimum, and in some cases placed in appendices, because comprehensive reviews are readily available elsewhere. (For the interested reader, a list of such additional readings is given in Chapter 3 of Section II.)

It is important to note that currently many first-line drugs prescribed to treat psychiatric disorders in children and adolescents are off-label/not FDA approved for the age or indication or both, although they are FDA approved for older individuals, usually adults, and for a more limited range of indications. This is because these newer drugs are often more effective or have fewer or less serious untoward/adverse effects, or both, than older FDA-approved drugs. For example, the selective serotonin reuptake inhibitor (SSRI) antidepressants and the atypical/second-generation antipsychotics were more frequently prescribed for non–FDA-approved indications in children and adolescents than the FDA-approved drugs, even prior to their approval in some cases. It is also interesting to note that the tricyclic antidepressants, which have been surpassed by the SSRIs in the total number of prescriptions written, were not approved for use in treating depression in children below age 12, even after fluoxetine, an SSRI, received approval for use in children aged 7 years and older. Medications that appear to be likely candidates for eventual FDA approval (if the necessary studies were funded and carried out) or which are beginning to be used in standard practice are emphasized. Because reviews of these medications are usually less readily available and some studies are very recent, relevant studies are summarized here. Although this emphasis on the literature of studies of drugs used for non–FDA-approved or off-label indications over FDA-approved drugs may seem paradoxical, it is deliberate and reflects current clinical practice. This is because a major difficulty occurs when patients do not respond with sufficient amelioration of symptoms to FDA-approved pharmacological treatments currently available, or even more importantly, no FDA-approved drug is approved for the treatment indication, or untoward effects prevent the drug's use in adequate doses. When the patient's symptoms prevent him or her from functioning in a psychosocial environment that will facilitate normal growth, maturation, and development, many clinicians use FDA-approved drugs for non–FDA-approved indications to treat their patients. Although this book does not proselytize for the use of medication for non–FDA-approved uses, it does present the clinician with possible alternative treatments for patients who are resistant to standard pharmacological treatments. In fact, the use of many of these medications for off-label indications is medically accepted in standard clinical practice, for example, the use of methylphenidate preparations in children below 6 years of age. As with FDA-approved treatments, the physician must consider, perhaps even more carefully, the risks versus the potential benefits of using any medication for non–FDA-approved indications. Medicolegal, ethical, and some practical issues of using drugs for non–FDA-approved indications are considered in appropriate sections of the book.

We emphasize that no book can substitute for a careful reading of the FDA-approved labeling (manufacturer's labeling/package insert) which contains additional information on all FDA-approved medications discussed in this book, unless it reprints them verbatim. No drug should be prescribed without the physician's having read and become familiar with its labeling information; to do so is a disservice to one's patient and renders one vulnerable to professional liability. This information, however, focuses on the drug's use for indications approved by the FDA and for many psychotropic drugs, there is little about the drug's use for non-approved indications in children and adolescents.

The package insert for many drugs is reprinted verbatim in the current *Physicians' Desk Reference* (PDR) and its supplements. The reader is reminded that the PDR, although convenient, includes products primarily marketed by their trade names. Once exclusive manufacturing rights have expired and the drug is marketed primarily or solely as a generic preparations, the PDR usually lists the drug with only the company of manufacture and dose forms available without giving detailed prescribing information. How this affects the prescribing practices of physicians to whom the PDR is distributed free of charge would be interesting to study. To obtain such information about older drugs such as chlorpromazine (Thorazine) or imipramine (Tofranil), one has to consult a source such as *Drug Information for the Health Care Professional, Volume 1* (United States Pharmacopeial Dispensing Information, 2005), a current psychopharmacology textbook, or the Web.

General Principles of Psychopharmacotherapy with Children and Adolescents

WILLIAM KLYKYLO

PSYCHIATRIC DIAGNOSIS AND PSYCHOPHARMACOTHERAPY

Psychopharmacotherapy should always be part of a comprehensive treatment plan arrived at after a thorough psychiatric evaluation that results in a diagnosis, or at least a working diagnosis. It is scientifically indefensible to initiate treatment without first attempting to formulate as clear an understanding of the clinical picture as possible. This will enable clinicians to institute the most appropriate and rational treatment(s) available in their therapeutic armamentaria for the situation at hand.

Current Psychiatric Diagnostic Nomenclature

A major difficulty with the official American Psychiatric Association (APA) nomenclature, the *Diagnostic and Statistical Manual of Mental Disorders*, Fourth Edition, Text Revision (DSM-IV-TR) (APA, 2000), and indeed with most current psychiatric nomenclatures, is that etiology is not usually taken into account in formulating a diagnosis. One reason for this is that, at our present state of knowledge, we do not know the etiologies of many conditions. Hence, we are often treating specific constellations of behavioral symptoms without adequately understanding their biological and genetic underpinnings and how they interact with their psychosocial and physical environments. For example, autistic disorder is not etiologically homogeneous but has a multitude of causes.

Theoretically, for a given psychiatric disorder, drugs may be effective by correcting the condition(s) leading to it (or them) or by influencing events somewhere along the usually complex pathways between the hypothesized abnormality(ies) and its subsequent psychological and/or behavioral consequences. Therefore, some psychoactive drugs may be effective in several dissimilar disorders because they influence or modify neurotransmitters and psychoneuroendocrine events in the brain along or near the end of these interacting, partially confluent, or final common pathways. Current research suggests that there are genetic bases for these phenomena (Cross-Disorder Group, 2013).

Other psychoactive drugs appear to exert their therapeutic effects through entirely different mechanisms in different diagnostic entities—for example, imipramine in depression, attention-deficit/hyperactivity disorder (ADHD), and enuresis.

Some patients with a specific diagnosis (e.g., ADHD, autistic disorder, or schizophrenia) will not have a satisfactory clinical response or will be refractory to a specific drug—even one known to be highly effective in statistically significant double-blind studies—or will even have a worsening of symptoms. This may reflect differences in genetic makeup or other biologically determined conditions, psychosocial environments, and/or internalized conflicts and the contributions each makes to the etiopathogenesis of each patient's psychiatric disorder.

Although diagnostic issues are not discussed specifically in this book, it is emphasized that an accurate diagnosis is of critical importance in choosing the correct medication. At times, the lack of expected clinical response to a medication should suggest to the clinician the possibility of an incorrect diagnosis and that a careful diagnostic reconsideration should be undertaken.

Other unfortunate clinical consequences may result from incorrect diagnoses. For example, antidepressants may precipitate an acute psychotic reaction when given to some individuals with schizophrenic disorder. Stimulant medications, too, may precipitate psychosis when given in sufficient doses to some children or adolescents with borderline personalities or unrecognized schizophrenia.

Wender (1988) noted that clinical experience suggested that some children diagnosed with ADHD were treated with stimulants and rapidly developed tolerance to them but were actually suffering from a major depressive disorder and that they responded to treatment with tricyclic antidepressants with remarkable improvement.

Changing diagnostic criteria may also complicate matters. For example, some of the controversy regarding the efficacy of stimulants in patients with development disabilities may have resulted from diagnostic issues. Until the publication of DSM-II (APA, 1968), there was no specific APA diagnosis for what was commonly known as the hyperactive child. There were various labels for this condition, including *hyperactive child, hyperkinetic syndrome, minimal brain dysfunction* (MBD), and *minimal cerebral dysfunction*. Intellectual disability was considered evidence of more than "minimal" dysfunction, and the various etiologies were thought to be biological. Because of this concept, children with intellectual disabilities were excluded from the possibility of receiving a codiagnosis of MBD, hyperactive child, or an equivalent diagnosis, and some clinicians may not have tried stimulant medication in their patients who had even mild disabilities.

The situation changed with the publication of DSM-II, which noted that "in children, mild brain damage often manifests itself by hyperactivity, short attention span, easy distractibility, and impulsiveness" (APA, 1968, p. 31). It also suggested that unless there are significant interactional factors (e.g., between child and parents) that appear to be responsible for these behaviors, the disorder should be classified as a nonpsychotic, organic brain syndrome and not as a behavior disorder.

In DSM-III (APA, 1980a), the diagnosis of attention-deficit disorder with hyperactivity (ADDH) was based on the presence of a specific constellation of symptoms, and no etiology was hypothesized. Hence, children of any intelligence could exhibit such features. DSM-III additionally notes that mild or moderate mental retardation may predispose one to the development of ADDH and that the addition of this diagnosis to the severely and profoundly retarded child is not clinically useful because these symptoms are often an inherent part of the condition.

DSM-III-R redefines ADDH somewhat, renames it (ADHD), and refines its relation with mental retardation. It notes that many features of ADHD may be present in mentally retarded people because of the generalized delays in intellectual development. DSM-III-R (APA, 1987), DSM-IV (APA, 1994), and DSM-IV-TR (APA, 2000) note that a child or adolescent with an intellectual disability should be additionally diagnosed with ADHD only if the relevant symptoms significantly exceed those that are compatible with the child's or adolescent's mental age. These changes in diagnostic criteria, although directed toward greater precision in identification and classification of disorders, have often complicated the process of treatment planning for clinicians.

DIAGNOSIS AND TARGET SYMPTOMS

In making the decision about which psychoactive medication to select initially, two major issues should be addressed: diagnosis and target symptoms. Both are important and are often interrelated. It is important to make the most accurate diagnosis possible using the available data and to identify and quantify target symptoms in order to choose an efficacious drug and to assess the results of medication. The target symptoms must be of sufficient severity and must interfere so significantly with the child's or adolescent's current functioning and future maturation and development that the potential benefits of the drug will justify the risks concomitant with its administration.

The initial medication may be chosen with respect to either diagnosis or target symptoms or both. Sometimes the decision is not difficult because the same medication is appropriate for both the target symptoms and the diagnosis. For example, antipsychotics are the drugs of first choice for treating schizophrenia and are appropriate for most of the significant target symptoms (e.g., hallucinations, thought disorder, and delusions). The symptom "hyperactivity," however, is present in numerous childhood psychiatric disorders, but all hyperactivity is not the same (Fish, 1971). The clinician should be fully aware of the diagnosis in treating this symptom. Hyperactivity in a youngster with ADHD would be expected to respond favorably to the administration of a stimulant, whereas a schizophrenic youngster who is in relative remission but exhibits marked hyperactivity would have a risk of having his or her psychotic symptoms reexacerbated if stimulant medication were used. Stimulant drugs, the drugs of choice in ADHD, are sometimes considered to be relatively contraindicated in schizophrenia and may cause worsening of psychotic symptoms. More recently, however, clinicians have prescribed stimulants to psychotic children who are being maintained on antipsychotic medication but have the remaining symptoms of hyperactivity, distractibility, and inattention, with resulting further clinical improvement.

Medication can also be prescribed to treat specific diagnoses. Lithium, for example, has a certain specificity for treatment of mania in patients diagnosed with bipolar disorder, manic, but also appears to have an antiaggressive action that cuts across various diagnoses. Lithium has been used effectively to treat aggression directed against others or self-injurious behavior in children and adolescents diagnosed with conduct disorder, mental retardation with disturbance of behavior, and autistic disorder.

SPECIAL ASPECTS OF CHILD PSYCHOPHARMACOTHERAPY
Maturational/Developmental Issues
Physiologic Factors

The relation between biological developmental issues and psychopharmacotherapy has been long recognized and emphasized by Popper (1987b), Geller (1991), and many other authors. Children and adolescents may require larger doses of psychoactive medication per unit of body weight compared with adults to attain similar blood levels and therapeutic efficacy. It is usually assumed that two factors explain this situation: more rapid metabolism by the liver and an increased glomerular filtration rate in children compared with that in adults. The latter suggests a greater renal clearance for some drugs, including lithium, which helps in explaining the fact that therapeutic dosages of lithium in children usually do not differ from those in adults (Campbell et al., 1984a).

Teicher and Baldessarini (1987) pointed out that children may respond to drugs differently compared with adults because of pharmacodynamic factors (drug-effector mechanisms) that are caused by developmental changes in neural pathways or their functions (e.g., Geller et al. [1992] reported that prepubescent subjects treated with the tricyclic antidepressant nortriptyline reported almost no anticholinergic adverse effects; especially noteworthy was the lack of any prominent dry mouth frequently reported by adults) or because of pharmacokinetic factors caused by developmental changes in the distribution, metabolism, or excretion of a drug.

Jatlow (1987) has noted that, although the rapid rate of drug disposition may decrease gradually throughout childhood, there may be an abrupt decline around puberty. Drug disposition usually reaches adult levels by middle to late adolescence. Clinically, this would indicate that the clinician should be especially alert to possible changes in pharmacokinetics during the time period around puberty and be ready to adjust dose levels if necessary. When they are available, it may be useful to obtain plasma concentration levels if there appears to be a change in the clinical efficacy of a drug as a child matures into an adolescent.

Puig-Antich (1987) summarized some of the evidence that catecholamine (norepinephrine, epinephrine, and dopamine) systems are not fully anatomically developed and operationally functional until adulthood. The fact that younger children may respond to stimulant medication differently from older adolescents and adults may be explained by the immaturity of the catecholamine systems (Puig-Antich, 1987); they can also be considered to result from developmental pharmacodynamic factors.

The pharmacokinetics of many drugs have been observed to change over the course of life. For example, children and adolescents below 15 years of age treated with clomipramine had significantly lower steady-state plasma concentrations for a given dose than did adults (*Physicians' Desk Reference* [PDR], 1990). Rivera-Calimlim et al. (1979) reported that children and adolescents 8 to 15 years of age required larger doses of chlorpromazine than those required by adults to attain similar plasma concentrations.

There may also be differences between acute and chronic pharmacokinetics. For example, Rivera-Calimlim et al. (1979) reported a decline in plasma chlorpromazine levels in most of their child and adolescent patients who were on a fixed dose and suggested it might be due to autoinduction of metabolic enzymes for chlorpromazine during long-term treatment, as had been previously reported in adults. The consequences of autoinduction and its cellular basis have been extensively reported (Bonate and Howard, 2005).

A clear relationship between plasma concentrations and clinical response to imipramine was noted for prepubescent subjects and older adults with endogenous depression but not for adolescents and young adults (Burke and Puig-Antich, 1990). The authors hypothesized that the relatively poor clinical efficacy of tricyclic antidepressants in postpubescent adolescents and young adults compared with the clinical response of prepubescent children and older adults is secondary to a negative effect of increased sex hormone levels on the antidepressant action of imipramine.

Herskowitz (1987) reviewed the developmental neurotoxicity of pharmacoactive drugs. Developmental neurotoxicity is concerned with stage-specific, drug-induced biochemical or physiologic changes, morphologic manifestations, and behavioral symptoms. For example, stimulant medication may adversely affect normal increases in height and growth, at least temporarily, in some actively growing children and adolescents. Some psychoactive drugs taken during early pregnancy have significant potential for damaging the fetus (e.g., lithium may cause cardiac malformations).

Cognitive/Psychological/Experiential Factors

The maturation and development of the central nervous system as well as the life experiences accumulating since infancy determine much of the specific level of functioning of a given child or adolescent. Although detailed knowledge of these factors is essential to evaluate any child or adolescent psychiatrically, this book addresses only their specific relevance to psychopharmacotherapy.

In general, the younger the patient, the less the verbal facility available to convey information to the clinician and, reciprocally, the less the cognitive ability available to understand information the clinician wishes to impart. Part of the psychiatric evaluation leading to a decision that psychotropic medication is indicated will provide the clinician with an assessment of the level of the patient's ability to communicate his or her emotional status and of his or her cognitive/linguistic ability to understand the proposed treatment and reliably report the effect of the treatment.

In the very young child or the child with no communicative language, the clinician can only observe behavioral effects of medication directly or learn of them as reported by others. The younger the child, the fewer the compliments or complaints about the beneficial or adverse effects. Also, the young child has less-differentiated emotions and more limited experience with feelings and emotions and with communicating them to others than do older children. In addition, some chronically depressed or anxious children may not have had a sufficiently recent normal emotional baseline with which they can compare their present mood. Such children may experience a depressed mood as their normal, usual state of being and, therefore, do not have a normal baseline frame of reference upon which to draw in describing how they feel.

The younger the child, the less accurate his or her time estimates. Until approximately 10 years of age, concepts of long periods of time are often not easily understood. It can be very useful and at times essential to use concrete markers of time in discussing time concepts and chronology of events with children. For example, the clinician may enquire whether something occurred before or after the last birthday, specific holidays (e.g., Christmas, Thanksgiving, or Halloween), specific events (e.g., separation or divorce of parents, when the family moved to another home, an operation, a relative's death, or the birth of a sibling), the seasons or weather (e.g., winter, snow, cold, or summer, hot), or the school year (e.g., specific teacher's name or grade, or Christmas, spring or Easter, or summer vacation).

Concepts such as concentration, distractibility, and impulsivity may be beyond the understanding of some early latency-age children. Different children may use different words or expressions to mean the same concept. It is important to be certain that a child knows the meaning of a specific word and not assume an understanding because the child responds to a question. If there is any doubt, ask what something means or explain it in another way. It can be very useful to ask the same thing in several different ways.

In the final analysis, once the patient's psychopathology and his or her developmental experiential factors are taken into account, it is the quality of the relationship between the clinician and the child or adolescent that becomes paramount in determining the usefulness of information shared.

Relationship to the Patient's Family or Caregivers

Diagnosis, Formulation, and Development of the Treatment Plan

A complete psychiatric assessment, including appropriate psychological tests, resulting in a working diagnosis and comprehensive treatment plan; appropriate physical and laboratory examinations; and baseline behavioral measurements should be completed as minimum prerequisites before the initiation of psychopharmacotherapy. The treatment plan should be developed in conjunction with either the parent(s) or the primary caretaker and should include participation of the child or adolescent as appropriate to his or her understanding. Treatment with psychoactive drugs should always be part of a more comprehensive treatment regimen and is rarely appropriate as the sole treatment modality for a child or adolescent.

At variance with this traditional wisdom, however, are the results of several studies comparing the treatment of hyperactive children with stimulant medication alone versus stimulant medication combined with other interventions, such as cognitive training, attention control, social reinforcement, and parent training. A review of these studies concluded that "the additional use of various forms of psychotherapies (behavioral treatment, parent training, cognitive therapy) with stimulants has not resulted in superior outcomes than medication alone" (Klein, 1987, p. 1223). One possible factor contributing to this result is that in several studies children who were treated with methylphenidate alone showed improvement in social behavior. Following this course of treatment, adults—both parents and teachers—related to the children more positively (Klein, 1987). The Multimodal Treatment Study Group of Children with Attention-Deficit/Hyperactivity Disorder (MTA) Cooperative Group also found that stimulant medication was the most important factor in improving ADHD symptoms. This is further discussed in Chapter 4 (MTA Cooperative Group, 1999a, 1999b).

It seems clinically unlikely, however, that all the difficulties of ADHD children are secondary to the target symptoms that improve with psychostimulants. Those difficulties that result from other psychosocial problems, including psychopathological familial interactions and long-standing maladaptive behavioral patterns, would be expected to benefit from additional interventions; until it is possible to differentiate those children whose difficulties arise from their attention deficit *per se* from children whose symptoms are of multidetermined origin, a comprehensive treatment program is recommended for all children. Obviously, this same principle applies to all psychiatric disorders, regardless of their responsiveness to medications.

The legal guardian/caregiver and the child or adolescent patient, to the degree appropriate for the patient's age and psychopathology, should participate in formulating the treatment plan. The use of medication, including expected benefits and possible short- and long-term adverse effects, should be reviewed with the caregivers/parents and patient in understandable terminology. It is essential to carefully assess the attitude and reliability of the persons who will be responsible for administering the medication. Unless there is a positive or at least honestly neutral attitude toward medication and some therapeutic alliance with the parents, it will be difficult or infeasible to make a reliable assessment of drug efficacy and compliance. Likewise, to store and administer medication safely on an outpatient basis requires a responsible adult, especially if there are young children in the home or if the patient is at risk of suicide.

It should be explained to parents that, even if medication helps some biologically determined symptoms (e.g., in some cases of ADHD), the disorder's presence may have caused psychological difficulties in the child or adolescent as well as disturbances in familial and social relationships. Controlling or ameliorating the biological difficulty does not usually correct the long-standing internalized psychological or interpersonal problems and long-standing maladaptive patterns of behavior immediately. Resolving these difficulties will take time and may often require concomitant individual, group, family, or other therapeutic intervention.

Compliance

Compliance is an issue of particular importance in child and adolescent psychiatry. Because the parents or other caretakers are usually interposed between the physician and patient, compliance is somewhat more complex than in adult psychiatry, in which the patient usually relates directly to the physician.

Obviously, for psychopharmacotherapy to be effective in the disorder for which it is prescribed, the drug should be taken following the prescribed directions. Erratic compliance or running out of medication may cause the patient to undergo what is in effect an abrupt withdrawal of medication. Withdrawal syndromes may sometimes be confused with adverse effects, worsening of the clinical condition, or inadequate medication levels. In some cases, such as when an antipsychotic is used, the patient is at increased risk for an acute dystonic reaction if the physician starts at the optimal dose after the drug has been discontinued for several days or more. In addition, when medication is stopped, it may sometimes require a higher dose of medication to regain the same degree of symptom control. For example, Sleator et al. (1974) found that 7 of 28 hyperactive children who showed clinical worsening during a month-long placebo period after having received methylphenidate for 1 to 2 years required an increase in dose to regain their original clinical improvement. Hence, it is very important to emphasize to parents that running out of medication is to be avoided.

Many factors may interfere with compliance. Some parents will at times withhold medication if their child appears to be doing well, or, conversely, increase the medication without the physician's approval if behavior worsens, or even administer the drug to the child as a punishment.

When parents or legal guardians seek treatment for their children primarily because of pressure from others such as a school, a child welfare agency, or a court, there may be considerable resistance to both treatment and medication. Some of these parents may delay filling the prescription, lose it, or simply not fill it. Other parents consider it something to be done when convenient, especially if they have to travel any distance to get the prescription filled. If money is involved, even the amount necessary for travel to the pharmacy or to pay for the medication, some families, especially those on public assistance or very limited budgets, may have to delay purchasing the medication for legitimate financial reasons. These issues may come into play each time the prescription is renewed; additionally, it is common in many clinics for parents to miss appointments, including those when medication is to be renewed.

At times, some children and adolescents, both outpatients and inpatients, may actively try to avoid ingesting medication. Their techniques include pretending to place the pill in their mouths and later discarding it, and placing the pill under the tongue or between teeth and the cheek when swallowing and later spitting it out. Compliance in these cases may be improved if the person administering the medication observes it in the mouth and watches the patient swallow it. Crushing the medication may be helpful in some cases, but one must be certain that absorption rates will not be so significantly altered as to cause decreased clinical efficacy or adverse or toxic effects. If available, switching to a liquid form of the drug may be indicated for some patients.

Another factor that influences compliance, particularly in older children and adolescents, is related to adverse effects. For example, if they feel "funny" or different or if they develop a stomachache, they may be more reluctant to take medication. Adolescents may be especially sensitive to adverse effects affecting their sexual functioning. The more responsible a child or adolescent is for administering his or her own medication, the more likely, in general, that unpleasant, adverse effects will interfere with compliance. Richardson et al. (1991) reported that children and adolescents who developed parkinsonism while receiving neuroleptics were very aware of the symptoms and described them as "zombie-like" and a reason for noncompliance with outpatient treatment. These and other adverse effects can have similar influences on children and adolescents.

Noncompliance may be lessened sometimes if an adequate, understandable explanation of the simple pharmacokinetics of the drug is given to parents and patients when initially discussing medication. For example, the importance of keeping blood levels fairly constant by taking the medication as prescribed can be emphasized and reviewed again if lack of compliance becomes important. Conversely, when parents continue to sabotage treatment consciously, unconsciously, because of their own psychopathology, or for other reasons, and this behavior seriously interferes with the psychiatric treatment of a child or adolescent, it may be necessary to report the patient to a government agency as a case of medical neglect and request legal intervention. Likewise, it may be necessary to discontinue medication if compliance is very poor or so unacceptably erratic as to be potentially dangerous.

Explaining Medication to the Child or Adolescent

The clinician should discuss the medication with the child or adolescent as appropriate to the patient's psychopathology and ability to understand. Giving the patient an opportunity to participate in his or her treatment is helpful for many reasons.

The patient can feel like an active partner in the treatment. This can alleviate feelings of passivity (i.e., that treatment is something over which the patient has no control). Letting the patient know that he or she should pay attention to the effects of the medication in order to report them to the therapist, that the patient will be listened to, and that the information the patient conveys will be considered seriously in regulating the medicine also helps the therapeutic relationship. The patient can also be informed that although medication may provide some relief or help, it cannot do everything, and he or she must still contribute effort toward reaching the treatment goals. This can be particularly important during adolescence, when issues of autonomy and control over one's own body are normal developmental concerns.

Because the patient is experiencing firsthand the disorder being treated, in many cases valuable information necessary for regulating the medication can be obtained directly. Some fairly young children can express whether the medicine makes them feel better, more calm, or quiet; less mad or less like fighting; happier or sadder; less afraid, upset, nervous, or anxious; or worse, sleepy, tired, more bored, "madder," or harder to get along with; and so on. Although parents or caretakers can provide much useful information, they may be unaware of some information that the patient can provide if time is taken to learn the words or expressions that the child uses to communicate feelings and experiences.

Adverse effects should be explained so that the child or adolescent understands them. The patient's awareness that adverse effects may be transient (e.g., that tolerance for sedation may develop) or reversible with dose reduction may be helpful in gaining cooperation during the titration period. Foreknowledge also increases the sense of control and can decrease fear of some adverse effects. For example, if an acute dystonic reaction is a possibility, it is important to realize how frightening this can be to some patients (and their parents). Explaining beforehand that if this reaction occurs, medicine will help, and the condition will go away can make the experience less frightening. Also, if a rapidly effective oral medication such as diphenhydramine, an antihistamine with anticholinergic properties, is made available and patients and parents are aware of what is happening, the medication may be administered earlier in the process, frequently aborting a potentially more severe reaction.

Children who ride bicycles and adolescents who drive a car, motor bike, or motorcycle, or operate potentially dangerous machinery should be cautioned if a medication may cause sedation or other impairment. They should be told to wait until they are sure how they are reacting to the medication before engaging in these activities. Similarly, if an adolescent is likely to use alcohol or other psychoactive drugs, he or she should be warned of possible additive or other adverse effects. Drugs like monoamine oxidase inhibitors are too risky to recommend except in very cooperative patients who are able to follow the necessary strict dietary restrictions to avoid a potential hypertensive crisis.

Medicolegal Aspects of Medicating Children and Adolescents

Medicolegal issues usually involve concerns about the clinician's clinical competence or performance. These issues arise primarily when something goes wrong. Incidentally, that "wrong something" may have nothing to do with the clinician's specific treatment or competence but may, for example, be an outcome that displeases the patient or guardian. Even then, for a medicolegal issue to arise, someone who has become aware of it must decide to pursue the matter legally.

The importance of these issues is that the clinician's relationship with the patient and his or her family or caretakers can either increase or decrease the likelihood of legal proceedings. As a general rule, the better the quality of the relationship and rapport between the physician and the patient and his or her family, the less is the likelihood for legal proceedings to occur. Parents who are angry at their child's physician, who feel neglected or not cared about, are more likely to institute legal proceedings. Taking time to explain what the medicine may and may not do is important; no medication can be guaranteed to be clinically effective and safe for every patient.

If there is a risk that a depressed patient may attempt suicide but the patient is not hospitalized, this should be discussed with all concerned parties. Public perception of the association of suicidal ideation with a number of psychotropic agents has intensified the importance of these concerns. The patient may be asked to commit verbally or in writing to a contract to contact the clinician before any attempt to take his or her own life. Legal guardians should be informed of and concur with the decision that their child or ward will not be hospitalized and that, although there is a risk, the degree of risk is acceptable to avoid hospitalization. The guardians should be asked to provide more formal supervision until the depression improves sufficiently. If such measures are carried out and documented and a working rapport established, the risk of legal action and/or liability will be lessened should a suicide attempt, successful or otherwise, occur.

The clinician should make a genuine effort to establish a working rapport with parents who have consented under duress to the treatment of their child or adolescent (e.g., if their child has been removed from their care by a governmental agency because of abuse or neglect or where medication may be a prerequisite for remaining in a particular educational program), although this is frequently difficult.

Holzer (1989) noted that most, if not all, malpractice claims occur in cases with either an unexpected clinical outcome or an event that is perceived by the patient (or parents) as avoidable or preventable. The aspects of psychopharmacotherapy that have potential for medicolegal implications parallel this book's entire section on general principles of psychopharmacotherapy. Lawsuits are most frequently brought if something is omitted or if something goes wrong that could reasonably have been prevented. It should be emphasized that proper documentation in the clinical record is essential. If this is not done, the clinician's position is precarious if legal difficulties arise. The ascendancy of electronic health records (EHRs) has made it possible for physicians to document more fully their assessments and interventions; but electronic health records have made every aspect of patient care easily discoverable. Particular areas of concern are discussed later.

For a comprehensive overview of malpractice issues in child psychiatric practice, see Benedek et al. (2010).

Ethical Issues in Child and Adolescent Psychopharmacology

Ethical concerns are paramount in the practice of psychiatry, and especially with children, because of their inherent vulnerability and their special reliance upon others and their environment. Contemporary medical ethics rests upon a set of major principles (Veatch, 1991): beneficence, maleficence, autonomy, veracity, fidelity, and avoidance of killing. These principles are often designated consequentialist (beneficence and nonmaleficence—having to do with good outcome) and nonconsequentialist (having to do with inherent morality—autonomy, fidelity, veracity, avoidance of killing, and justice). Although many today assign a higher lexical ranking to the nonconsequentialist principles, this stance may be questioned in view of the vulnerability of children and their inherent lack of autonomy. In any case, it is the duty of the practitioner to recognize and balance appropriately the application of these principles.

The consequentialist principles of beneficence and nonbeneficence are usually the instinctive first consideration of clinicians. All medications that we use have both desirable and adverse effects, and each prescription represents an attempt to balance these effects for an individual patient. The history of psychopharmacology is replete with misapprehensions of these. The neuromuscular and metabolic effects of neuroleptics compared with their limited effectiveness in many off-label uses are a prime example.

Another such example would be the use of a psychostimulant in the child whose inattentive behavior in school results not from an attention deficit disorder but from a language-based learning disability. The child would demonstrate less activity when receiving the medication to the possible satisfaction of adults; however, this child would not be adequately educated, and the occurrence of dysphoria or other adverse effects might hurt the child.

It is an intrinsic duty (based on the principle of fidelity) for a physician to pursue beneficence and avoid maleficence. It is obvious that a physician can do so only with a comprehensive biopsychosocial diagnostic understanding of the child patient. The physician must also have as full a familiarity as possible with the effects of any agents to be considered. Ignorance is unethical.

The consequentialist principles present a more nuanced challenge. Avoiding killing is a clearly defined and almost universally accepted principle among physicians, despite concerns about euthanasia. Fidelity, the adherence to behavioral and professional standards, in the context of a doctor–patient relationship based on a social contract, is universally accepted. Justice in the context of medical ethics refers to the allocation of resources among a larger population; its application involves a range of political and cultural issues that are constantly debated.

Veracity in today's context requires not only the avoidance of falsehoods but the telling of the "whole truth." Two complications arise here. First of all, doctors and patients considering pharmacologic treatment face an intimidating volume of information. The pages of fine print in the *Physicians' Desk Reference* are intimidating to many patients and families and contain information of varying relevance to physicians. The full possibility of adverse effects from any agent can never be absolutely known. In this situation, physicians should offer as much information as they judge families can digest at a given time, with the added proviso that other information is available, that it can be acquired from the physician and other sources, and that no other information can be absolutely complete. At times, physicians fear that information may be daunting to families and will discourage the acceptance of beneficial agents. Parents almost always do have the autonomous right to refuse to give psychotropic agents to their children, despite the concerns of physicians. Coercion is usually unethical and seldom successful. These issues can be resolved only through communication, and the ability to communicate with authority, empathy, and clarity is as essential as skill and psychopharmacology as is scientific knowledge (Krener and Mancina, 1994).

The second complication of veracity is the cognitive level of the child patient. One must provide a clear and developmentally appropriate explanation of risks, benefits, and possible adverse effects of medication; this is important not only from an ethical standpoint but also to assure that the child can recognize positive and/or adverse effects and report them.

Autonomy is the most complicated ethical issue in child psychopharmacology. In general, parents have absolute authority in decisions related to the treatment of minor children. Concurrently, however, children, despite their intrinsically limited autonomy, are seen as having the right to assent or refuse treatment. Assent is "agreement obtained from those who are unable to enter a legal contract" (Ford et al., 2007). Dockett and Perry (2011) describe assent as "a relational process whereby children's actions and adult's responses taken together reflect children's participation in decisions"; this is an interactive process. In their masterful review, Krener and Mancina (1994) describe various models for decision making and demonstrate that autonomy in child patients, as well as compliance, is engendered by a communicative rather than an authoritative or prescriptive stance.

This same principle is obtained in addressing the autonomy of parents or guardians. In rare cases, this autonomy may be superseded by legal interventions as in overt abuse or neglect; however, this almost never occurs regarding issues of psychopharmacology. Consequently, for both ethical and pragmatic reasons, the clinician must respect the nearly total autonomy of parents. Krener and Mancina provide models and examples for decision making. In all of these cases, there is a framework of communication that is respectful, empathetic, and complete.

The most specific application of autonomy arises in informed consent. Today, most physicians are aware of the absolute necessity for documentation of informed consent to all treatments, for legal as well as ethical reasons. Informed consent involves information and voluntariness. Patients and families are provided with diagnosis, the nature and purpose of a treatment, and the risks and benefits of a proposed treatment versus alternative treatments or no treatment (AMA, 2012). These principles have become accepted throughout much of the world (Malhotra and Subodh, 2009).

A special problem that involves all the principles of ethics arises from the use of psychotropic agents in the face of inadequate or inappropriate psychosocial services and environmental settings. This most often occurs with the intent of managing or attenuating aggressive behavior. At this writing, massive public attention is being directed toward the alleged misuse or overuse of psychotropic agents, notably neuroleptics among children in foster care (Kutz, 2011). Similar concerns have been raised for children in other treatment settings (MMDLN, 2011). It is charged that these medications have been given involuntarily (autonomy) and without full information (veracity) to children. Adverse effects have arisen (nonmaleficence) with few if any concurrent benefits (beneficence). Implicit and often explicit accusations are made that these agents are used for behavioral control in the absence of appropriate environments and psychosocial treatments (justice). Clinicians involved in these issues may be overwhelmed by massive numbers of needy children and very sparse treatment resources. In certain circumstances, they may opine that medications given even under the stated circumstances but in a resource-starved setting may constitute a more beneficent alternative than placement in more restrictive settings, multiple brief foster or residential placements, incarceration, or abandonment. The obvious answer to this ethical dilemma is the development of comprehensive environmental and treatment resources. In the absence of that blessed circumstance, clinicians must approach these questions with a broad awareness of all the ethical principles involved applying them with both rationality and sensitivity; this approach to ethics facilitates all medical practice. The Codes of Ethics and the Ethics Committees of the American Psychiatric Association and the American Academy of Child and Adolescent Psychiatry can provide assistance in assessing these dilemmas (Sondheimer and Klykylo, 2008).

Treatment Planning

Issues Concerning Diagnosis and Implications for Drug Choice and Premedication Workup

The areas of major concern are making a correct psychiatric diagnosis and being aware of any coexisting medical conditions. Taking accurate medical and psychiatric histories, including previous medications and the patient's response to them as well as adverse effects and allergic reactions, is essential. Nurcombe (1991) notes that if adverse reactions to a drug or drug interactions occur that could have been predicted by taking an accurate and adequate history, the physician may be held liable. History taking must be followed by a proper premedication workup; if the patient has a medical condition, the physician must consider how the psychotropic medication would affect that condition and whether there may be interactions with other medications the patient is taking. Some examples of this include the following: (a) making an incorrect diagnosis and prescribing the wrong medication, or failing to detect or recognize coexisting conditions that would contraindicate the chosen medication; (b) prescribing a drug that will interact adversely with another medication the patient is taking or a drug to which the patient has previously been allergic; or (c) failing to perform a baseline and serial electrocardiograms (ECGs) or to monitor serum levels when tricyclics are used because of possible cardiotoxicity.

Issues Concerning Informed Consent

The treatment plan should be discussed and agreed to by the legal guardian and the patient as appropriate for his or her age and understanding. The diagnosis and the risks and benefits of the proposed treatment and alternative treatment possibilities should be reviewed. To give informed consent, a patient (or legal guardian) must be mentally competent, have sufficient information available, and not be coerced. Adolescents 12 years of age and older should participate formally in developing their treatment plans and in giving informed "assent." If this is not possible, it should be so stated in the clinical record. It is wise to have both the legal guardian and, when appropriate, the patient sign the treatment plan and/or an informed consent ("assent" for underage individuals) for medication. If this is not done, at a minimum the clinician must document the discussion of the treatment plan and the response of the patient and legal guardian in the clinical record.

Nurcombe (1991) recommends that the following be discussed:

1. The nature of the condition that requires treatment.
2. The nature and purpose of the proposed treatment and the probability that it will succeed.
3. The risks and consequences of the proposed treatment. (It should be noted, e.g., if the proposed medication is an off-label use and that possible rare or long-term treatment-emergent adverse events or unknown drug interactions may occur, especially for newer drugs where there is relatively little clinical experience. Also newer, postinitial drug marketing adverse events must be explained clearly and not minimized which could be interpreted as misleading in order to obtain consent, e.g., the recent warning for all antidepressant drugs that they increased suicidal thinking and behavior in short-term studies in children and adolescents with major depressive and other psychiatric disorders should not be downplayed. Another example would be to discuss possible prolactin increase, weight gain, and onset of type 2 diabetes with risperidone.)
4. Alternatives to the proposed treatment and their attendant risks and consequences.
5. Prognosis with and without the proposed treatment (p. 1132).

Popper (1987a) adds that it should be explicitly stated that there may be unknown risks in taking the medication, especially when using novel psychopharmacological treatments or treatments in which risks versus benefits are uncertain.

Involuntary medication of patients occurs primarily in emergency rooms and in inpatient wards. This is usually permissible in a true emergency, but Nurcombe (1991) cautions that even involuntary commitment to a hospital for psychiatric treatment permits involuntary medication only in narrowly defined circumstances. Administering medication forcibly without judicial approval in a nonemergency situation may be considered battery. Physicians should become thoroughly familiar with their state laws and local hospital policies governing these matters.

Issues Concerning the Administration of Medication

Issues that concern the administration of medication include justification for the decision to use medication in treating the psychiatric condition (risks vs. benefits), rationale for the initial drug chosen, and administration of the drug by the appropriate route, usually orally, and in a clinically efficacious dose. If a patient is suicidal, the prescribing physician should ascertain to the best of his or her ability and document that only sublethal amounts of medication are accessible to the patient. It is best to have a responsible adult, usually a parent, have control of the medication—keeping it where the patient does not have access to it and dispense it to the patient as directed. The medication should be completely or nearly finished before more is prescribed. The clinician must monitor the medication adequately for the duration of the therapy and should either discontinue the medication or attempt to do so at appropriate intervals, or document in the clinical record the reasons for the decision not to follow this protocol.

Examples of behavior that may increase medicolegal risk include failing to prescribe medication for a condition for which most practitioners would, prescribing a medication without personally evaluating the patient (e.g., based on another physician's report), prescribing an inappropriate drug for the diagnosis (e.g., amphetamines to a drug abuser), using an unsatisfactory rationale to justify the choice of drug, administering an inappropriate dosage for the disorder (e.g., subtherapeutic levels), or administering medication by an inappropriate route (e.g., continuing to give medication intramuscularly when it is no longer indicated or necessary). A patient's use of prescribed medication to attempt or successfully complete a suicide may also result in legal action.

Off-label Prescribing/Deviating from a Manufacturer's Labeling of a Drug

This book discusses many uses of psychoactive medications that are different from those formally recommended by the manufacturer or approved by the U.S. Food and Drug Administration (FDA) for advertising as safe and effective. Many of these off-label uses are medically accepted, but others are not yet common medical practice. Deviating from the usual clinical practice may increase the risk of legal action. Although legally permissible, using FDA-approved drugs for non–FDA-approved indications and using FDA-approved drugs for approved indications in children below the age limit for which they are approved may increase the potential for liability. Similarly, not adhering to the recommendations of the drug manufacturer (in the package insert or as reprinted in the *PDR*)—for example, exceeding recommended dosages—should alert the clinician to carefully document the rationale for doing so. In general, however, clinicians are on solid ground if they have assessed the risk–benefit ratio for prescribing a medication for a non–FDA-approved indication and have documented a scientifically reasonable rationale for choosing a particular drug over other possible treatments in the medical record.

It should be clear that the preceding discussion of off-label use applies primarily to situations where data were lacking at the time of application for approval by the FDA and subsequent research and clinical practice support a rationale for their use. Most frequently, there were insufficient data to determine efficacy and safety in the pediatric age-group or the drug was being used for a diagnosis not initially studied. It should be clear that ignoring specific safety recommendations contained in the package insert that are based on verifiable data is an entirely different situation and is not condoned.

In clinical practice, standard treatments and off-label (non–FDA-approved) but clinically accepted treatments that may be efficacious with less risk almost always should be tried before less clinically accepted or riskier medications. Concurrence of a consultant and appropriate psychopharmacological references supporting such use may be helpful when the off-label use is not commonly accepted (Nurcombe, 1991). As a general principle, the more novel the treatment or uncertain the risk–benefit ratio, the more severely disabling the condition should be for which it is used.

Issues Concerned with Documenting Ongoing Appropriate Attention to Medication and Related Matters in the Clinical Record

The patient's clinical record should reflect continued appropriate monitoring of the medication's efficacy; monitoring for the presence or absence of adverse effects, including tardive dyskinesia; results of laboratory tests or other procedures (e.g., ECG) performed at appropriate intervals to monitor adverse effects; justifications for increases or decreases in dosage or changes in times of administration; decisions to employ a drug holiday or discontinue medication; and consequences of discontinuing medication, including any change in symptomatology, reexacerbation of symptoms, rebound effects, or withdrawal syndromes such as a withdrawal dyskinesia.

When patients are hospitalized, it is important for the clinician to address in the medical record not only his or her own observations of the patient but also those of other professionals who have reported or recorded behaviors or symptoms that may indicate adverse effects of medication (e.g., unsteadiness of gait reported by a nurse or falling asleep in class reported by a teacher).

Most authorities recommend that children and adolescents who are receiving psychoactive medication should have it discontinued or at least tapered down periodically, typically within 6 months to at most 1 year, to ascertain whether it is still needed or whether a lower dose might be sufficient. That this has been done should be documented in the chart, and if the clinician delays this tapering excessively, the reason should be clearly explained in the chart (e.g., the previous attempt resulted in a severe relapse of symptoms that were difficult to control in a schizophrenic adolescent or a clinical decision has been reached to delay an attempt to lower or discontinue medication until the completion of the school year because functioning has been marginal although somewhat improved with medication). Decisions such as these should also be discussed with the parents and the patient and their agreement documented as part of the treatment plan.

The reviews of Nurcombe (1991), Nurcombe and Partlett (1994), and Benedek et al. (2010) of medicolegal aspects of the entire practice of child and adolescent psychiatry, including specific court cases and decisions, are recommended to the interested reader. Popper (1987a) has written a chapter that remains relevant on ethical considerations of the relationship between obtaining consent for the use of medication from parents and children and adolescents and incomplete or unknown medical knowledge of the risks and long-term effects of psychoactive medication used during childhood and adolescence.

BASELINE ASSESSMENTS PRIOR TO INITIATION OF MEDICATION

All patients should have a complete medical history and physical and neurologic examinations. These examinations are essential to identify any organic factors contributing to the psychiatric symptomatology and any coexisting medical abnormalities. In addition, all drugs may cause adverse physical and psychological effects; hence, a baseline examination prior to the initiation of psychopharmacotherapy should be mandatory.

Although there is considerable information available for stimulant medications, relatively little information is available concerning the long-term adverse effects of psychoactive drugs on the growth and development of children and adolescents. Because of this fact as well as the potential medicolegal ramifications, particularly when drugs are used for non–FDA-approved indications, it is recommended that the premedication workup be reasonably comprehensive. The reader who wishes a more detailed review of laboratory tests and diagnostic procedures applicable to general psychiatry than that provided in the subsequent text is referred to the review of Realmuto (2012).

Physical Examination

The physical examination should include recording baseline temperature, pulse and respiration rates, and blood pressure. Height and weight should be entered on standardized growth charts, such as the National Center for Health Statistics Growth Charts (Hamill et al., 1976), so that serial measurements and percentiles may be plotted over time. In their recent review, Correll and Carlson (2006) have indicated that the relative potency of atypical/second-generation antipsychotic drugs in inducing weight gain and increasing the risk for developing the metabolic syndrome is approximately: clozapine = olanzapine >> risperidone ≥ quetiapine > ziprasidone ≥ aripiprazole.

Laboratory Tests and Diagnostic Procedures

The following are frequently recommended premedication laboratory tests and diagnostic procedures. Some of these tests may have already been done as a part of the pediatric/medical evaluation that should be a part of any comprehensive psychiatric evaluation. These tests will be addressed more specifically under each class of medications or, if appropriate, for specific drugs when they are discussed. Obviously, the premedication workup will be influenced by and should be modified to accommodate any particular abnormal findings in the medical history or examination, such as renal, thyroid, and cardiac abnormalities, or by any initial abnormal laboratory results themselves.

Laboratory tests routinely or frequently recommended as part of a comprehensive, complete, pediatric examination, and/or premedication workup include the following:

1. Complete blood cell count (CBC), differential, and hematocrit
2. Urinalysis
3. Blood urea nitrogen (BUN) level
4. Serum electrolyte levels for sodium (Na^+), potassium (K^+), chloride (Cl^-), calcium (Ca^{2+}), and phosphate (PO_4^{3-}), and carbon dioxide (CO_2) content
5. Liver function tests: aspartate aminotransferase (AST) or serum glutamic oxaloacetic transaminase (SGOT), alanine aminotransferase (ALT) or serum glutamic pyruvic transaminase (SGPT), alkaline phosphatase, lactic dehydrogenase (LDH), and bilirubin (total and indirect)
6. Blood glucose, especially when second-generation antipsychotics will be prescribed, as they can cause metabolic syndrome and cause or exacerbate type 2 diabetes. The American Diabetes Association has published, in collaboration with the APA, a protocol for monitoring adult patients who will be treated with second-generation antipsychotics. Fasting plasma glucose and a fasting lipid profile are recommended (American Diabetes Association and American Psychiatric Association, 2004)
7. Lipid profile: hyperlipidemia with elevated triglyceride and cholesterol serum levels have been reported as an adverse effect of some second-generation antipsychotics. Sheitman et al. (1999) reported an increase of almost 40% in serum triglycerides in adults taking olanzapine
8. Serum lead level determination in children below 7 years of age and in older children when indicated
9. If substance abuse (alcohol or drugs) is suspected, screening of urine and/or blood is usually indicated

Other laboratory tests may be recommended prior to using specific psychoactive medications.

Pregnancy/Pregnancy Test

Because drugs may have known or unknown adverse effects on the developing fetus, a serum beta human chorionic gonadotropin test for pregnancy should be considered for any adolescent capable of becoming pregnant, at a time as close to beginning the medication as convenient and reasonable. A related issue is that, if an adolescent is considered to be at significant risk for becoming pregnant despite birth control counseling, certain medications (e.g., lithium) should not be prescribed if at all possible, as the embryo would usually be exposed to the drug before pregnancy was detected.

Risk versus benefit must be carefully considered for both the patient and the (potential) embryo/fetus if a woman is on medication and has unprotected sexual relations or attempts to become pregnant. As is also well known, pregnancies do occur at times even with "protected" sex. Once pregnancy is verified, serious concerns about teratogenic risk to the embryo/fetus arise. "A pregnant woman should not take any drug unless it is necessary for her own health or that of her fetus" (Friedman and Polifka, 1998, p. ix). Additional concerns occur when mothers who are taking medication wish to breast-feed their infants, as some drugs and/or their metabolites are secreted in breast milk.

Discussion of these very important issues on a drug-by-drug basis is beyond the scope of this book. In addition to the package insert, the reader who needs more information is referred to an excellent overview of the management of pregnant psychiatric patients on medication and a compendium of psychiatric drugs with their known risks and teratogenic effects and the risks related to breast feeding (Friedman and Polifka, 1998).

Thyroid Function Tests

There is a strong association between clinical thyroid disease and psychiatric disorders, particularly mood disorders (Esposito et al., 1997). Thyroid function tests (thyroxine [T_4], triiodothyronine resin uptake [T_3RU], and thyroid-stimulating hormone or thyrotropin) are recommended prior to the use of tricyclic antidepressants and lithium. Abnormal thyroid function can aggravate cardiac arrhythmias that may occur as an adverse effect of tricyclic antidepressants (*PDR*, 1995). Lithium has been reported to cause hypothyroidism with lower T_3 and T_4 levels and elevated ^{131}I uptake.

Kidney Function Tests

Many drugs are excreted at least partially through the kidney and in the urine. Because of reported adverse effects of lithium carbonate on the kidney, baseline evaluation of kidney function should be determined. Jefferson et al. (1987) suggest that a baseline serum creatinine and urinalysis are usually adequate and that more extensive testing (e.g., creatinine clearance, 24-hour urine volume, and maximal urine osmolality) is not practical or necessary for most patients.

Prolactin Levels

Prolactin is a polypeptide protein hormone synthesized and secreted by lactotrophs of the anterior pituitary gland. Prolactin stimulates breast tissue development and production of milk and lactation. Prolactin secretion is controlled by the tuberoinfundibular dopamine pathway and the inhibitory action of dopamine on D_2 receptors located on the surface of pituitary lactotrophs (Ayd, 1995; Stahl, 2000). Drugs that antagonize dopamine D_2 receptors, that is, with D_2 blocking action such as antipsychotics and cocaine, as well as drugs that may indirectly influence

dopaminergic function such as fluoxetine, therefore have the capability of causing elevated prolactin levels (hyperprolactinemia) that have been associated with
inhibition of gonadotropin secretion, with galactorrhea and amenorrhea in women
and with gynecomastia, decreased testosterone level, and impotence in men (Kane
and Lieberman, 1992). In their seminal review, Correll and Carlson (2006) have
indicated that the relative potency of antipsychotic drugs in inducing hyperprolactinemia is approximately: risperidone > haloperidol > olanzapine > ziprasidone >
quetiapine > clozapine > aripiprazole.

The long-term clinical implications/effects of hyperprolactinemia on the general
maturation and development of children and adolescents, and, in particular, on
their endocrine and central nervous systems, are uncertain. However, the review
of Correll (2008) suggests that there may be multiple adverse consequences associated with this condition, including pituitary tumors. Because of this, a baseline
prolactin level may be useful prior to initiating treatment with a drug known to
affect prolactin secretion.

Wudarsky et al. (1999) reported prolactin levels in 35 subjects (22 males,
13 females; mean age 14.1 ± 2.3 years, age range 9.1 to 19 years) diagnosed
with schizophrenia ($N = 32$) or psychotic disorder not otherwise specified (NOS)
($N = 3$) before age 13 who were treated with haloperidol, olanzapine, and/or clozapine for 6 weeks. Reference normal plasma prolactin values used for this study
were as follows: adult range (combined male and female), 1.39 to 24.2 ng/mL;
mean for adult males, 5.6 ng/mL (range, 1.61 to 18.77 ng/mL), and for adult females, 7.97 (range, 1.39 to 24.2). Conventional normal reference values for prepubescent males are 4.0 ± 0.5 ng/mL and for prepubescent females, 4.5 ± 0.6 ng/mL.

Mean baseline prolactin levels were measured after a mean washout period
of 3 weeks and were below normal limits. Prolactin levels during the sixth
week were significantly elevated from baseline for all three drugs (haloperidol,
9.0 ± 4.2 ng/mL vs. 47.8 ± 30.6 ng/mL [$P < .001$]; clozapine, 9.0 ± 3.4 ng/mL vs.
11.2 ± 4.0 ng/mL [$P < .007$]; olanzapine, 10.0 ± 4.7 ng/mL vs. 23.7 ± 7.7 ng/mL
[$P < .003$]). The mean plasma prolactin level for the 10 subjects on haloperidol
was above the upper limit of normal (ULN), and 9 subjects had levels above the
ULN. The mean plasma prolactin value for the 15 subjects on clozapine, although
significantly elevated from baseline, remained within the ULN, and plasma prolactin levels remained within the normal range for all 15 subjects. The mean plasma
prolactin level for the 10 subjects on olanzapine was above the ULN, and 7 of
the subjects had plasma prolactin levels above the ULN. The authors noted that
plasma prolactin levels usually returned to baseline values within a few days after
medication was discontinued but persisted for up to 3 weeks in a few cases. When
compared with adults, these younger subjects had more robust increases in plasma
prolactin levels on haloperidol and olanzapine but not clozapine, perhaps because
of a greater number or sensitivity of dopamine receptors in the tuberoinfundibular systems of children and adolescents. The authors called for additional studies
of prolactin response to various medications in this age group and the effects of
hyperprolactinemia on their development and maturation (Wudarsky et al., 1999).

Saito et al. (2004) conducted a prospective study of 40 subjects (22 males,
18 females; mean age, 13.4 years, age range 5 to 18 years) that examined the
change in prolactin levels from baseline to a mean of 11.2 weeks of treatment
with risperidone ($N = 21$), olanzapine ($N = 13$), or quetiapine ($N = 6$). Primary
diagnoses were schizophrenia/psychosis ($N = 14$); mood disorder ($N = 14$); disruptive behavior disorder ($N = 9$); intermittent explosive disorder ($N = 1$); pervasive
developmental disorder NOS ($N = 1$); and eating disorder NOS ($N = 1$); 80%
of the subjects were taking two or more psychotropic medications. The authors
hypothesized that, because of risperidone's relatively high affinity for D_2 receptors in the pituitary, children and adolescents receiving risperidone would develop
hyperprolactinemia to a greater extent than those subjects receiving olanzapine

and quetiapine. Baseline prolactin levels were drawn before beginning the atypical antipsychotic in 17 (43%) subjects and within 1 week after beginning treatment in 23 (57%). The reference range for normal was 3.9 to 25.4 ng/mL for all children, 4.1 to 18.4 ng/mL for males, and 3.4 to 24.1 ng/mL for females. Baseline prolactin levels, pubertal status, and gender were not significantly different among the three groups. Hyperprolactinemia was present in 53% of the subjects at end point. A greater percentage of subjects receiving risperidone (15/21 or 71%) had elevated prolactin levels (group mean end-point level 46.8 ± 33.3 mg/mL) than subjects receiving olanzapine (5/13 or 38%) with a group mean end-point level of 24.5 ± 17.8 ng/mL or subjects receiving quetiapine (1/6 or 17%) with a group mean end-point level of 16.7 ± 10.1 ng/mL. The end-point level of risperidone was significantly higher than that of olanzapine ($P = .008$) and that of quetiapine ($P = .027$). Prolactin levels in the olanzapine and quetiapine groups were not significantly different from each other. Regarding end-point prolactin levels, there were no significant gender differences, and postpubertal females did not have significantly different levels from the entire group. In addition, end-point prolactin levels were not associated with changes in weight. Interestingly, 25% (seven women and three men) of the entire group reported sexual adverse effects: breast tenderness ($N = 4$), irregular menses ($N = 3$), decreased libido ($N = 3$), erectile dysfunction ($N = 3$), galactorrhea, and amenorrhea ($N = 1$); the authors suggested that this rather high level resulted from their asking specific questions rather than recording only spontaneous reports. There was no association between the drug taken and sexual side effects; five of these subjects were on risperidone; three were on olanzapine; and two were on quetiapine. The authors also noted that the lower incidence of hyperprolactinemia in their study compared with that of Alfaro et al. (2002) is likely because the doses they employed were only approximately one half those used in the Alfaro et al. study. This study also suggested that children and adolescents may be more likely than adults to develop hyperprolactinemia at a specific dose of atypical antipsychotic.

Pappagallo and Silva (2004) reviewed the literature through 2003 on the effect of atypical antipsychotic drugs in children and adolescents. They identified 14 studies with a total of 276 subjects. The authors concluded that, of the atypical antipsychotics, risperidone has been more frequently associated with hyperprolactinemia and clozaril, the least; however, they noted that aripiprazole, which has been recently approved, has partial D_2 agonist properties and may result in smaller increases in prolactin levels; to date, studies in adults have shown no significant prolactin elevations; values in children and adolescents had not been reported. The authors note that there is some evidence that prolactin levels may decrease over time without dose reduction. When prolactinemia is present, the authors suggest that other possible causes, including oral birth control pills, opiates, and pregnancy, be considered. If the increase in prolactin is mild and adverse effects associated with prolactin are not troublesome, one can elect to continue to administer the medication with close monitoring of clinical effects and periodic prolactin levels. It is noted that data which elucidate the long-term effects of hyperprolactinemia on the physical and emotional development of such children and adolescents are not yet available.

Croonenberghs et al. (2005) conducted an international multisite 1-year open-label trial of risperidone with 504 patients (419 males, 85 females; mean age 9.7 ± 2.5 years, range 4 to 14 years). Mean serum prolactin levels at baseline were 7.7 ± 7.1 ng/mL for boys (ULN 18 ng/mL) and 10.1 ± 8.1 ng/mL for girls (ULN 25 ng/mL). Prolactin levels rose rather sharply and peak average prolactin levels occurred at week 4 in both boys and girls and were above normal limits for both (boys, 28.2 ± 14.2 ng/mL and girls, 35.4 ± 19.1 ng/mL). Prolactin levels then gradually decreased until by the ninth month of treatment; they were again within normal limits for both and remained there for the duration of the study although they remained higher than baseline. The following adverse effects, which could possibly be related to hyperprolactinemia, were noted: mild to moderate gynecomastia in 25 subjects (22 men, 3 women); menstrual disturbances in 6 subjects; galactorrhea in 1 patient; and moderately severe menorrhagia in 1 patient. However, as these symptoms can occur in normal populations, it is impossible to assess the added risk attributed by risperidone as there is no control group.

Electrocardiogram

Many psychiatric medications may have adverse effects on the cardiovascular system, on both the electroconductivity of the heart, as evidenced by the ECG, and on hemodynamics (e.g., blood pressure). A baseline ECG is recommended as part of the complete physical examination of every child prior to prescribing psychoactive medication; it should be mandatory in any person with a history of, or clinical findings suggestive of, cardiovascular disease. ECGs are noninvasive and relatively inexpensive. It is not rare to detect an unsuspected cardiac abnormality.

The American Heart Association has issued useful guidelines regarding the cardiovascular monitoring of children and adolescents receiving psychotropic drugs (Gutgesell et al., 1999 [note that the reprint of this article in the *Journal of the American Academy of Child & Adolescent Psychiatry* appears to have inadvertently omitted the anticonvulsants from Table I]). Although helpful, these guidelines are conservative; for example, they state that no ECG monitoring is necessary when prescribing alpha-2-adrenergic agonists such as clonidine and guanfacine, while Kofoed et al. (1999) present data supporting a cogent argument that pretreatment ECGs are necessary to assist in distinguishing drug-induced changes from variability unrelated to the drug effects of clonidine. In addition, the list of psychotropic agents included in the guidelines is not up to date; all the atypical antipsychotics as well as the newer antidepressants are missing.

It also frequently occurs that if the response to a particular drug is not clinically satisfactory, it is discontinued and another drug is prescribed or another drug may be added to the initial drug. In some such cases, the new drug or combination of drugs would make an ECG necessary for optimal clinical practice.

A baseline ECG should be recorded prior to the administration of tricyclic antidepressants to determine any preexisting conduction or other cardiac abnormality because clinically important cardiotoxicity may occur, especially at higher serum levels. The ECG should be monitored with dose increases and periodically thereafter if tricyclics are used (this is discussed in detail in Chapter 7 under "Tricyclic Antidepressants and Cardiotoxicity").

Most of the antipsychotics, both standard and atypical, may cause ECG changes, including prolongation of the QTc interval. Lithium may also cause cardiac abnormalities, and an ECG is recommended prior to initiating therapy. Carbamazepine may also prolong the QTc interval.

Polypharmacy may also cause drug–drug interactions; of particular importance are interactions where one drug may affect the metabolism of a second drug (e.g., by inhibiting metabolism by the cytochrome P450 enzyme system). For example, two sudden deaths were reported when clarithromycin, which inhibits the cytochrome P450 enzyme system, and pimozide, which is metabolized by the P450 enzyme system, were administered simultaneously, giving rise to the possibility that their interaction was a contributing or causal factor.

Electroencephalogram

An electroencephalogram (EEG) may be considered for patients to whom antipsychotics, tricyclic antidepressants, or lithium will be administered, because all these drugs have been associated with either lowered threshold for seizures or other EEG changes. This group would include patients who have a history of seizure disorder, who are on an antiepileptic drug for a seizure disorder, or who may be at risk for seizures (e.g., following brain surgery or head injury).

Blanz and Schmidt (1993) reported a significant increase in pathologic EEG findings (short biphasic waves) in child and adolescent patients receiving clozapine. Similarly, Remschmidt et al. (1994) reported EEG changes in 16 (44%) of 36 adolescents being treated with clozapine. Baseline EEG and periodic monitoring of EEG while on clozapine should be mandatory.

Baseline Behavioral Assessment

Clinical Observations

Baseline observations and careful characterizations of both behavior and target symptoms must be recorded in the clinical record. These should include direct observations by the clinician in the waiting room, office, playroom, and/or ward, as well as those reported by other reliable observers in other locations, such as the home and school. It is important to include usual eating and sleeping patterns, because these may be altered by many drugs. These observations should be described both qualitatively and quantitatively (amplitude and frequency), and the circumstances in which they occur should be noted in the clinical record.

It is also essential to record an accurate baseline rating in the clinical record before beginning psychopharmacotherapy in children or adolescents who have existing abnormal movements or who are at risk of developing them (e.g., patients diagnosed with autistic disorder or severe mental retardation and/or patients who will be treated with antipsychotics). This documentation is necessary both to follow the patient's clinical course and to be able to differentiate among recrudescence of preexisting involuntary movements, stereotypies, and mannerisms and any subsequent withdrawal dyskinesias or new stereotypies that may occur when medication, particularly an antipsychotic, is discontinued. The availability of these longitudinal data becomes even more critical if the treating physician changes. Although the baseline data can be documented in the clinician's records, the use of a rating scale such as the Abnormal Involuntary Movement Scale (AIMS) (Rating Scales, 1985) or the Extrapyramidal Symptom Rating Scale (ESRS) (Gharabawi et al., 2005) that assesses abnormal movements is strongly recommended.

To be able to assess the efficacy of a specific medication, a baseline observation period, with reasonably stable or worsening target symptoms, is necessary. Other than in emergency situations (e.g., a violent, physically assaultive, and/or severely psychotic individual), observation of the patient for a minimum of 7 to 10 days is recommended before initiating pharmacotherapy. For inpatients, this will permit assessment of the combined effects of hospitalization and a therapeutic milieu and the removal of the identified patient from his or her living situation on the patient's psychopathology and symptoms. For outpatients, this observation period will give the clinician an opportunity to see the effect of the clinical contact and assessment on the symptom expression of the patient and the psychodynamic equilibrium of the family. During this observation period, some children and adolescents, both inpatients and outpatients, will improve enough that psychopharmacotherapy will no longer be indicated. Unfortunately, because of the high cost of inpatient hospitalization and pressure by various managed care organizations, patients are often medicated before there is time to assess their responses to the inpatient environment.

Rating Scales

Rating scales are an essential component of psychopharmacological research. They provide a means of recording serial qualitative and quantitative measurements of behaviors, and their interrater reliability can be determined. Two early influential publications concerning rating scales and psychopharmacological research in children were the *Psychopharmacology Bulletin's* special issue *Pharmacotherapy of Children*

(1973) and its 1985 issue featuring "Rating Scales and Assessment Instruments for Use in Pediatric Psychopharmacology Research" (Rating Scales, 1985). These remain relevant but many comprehensive reviews and lists are now available, notably from the American Academy of Child and Adolescent Psychiatry (AACAP, 2010).

Although rating scales are valuable in nonresearch settings, they tend to be used less in clinical practice. Perhaps those most frequently used are the various Conners rating instruments: Conners Teacher Questionnaire (CTQ), Conners Parent–Teacher Questionnaire (CPTQ), and Conners Parent Questionnaire (CPQ) (*Psychopharmacology Bulletin,* 1973). The abbreviated CPTQ, reproduced as Table 2.1, is useful in helping to identify patients who have ADHD and to record serial ratings that provide good periodic estimates of the clinical efficacy of medication in the classroom and home environments. The CPTQ can be completed in a short time because it has only 11 items. The first 10 items are common to the CTQ and the CPQ; the 11th item is an overall estimate of the degree of seriousness of the child's problem at the time of the rating; that item is not included in the following discussion of scoring. A total score of 15 on the first 10 items has been widely used in research as the cut-off for two standard deviations above the mean, and subjects scoring 15 or more points have been considered hyperactive (Sleator, 1986). The mean value of the 10 items of the CPTQ yields a score comparable to factor IV, the hyperactivity index, of the CTQ, and a 0.5-point or more decrease in the mean (or a decrease of 5 points in the total score on the first 10 items of the CPTQ) generally indicates that medication is effecting a meaningful improvement (Greenhill, 1990).

The AIMS (Table 2.2) is a 12-item scale designed to record in detail the occurrence of dyskinetic movements. Abnormal involuntary movements are rated on a

---

TABLE 2.1 » Conners Parent–Teacher Questionnaire

INSTRUCTIONS: Listed below are items concerning children's behavior or the problems they sometimes have. Read each item carefully and decide how much you think this child has been bothered by this problem at this time: *Not at All, Just a Little, Pretty Much,* or *Very Much.* Indicate your choice by circling the number in the appropriate column to the right of each item.

Answer All Items	Not at All	Just a Little	Pretty Much	Very Much
1. Restless (overactive)	0	1	2	3
2. Excitable, impulsive	0	1	2	3
3. Disturbs other children	0	1	2	3
4. Fails to finish things he starts (short attention span)	0	1	2	3
5. Fidgeting	0	1	2	3
6. Inattentive, distractible	0	1	2	3
7. Demands must be met immediately; frustrated	0	1	2	3
8. Cries	0	1	2	3
9. Mood changes quickly	0	1	2	3
10. Temper outbursts (explosive and unpredictable behavior)	0	1	2	3
	None	Minor	Moderate	Severe
How serious a problem do you think this child has at this time?	0	1	2	3

Modified from Department of Health, Education, and Welfare, Health Services and Mental Health Administration, National Institutes of Health.

TABLE 2.2 » Abnormal Involuntary Movement Scale (AIMS)

INSTRUCTIONS: Complete Examination Procedure before making ratings. MOVEMENT RATINGS: Rate highest severity observed. Rate movements that occur upon activation one less than those observed spontaneously

		(Circle One)				
FACIAL AND ORAL MOVEMENTS	1. **Muscles of facial expression** (e.g., movements of forehead, eyebrows, periorbital area, cheeks; include frowning, blinking, smiling, grimacing)	0	1	2	3	4
	2. **Lips and perioral area** (e.g., puckering, pouting, smacking)	0	1	2	3	4
	3. **Jaw** (e.g., biting, clenching, chewing, mouth opening, lateral movement)	0	1	2	3	4
	4. **Tongue:** Rate only increase in movement both in and out of mouth, NOT inability to sustain movement	0	1	2	3	4
EXTREMITY MOVEMENTS	5. **Upper** (arms, wrists, hands, fingers): Include choreic movements (i.e., rapid, objectively purposeless, irregular, spontaneous), athetoid movements (i.e., slow, irregular, complex, serpentine). Do NOT include tremor (i.e., repetitive, regular, rhythmic)	0	1	2	3	4
	6. **Lower** (legs, knees, ankles, toes): For example, lateral knee movement, foot tapping, heel dropping, foot squirming, inversion and eversion of foot	0	1	2	3	4
TRUNK MOVEMENTS	7. **Neck, shoulders, hips** (e.g., rocking, twisting, squirming, pelvic gyrations)	0	1	2	3	4

GLOBAL JUDGMENTS	8. **Severity of abnormal movements**	None, normal	0
		Minimal	1
		Mild	2
		Moderate	3
		Severe	4
	9. **Incapacitation due to abnormal movements:** Rate only patient's report	None, normal	0
		Minimal	1
		Mild	2
		Moderate	3
		Severe	4
	10. **Patient's awareness of abnormal movements:** Rate only patient's report	No awareness	0
		Aware, no distress	1
		Aware, mild distress	2
		Aware, moderate distress	3
		Aware, severe distress	4
DENTAL STATUS	11. **Current problems with teeth and/or dentures**	No	0
		Yes	1
	12. **Does patient usually wear dentures?**	No	0
		Yes	1

EXAMINATION PROCEDURE

Either before or after completing the Examination Procedure, observe the patient unobtrusively at rest (e.g., in waiting room).

The chair to be used in this examination should be a hard, firm one without arms.

1. Ask patient whether there is anything in his/her mouth (gum, candy, etc.) and, if there is, to remove it.

2. Ask patient about the current condition of his/her teeth. Ask patients if he/she wears dentures. Do teeth or dentures bother patient now?

(continued)

TABLE 2.2 » Abnormal Involuntary Movement Scale (AIMS) (Continued)

EXAMINATION PROCEDURE

3. Ask patient whether he/she notices any movements in mouth, face, hands, or feet. If yes, ask to describe and to what extent they currently bother patient or interfere with his/her activities.

4. Have patient sit in chair with hands on knees, legs slightly apart, and feet flat on floor. (Look at entire body for movements while in this position.)

5. Ask patient to sit with hands hanging unsupported. If male, between legs, if female and wearing a dress, hanging over knees. (Observe hands and other body areas.)

6. Ask patient to open mouth. (Observe tongue at rest within mouth.) Do this twice.

7. Ask patient to protrude tongue. (Observe abnormalities of tongue movement.) Do this twice.

8. Ask patient to tap thumb, with each finger, as rapidly as possible for 10–15 seconds; separately with right hand, then with left hand. (Observe facial and leg movements.)[a]

9. Flex and extend patient's left and right arms (one at a time). (Note any rigidity and rate on DOTES.)

10. Ask patient to stand up. (Observe in profile. Observe all body areas again, hips included.)

11. Ask patient to extend both arms outstretched in front with palms down. (Observe trunk, legs, and mouth.)[a]

12. Have patient walk a few paces, turn, and walk back to chair. (Observe hands and gait.) Do this twice.[a]

DOTES = Dosage and Treatment Emergent Symptoms Scale (Guy, 1976a).
Code: 0 = none; 1 = minimal, may be extreme normal; 2 = mild; 3 = moderate; 4 = severe.
[a]Activated movements.
Modified from Department of Health, Education, and Welfare. Public Health Service. Alcohol, Drug Abuse, and Mental Health Administration, National Institute of Mental Health.

5-point scale from 0 to 4, with 0 being none, 1 being minimal or extreme normal, 2 being mild, 3 being moderate, and 4 being severe. If a procedure is used to activate the movements (e.g., having the patient tap his or her thumb with each finger as rapidly as possible for 10 to 15 seconds separately with the right and then the left hand), movements are rated one point lower than those occurring spontaneously. Seven of the items rate abnormal involuntary movements in specific topographies: four items concern facial and oral movements, two items concern extremity movements, and one item concerns trunk movements. Three items are global ratings: two by the clinician concern the overall severity of the abnormal movements and the estimated degree of incapacity from them and a third records the patient's own degree of awareness of the abnormal movements. Using the AIMS will also make it less likely that an area that should be assessed will be omitted inadvertently and will also provide quantitative ratings for following the clinical course. Having a baseline and subsequent AIMS ratings available is most helpful to the initial treating physician in assessing any changes in baseline abnormal involuntary movements increases, decrements, or changes in topography during the course of active treatment with psychoactive medication, as well as during periods of withdrawal from medication. These ratings are often essential to differentiate preexisting abnormal involuntary movements from withdrawal dyskinesias. Such ratings are even more helpful when other physicians may assume the treatment of the patient at a future time.

Medicating the Patient: Selecting the Initial and Subsequent Medications

In general, it is recommended that a drug approved by the FDA—for the patient's age, diagnosis, and target symptoms—be chosen initially unless other, off-label drugs which are equally or more clinically effective and safer regarding adverse effects are available and are regularly used in the practice of child and adolescent psychopharmacology (e.g., the atypical antipsychotics). Factors such as selecting the drug with the least risk of serious adverse effects; known previous response(s) of the patient to psychotropic medication; the responses of siblings, parents, and other relatives with psychiatric illnesses to psychotropic medication; family history (e.g., a history of Tourette's disorder); and the clinician's previous experience in using the medication should also be weighed in choosing the initial and, if necessary, subsequent drugs.

The Texas Children's Medication Algorithm Project published algorithms for the treatment of childhood major depressive disorder (Emslie et al., 1997; Hughes et al., 1999) and childhood ADHD with and without common comorbid disorders (Pliszka et al., 2000a, 2000b, 2006) diagnosed by DSM-IV (APA, 1994) criteria. The algorithms and guidelines for their use were developed using expert consensus methodology based on scientific evidence, when available, and clinical experience and opinion, when necessary, with the goal of synthesizing research and clinical experience for clinicians in the public health sector and thereby increasing the quality and consistency of their treatment strategies.

Three of the Texas Children's Medication Algorithms are reproduced in Figures 2.1 to 2.3 as examples of the current state of the art in child and adolescent psychopharmacology research. To fully appreciate the thinking behind these and before using them, the complete publications should be read carefully. Algorithms serve only as a guide and these are presented as an example; clinicians will modify them to suit the individual clinical needs of their patients. Note that in Figure 2.2, magnesium pemoline is no longer an option as all drug companies manufacturing and distributing this drug in the United States have stopped doing so because the risk of acute hepatic failure is considered greater than the potential benefits. There-fore, clinicians will skip this stage and proceed directly to stage 4. In the ADHD with comorbid tic disorder, the authors administer a stimulant and alpha agonist together, which some clinicians would not feel comfortable about, given the con-troversy about coadministering methylphenidate and clonidine. Psychotherapeutic and psychosocial interventions, which are important to varying degrees with different patients, are not specifically integrated with these algorithms but remain essential components of any comprehensive treatment program.

Generic versus Trade Preparations

There has been controversy in the literature on the merits of brand-name drugs, usually the initial, patented preparations of a medication, and generic prepara-tions, which typically enter the market after exclusive patent rights expire and cost considerably less than the brand-name product. Although the active ingredients in the various preparations should be pharmaceutically equivalent, the inert ingredi-ents and the manufacturing processes may vary; therefore, the bioavailability of a drug may be significantly different among various preparations.

Many states now permit substitution of generic drugs for drugs prescribed by the brand name under specified conditions. New York State, for example, requires all prescription forms to have imprinted on them the following: "This prescription will be filled generically unless prescriber writes 'daw' [dispense as written] in the box below." Pharmacists are directed to "substitute a less expensive drug product containing the same active ingredients, dosage form and strength" as the drug originally prescribed, if available (New York State Department of Health, 1988, p. iii). The book recognizes the differences in bioavailability among products.

The FDA Center for Drug Evaluation and Research publishes a book, *Approved Drug Products with Therapeutic Equivalence Evaluations* (the "Orange Book"), which lists drugs, both prescription and nonprescription, approved by the FDA on the basis of safety and effectiveness. The list gives the FDAs evaluations of the therapeutic equivalence of prescription drugs that are available from multiple sources. It classifies drug preparations into two basic categories: A and B ratings. A ratings are given to drug products that the FDA considers to be therapeutically equivalent to other pharmaceutically equivalent products for which there are no

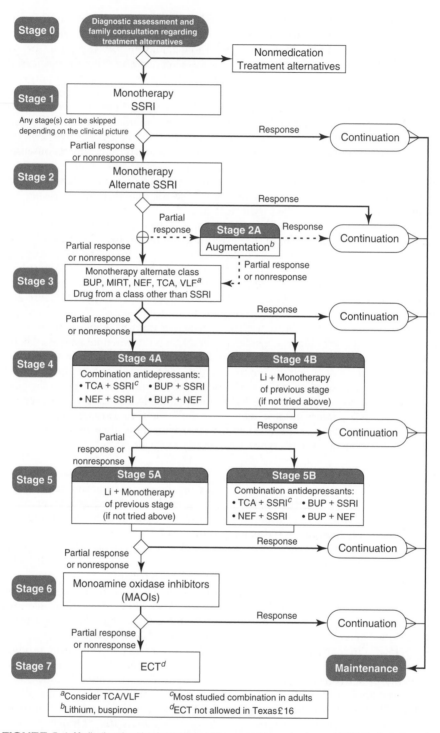

FIGURE 2.1 Medication algorithm for treating children and adolescents who meet DSM-IV criteria for major depressive disorder. SSRI, selective serotonin reuptake inhibitor; BUP, bupropion; MIRT, mirtazapine; NEF, nefazodone; TCA, tricyclic antidepressant; VLF, venlafaxine; MAOIs, monoamine oxidase inhibitors; ECT, electroconvulsive therapy. (Adapted from Crismon et al. 1999.)

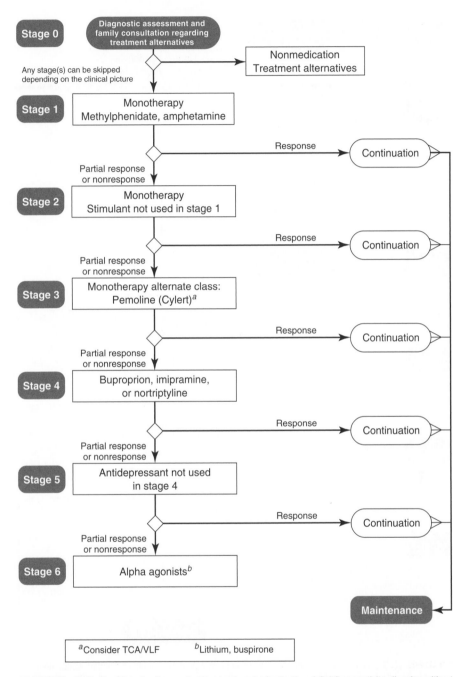

FIGURE 2.2 Algorithm for the medication treatment of attention-deficit/hyperactivity disorder without comorbid psychiatric disorder. Note, since this algorithm was published, pemoline has been withdrawn from the market. [a]Plus liver function monitoring and substance abuse history. [b]Cardiovascular side effects. (Adapted from Pliszka SR, Greenhill LL, Crismon ML, et al. Texas Consensus Conference Panel on Medication Treatment of Childhood Attention-Deficit/Hyperactivity Disorder. The Texas children's medication algorithm project: report of the Texas consensus conference panel on medication treatment of childhood attention-deficit/hyperactivity disorder: part I. *J Am Acad Child Adolesc Psychiatry.* 2000a;39:908–919.)

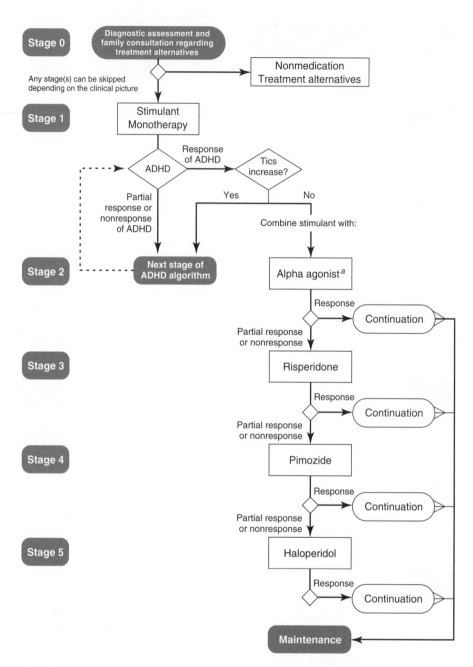

FIGURE 2.3 Algorithm for the medication treatment of ADHD with comorbid tic disorder. ADHD, attention-deficit/hyperactivity disorder. [a]Caution: cardiovascular side effects. (Adapted from Pliszka SR, Greenhill LL, Crismon ML, et al. Texas Consensus Conference Panel on Medication Treatment of Childhood Attention-Deficit/Hyperactivity Disorder. The Texas children's medication algorithm project: report of the Texas consensus conference panel on medication treatment of childhood attention-deficit/hyperactivity disorder: part I. *J Am Acad Child Adolesc Psychiatry.* 2000a;39:908–919.)

known or suspected bioequivalence problems or for which actual or potential problems are thought to have been satisfactorily resolved. B ratings are given to drug products that the FDA does not at this time consider to be therapeutically equivalent to other pharmaceutically equivalent products.

These differences can have great clinical significance. For example, Dubovsky (1987) reported a case of severe nortriptyline intoxication due to changing from a generic to a trade preparation, which seemed to result from the significantly greater bioavailability of the trade preparation.

These comments are not a recommendation for any preparation over any other but are meant to inform the clinician that different preparations of the same medication of the same strength may have different bioavailabilities and that when they are substituted for one another, there is a potential for significant clinical repercussions. If prescriptions are written that may be filled with various generic preparations, it is prudent for the physician to inform the patient or responsible adult that if the medication is different when refilled, to inform him or her and to note any changes in symptoms or feelings after switching to a new preparation. Although changes in manufacturer may occur at times even when prescriptions are filled at the same pharmacy, the likelihood of a change in manufacturer increases when different pharmacies are used. If a patient runs out of medication while traveling and must obtain the drug(s) from a new source, a change of manufacturer may be more likely. Hence, it is worthwhile to remember to ascertain that a patient has sufficient medication before going to summer camp or traveling.

Standard (FDA-approved) and Nonstandard (Off-label) Treatments

In this book, those treatments that have been approved by the FDA for advertising and interstate commerce will be considered standard treatments. This implies that the drug has demonstrated clinical efficacy and that its use is substantially safe. The FDA's legal authority over how marketed drugs are used, the dosages employed, and related matters is limited to regulating what the manufacturer may recommend and must disclose in the package insert or labeling. "The prescription of a drug for an unlabeled (off-label) indication is entirely proper if the proposed use is based on rational scientific theory, expert medical opinion, or controlled clinical studies" (American Medical Association, 1993, p. 14).

Over the past five decades, a substantial body of clinical and investigational data has accumulated on using FDA-approved drugs to treat children below the recommended age (e.g., imipramine to treat major depressive disorder in children below 12 years of age), using FDA-approved drugs to treat children and adolescents for non–FDA-approved (off-label) indications (e.g., lithium to treat aggressive conduct disorder in any age-group and tricyclic antidepressants to treat ADHD), and using drugs before they were approved by the FDA for any indication (investigational drugs) to treat psychiatric disorders in children and adolescents (e.g., clomipramine and fluvoxamine maleate).

Selective serotonin reuptake inhibitor (SSRI) antidepressants and atypical antipsychotics are at present the most clinically important FDA-approved drugs used for nonapproved (off-label) indications in children and adolescents, although some SSRIs are approved for some indications in this age-group. There is a growing consensus among child psychiatrists that the benefit/risk ratio of their use for non–FDA-approved indications is often preferable to that of some currently approved medications (e.g., a decreased risk of developing tardive dyskinesia). This will be discussed in more detail in the specific drug section of the book.

Drug Interactions

Many psychoactive drugs have significant interactions with other medications. It is essential to be aware of any drug, prescription or otherwise, that the patient may be taking concurrently and to evaluate the potential interaction.

As part of the medical history, enquiries should be made about all medications, including those prescribed by other physicians; over-the-counter drugs; dietary supplements; and herbal preparations used even occasionally by the patient; and, as appropriate, alcohol and illicit or recreational drug use. Parents or caretakers and patients, as appropriate to their age and mental abilities, should be instructed to inform any physician who may treat them of the psychoactive medication(s) currently being taken. Similarly, patients whom the clinician is treating with psychoactive medication should be instructed to report at the next appointment whenever another physician prescribes any other medication for them or if they take any other drugs, over the counter or illicit, on their own initiative.

If substance abuse is known or suspected, screening of urine and/or blood for toxic substances may be indicated.

Drug interactions are discussed for each of the classes of psychoactive drugs. An attempt has been made to emphasize the most important interactions and those interactions most likely to be encountered by the physician who is treating psychiatrically disturbed children and adolescents.

It is beyond the scope of this book to review all possible drug interactions. It is the prescribing physician's responsibility to attempt to determine any other drugs his or her patient is taking and to assess any potentially adverse interactions of the medications before prescribing a new medication. The package insert, current *PDR*, current *Drug Interactions and Side Effects Index*, *Drug Facts and Comparisons*, *Drug Interactions in Psychiatry* (Ciraulo et al., 1989), or other suitable reference should be consulted. When appropriate and with the patient's consent, any other physicians treating the patient should be contacted so that a comprehensive treatment regimen that addresses both the psychiatric and the medical disorders of the patient safely may be mutually developed.

Regulating the Medication

Selecting the Initial Dosage

It is recommended in most cases that the treating physician initially prescribe a low dose, which will be either ineffective or inadequate for most patients. Although this cautious approach may lengthen the time necessary to reach a therapeutic dose, it is worthwhile for several reasons. First, pharmacokinetics vary not only among various age groups but also among individuals of a specific age. For genetic and other reasons, some individuals, for example, slow metabolizers, may be highly sensitive and responsive to a given medication whereas others, namely, rapid metabolizers, may be relatively resistant or nonresponsive. By beginning with a low dose, the physician will avoid starting at a dose that is already in excess of the optimal therapeutic dose for a few patients, and those children and adolescents who are good responders at low dosages of medication will not be missed. If the initial dose is too high, the therapeutic range for these low-dose responders will not be explored and only adverse effects, which may at times even be confused with worsening of target symptoms, will be seen. Hence, a potentially beneficial medication may be needlessly excluded. For example, first, with stimulants a worsening of behavior may occur when optimal therapeutic doses for a specific patient have been exceeded. Second, with some drugs (e.g., methylphenidate), there is no significant relationship between the serum level and clinical response. Third, excessive initial dosage may also cause behavioral toxicity, particularly in younger children. Behavioral toxicity has long been known to occur often before other adverse effects and includes symptoms such as worsening of target symptoms, hyperactivity or hypoactivity, aggressiveness, increased irritability, mood changes, apathy, and decreased verbal productions (Campbell et al., 1985). Fourth, some adverse effects of the drug may be eliminated or minimized; for example, acute dystonic reactions of antipsychotics and some adverse effects of lithium carbonate appear to be related in many cases to both serum levels and the rapidity of increase in serum level, and sedation may be less of a problem if dosage is increased gradually (Green et al., 1985).

The primary exceptions to gradual titration occur when an emergency situation exists, most often where there is danger or potential danger for injury to self, others, or property, and acute agitation or psychosis must be controlled as soon as possible.

Timing of Drug Administration

Scheduling Dosages

Times chosen for administration of the drug and the number of times the drug is administered per day should be related to the pharmacokinetics of the drug; for example, stimulants are most frequently given around breakfast and lunch, whereas antipsychotics may initially be given three or four times daily to reduce the risk of sedation and acute dystonic reactions. Once dosage has been stabilized, it may be clinically more convenient and may sometimes increase compliance if medications that have longer half-lives are administered only once or twice daily. Over the past 15 years, the number of long-active, controlled, sustained, or extended-release preparations of drugs has increased significantly. Prescription of such has likewise increased with increased convenience to the patient. This has been especially helpful in that many school children taking stimulant medication for ADHD no longer need to take it in school.

Pharmacokinetics and developmentally determined pharmacodynamic factors must still take precedence over convenience. For example, it may be possible to give the entire daily dose of an antipsychotic at bedtime to children and adolescents, whereas because younger children metabolize tricyclic antidepressants differently compared with adolescents and adults and they may be more sensitive to cardiotoxic effects, it is recommended that these drugs continue to be administered to children and younger adolescents in divided doses.

Drug Holidays

Because of the adverse effects of medications and their known and unknown effects on the growth, maturation, and development of children and adolescents, it is universally agreed that it is prudent to use medication in as low a dose and for as short a time as is clinically expedient. For some children, "drug holidays" may be a useful means of minimizing the cumulative amount of medication taken over time. The feasibility and type of drug holidays vary with the diagnosis and the severity of the disorder.

When stimulant medication is needed primarily to improve classroom functioning (increase attention span and decrease hyperactivity and sometimes conduct problems), as with some ADHD children, it is often possible to withhold medication on weekends and on school holidays and vacations, including the entire summer. This is particularly important if there appears to be evidence of any suppression of height and weight percentiles, because there may be catch-up or compensatory growth following discontinuation of stimulant medication.

Sometimes parents find that their hyperactive child is not a serious management problem without medication at home but that difficulties arise when the child accompanies them on a shopping excursion or goes to a birthday party. In cases like this, when the parents' judgment can be trusted and medication is not used as a punishment, an understanding with the parents and child that medication may be used occasionally on weekends or vacations in situations that are particularly difficult for the child may be therapeutically indicated.

There is reasonable concern about the possibility of the development of an irreversible tardive dyskinesia in children and adolescents who receive long-term therapy with antipsychotic medication. There is some evidence that the development of tardive dyskinesia may be associated with both the total amount of antipsychotic drug ingested and the duration of treatment, although constitutional vulnerabilities to developing tardive dyskinesia also appear to play an important role (Jeste and Wyatt, 1982). Consequently, possible means of reducing the total amount of an antipsychotic drug ever taken may be clinically important in reducing the likelihood of developing tardive dyskinesia.

Newton et al. (1989) and Perry et al. (1989) both reported studies of patients receiving first-generation antipsychotic medications, among whom drug holidays were not associated with differences either in symptom severity or adverse effects. Drug holidays require continued maintenance of clinical supervision and of observation by parents and caretakers, to document clinical changes and to circumvent relapses.

Dosage Increases

Changes in medication level should be based on the clinical response of the patient, and the rationale for each change should be documented in the clinical record. Knowledge of the characteristic time frame of response for a particular drug and diagnosis should influence these decisions. Therefore, the clinician may increase dosage once or twice weekly in some cases, when using stimulants or neuroleptics. On the other hand, the clinical efficacy of antidepressants may not be fully apparent for several weeks when used to treat a major depressive disorder. Once the total daily dose of an antidepressant has reached a level that is usually associated with clinical response, increasing the dose because of a failure to respond during the first 2 or 3 weeks of treatment is not sound psychopharmacologic practice unless serum drug levels are being monitored and are thought to be in the subtherapeutic range.

Titration of Medication

The goal of the clinician is to achieve meaningful therapeutic benefits for the patient with the fewest possible adverse effects. Here again, it is recommended that risks versus benefits be assessed. To do so scientifically, however, it is necessary to explore the dose range of a patient's response. Unless there are extenuating circumstances, it is usually advisable to continue raising the dose level until one of the following events occurs:

1. Entirely adequate symptom control is established.
2. The upper limit of the recommended dosage (or higher level if commonly accepted) has been reached.
3. Adverse effects that preclude a further increase in dose have occurred.
4. After a measurable improvement in target symptoms, a plateau in improvement or a worsening of symptoms occurs with further increases in dose.

Unless this procedure is followed, an injustice may be done to the patient. This occurs most frequently when there is some behavioral improvement and the treating clinician stabilizes the dosage at that point. Further significant improvement that might have occurred had a higher dose been given is missed. It is recommended that the next higher dose be explored. If there is significant additional improvement, the therapist, in consultation with the patient and his or her parents, can make a judgment regarding whether the benefits outweigh the risks from the additional dosage.

Determining the Optimal Dose

Once the titration of the therapeutic dose to maximum clinical benefit has been achieved for a specific patient, the lowest possible dose that produces those desired effects should be determined. This is considered the optimal dose for a specific patient. In clinical practice, this may sometimes require a compromise, and amelioration of target symptoms to an acceptable degree may occur only when some adverse effects are also present.

In those cases in which either no significant therapeutic benefit occurs or adverse effects prevent the employment of a clinically meaningful therapeutic dose, trial of a different medication must be considered. If there is a partial but meaningful clinical response, some clinicians would consider adding an additional medication (polypharmacy) rather than discontinuing the drug and administering another. Whatever the case, clinicians should not continue to prescribe medication in doses that do not result in significant clinical improvement.

Adverse Effects (Side Effects)

All drugs, including placebos, have adverse effects, or side effects. Actually, if one excludes allergic and idiosyncratic reactions, adverse effects are as much a characteristic of the pharmacologic makeup of a specific drug and are as predictable as the drug's therapeutic effects. Simply put, drugs have effects: some effects are desirable and some are not. Individual patients may vary as much in their experience of adverse effects of a drug as in their therapeutic responses to it. Adverse effects are important not only because of the immediate problematic effects they cause but also because they may be intimately related to issues of compliance, as discussed in the preceding text.

It is sometimes useful to think of adverse effects as the "unwanted effects" of the drug for the specific patient and therapeutic indication. For a different patient and situation, an adverse or side effect will actually become the desired therapeutic action of the drug. For example, sedation, which may be an adverse effect when a benzodiazepine is prescribed for anxiolysis, is the desired result when a benzodiazepine is prescribed as a soporific. Similarly, appetite suppression is usually an undesired effect of stimulants prescribed for ADHD but the action of choice when used in treating exogenous obesity.

Many adverse effects are related to dose or serum levels, but others are not. They may occur almost immediately (e.g., an acute dystonic reaction) or be delayed for years (e.g., tardive dyskinesia). They may be life threatening or fatal, or relatively innocuous. The adverse effects of a specific drug may differ according to the age and/or diagnosis of the subjects. For example, haloperidol produced excessive sedation in hospitalized school-age aggressive-conduct-disordered children on doses of 0.04 to 0.21 mg/kg/day (Campbell et al., 1984b) but not in preschoolers with autistic disorder on doses of 0.019 to 0.217 mg/kg/day (Anderson et al., 1984).

A thorough knowledge of the most important and frequent adverse effects of the medications considered is essential and will often play a decisive role in which medication is selected and/or when dosage is scheduled. For example, if a schizophrenic youngster has insomnia, the clinician may select a low-potency antipsychotic drug and adjust the dosage schedule so that any sedation will aid the child in falling asleep. As an added benefit, the risk of an acute dystonic reaction is lower than if a high-potency antipsychotic drug had been chosen.

Likewise, the management of adverse effects is a vital component of pharmacotherapy. In clinical practice, careful attention to adverse effects and flexibility about the time and amounts of specific doses may enable one to obtain a satisfactory clinical result with a minimal or acceptable level of adverse effects that is not possible if a fixed dosage schedule is used, as in some research protocols. Therefore, one can adjust medication levels slowly and in small increments or divide doses unequally over the day (e.g., giving more in the morning, more before bed, or the entire daily dose at bedtime).

The clinician must remember that the ability to understand adverse effects and verbalize unusual sensations, feelings, or discomfort not only varies among individual children but is also developmentally determined. Younger children spontaneously report adverse effects less frequently than do older children. Hence, the younger the child, the more essential it becomes for caretakers to be actively looking for adverse effects and for the physician to ask the patient about adverse effects using language appropriate to the child's level of understanding.

Many psychotropic drugs may cause treatment-emergent sexual dysfunction–related adverse effects which are of significant concern to adolescents, especially those who may be sexually active. As many adolescents are uncomfortable in discussing such matters and do not spontaneously report them, it is particularly important for the clinician to routinely ask about such symptoms in a nonjudgmental, nonthreatening way.

It is essential that the clinician examine the patient frequently for the development of adverse effects during the period when the medication is being regulated, at regular intervals during maintenance therapy, and during scheduled periodic withdrawals of the medication. For example, with antipsychotic drugs, one should look particularly for sedation and extrapyramidal side effects, the development of abnormal movements, and, during drug withdrawal periods, any evidence of a withdrawal dyskinesia. Completion of the AIMS, as described earlier, is recommended as an aid in quantifying and following abnormal movements over time.

Monitoring of Serum Levels of Drugs and/or of Their Metabolites

Morselli et al. (1983) and Gualtieri et al. (1984a) reviewed the pharmacokinetics of psychoactive drugs used in child and adolescent psychiatry and the clinical relevance of determining their serum or blood levels. Determining the blood or plasma levels of drugs and/or their metabolites is most useful when accurate measurements of all significant active metabolites of a drug are available and there is a known relationship between the clinical effects of the drug and serum concentration (Gualtieri et al., 1984a). Obviously, monitoring levels of drugs whose toxicity is level-related, such as tricyclic antidepressants, lithium, and mast anticonvulsants is crucially important for patient safety.

For many of the drugs in current use in child and adolescent psychopharmacology, serum levels are not as clearly related to clinical effects or toxicity. Consequently, serum levels of stimulant drugs, selective serotonin and norepinephrine reuptake inhibitors, and second-generation neuroleptics are not as commonly measured as those of older drugs and are often of uncertain clinical utility. Still, there is a role for these measurements in some situations, especially when compliance is in question.

Clinically, the monitoring of serum levels is useful to verify compliance and to be certain that adequate therapeutic serum levels are available (i.e., that values fall within the therapeutic window) and thereby avoid discontinuing a trial of medication before clinically effective serum levels have been reached or, conversely, avoid inadvertently reaching toxic serum levels.

School-aged children often have more efficient physiologic systems for drug metabolism and excretion than adults. As a result, doses comparable to those administered to adults, either on a total daily dose or on a dose-per-unit-weight basis, may result in subtherapeutic serum levels in children and younger adolescents. This could be one factor contributing to the clinical observation that children with schizophrenia, as a group, appear to show less dramatic clinical improvement than adolescents and adults when administered neuroleptics (Green, 1989). It will be necessary to measure antipsychotic serum levels to determine if this lack of improvement is due to subtherapeutic levels in some cases, because some children may also show clinical improvement at lower serum levels than do adults (Rivera-Calimlim et al., 1979).

Meyers et al. (1980) reported the case of a 13-year-old prepubescent boy diagnosed as having schizophrenia who required a dose of haloperidol of at least 30 mg/day to reach therapeutic serum neuroleptic levels. Monitoring serum levels of antipsychotic drugs may therefore yield clinical information that is, at times, extremely useful. If a child or adolescent does not have a satisfactory response to usual doses of antipsychotic drugs, serum neuroleptic levels should be determined, if available, before deciding to discontinue the drug.

In addition to age-related differences in pharmacokinetics, remarkable interindividual variations occur. For example, Berg et al. (1974) reported that a 14-year-old girl with bipolar manic-depressive disorder required up to 2,400 mg of lithium daily to maintain serum lithium levels of 1 mEq/L. Her father had the same disorder and also required unusually high doses of lithium to reach therapeutic levels.

Currently, regular determinations of serum levels should be considered mandatory when lithium carbonate, antiepileptic drugs, or tricyclic antidepressants are used in treating children and adolescents. In current practice, for example, monitoring of drug and metabolite serum levels is of considerable practical importance in the use of the tricyclic antidepressants. This monitoring is needed because there is minimal correlation between the dose and serum level, and serum levels are correlated significantly with the clinical response and/or potentially serious adverse effects (e.g., cardiotoxicity). For example, Puig-Antich et al. (1987) have emphasized that they found no predictors of total maintenance plasma levels, including dosage, in their prepubertal subjects treated with imipramine for major depressive disorder. They also reported that positive therapeutic response to imipramine in prepubertal children was strongly correlated with serum levels above 150 ng/mL.

Similarly, Biederman et al. (1989b) reported that desipramine serum levels varied an average of 16.5-fold at four different dose levels in 31 children and adolescents diagnosed with attention-deficit disorder. These authors, however, found no significant linear relationship between the total daily dose or weight-corrected (mg/kg) daily dose and the steady-state serum desipramine level and any outcome measure, including clinical improvement. There was a tendency for serum desipramine levels in subjects who were rated very much or much improved on the Clinical Global Improvement Scale to average 60.8% higher than in unimproved subjects.

Morselli et al. (1983) also emphasized that monitoring drug plasma levels of haloperidol, chlorpromazine, imipramine, and clomipramine is particularly helpful in optimizing long-term treatment with these agents.

On the other hand, a detailed review of the pharmacokinetics and actions of methylphenidate concluded that "blood MPH [methylphenidate] levels are not statistically related to clinical response, nor are they likely to prove clinically helpful until this lack of correlation is understood" (Patrick et al., 1987, p. 1393).

Serum levels are also mandatory when antiepileptic drugs are being used for control of seizures, although this use is not reviewed in this book. When antiepileptic drugs are used for other psychiatric indications, such as control of aggression or as mood stabilizers, effective serum levels are thought to be in the same range as when they are used to control seizures. Monitoring of serum levels (both drug and significant metabolites) will become increasingly important for other drugs used in child and adolescent psychiatry if and when their determinations become more readily available and correlations with clinical efficacy and adverse effects are established.

Length of Time to Continue Medication

Children and adolescents are immature, developing individuals progressing toward adulthood. Because of concerns about long-term adverse effects such as tardive and withdrawal dyskinesias and growth retardation as well as our inadequate knowledge of other long-term adverse effects of psychopharmacological agents on their biological and psychological maturation, there is virtually unanimous agreement that medication should be given for as short a period as possible.

The vicissitudes of the natural courses of psychiatric illnesses in children and adolescents are often not predictable for specific individuals. It is to be hoped, especially when there is a significant psychosocial etiologic factor, that medication will augment the child's response to other therapeutic interventions and enhance his or her social and academic functioning, maturation, and development. Once real gains are made and internalized, the cycle of failures broken, and the maladaptive patterns replaced with more appropriate ones, it may be possible to discontinue the drug and maintain therapeutic gains. Even in chronic conditions with strong biological underpinnings, such as pervasive developmental disorder, schizophrenia, and depression, the clinical course may spontaneously vary so that in some patients psychoactive medication may be reduced or even discontinued.

Periodic Withdrawal/Tapering of Medication

It is often considered advisable to discontinue psychotropic medications (or to attempt to do so) in child and adolescent patients on a regular basis, certainly no less frequently than every 6 months to 1 year. There may be occasional exceptions to this (e.g., the long-term prophylactic use of lithium carbonate or an antidepressant to prevent recurrences of mood disorders or not withdrawing an antipsychotic in a child or adolescent being treated for schizophrenia who has experienced serious relapses during prior withdrawal attempts). Whenever medication is continued beyond 6 to 12 months, it is important to document the clinical reasons for doing so in the medical record.

Discontinuation/Withdrawal Syndromes

Rapidly metabolized drugs such as methylphenidate and amphetamines may be discontinued abruptly. However, with these drugs, which have short half-lives, there may be some rebound effect during routine daily administration of the drug as serum levels decline during late afternoon or evening.

To minimize the likelihood of developing withdrawal syndromes, it is recommended that most medications be gradually reduced rather than stopped abruptly. The clinician should continue to complete the AIMS in patients who had preexisting abnormal movements prior to the initiation of medication that may have been masked or ameliorated or who are otherwise at risk for developing abnormal movements following withdrawal. If a withdrawal dyskinesia emerges upon discontinuing an antipsychotic drug, effort should be made to keep the patient off antipsychotics. Any abnormal movements should continue to be recorded on the AIMS.

Gualtieri et al. (1984b) reported both physical withdrawal symptoms (e.g., decreased appetite, nausea and vomiting, diarrhea, and sweating) and acute behavioral deterioration in approximately 10% of children and adolescents after their withdrawal from long-term treatment with first-generation antipsychotics. Both types of withdrawal symptoms ceased spontaneously within 8 weeks. It is extremely important that the clinician recognize that such symptoms may be expected withdrawal effects and that they are not necessarily a return of premedication symptoms. The symptoms must be monitored qualitatively and quantitatively over a sufficient period to see if they diminish, as would be expected with a withdrawal syndrome, or if they indicate that the underlying psychiatric disorder still requires medication for symptom amelioration.

When tricyclics are withdrawn abruptly or too rapidly, some children experience a flu-like withdrawal syndrome resulting from cholinergic rebound. This characteristically includes gastrointestinal symptoms such as nausea, abdominal discomfort and pain, vomiting, and fatigue. Tapering the medication down over a 10-day period rather than abruptly withdrawing it will usually avoid this effect or significantly diminish the withdrawal syndrome. The clinician is cautioned that in patients with poor compliance, who in essence may undergo periodic self-induced acute withdrawals, the withdrawal syndrome may be confused with adverse effects, inadequate dose levels, or worsening of the underlying psychiatric disorder.

A withdrawal or discontinuation syndrome has also been identified for the SSRIs. Rosenbaum et al. (1998) reviewed the literature on discontinuation-emergent symptoms in adults taking SSRIs and noted that dizziness, headache, nausea, vomiting, diarrhea, movement disorders, insomnia, irritability, visual disturbances, lethargy, anorexia, tremor, electric shock sensations, and lowered mood have all been reported following SSRI discontinuation. There appeared to be a relationship between half-life and the development of discontinuation-emergent symptoms. Patients abruptly discontinued from drugs with longer half-lives, for example, fluoxetine, developed fewer clinically significant effects than did patients who abruptly discontinued drugs with short half-lives, for example, paroxetine or sertraline. Similar data are now emerging for children (Diler and Avci, 2002).

Similarly, it is recommended that the alpha-adrenergic agonists, clonidine hydrochloride and guanfacine hydrochloride, be tapered gradually to reduce the likelihood of a hypertensive reaction and other symptoms, such as headache, nervousness, and agitation. This is more important for clonidine, as its half-life is significantly shorter than that of guanfacine.

In significant numbers of cases, after an initial treatment period of varying duration, medication may no longer be required or adequate symptom control can be maintained on a lower maintenance dose. In contrast, over time some patients may require higher doses to maintain gains. This may reflect a worsening of the psychiatric disorder *per se* or a developmental/maturational effect, as in a child with autistic disorder who becomes both stronger and more aggressive as he or she enters adolescence. In other cases, the need for increased medication may be a consequence of an individual's normal physiologic maturation altering the drug's pharmacokinetics and/or normal or excessive weight gain. In any case, ongoing regular clinical supervision of any child on medication is essential. This is both the responsibility and the privilege of the child and adolescent psychiatrist.

SECTION TWO
Specific Drugs

CHAPTER 3

Introduction

WILLIAM KLYKYLO

Child psychopharmacology is a relatively new field. The 1937 publication by Charles Bradley reporting the effects of administering racemic amphetamine sulfate (Benzedrine) to 30 children 5 to 14 years of age with various behavioral disturbances is usually considered to mark the beginning of the modern era of child psychopharmacology.

More than 20 years later, the first book concerned exclusively with psychopharmacologic research in child psychiatry, *Child Research in Psychopharmacology*, evolved out of the 1958 Conference on Child Research in Psychopharmacology sponsored by the National Institute of Mental Health (Fisher, 1959). The book contains an annotated list of 159 references of studies of the effects of psychopharmacologic agents administered to children with psychiatric problems, beginning with Bradley's 1937 publication. Interestingly, M. Molitch and coworkers also published, in 1937, three papers concerning the use of amphetamine sulfate in children, including two placebo-controlled studies (Molitch and Eccles, 1937; Molitch and Poliakoff, 1937; Molitch and Sullivan, 1937). Two of the studies found that amphetamine sulfate improved scores of children on intelligence tests, and one reported that 86% of 14 enuretic boys who had not responded to placebo were dry when given increasing doses of amphetamine sulfate and reverted to bedwetting within 2 weeks after the drug was discontinued.

In the 1950s, the classes of drugs currently most important in general psychiatry were introduced: the antipsychotics (chlorpromazine and other compounds), the antidepressants, and lithium carbonate. The benzodiazepines, in particular diazepam and chlordiazepoxide, were introduced into clinical psychiatric practice in the early 1960s. Then in the late 1980s and throughout the 1990s, the selective serotonin reuptake inhibitor (SSRI) antidepressants and the atypical antipsychotics, now referred to as second-generation antipsychotics, began to be introduced. Because of increased difficulties in conducting psychopharmacologic research and in obtaining FDA approval of the safety and efficacy of psychoactive drugs in children and younger adolescents, the investigation and introduction into clinical practice of psychoactive drugs in children have always lagged somewhat behind that for adults. Weiner and Jaffe (1985) have written a brief but interesting overview of the earlier history of child and adolescent psychopharmacology.

Texts focusing entirely or significantly on child and adolescent psychopharmacology include those by Aman and Singh (1988), Bezchlibnyk-Butler and Virani (2004), Campbell et al. (1985), Gadow (1986a, 1986b), Klein et al. (1980), Kutcher (1997, 2002), Martin et al. (2003), Riddle (1995a, 1995b), Rosenberg et al. (1994, 2002), Walsh (1998), Weiner (1985), Werry (1978), Werry and Aman (1999), Trivedi and Chang (2012), and McVoy (2012). The reader who wishes an in-depth review of major issues of the recent past is referred to *Neuropsychopharmacology: The Fifth Generation of Progress* (Davis et al., 2002) and the fascinating *An Oral History of Neuropsychopharmacology: The First Fifty Years, Peer Interviews (Volumes 1-10)* (Ban, 2011). A review of these texts, and indeed their very proliferation, documents the massive growth of psychopharmacology as a component of the medical care of children and adolescents.

In most instances, reviews of the literature establishing the clinical efficacy and safety of earlier FDA-approved treatments for the psychiatric disorders of children and adolescents are not included in this book. Readers who wish to review the research data establishing these standard treatments will find such information to be accessible in the texts cited above.

Section II of this book not only summarizes the standard treatments but also focuses in greater detail on research into new and not yet approved uses of drugs in child and adolescent psychiatry and reviews these studies. Some knowledge of psychopharmacologic research principles and techniques is essential to critically evaluate the data that appear in the psychiatric literature and to make informed clinical decisions about whether a trial of a particular drug is warranted for a particular patient.

Most important psychopharmacologic research designs include comparison of the drug being investigated with either placebo or a drug approved as a standard treatment for the psychiatric disorder in question. Hence it is important to have a basic understanding of placebos.

PLACEBOS

According to the *Oxford English Dictionary* (OED) (1989), the English word *placebo* was directly adopted from the Latin word meaning "I shall be pleasing or acceptable." By 1811, it was defined in *Hooper's Medical Dictionary* (OED, 1989) as "an epithet given to any medicine adapted more to please than benefit the patient." In 1982, the OED added the following definition of *placebo*, which fairly accurately described its current use in psychopharmacologic research: "A substance or procedure which a patient accepts as a medicine or therapy but which actually has no specific therapeutic activity for his condition or is prescribed in the belief that it has no such activity." Although placebos are often composed of substances thought to be inert, in psychopharmacologic research, placebos may also contain active ingredients chosen to simulate adverse effects of the drug to which the placebo is being compared. The purpose of this is to keep all participants "blind" by making it more difficult for patients and observers to distinguish between drug and placebo based solely on the drug's adverse effects.

Placebos play a crucial role in clinical psychopharmacologic research by providing nonspecific treatment effects for comparison with the drug under investigation. These nonspecific psychological and physiologic changes are not drug specific and may be measured by rating scales (Prien, 1988). These changes include both beneficial and adverse effects produced by the expectations the patient or observers have about the drug, natural fluctuations in the clinical course of the disease, and spontaneous alterations in the patient's condition that may have nothing to do with the illness under consideration; effects of the relationship among the patient, therapist, and other medical staff; and other unknown effects.

Because of these nonspecific effects, even "inert" placebos have side effects. These may commonly include such symptoms as fatigue, tiredness, anxiety, muscle aches, nausea, diarrhea, constipation, dry mouth, dysmenorrhea, and behavioral changes such as increased or decreased aggressiveness, impulsiveness, attention span, or irritability. These are often symptoms that might appear periodically in the general population. It is the difference in incidence and severity of these unwanted effects between placebo and drug that is important.

The psychological consequences of placebos have long been recognized. Recent research has explored the possibility that some placebo effects may be mediated by detectable neurobiological processes, including endorphin activity (Zubieta et al., 2005). Finniss et al. (2010) have produced a masterful review of the scientific and ethical consequences of our increased understanding of these issues.

The most methodologically sound use of a placebo for testing a new medication is a double-blind, randomized, parallel-groups design (Prien, 1988). Stanley (1988) has written an interesting article concerning ethical and clinical considerations in the use of placebos that evaluated such factors as withholding medication during a placebo period and whether treatment may be ethically withheld in a placebo-controlled trial when a known treatment is available.

Head-to-head studies compare a new drug to a drug already recognized as effective and safe. This strategy/design can avoid the ethical conundrum of denying treatment to patients who would have been assigned placebo in a placebo-controlled study and is important when delay of treatment known to be effective for a given diagnosis could result in serious harm to the patient. Prien (1988) offered six alternative study designs for use when it is not possible to use a double-blind, randomized, parallel-groups design and discussed some of their limitations. White et al. (1985) edited a fascinating book concerning the theory, ethics, use in research and clinical practice, and mediating mechanisms of placebos.

EVALUATING RESEARCH STUDIES

Efficacy and safety are determined by a statistically significant benefit with acceptable adverse effects of the new medication compared with placebo. Statistics, however, inform us about groups of patients, not individuals. Hence if etiologically dissimilar groups are subsumed under the same diagnosis, a few patients may truly benefit, but their improvement could be so diluted by the larger majority who did not benefit that the drug might show no statistically significant benefit. Some researchers now note whether there are strong individual responders in a drug study even when there is no statistical difference between experimental and control groups. Therefore, individual case reports, studies of relatively small numbers, and open studies should not be summarily dismissed.

In evaluating the literature on child and adolescent psychopharmacology, it is important to remember that a drug that is statistically and significantly better than another drug or placebo does not necessarily mean that the drug is the optimal treatment for a given condition or for a specific child or adolescent. The drug may be effective only in certain environments (e.g., a laboratory) and cannot be generalized to more ordinary circumstances, or it may improve only certain symptoms but not affect other major target symptoms to a clinically meaningful degree, or the overall improvement may be relatively modest with significant symptoms or deficits remaining. For example, Sprague and Sleator (1977) found that 0.3 mg/kg of methylphenidate produced optimal enhancement of learning short-term memory tasks in hyperkinetic children in the laboratory, but 1 mg/kg of methylphenidate produced the maximum improvement of social behavior in the classroom as shown by ratings on the Abbreviated Conners Rating Scale. Another example is that although children with autistic disorder have shown statistically significant improvements with several drugs, the degree of their improvement is typically modest, with marked residual deficits remaining, and at present no drug is satisfactory for treatment of this condition (Green, 1988).

In evaluating research, diagnostic criteria and the diagnostic heterogeneity/homogeneity of the sample, and both the severity of the patients included and the clinical setting in which the drug was given, must be evaluated. Therefore, until the formalization by DSM-III (American Psychiatric Association, 1980a) of diagnostic distinctions between schizophrenia with childhood onset and autistic disorder (or their equivalents), both were subsumed under the diagnosis of schizophrenia, childhood type; many studies included diagnostically heterogeneous samples or the composition of the sample could not be determined, rendering interpretation of the studies difficult or impossible (Green, 1989).

Gadow and Poling (1988) provide another relevant example. They noted that stimulant medication is not commonly prescribed for persons with intellectual disabilities in residential facilities where most of the residents are usually severely or profoundly disabled. They pointed out that some reviews of the use of stimulants among those falling into these diagnostic categories suggested that stimulants might not be useful in treating behavior disorders and could even exacerbate attention deficit in these patients. They noted that the large majority of these individuals are not in institutions and that they are prescribed stimulants for management of disturbed behavior, particularly hyperactivity, much more frequently and with more favorable results than one might expect from reading the literature. In fact, these authors concluded that stimulants were highly effective in diminishing conduct problems and hyperactivity for some individuals with intellectual disabilities, whatever their IQs.

As psychiatric nosology and diagnosis become more refined and the etiopathogeneses of more homogeneous subgroups are delineated, more focused research may be undertaken and more specific and rational psychopharmacology will inevitably follow.

SPECIFIC DRUG TREATMENTS

In this section of the book, psychopharmacologic agents are organized and discussed by class rather than according to the psychiatric diagnoses for which they are treatments. The rationale for this organization is related to several of the issues discussed in the first part of the book. At the present time, most diagnoses are based on phenomenology (i.e., constellations of clinical symptoms) rather than on any basic understanding of the etiopathogenesis of the condition. Therefore, a given drug may be used to treat several psychiatric diagnoses. Hence, repetition of facts under each diagnostic category and extensive cross-referencing are avoided.

Each class of drugs is introduced with some general comments, including indications for use, contraindications, interactions with other drugs, and the most common untoward effects. The basic pharmacokinetics, including approximations of time of peak serum levels and the drug's serum half-life, major metabolites, and excretion, are discussed. Unless otherwise noted, all dosage recommendations are for oral administration.

Specific drugs of each class are reviewed individually. Traditional or standard, FDA-approved treatments are discussed, but additionally many treatments not approved for advertising by the FDA but reported to be efficacious in the literature and used clinically by practitioners are discussed as well.

Most of the studies cited in this book either illustrate a particular point or provide the reader with some of the evidence for using off-label treatments. This evidence ranges from convincing to merely suggestive of a possible alternative for a seriously disturbed patient who has not responded satisfactorily to any prior treatment attempts. Excellent and extensive literature reviews of the standard psychopharmacologic treatments discussed later are readily accessible in the additional earlier texts on child and adolescent psychopharmacology referenced earlier in this chapter.

Although always important, informed consent, preferably written, is particularly important if FDA-approved drugs are used for nonapproved indications. If standard approved treatments for a seriously disabling disorder have been tried with little or no success, a clinical trial of a nonapproved or even an investigational medication is much more easily justified. The physician has the responsibility to become thoroughly familiar with the official package labeling information provided by the manufacturer of the drug or the relevant entry in the latest edition and supplements of the *Physicians' Desk Reference* before prescribing any drug.

Table 3.1 lists the most common psychiatric diagnoses in children and younger adolescents for which psychopharmacotherapy may be therapeutically indicated and the medications that have been used in treating that disorder. Whenever a specific drug or class of drugs is generally preferred for a particular condition, an attempt has been made to rank them in order of usual preference if possible; however, for some diagnoses there are many drugs for which there is no clear order of preference. The listing of a medication indicates that it is discussed or reports of interest are summarized in the text; such a listing does not necessarily imply that the drug is a recommended treatment.

TABLE 3.1 » Diagnoses in Childhood and Adolescence for Which Psychopharmacotherapy May Be Therapeutically Indicated and Drugs Discussed in the Text

Attention-deficit/hyperactivity disorder
    Methylphenidate preparations
    Amphetamine preparations
    Atomoxetine
    Clonidine
    Guanfacine
    Bupropion
    Tricyclic antidepressants
    Haloperidol[a]
    Atypical/second-generation neuroleptics[a]
    Fluoxetine[a]
    Clomipramine[a]
    MAOIs[a]
    Venlafaxine[a]
Bipolar disorder/mania
    Lithium
    Valproic acid
    Carbamazepine
    Risperidone
    Oxcarbazepine
    Topiramate
    Phenytoin (diphenylhydantoin)[a]
    Gabapentin[a]
    Lamotrigine[a]
Conduct disorder (severe, aggressive)
    Atypical/second-generation antipsychotics
    Haloperidol; other first-generation antipsychotics
    Methylphenidate
    Lithium
    Buspirone
    Propranolol
    Valproic acid
    Carbamazepine
    Trazodone
    Clonidine
    Molindone

(continued)

TABLE 3.1 » Diagnoses in Childhood and Adolescence for Which Psychopharmacotherapy May Be Therapeutically Indicated and Drugs Discussed in the Text (Continued)

Encopresis
    Lithium
Enuresis
    DDAVP
    Imipramine
    Benzodiazepines
    Carbamazepine
    Amphetamines
    Clomipramine
    Desipramine
Generalized anxiety disorder (overanxious disorder of childhood)
    Benzodiazepines
    Diphenhydramine
    Fluoxetine
    Buspirone
    Hydroxyzine
Intermittent explosive disorder
    Propranolol
Major depressive disorder
    Antidepressants
    Lithium augmentation
    Lithium for prophylaxis
Manic episode
    Lithium
    Valproic acid
    Atypical/second-generation antipsychotics
Intellectual disability (with severe behavioral disorder and/or self-injurious behavior)
    Atypical/second-generation antipsychotics
    Haloperidol
    Chlorpromazaine
    Lithium
    Propranolol
    Naltrexone
Obsessive-compulsive disorder
    Sertraline
    Fluoxetine
    Paroxetine
    Fluvoxamine
    Clomipramine
    Clonazepam
Panic disorder
    Sertraline
    Paroxetine
    Alprazolam
    Clonazepam
    Tricyclic antidepressants
Pervasive developmental disorders, accompanied by agitation or aggression
    Risperidone and other atypical/second-generation antipsychotics
    Haloperidol
    Fluphenazine
    Naltrexone

TABLE 3.1 » Diagnoses in Childhood and Adolescence for Which Psychopharmacotherapy May Be Therapeutically Indicated and Drugs Discussed in the Text (Continued)

    Methylphenidate preparations
    Amphetamines preparations
    Clomipramine
    Buspirone
    Clonidine
Posttraumatic stress disorder
    Sertraline
    Propranolol
Schizophrenia
    Atypical/second-generation antipsychotics
    First-generation antipsychotics
Selective mutism
    Fluoxetine
    Sertraline
Separation anxiety disorder
    Fluoxetine
    Chlordiazepoxide
    Alprazolam
    Buspirone
    Clomipramine
    Imipramine
    Clonazepam
Sleep disorders
    Primary insomnia
        Benzodiazepines
        Diphenhydramine
        Hydroxyzine
        Clonidine
    Circadian-rhythm sleep disorder
        Benzodiazepines
        Diphenhydramine
        Hydroxyzine
    Sleep terror disorder
        Diazepam
        Alprazolam
        Imipramine
        Carbamazepine
    Sleepwalking disorder
        Diazepam
        Imipramine
    Tourette disorder
        Haloperidol
        Pimozide
        Clonidine
        Desipramine
        Guanfacine
        Bupropion
        Nortriptyline
        Fluoxetine

[a]These are agents for which there are limited clinical data, which have problematic untoward effects, or which are otherwise seldom used.

Sympathomimetic Amines, Central Nervous System Stimulants, and Executive Function Agents

RICK BOWERS and RYAN MAST

Note: The U.S. Food and Drug Administration (FDA) has directed that a Black Box Warning be added to the labeling of amphetamine and methylphenidate products stating, "Stimulants have a high potential for abuse. Administration of stimulants for prolonged periods of time may lead to drug dependence, particular attention should be paid to the possibility of subjects obtaining stimulants for nontherapeutic use or distribution to others and the drugs should be prescribed or dispensed sparingly. Misuse of stimulants may cause sudden death and serious cardiovascular adverse events." These agents should be given cautiously to patients with a history of drug dependence or alcoholism. Chronic, abusive use can lead to marked tolerance and psychological dependence with varying degrees of abnormal behavior. Frank psychotic episodes can occur, especially with parenteral abuse. Careful supervision is required during drug withdrawal from abusive use since severe depression may occur. Withdrawal following chronic therapeutic use may unmask symptoms of the underlying disorder that may require follow-up.

Sudden death has been reported in association with central nervous system (CNS) stimulant treatment at usual dosages in children and adolescents with structural cardiac abnormalities or serious heart problems. It is noted specifically for Adderall XR, "Its misuse is associated with serious cardiovascular adverse events and may cause sudden death in patients with preexisting cardiac structural abnormalities." The FDA does not recommend general use of stimulants in children or adults with structural cardiac abnormalities, or other serious cardiac problems that may place them at increased vulnerability. It is recommended that a doctor be called right away if a child has any sign of heart problems such as chest pain, shortness of breath, or fainting while taking stimulant medications.

INTRODUCTION

Sympathomimetic amines and central nervous system (CNS) stimulants are commonly referred to as stimulants. Two of these agents, methylphenidate (MPH) and amphetamine, are the drugs of choice for treating attention-deficit/hyperactivity disorder (ADHD). Particularly, the extended-release formulations of these medications may be preferable in variables such as med compliance and potential for abuse. Magnesium pemoline, which also falls into this category of drugs, was withdrawn from the market in 2005 by manufacturers because the increased risk of acute hepatic failure was unacceptable. Atomoxetine, a selective norepinephrine reuptake inhibitor (SNRI), is also approved by the FDA to treat ADHD; however, head-to-head comparisons suggest that stimulants are more effective than atomoxetine in improving hyperactivity, impulsivity, and inattention in such subjects (Starr and Kemner, 2005; Wigal et al., 2005; National Medical Association, FOCUS presentation, 2005; this is reviewed under the section "Atomoxetine versus Stimulants in the Treatment of Attention-Deficit/Hyperactivity Disorder in Children and Adolescents"). Long-acting forms of the alpha-adrenergic agonists guanfacine and clonidine are now approved by the FDA for the treatment of ADHD as monotherapy and as adjunctive therapy to stimulant medications. Amantadine (AMT) is a novel agent whose actions on the dopamine system are indirect and appear to be involved more as a modulator of dysfunction in the dopamine system. AMT seems to have utility for individuals with brain injury from various causes who have moderate to severe mental retardation and exhibit behavioral problems.

The most useful recent comprehensive review of the use of stimulants in treating ADHD is "Practice Parameter for the Use of Stimulant Medications in the Treatment of Children, Adolescents, and Adults" (Greenhill et al., 2002).

Bradley's (1937) report on the use of racemic amphetamine sulfate (Benzedrine) in children having behavioral disorders is usually cited as the beginning of child psychopharmacology as a discipline. Since this initial report, more research has been published on the stimulants and on ADHD than on any other childhood disorder. Double-blind, placebo-controlled studies have consistently found that stimulants are significantly superior to placebo in improving attention span and in decreasing hyperactivity and impulsivity. Although most of the earlier studies were in children, two double-blind studies have confirmed the clinical efficacy of MPH in treating adolescents diagnosed with attention-deficit disorder (ADD) who also had ADD as children (Klorman et al., 1988a, 1988b). Since then, many more studies on the use of stimulants, particularly the use of extended-release formulations, in adolescents and adults have been published.

Several investigators have reported that MPH also improved academic performance and/or peer interactions (e.g., Pelham et al., 1985, 1987; Rapport et al., 1994). Whalen et al. (1987) reported on 24 children between 6 and 11 years of age who were diagnosed with ADD or attention-deficit disorder with hyperactivity (ADDH) and who received either placebo, 0.3 mg/kg MPH daily, or 0.6 mg/kg MPH daily, in random order so that all children received each dosage level for a total of 4 days. The authors reported that all children showed decrements in negative social behaviors when rated during relatively unstructured outdoor activities at the 0.3-mg/kg level, compared with placebo. The youngest 12 children showed further improvement in social behavior at the higher dose.

Rapport et al. (1994) evaluated the acute effects of four dose levels (5, 10, 15, and 20 mg) of MPH on classroom behavior and academic performance of 76 children diagnosed with ADHD in a double-blind, placebo-controlled, within-subject (crossover) protocol. Compared with baseline, the subjects showed a nearly linear increase in normalization of behavior as the dose of MPH increased. On the Abbreviated Conners Teacher Rating Scale (CTRS), scores improved in 16% and normalized in 78% of the subjects. Attention, measured by on-task behavior, improved in 4% and normalized in 72% of the subjects. Academic efficiency, measured by the percentage of academic assignments completed correctly, improved in 3% and nor-malized in 50% of the subjects. Hence, there are several different clinically signifi-cant subsets of children: those who improve in all domains, those who improve in the behavioral and attention domains but do not improve in the academic domain and require additional interventions (e.g., tutoring), those who show behavioral improvement but no significant improvement in attention or academic ratings, and a fourth subset who do not benefit from MPH in any of the three domains.

In a double-blind, placebo-controlled study of 40 children (age range, 6 to 12 years; mean, 8.6 ± 1.3 years) who were diagnosed with ADHD and treated with MPH, DuPaul et al. (1994) found that subjects ($N = 12$) who had additional internal-izing symptoms such as anxiety or depression and who had high scores on the inter-nalizing scale of the Child Behavior Checklist (CBCL) were significantly less likely to benefit from MPH at three different doses (5, 10, and 15 mg) in school, as evidenced by teachers' ratings and in the clinic setting compared with subjects with borderline ($N = 17$) or low ($N = 11$) scores on the CBCL. There was a significant deterioration in functioning on MPH among some children. In particular, 25% of the subjects in the high internalizing group were rated on the Teacher Self-Control Rating Scale as showing a worsening in classroom behavior, compared with 9.1% in the low and none in the borderline internalizing groups. On the same scale, however, 50% of the high, 93.75% of the borderline, and 72.7% of the low internalizing groups were rated as improved or normalized. It appears that the presence of anxiety or depres-sion may hinder the effectiveness of stimulant treatment or even worsen behavior.

ADHD and conduct disorder may frequently coexist; in fact, DSM-IV-TR (American Psychiatric Association [APA], 2000) notes that if either diagnosis is present, the other diagnosis is commonly found. Psychostimulants also reduce some forms of aggression present in children diagnosed with ADDH (Allen et al., 1975; Klorman et al., 1988b). Amery et al. (1984) compared dextroamphetamine and placebo in 10 boys diagnosed with ADDH with a mean age of 9.6 ± 1.6 years. Dextroamphetamine was adminis-tered in doses of 15 to 30 mg/day. The authors reported that scores on the Thematic Apperception Test Hostility Scale and Holtzman Inkblot Test Hostility Scale, and observations of overt aggression in a laboratory free-play situation, were reduced sig-nificantly ($P < .05$) during a 2-week period on dextroamphetamine, compared with a similar period on placebo. These data are important, as ADHD and conduct disorder frequently coexist and stimulants are often not considered in treating children whose conduct disorders are the primary consideration.

Approximately 75% of children with ADHD treated with stimulants will show favorable responses (Green, 1995). Among these favorable responses, there will be a spectrum. Some children will respond extremely well; others will benefit but to a lesser degree. Also, some children with ADHD (or an earlier equivalent diagnosis) will respond favorably to one stimulant drug but less favorably, not at all, or unfavorably to another. For example, Arnold et al. (1976) conducted a double-blind crossover study of D-amphetamine, L-amphetamine, and placebo in 31 children with minimal brain dysfunction (MBD). Both isomers were statistically superior to placebo and did not differ significantly from each other. Interestingly, of the 25 children with positive responses, 17 responded well to both isomers, 5 responded favorably to the D-isomer only, and three responded favorably to the L-isomer only (Arnold et al., 1976).

In a double-blind crossover study, Elia et al. (1991) compared MPH, dextro-amphetamine, and placebo in treating 48 males (age range, 6 to 12 years; mean, 8.6 ± 1.7 years) with a history of hyperactive, inattentive, and impulsive behaviors that interfered with functioning both at home and at school. Following a 2-week baseline period, subjects were assigned randomly for 3-week periods during each week of which the dosage was increased, unless untoward effects prevented it, to one of three regimens: (a) MPH doses were given at 9 AM and 1 PM: subjects weighing <30 kg received during week 1, 12.5 mg; week 2, 20 mg; and week 3,

35 mg. Subjects weighing 30 kg or more received during week 1, 15 mg; week 2, 25 mg; and week 3, 45 mg. The actual mean dosage for all subjects for week 1 was 0.9 mg/kg; week 2, 1.5 mg/kg; and week 3, 2.5 mg/kg. (b) Dextroamphetamine doses were given at 9 AM and 1 PM: subjects weighing <30 kg received during week 1, 5 mg; week 2, 12.5 mg; and week 3, 20 mg. Those weighing 30 kg or more received during week 1, 7.5 mg; week 2, 15 mg; and week 3, 22.5 mg. The actual mean dosage for all subjects during week 1 was 0.4 mg/kg; week 2, 0.9 mg/kg; and week 3, 1.3 mg/kg. (c) Placebo dosage was held at the preceding week's level, increased to a lower dosage than mandated by the next level, or decreased because of untoward effects in 19 subjects (40%), including seven on MPH, seven on dextroamphetamine, and five on both drugs. The authors reported that 38 (79%) subjects responded to MPH and that 42 (88%) responded to dextroamphetamine; overall, 46 (96%) of the 48 subjects had a positive clinical response to one or both stimulants as rated on the Clinical Global Impressions (CGI) Scale and, in particular, for restless and inattentive behaviors. Eight subjects did not respond to MPH, four did not respond to dextroamphetamine, and two did not respond to either drug. Elia et al. (1991) distinguished between behavioral nonresponse and untoward effects, which few investigators have done. They noted that, although behavioral nonresponse to stimulants is rare, when a wide range of doses is given, most subjects had some untoward effects. During week 2 or 3 of treatment, untoward effects required that for 19 (40%) of the subjects, the dose be only partially increased in 15 (6 on MPH, 4 on dextroamphetamine, and 5 on both), held constant in 2 (1 on each medication), and decreased in 2 subjects receiving dextroamphetamine. When behavioral nonresponders were combined with subjects having untoward effects, the rate of nonresponse was similar to that reported in the literature. The authors noted that making a definitive clinical decision regarding improvement was often difficult because behavioral improvements had to be balanced against untoward effects, and different symptoms responded independently to dosage, setting, and subject (Elia et al., 1991).

Wender (1988) notes that the development of tolerance to the therapeutic effects of stimulant medication is unusual and that when it occurs, it progresses gradually over a period of 1 or 2 years. If this occurs, a trial of another stimulant is suggested, because complete cross-tolerance among the stimulants does not occur (Wender, 1988). There is a suggestion that the efficacy of stimulants typically decreases with age (Taylor et al., 1987).

Gadow and Poling (1988) reviewed the literature on the use of stimulants in the mentally retarded and concluded that stimulants are highly effective in reducing symptoms of hyperactivity and conduct disorder in some individuals, regardless of the degree of their retardation.

Normal prepubertal boys and college-aged men reacted similarly to patients diagnosed with ADHD when given single doses of dextroamphetamine; they exhibited decreased motor activity and generally improved attentional performance (Rapoport et al., 1978a, 1980a). Hence, earlier teachings that stimulants have a paradoxical effect in hyperactive children are incorrect, and a positive response to stimulant medication cannot be used to validate the diagnosis of ADHD (Pliszka et al, 2007).

MPH AND ADHD

In 1999, the landmark studies of the authoritative Multimodal Treatment Study Group of Children with Attention-Deficit/Hyperactivity Disorder (MTA) Cooperative Group were published (MTA Cooperative Group, 1999a, 1999b). Its 14-month randomized, multisite, clinical trial of four different treatment strategies for 579 children, aged 7 to 9.9 years, diagnosed with ADHD combined type reaffirmed the treatment efficacy of the stimulants, when dosed in a t.i.d. fashion, especially MPH. Four types of treatment were compared: (a) medication management, (b) intensive behavioral treatment, (c) combined medication and intensive behavioral treatment, and (d) standard community care by community providers. All four groups improved, but for most ADHD symptoms children in the medication and combination groups improved significantly more than those in the intensive behavior treatment and standard community care groups. Core ADHD symptoms improved equally with the combined treatment or with medication alone; however, the combined therapy may have provided modestly better outcomes for non-ADHD symptoms (e.g., oppositional and aggressive symptoms) and positive functioning (MTA Cooperative Group, 1999a, 1999b).

PHARMACOKINETICS OF STIMULANTS

The stimulants undergo some metabolism in the liver but new data indicate stimulants may be metabolized primarily by gastrointestinal enzymes and are primarily excreted by the kidneys. Table 4.1 gives the site of metabolism, main metabolic products, time of peak plasma levels, serum half-lives, and routes of excretion of MPH and dextroamphetamine.

STANDARD STIMULANT PREPARATIONS COMPARED WITH LONG-ACTING OR SUSTAINED-RELEASE FORMS

Sustained-release preparations make once-daily dosage possible. One early report found the clinical efficacy of sustained-release MPH to occur approximately 1 hour later and to be less than the standard-release form of MPH on several important measures of disruptive behavior in two studies of 22 boys with ADHD (Pelham et al., 1987). These authors thought that if once-daily dosage was necessary, then slow-release dextroamphetamine would often be preferable to sustained-release MPH. Birmaher et al. (1989) noted that the maximum serum level takes longer to develop when sustained-release tablets are administered and that peak serum levels are lower compared with those for an equivalent dose of standard MPH. These authors suggested that the relative inefficacy of sustained-release MPH could result from differences in pharmacokinetics or absorption, or from tachyphylaxis.

Some subsequent studies, however, have reported significantly different results. Pelham et al. (1990) administered standard MPH, 10 mg every morning and noon; sustained-release MPH, 20 mg every morning; dextroamphetamine spansule (long-acting), 10 mg every morning; pemoline (pemoline has subsequently been withdrawn from the market), 56.25 mg every morning; and placebo in random

TABLE 4.1 » Some Pharmacokinetic Properties of Stimulant Drugs

Drug	Principal Metabolite(s)	Peak Serum Levels	Serum Half-Life	Principal Route(s) of Excretion
Methylphenidate (Ritalin)	Liver → 75% ritalinic acid, which is pharmacologically inactive	1.9 h (range, 0.3–4.4 h); Ritalin S-R, 4.7 h (range, 1.2–8.2 h)	2–2.5 h	Kidney excretes 70% to 80%, primarily as ritalinic acid, in 24 h
Dextroamphetamine sulfate (Dexedrine)	Liver P-hydroxylation, N-demethylation, deamination, and conjugation	2 h for tablet; 8–10 h for spansule	6–8 h in children, 10–12 h in adults	May be excreted unchanged by kidney Amount varies according to urinary pH—from 2% to 3% in very alkaline urine, to 80% in acidic urine

order for 3 to 6 days. Each double-blind, placebo-controlled, crossover study involved 22 boys, ages 8.08 to 13.17 years, diagnosed with ADHD. Midday placebos were given during the periods when long-acting drugs were administered. Subjects were rated on measures of social behavior and classroom performance and on a continuous performance task. All four medication conditions had similar time courses, with effects evident between 1 and 9 hours after ingestion, and they were significantly, and approximately equally, better than placebo. The effects of the three long-acting preparations were as great, or almost as great, at 9 hours as at 2 hours after ingestion. Only 15 (68%) of the 22 patients improved sufficiently for the authors to recommend that they continue to receive stimulant medication. For these 15 patients, dextroamphetamine spansules were recommended for 6, pemoline for 4, sustained-release MPH for 4, and standard MPH for 1. The clinical implications of this study are potentially very important because they suggest that the great majority (i.e., 14 [93.3%] of 15 children with ADHD) derive more overall benefit from long-acting forms than from standard-release forms of stimulants. At the time of the study over 20 years ago, it was estimated that approximately 90% of children receiving medication for ADHD were prescribed MPH, and, of these, only approximately 10% received the sustained-release form. It should be noted that early forms of long-acting MPH such as Ritalin SR used an inferior waxbead delivery system and were inconsistent in delivery and results. Later MPH preparations such as Ritalin LA, Metadate CD, Focalin XR, and Concerta utilized more sophisticated delivery systems that seemed to provide more consistent and prolonged stimulant effect.

Fitzpatrick et al. (1992) compared the efficacy of standard and sustained-release MPH, and a combination of the two forms, in a double-blind, placebo-controlled study of 19 children (17 males and 2 females; age range, 6.9 to 11.5 years) diagnosed with ADD. Dosage of sustained-release MPH was 20 mg/day for all patients. Patients weighing <30 kg and >30 kg received 7.5 and 10 mg, respectively, in the morning and at noon, when on standard MPH only, and 5 and 7.5 mg, respectively, in the morning and at noon, when receiving standard MPH in combination with sustained-release MPH. Patients were rated on several scales by parents, teachers, and clinicians. All three active drug conditions were significantly better than placebo and were approximately equivalent in efficacy.

These studies, in which the medications were administered for relatively short periods, have relatively small numbers of subjects and need to be replicated with larger populations. They do, however, alert the clinician to the likelihood that sustained-release preparations are more efficacious than thought initially, and they may be the preferred dosage forms for most children with ADHD, especially when considering compliance issues and abuse potential.

Since the preceding studies were published, several new stimulant preparations with increased duration of action have appeared in the market. Adderall XR, which is a preparation of four amphetamine salts, has a duration of action that increases significantly with increases in dose and is compared to MPH and reviewed later under the discussion of amphetamines; Vyvanse, a D-isomer amphetamine pro-drug, has also been released. Extended-release forms of MPH in tablet, beaded-capsules, a patch, and an extended-release MPH preparation that uses an osmotic release oral system (OROS) of medication delivery combined with a semipermeable membrane to achieve a reported 12-hour duration of effect, have all been marketed. These drugs are further discussed later.

CONTRAINDICATIONS FOR STIMULANT ADMINISTRATION

Known hypersensitivity to the medication and glaucoma are significant contraindications. There are several other conditions such as tics, seizures, autism, and psychosis that were once considered absolute contraindications to the implementation of psychostimulant therapy. Indeed such warnings are still cited in the manufacturers' product information (PIs) literature that accompanies most psychostimulant products. However, more recent literature tends to qualify such conditions as relative *contraindications based on the clinical findings that many patients with these conditions still benefit markedly by the utilization of these agents even when these conditions are a comorbid health issue.* Today, a review of the relevant literature suggests that if risks and benefits are carefully assessed and explained to the patient, it is reasonable to proceed with a trial of a psychostimulant while carefully monitoring the patient. The following discussions of the literature will further clarify the "relative" nature of these contraindications as they apply to various comorbid conditions.

Stimulants may cause stereotypies, tics, and psychosis *de novo* in sensitive individuals or if given in high-enough doses. Stimulants are relatively contraindicated in children and adolescents with a history of schizophrenia or other psychosis, pervasive developmental disorders, or borderline personality organization, because they appear to worsen these conditions in some cases. However, stimulants have been given to some patients with these diagnoses under conditions of close scrutiny with very beneficial results. If the patients are also being treated simultaneously with mood-stabilizer medications, the above risks may be diminished.

There is controversy over whether the stimulants should be given to children and adolescents with tic disorder, Tourette syndrome (TS), or a family history of such. Their use in pervasive developmental disorders and in TS or with tic disorders is discussed in greater detail later.

Stimulants may aggravate symptoms of marked anxiety, tension, and agitation and are contraindicated when these symptoms are prominent (*PDR*, 2005, p. 2353). Stimulants also have the potential to cause hypertensive crises when used with monoamine oxidase inhibitors (MAOIs). They should not be used concomitantly with an MAOI or within 14 days of an MAOI being discontinued.

Stimulants have a potential to be abused. They should not be prescribed to patients who have a history of drug abuse or when there is a likelihood that family members or friends would abuse the medication. In some cases in which the family is unreliable but stimulants are the drug of choice, it is worthwhile to attempt to work out a way to dispense and store all the stimulant medication at school because, for most children, coverage during the time in school is the foremost consideration.

Magnesium pemoline was withdrawn from the market in 2005 because its potential risks were greater than its potential benefits. Reports of acute hepatic failure, some of which were fatal and others which necessitated liver transplants, were the reason for this. The reader who wishes to have information regarding magnesium pemoline may consult the prior editions of this book.

INTERACTIONS OF STIMULANTS WITH OTHER DRUGS

Stimulants should not be administered with MAOIs or until at least 14 days after MAOIs were last ingested, to avoid possible hypertensive crises.

In combination with tricyclic antidepressants, the actions of both may be enhanced.

Stimulants potentiate sympathomimetic drugs (including street amphetamines and cocaine) and may counteract the sedative effect of antihistamines and benzodiazepines.

Lithium may inhibit the stimulatory effects of amphetamines.

Amphetamines may act synergistically with phenytoin or phenobarbital to increase anticonvulsant activity.

Many other drug interactions, which are less likely to be encountered in child and adolescent psychiatry than those mentioned in the preceding text, may occur.

MPH and Clonidine

On July 13, 1995, a National Public Radio broadcast reported that sudden deaths had occurred in three children taking a combination of MPH and clonidine. The ramifications of this are discussed later in the section "Interactions of Clonidine Hydrochloride with Other Drugs."

ADVERSE EFFECTS OF STIMULANTS

There is some evidence that, overall, the untoward effects of MPH occur less frequently and with less severity than those from dextroamphetamine (Conners, 1971; Gross and Wilson, 1974). Gross and Wilson (1974) noted that side effects were infrequently severe enough to necessitate immediate discontinuation of the medication (1.1% of 377 patients for MPH and 4.3% of 371 patients for dextroamphetamine).

The most frequent and troublesome immediate untoward effects include insomnia, anorexia, nausea, abdominal pain or cramps, headache, thirst, vomiting, lability of mood, irritability, sadness, weepiness, tachycardia, and blood pressure changes. Many of these symptoms diminish over a few weeks, although the cardiovascular changes may persist.

Since 1972, disturbances in growth—decrements in both height and weight percentiles—have been reported for both MPH and dextroamphetamine, and the long-term untoward consequences of these effects have been of particular concern (Safer et al., 1972). There has been controversy about the significance of these changes. Mattes and Gittelman (1983) reported significant decreases in height and weight percentiles over a 4-year period. A subsequent controlled study found a significant reduction in growth velocity during the period when stimulants are actively administered (Klein et al., 1988). Despite this adverse effect on growth during the active treatment phase, it appears that an accelerated rate of growth or growth rebound occurs once the stimulant is discontinued and that there is usually no significant compromise of ultimate height attained (Klein and Mannuzza, 1988). It seems likely, however, that some children are at greater risk for growth suppression than others, and serial heights and weights of any child receiving stimulant medication should be plotted carefully on a growth chart (e.g., the National Center for Health Statistics Growth Chart) (Hamill et al., 1976).

Vincent et al. (1990) reported no significant deviations from expected height and weight growth velocities in 31 adolescents diagnosed with ADHD who had received MPH continuously for a minimum of 6 months to a maximum of 6 years after their 12th birthdays. Mean age at the beginning of the study was 12.9 ± 0.8 years. The mean daily dose was 34 ± 14 mg or 0.75 ± 0.29 mg/kg and did not differ significantly with age or sex. The results suggested that early adolescent growth is not significantly adversely affected by MPH.

Faraone et al. (2005) reported on the long-term effects of extended-release mixed amphetamine salts extended release (MAS XR) on growth in 568 children (mean age, 8.7 ± 1.8 years; age range, 6 to 12 years; 78% male, 73% White, 12% Black, 9% Hispanic), in a multicenter, open-label study. Subjects received doses of 10 to 30 mg/day for a period of 6 to 30 months. Based on the Centers of Disease Control norms, subjects experienced decreases in weight, body mass index (BMI), and height percentiles over the period of study; these decrements were greatest for the heaviest and tallest children; these deficits occurred primarily during the first year, and decreases in weight, BMI, and height were not significant during the second year on medication. The height deficit was significant for subjects whose baseline heights were greater than the 25th percentile ($P = .001$ for the second quartile and $P < .0001$ for the third and fourth quartiles). The height loss was only 1.2 percentile points for the shortest children at baseline, whereas the tallest children at baseline experienced a 10 percentile decrease in height at the end of the study. The authors noted that monitoring growth parameters was essential but that for most children, the decreases caused by MAS XR was not likely to be of clinical concern.

Charach et al. (2006) followed up 79 subjects, age range 6 to 12 years, who were diagnosed with ADHD by DSM-III-R criteria (APA, 1980a) and maintained on stimulant medication, annually for up to 5 years to determine the long-term effects of stimulants on their heights and weights. Subjects were taking various preparations of amphetamine and MPH, which were converted to an equivalent daily dose of MPH in mg/kg/day based on their potency. Small but statistically significant effects were found. Based on a statistical model, patients receiving >1.5 mg/kg/day of MPH show a decrease in expected weight gain after 1 year and subjects receiving >2.5 mg/kg/day have a decrease in expected height after 4 years on medication; the higher the dose, the greater the decrease in expected weight or height. Regular monitoring of height and weight is indicated for children and adolescents administered stimulants as a long-term treatment.

A few children treated with stimulants may develop a clinical picture resembling schizophrenia. This condition occurs most frequently when untoward effects such as disorganization are misinterpreted as a worsening of presenting symptoms and the dosage is further increased until prominent psychotomimetic effects occur. It may also occur when stimulants are administered to children with borderline personality disorders or schizophrenia, conditions in which stimulants are relatively contraindicated. In most such cases, the psychotic symptomatology improves rapidly after discontinuation of the drug (Green, 1989).

Some parents express concern that treatment with stimulants will predispose their child to later drug abuse or addiction. Most available evidence indicates that this is not the case. Although drug abuse itself is of major concern in our culture, children diagnosed with ADHD who have been treated with stimulants appear to be at no greater risk for drug or alcohol abuse as teenagers and adults than controls (Weiss and Hechtman, 1986). Past research looking for a link between ADHD medications and substance abuse has produced conflicting conclusions from no association, a protective effect and an increased risk. But many of those studies had methodological limitations to varying degrees, and not all of the studies followed their samples a sufficient period of time into late adolescence and early adulthood. A National Institutes of Health funded study at the Massachusetts General Hospital attempted to overcome the deficiencies of previous studies (Biederman et al., 2008). This was accomplished by following the study subjects up to a median age of about 22, including an assessment for psychiatric problems such as conduct disorder that are associated with substance abuse, and applying rigorous methods to accurately analyze the data. The research study team interviewed 112 young men (ranging in age from 16 to 27), previously diagnosed with ADHD, over a span of a decade about their use of alcohol, tobacco, and other psychoactive drugs. Seventy-three percent of the subjects had been medicated with stimulants at some time in their treatment, but only 22% were currently taking the stimulant medications. The study found no relationship between having ever received stimulant treatment and the risk of future alcohol or other substance abuse. The age at which stimulant treatment began and how long it continued also had no impact on substance use. The study demonstrated that the use of psychostimulant treatments in ADHD children does appear to increase the risk for substance abuse in adulthood, but unfortunately also suggests there is no protective effect as well. Such data indicating low compliance of stimulant therapy during these critical years of late adolescence and young adulthood, however, begs the question. If stimulant med compliance into young adulthood was greater, would substance abuse be less?

For children (6 to 12 years of age) taking OROS MPH in doses up to 54 mg daily, the most frequent adverse events (AEs) were headache (14%), upper respiratory tract infection (8%), abdominal pain (7%), vomiting (4%), loss of appetite (4%), insomnia (4%), increased cough (4%), and pharyngitis (4%). The most frequent AEs for adolescents taking OROS MPH in doses up to 72 mg daily were headache (9%), accidental injury (6%), and insomnia (5%) (*PDR*, 2006).

REBOUND EFFECTS OF STIMULANTS

Rebound effects may occur beginning approximately 5 hours after the last dose of short-acting MPH. Behavioral symptoms of rebound are often identical to those of the ADHD being treated and, in some cases, may even exceed baseline levels prior to administration of stimulants.

Rapoport et al. (1978a) reported that normal children who received short-acting dextroamphetamine experienced behavioral rebound approximately 5 hours after a single acute dose. Symptoms included excitability, talkativeness, overactivity, insomnia, stomachaches, and mild nausea. Long-acting formulations of stimulants may reduce the risk of rebound effects but may still occur albeit much later in the day when serum concentrations taper off approximately 8 to 12 hours after dosing.

STIMULANTS' RELATIONSHIP TO TICS AND TOURETTE SYNDROME

Stimulants can exacerbate existing tics and precipitate tics and stereotypies *de novo*. Because of this, manufacturers state its use is contraindicated in patients with motor tics, a diagnosis of TS or a family history of TS. There is some disagreement among experts regarding whether stimulants should be given to persons with tics, TS, or a family history of either condition.

In a study of 1,520 children diagnosed with ADDH and treated with MPH, Denckla et al. (1976) reported that existing tics were exacerbated in 6 cases (0.39%) and tics developed *de novo* in 14 cases (0.92%). After the discontinuation of MPH, all 6 of the tics that had worsened returned to their premedication intensity, and 13 of the 14 new tics completely remitted.

Shapiro and Shapiro (1981) reviewed the relationship between treating ADDH with stimulants and the precipitation or exacerbation of tics and Tourette syndrome (TS). They also noted that they had treated 42 patients for symptoms of both MBD and TS with a combination of MPH and haloperidol. Dosage of MPH ranged from 5 to 60 mg/day and was individually titrated for each patient. The authors also used MPH (dose range, 5 to 40 mg/day) in 62 additional patients with TS to counteract the untoward effects of haloperidol, such as sedation, amotivation, dysphoria, cognitive impairment, and dullness. Shapiro and Shapiro (1981) concluded that the evidence suggests that stimulants do not cause or provoke TS, although high doses of stimulants can cause or exacerbate tics in predisposed patients. Clinically, they noted that tics seemed less likely to be exacerbated by stimulants in patients who were also taking haloperidol for TS; when tics did increase in intensity, they remitted within 3 to 6 hours, the approximate duration of the usual clinical effects of MPH.

Lowe et al. (1982) reported on a series of 15 patients diagnosed with ADDH who were treated with stimulant medications, including MPH, dextroamphetamine, and pemoline. These patients subsequently had tics develop *de novo*, or had existing tics worsen, sometimes into full-blown cases of TS. Nine subjects had existing tics; eight had family histories of tics or TS. Twelve of the 15 cases eventually required medication for control of the tics. The authors considered the presence of TS or tics to be a contraindication to stimulant medication and that stimulants should be used with great caution in the presence of a family history of tics or TS. They also considered the development of tics after treatment with stimulants sufficient reason to discontinue the use of stimulant medication.

Lowe et al. (1982) noted that the early clinical signs of TS may be difficult to differentiate from ADDH. Shapiro and Shapiro (1981) noted that approximately 57% of children with tics or TS had concomitant minimal brain dysfunction, although most children with MBD do not develop either tics or TS.

Comings and Comings (1984) investigated the relationship between TS and ADDH. They found that ADDH was present in 62% of 140 males <21 years of age diagnosed with TS. A study of their family pedigrees suggested that the TS gene could be expressed as ADDH but without tics. The authors thought that their data implied that patients diagnosed with ADDH and treated with stimulants who subsequently developed tics had ADDH as a result of the TS gene and probably would have developed tics or TS even if they had not received stimulants. It is unclear whether stimulant medication might hasten the expression of such symptoms.

Gadow et al. (1992) treated 11 boys, aged 6.1 to 11.9 years (mean, 8.3±1.96 years), diagnosed with comorbid tic disorder and ADHD, with MPH. The drug was administered under double-blind conditions; each subject was assigned to random 2-week periods of placebo and MPH in doses of 0.1, 0.3, and 0.5 mg/kg/day. The authors noted that MPH significantly decreased hyperactive and disruptive behaviors in class and reduced physical aggression on the playground. Vocal tics were also significantly reduced in the lunchroom and classroom. Based on this and other studies cited in their report, the authors concluded that MPH is a safe and effective treatment for some children with comorbid ADHD and tic disorder over a short-term period; however, they cautioned that a risk of protraction or irreversible worsening of tics may exist for some individuals and that the consequences of long-term treatment of such patients are unknown.

Gadow et al. (1995) conducted a double-blind, placebo-controlled, 8-week study in which 34 prepubertal children, 31 males and 3 females, 6.08 to 11.9 years of age, diagnosed by DSM-III-R (APA, 1987) criteria with ADHD and comorbid chronic motor tic disorder or TS were treated with placebo and MPH in doses of 0.1, 0.2, and 0.5 mg/kg given twice daily (usually before leaving for school and at noon) for 2 weeks for each condition. Most children were additionally diagnosed with opposition defiant or conduct disorder. Tics were rated on five different scales by one of the authors and on the Global Tic Rating Scale by parents and teachers.

All 34 subjects responded with dramatic clinical improvement in hyperactivity and inattentive, disruptive, oppositional, and aggressive behaviors when treated with MPH. Teachers noted significant improvement in symptoms on the 0.1 mg/kg dose. There were no statistically or clinically significant adverse effects on the severity of tics with MPH treatment, but in the classroom, there was an increased frequency of motor tics on the 0.1 mg/kg/dose compared with placebo and in the physician's 2-minute motor tic count on the 0.5 mg/kg/dose. Teachers rated vocal tics as significantly less frequent on all three doses of MPH than placebo. The authors concluded that MPH was a safe and effective treatment for most children diagnosed with comorbid ADHD and tic disorder. They also cautioned that it can be extremely difficult to determine whether MPH or natural fluctuations are responsible for observed changes in the frequency or intensity of tics and that MPH is reported to have a negative effect on tics in some children (Gadow et al., 1995).

Gadow et al. (1999) continued to follow prospectively the 34 children who participated in their 1995 study at 6-month intervals for an additional 2 years of open treatment with MPH. There was no significant change in mean group scores rating severity or frequency of motor or vocal tics during the 2-year maintenance period compared with baseline or double-blind placebo ratings. Direct observations in the simulated classroom were almost identical at baseline, during the double-blind placebo protocol and the 2-year follow-up. Although there was no evidence that MPH maintenance therapy for up to 2 years exacerbated vocal or motor tics for their subjects as a group, the authors cautioned that their results do not rule out the possibility of this occurring in specific individuals. Behavioral improvements in ADHD symptomatology were maintained during the 2-year follow-up; however, behavioral problems associated with oppositional defiant and conduct disorders did not maintain their gains. Over the 2-year period, there was a significant increase of approximately 10 beats per minute in heart rate, which was not felt to be clinically significant, and slightly less weight gain (0.72 kg) and less height gain (0.67 cm) than expected, both of which are so small as to not be of concern for most children.

Castellanos et al. (1997) conducted a 9-week, double-blind crossover, placebo-controlled treatment protocol (in three separate cohorts) with a total of 20 males (mean age 9.4 ± 2.0 years, range 6 to 13 years) diagnosed with comorbid ADHD and TS comparing MPH, dexedrine (DEX), and placebo at various doses. Doses of stimulants were quite high at the upper range (e.g., 45 mg/dose [90 mg/day] for MPH and 22.5 mg/dose [45 mg/day] for DEX). Efficacy was determined by ratings on the Tourette Syndrome Unified Rating Scale and the Conners teachers' hyperactivity ratings. Medication was administered at breakfast and lunch daily. Because of the three separate cohorts, only a summary of the overall findings will be given here. Target ADHD behaviors of all subjects improved on teachers' ratings on stimulants, and there was no significantly greater improvement at the higher doses. At the lowest dose (12.5 or 15 mg/dose for MPH and 5 or 7.5 mg/dose for DEX), there was no significant change of tic severity. At highest drug doses, tic severity was significantly increased but DEX increased the severity significantly more than MPH or placebo. Of particular clinical interest was the finding that the increases in tics that occurred at higher doses of MPH tended to diminish over time and return to placebo levels when MPH was maintained or increased; this occurred in 17 of the 20 subjects. This diminution in tic severity also occurred with DEX but less significantly (in 9 of 20 subjects, $P < .01$). The authors concluded that stimulants (usually MPH is preferred) at the lowest effective dose should be considered as a possible treatment for children with comorbid ADHD and TS. Some clinicians would advocate that the purified D-isomer of MPH, which is available in short- and long-acting formulations, may have theoretical and true clinical benefit in providing a less tic-promoting effect than D- and L-MPH formulations.

To further investigate whether treatment with MPH causes tics *de novo* or worsens preexisting tics in children diagnosed with ADHD, Law and Schachar (1999) conducted a 1-year-long randomized, placebo-controlled, prospective study of 91 such children who had never received medication for ADHD or tics. Inclusion criteria included the following: presence of at least 8 of the 14 DSM-III-R (APA, 1987) criteria for the diagnosis of ADHD in either the school or the home setting and a minimum of 5 such criteria in the other setting; ADHD symptoms beginning before age 7 and of at least 6 months duration; Full Scale Intelligence Quotient (FSIQ) >80 (based on the Block Design and Vocabulary subtests of the WISC-III) (Wechsler, 1974); and no primary anxiety of affective disorder. Exclusion criteria were as follows: severe motor or vocal tic disorder or TS, as it was assumed that MPH would exacerbate such tics, but subjects with mild to moderate tics were permitted, as the authors assumed the risk of their worsening would be less and they would be more easily managed if they did occur.

Subjects were recruited from 302 consecutive referrals to an ADHD program in an urban pediatric hospital. Admission criteria were met by 105 children, and 91 elected to participate in the study. Mean age was 8.35 ± 1.55 years. Of the 46 randomly assigned to the MPH group, 11 (23.9%) had preexisting tics; of the 45 randomly assigned to the placebo group, 16 (35.6%) had preexisting tics. Study medication was begun at doses of 5 mg at breakfast and at noon on schooldays; the use of weekend and holiday medication was decided by the caregiver. Medication was increased by 10 mg weekly (each dose increased by 5 mg) until a target dose of 0.7 mg/kg/day was achieved or untoward effects precluded further increase. If families elected to switch to the alternative medication, which was an option, another blinded titration to reach the target goal was performed. Tics were rated on a 10-point scale: 0 = no tics, 1 to 3 = mild tics, 4 to 6 = moderate tics, and 7 to 9 = severe tics.

If tics developed during the treatment, the current dose of medication was continued for 1 week. If the tic did not diminish, medication was decreased by 5-mg amounts until the tic was rated as mild or disappeared. In most cases of mild tic, parents and children elected to continue with the protocol, as the clinical improvement outweighed the impact of mild tics. During the 1-year protocol, 27 (60%) of the subjects on placebo requested to change to the alternative medication because of inadequate clinical improvement; none switched because of onset of a tic disorder. No patient receiving MPH elected to switch medications. At the end of 1 year for a total of 72 subjects, there remained 18 subjects in the placebo group; the MPH group was increased by the 27 subjects who switched from placebo and decreased by one subject because of follow-up difficulties.

The mean dose of MPH at the end of dose titration was 0.5 mg/kg/day. The target of 0.7 mg/kg/day was not reached for many subjects because of untoward effects, both physiologic (insomnia, dizziness, decreased appetite, headache, and daytime drowsiness) and behavioral (staring and preoccupations), and development or worsening of tics. Because of the switches from placebo to MPH, the final distribution of subjects whose tics predated the study's onset was 21 (29.2%) of the 72 subjects in the MPH group and 6 (33.3%) of the 18 subjects in the placebo group.

By the end of the study, 10 (19.6%) of the 52 subjects with *no preexisting tics* who received MPH and 2 (16.7%) of the 12 subjects remaining in the placebo group had developed clinically significant tics that were of moderate intensity or worse, including one child in the MPH group who developed Tourette-like symptoms. There was no significant difference in the development of tics *de novo* between the groups ($P = .59$). The 12 subjects who developed tics were managed by maintaining the dose of MPH at the level when tics emerged in 8 cases, reducing the MPH dose in 3 cases, and adding clonidine in 1 case. Among the 27 subjects with preexisting tics, 7 (33.3%) of the 21 receiving MPH had worsening of their tics, including 1 boy who developed Tourette-like symptoms; 2 (9.2%) experienced no change in their tics; 5 (23.8%) experienced improvement; and 7 (33.3%) had complete remission of their tics. Of the 6 such patients in the placebo group, 2 (33.3%) had worsening of tics and 4 had complete remission of their tics. Hence, in both the MPH group and the placebo group, 66.7% (14/21 and 4/6) of the subjects with preexisting tics experienced improvement or no change in their tics, and tics worsened in 33.3% of the subjects (7/21 and 2/6). There was no significant difference between the groups ($P = .70$).

Tics *de novo* developed throughout the 1-year treatment in both groups. In the MPH group, 20 subjects developed new tics: 12 (60%) within 4 months, 6 (30%) between 4 and 8 months, and 2 (10%) between 8 and 12 months. In the placebo group, 9 subjects developed new tics: 1 (11.1%) within 4 months, 5 (55.6%) between 4 and 8 months, and 3 (33.3%) between 8 and 12 months. Only 12 of these 29 subjects who developed new tics were reported to still have tics at the end of the study, illustrating both the waxing and waning natural course of tics as well as the response to decreasing the dose of MPH in some cases. Law and Schachar (1999) concluded that titration of MPH to an optimal average maintenance dose of 0.5 mg/kg/day does not cause tics *de novo* or worsen preexisting tics of moderate severity or less, more often than placebo in children being treated for ADHD for up to 1 year.

Sverd (2000) recently reviewed the use of MPH to treat children with comorbid ADHD and tic disorders. Sverd concluded that the literature supports that ADHD is genetically related to TS in a substantial proportion of cases, that stimulants cause tics *de novo* or exacerbation of tics relatively infrequently, and that MPH may be safely used to treat children diagnosed with ADHD and comorbid tic disorder.

Currently, a conservative approach would consider the stimulants relatively contraindicated in treating children and adolescents with tics or TS, and a reason for caution in the presence of family history of such. In fact, two manufacturers of MPH products state that it is contraindicated in patients with motor tics or with a family history or diagnosis of TS. A review of the relevant literature, however, suggests that if risks and benefits are carefully assessed, it is reasonable to attempt a trial with MPH or amphetamine (there are more data for MPH) in such patients if they are carefully monitored.

STIMULANT DRUGS APPROVED FOR USE IN CHILD AND ADOLESCENT PSYCHIATRY

The stimulants are the most frequently prescribed psychiatric drugs during childhood. In 1977, more than half a million children were being treated with MPH in the United States alone (Sprague and Sleator, 1977). By 1987, it was conservatively estimated that in the United States, 750,000 youth were being treated with medication for hyperactivity or inattentiveness (Safer and Krager, 1988). In Baltimore County, 6% of all public elementary school students were receiving such medication; MPH accounted for 93% of the drugs prescribed, and other stimulants accounted for another 6% (Safer and Krager, 1988). In more recent times with the development of improved long-acting formulations of MPH and amphetamine-based products, there is much greater balance in the prescription of MPH versus amphetamine products.

MPH Stimulant Drugs Approved for Use in Child and Adolescent Psychiatry

D-L-*Methylphenidate Hydrochloride (Ritalin, Ritalin LA, Ritalin SR, Methylin, Methylin ER, Metadate, Metadate ER, Metadate CD, Concerta, Daytrana)*

Pharmacokinetics of D-L-Methylphenidate Hydrochloride

Administration of short-acting MPH with meals does not appear to adversely affect its absorption or pharmacokinetics and may diminish problems with appetite suppression (Patrick et al., 1987). Long-acting stimulant formulations may be affected by high-fat meals resulting in lower peak serum levels.

An improvement of target symptoms can be seen in as few as 20 minutes after a therapeutically effective dose of standard/immediate-release preparation MPH is given (Zametkin et al., 1985). Peak blood levels occur between 1 and 2.5 hours after administration of short-acting stimulants (Gualtieri et al., 1982), and the serum half-life is approximately 2.5 hours (Winsberg et al., 1982). Patrick et al. (1987) have reviewed the pharmacokinetics of MPH in detail. The major metabolite produced in the liver is ritalinic acid, which is pharmacologically inactive. Between 70% and 80% of the radioactivity of radiolabeled MPH, >75% of which is ritalinic acid, is recovered in the urine within 24 hours.

Because of these pharmacokinetics, the most frequent times to administer standard/immediate-release preparation MPH to children and adolescents are before leaving for school and during the lunch hour. This dosage schedule usually ensures adequate serum levels during school hours, which is the foremost consideration for most students.

Concerta was designed to have a 12-hour duration of effect and to be administered once daily in the morning. It is a long-acting MPH product that uses osmotic OROS drug-delivery technology to provide for the delivery of MPH at a controlled rate throughout the day. It has an osmotically active trilayer core surrounded by a semipermeable membrane that releases MPH gradually and an overcoating of rapidly available MPH producing an initial peak plasma concentration in approximately 1 to 2 hours. Plasma concentration then continues to gradually increase to an ultimate peak level in approximately 6 to 8 hours, following which levels gradually decline. Serum half-life is 3.5 ± 0.4 hours. Doses over 54 and 72 mg/day are not FDA approved for children and adolescents, respectively; however, small clinical trials have documented the safety and efficiency of dosages up to 108 mg in appropriate patients; doses >2 mg/kg/day are not recommended for any age.

Contraindications for the Administration of Methylphenidate Hydrochloride

MPH is contraindicated in patients with marked anxiety, tension, and agitation as it may worsen these symptoms. It is contraindicated in patients with known hypersensitivity to the drug, glaucoma or motor tics or a family history or diagnosis of TS. It is also contraindicated during treatment with MAOIs or within 14 days of discontinuing such medication.

Adverse Effects and Adjustment of Methylphenidate Hydrochloride Dose Schedule

Children who develop significant behavioral or attention difficulties in the late afternoon or early evening may do so because of a return-to-baseline behavior as serum levels decline into subtherapeutic levels and/or because of a rebound effect as the drug wears off (Rapoport et al., 1978a). A third dose of medication given in the afternoon may be helpful for some such children. Johnston et al. (1988), however, suggested that psychostimulant rebound effects are not clinically significant for most children.

Insomnia may also occur. It is clinically important to distinguish those children whose insomnia is an untoward effect of the drug from those whose insomnia may be due to the recurrence of behavioral difficulties as the medication effect subsides and/or a rebound effect. For the first group of children, a reduction in milligram dosage of the last dose of the day may be necessary. For the latter group, an evening dose or a dose approximately 1 hour before bedtime may be helpful. Chatoor et al. (1983) prescribed late afternoon or evening dextroamphetamine sustained-release capsules to seven children who had strong rebound effects as their medication wore off and who developed marked behavioral problems and difficulty settling down and sleeping at bedtime. Parents reported significant behavioral improvement and markedly less bedtime oppositional behavior and increased ease in falling asleep. The authors compared sleep EEGs in seven children recorded during periods on dextroamphetamine sustained-release capsules and on placebo. Compared with placebo, dextroamphetamine tended to delay onset of sleep slightly, significantly increased rapid eye movement (REM) latency (time to first REM period), and significantly decreased REM time (by approximately 14%) and the number of REM periods. Length of stage 1 and stage 2 sleep was significantly increased, and sleep efficiency (amount of time asleep during recording) decreased. Reduction in sleep efficiency was only 5%, which seemed minor compared with the significant behavioral improvement that occurred (Chatoor et al., 1983).

Stimulant Drugs as Proconvulsants and Anticonvulsants

As Gualtieri discusses, stimulants like almost all psychoactive drugs can affect the seizure threshold if the dose is sufficiently high or abruptly changed, but the patient's inherent predisposition to seizures is likely much more important than the effect of the drug. In high dosages, stimulants can cause seizures, but at typical therapeutic low dosages, stimulants usually raise the seizure threshold and improve seizure control (Gualtieri, 2002). Nonetheless, the manufacturer's package insert warns that there is some evidence that MPH may lower the convulsive threshold. McBride et al. (1986), however, found only a single case report in the literature in which a child who was previously seizure free had a seizure soon after treatment with MPH. The authors treated 23 children and adolescents, aged 4 to 15 years and diagnosed with ADD who had seizure disorders of various types ($N = 20$) or epileptiform EEG abnormalities ($N = 3$), with MPH. Fifteen of the children with documented seizure disorder received concomitant antiepileptic drugs. Individual doses of 0.33 ± 0.13 mg/kg were administered with total daily doses of 0.63 ± 0.25 mg/kg from 3 months to 4 years. The authors found no evidence of increased frequency of seizures following MPH treatment in 16 children with active seizure disorders or 4 children who had had active seizure disorders but who had been seizure free and off antiepileptic drugs from 2 months to 2 years. The 3 children with epileptiform abnormalities also did not develop seizures during the period they received MPH. This evidence suggests that MPH may not lower the seizure threshold to a clinically significant degree at usual therapeutic doses and that the presence of a seizure disorder in a child or adolescent with ADHD is not an absolute contraindication for a trial of MPH (McBride et al., 1986). Crumrine et al. (1987) also reported that they had administered MPH 0.3 mg/kg twice daily to 9 males 6.1 to 10.1 years of age who had diagnoses of ADHD and seizure disorder. The boys had been previously stabilized on anticonvulsant medication and experienced no seizures or changes in EEG background patterns or epileptiform activity during 4-week, randomized, double-blind crossover trials of MPH or placebo. Subjects improved significantly on the hyperactivity, inattention, and Hyperactivity Index factors on the Conners Teacher Questionnaire (Crumrine et al., 1987).

These reports suggest that when clinically indicated, it is not unreasonable to undertake a trial of MPH in children and adolescents with coexisting seizure disorders and ADHD. Clearly, frequency of seizures should be carefully monitored, and if their frequency increases or seizures develop *de novo*, the clinician may discontinue MPH.

Swanson et al. (1986) reported on six children who developed behavioral and cognitive tolerance to their usual doses of MPH during long-term treatment. To maintain satisfactory clinical response, their pediatricians had to titrate the total daily doses to levels of 120 to 300 mg administered in as many as five individual doses of 40 to 60 mg. These children performed a cognitive task better at their usual high dose (average, 60 mg three times daily) than at a lower dose (average, 30 mg three times daily), confirming cognitive tolerance. Overall, these children had high serum levels compatible with the high doses, suggesting that neither metabolic tolerance nor differential absorption was responsible for the behavioral tolerance.

Garfinkel et al. (1983) compared efficacy of MPH with placebo, desipramine, and clomipramine in a double-blind crossover study of 12 males (mean age, 7.3 years; range, 5.9 to 11.6 years) diagnosed with ADD who required day hospital or inpatient hospitalization because of the severity of their impulsivity, inattention, and aggressiveness. MPH was significantly better in improving symptoms on the Conners Scale as rated by teachers ($P < .005$) and program child care workers ($P < .001$).

Indications for Methylphenidate Hydrochloride in Child and Adolescent Psychiatry

FDA approved for treating ADHD and narcolepsy in patients at least 6 years of age.

Immediate-Release MPH Dosage Schedule

- *Children <6 years of age:* not approved for use.
- *Children at least 6 years of age and adolescents up to 17 years of age:* start with 5 mg once or twice daily (usually about 7:00 AM and noon) and raise dose gradually to 5 to 10 mg/week. Maximum recommended daily dosage is 60 mg. The usual optimal dose falls between 0.3 and 0.7 mg/kg administered two to three times daily (total daily dose range of 0.6 to 2.1 mg/kg) (Duncan, 1990).

(continued)

Indications for Methylphenidate Hydrochloride in Child and Adolescent Psychiatry (continued)

- *Adolescents at least 18 years of age and adults:* start with an initial daily dose of 5 mg two or three times daily, usually before meals, and titrate based on clinical response. Average dose is 20 to 30 mg/day with a range of 10 to 60 mg/day.

Immediate-Release D- and L-Methylphenidate Hydrochloride Dose Forms Available

Tablets: (Ritalin, Methylin): 5, 10 (scored), and 20 mg (scored)
Chewable tablets (Methylin chewable tablets): 2.5, 5, and 10 mg
Oral solution (Methylin oral solution): 5 mg/5 mL, 10 mg/5 mL

Extended/Sustained-Release MPH Dosage Schedule

- *Children <6 years of age:* not approved for use.
- *Individuals at least 6 years of age:* Methylphenidate hydrochloride sustained-release tablets and extended-release capsules are administered once daily in the morning. Their duration of action is approximately 8 hours. Start with an initial dose of 10 to 20 mg once daily and increase by a maximum of 10 mg weekly to a maximum total daily dose of 60 mg. If a patient is already receiving immediate-release MPH, an equivalent milligram dose of a sustained-release preparation may be substituted for the total dose of standard-release MPH used during the same period. Extended-release tablets must be taken whole and not crushed or chewed; sustained-release capsules may be opened and sprinkled on applesauce.

Extended/Sustained-Release Methylphenidate Hydrochloride Dose Forms Available

- *Sustained-release tablets (Ritalin SR 20 mg; Metadate ER 10 mg, 20 mg; Methylin ER 10 mg, 20 mg):* Sustained-release tablets of equivalent strength may be substituted for the total dose of the immediate-release form given over 8 hours.
- *D-and L-Methylphenidate extended-release capsules (Ritalin LA 10, 20, 30, and 40 mg; Metadate CD 10, 20, 30, 40, 50, and 60 mg):* The recommended initial dose is 20 mg once daily in the morning. Dosage may be titrated upward in 10 mg increments weekly. The maximum total daily dose recommended is 60 mg. The capsules may be opened and sprinkled on applesauce and consumed immediately without chewing, which is advantageous for some younger children or if there is a question of compliance (swallowing the capsule).
- *OROS (Osmotic Release Oral System) methylphenidate hydrochloride tablets (Concerta, OROS: 18, 27, 36, and 54 mg):* The maximum recommended once-daily dose is 54 mg in children and up to 72 mg/day (not to exceed 2 mg/kg/day) in adolescents. Concerta was designed to have clinical effects lasting approximately 12 hours. Swanson et al. (2000) have shown that OROS MPH can be initiated once daily at 18 mg/day and titrated weekly to a maximum recommended dose of 54 mg/day in children; that is, without prior titration on standard (immediate-release) MPH. Swanson et al. (2003) showed that OROS MPH remains clinically effective for at least 12 hours and that its efficacy is comparable to that of immediate-release MPH given three times daily.
- *MPH transdermal system (Daytrana, 10, 15, 20, and 30 mg patches):* Daytrana is approved for ages 6 to 17. Patch is to be applied by holding firmly in place with palm of hand for 30 seconds to clean dry skin in hip area (alternating daily) 2 hours before effect is needed and should be removed in 9 hours after application or 3 hours before bedtime (to allow decrease in serum MPH concentrations so as not to disrupt sleep onset). Daytrana patches may be removed earlier than 9 hours if a shorter duration of effect is desired. This allows for variable control of duration of effect to accommodate for changing patient schedules. The recommended initial dose is the 10-mg patch increasing to the next patch size weekly if clinically indicated and tolerated. The maximum FDA-approved dosage is the 30-mg patch daily. The patch has the typical stimulant side-effect profile in addition to not infrequent skin erythema at patch site to some degree with accompanying pruritus, especially during the winter months.

Reports of Interest

OROS Methylphenidate Hydrochloride in the Treatment of ADHD

Wilens et al. (2005) conducted a long-term open-label study of OROS MPH in the treatment of 407 children (age range 6 to 13 years, mean age 9.2 ± 1.8 years). Of those enrolled, 229 subjects continued treatment to the 21/24-month endpoint. Subjects were prescribed 18 to 54 mg daily; the mean daily dose at baseline was 35.2 mg and at endpoint was 44.2 mg. Using last observation carried forward

(LOCF) analyses, 85% of parents/caregivers and 92% of investigators rated a good "2" or excellent "3" response on the Global Assessment of Effectiveness. Regarding AEs, 282 (69.3%) reported at least one AE that investigators thought to be probably due to OROS MPH. The most frequent were headache (30.2%), insomnia (19.9%), decreased appetite (18.7%), abdominal pain (11.1%), and tics (0.8%). The authors concluded that OROS MPH was effective and tolerable in this population for up to 2 years.

Methylphenidate Hydrochloride in the Treatment of ADHD in Preschoolers

In a double-blind, placebo-controlled comparison of two doses (0.3 and 0.5 mg/kg/day) of MPH and placebo, Musten et al. (1997) treated 31 preschoolers (26 males, 5 females, mean age 58.07 ± 6.51 months, range 48 to 70 months) diagnosed with ADHD by DSM-III-R (APA, 1987) criteria. Twenty-six (84%) of the subjects were also diagnosed with comorbid oppositional defiant disorder (ODD) and six (19%) with conduct disorder. Bilingual children had a score of ≥72 and English-only-speaking children of ≥80 on the Peabody Picture Vocabulary Test. Efficacy was evaluated by ratings on the Gordon Diagnostic System Delay and Vigilance Tasks (for attention and impulsivity), and the Conners Parent Rating Scale–Revised (CPRS-R). Subjects were randomly assigned to each of the three conditions for a period of 7 to 10 days.

MPH significantly improved impulsivity on the Gordon Delay Task. Subjects made more correct responses on MPH than on placebo ($P < .05$) and there was no difference between the two doses of MPH. On the Gordon Vigilance Task (assessing sustained attention and impulsivity under conditions of high arousal and low feedback), there was significantly better performance on MPH than on placebo ($P < .01$) and there were no significant differences between the two doses of MPH. Parents ratings on the three subscales of the CPRS-R (Learning, Conduct, and Hyperactivity Index) all showed MPH to be significantly better than placebo ($P = .001$). There was no difference in the two MPH doses for the Conduct or Hyperactivity Index, but MPH 0.5 mg/kg/day was significantly better than MPH 0.3 mg/kg/day on the learning subscale. There was no evidence of improvement with MPH in children's compliance with parental directives on three laboratory tasks; however, MPH significantly improved the children's ability to stay on task in the 0.5 mg/kg dose but not in the 0.3 mg/kg dose. Subjects' productivity in a "cancellation task" was significantly improved on the 0.5 mg/kg dose only. Compared with placebo, parents reported significantly more untoward effects of greater severity with MPH 0.5 mg/kg/day but not with MPH 0.3 mg/kg/day. The authors concluded that the treatment of their subjects with MPH resulted in improvement similar to that reported for older children. It significantly improved attention and parent-rated behaviors. Overall, the results on using 0.5 mg/kg/day were superior to using the lower dose and supported using an initial dose of 0.5 mg/kg/day in this age group. The authors also noted that their protocol had fixed doses and that optimal doses for some subjects may have been higher and resulted in further improvement (Musten et al., 1997).

In their review of stimulant medication, Wilens and Spencer (2000) reviewed seven earlier placebo-controlled studies of MPH in a total of 187 preschoolers, with mean age of 4.9 years and age range of 1.8 to 6 years. The studies were 3 to 9 weeks long; total mean MPH daily dose was 5 to 20 mg/day or 0.3 to 1.0 mg/kg/day. Overall, there was mild to moderate improvement in ADHD symptomatology in all the studies. They noted that subjects' compliance increased with higher doses, which tended to improve the mother–child relationship.

MPH in the Treatment of Mentally Retarded Children Diagnosed with ADHD

Handen et al. (1999) reported a 3-week, double-blind, placebo-controlled study of MPH in treating 11 preschool children (9 males, 2 females; mean age,

58.9 ± 8.2 months; age range, 4.0 to 5.9 years), 9 were diagnosed with ADHD by DSM-III-R (APA, 1987) criteria and the other 2 had long-standing difficulty with inattention and overactivity. Two of the subjects with ADHD were diagnosed with comorbid ODD. Most subjects had intelligence quotients (IQs) in the mentally retarded range (mean IQ, 60.0 ± 11.6; IQ range, 40 to 78). Receptive/expressive language functioning was consistent with IQ in most subjects, and no subjects had diagnoses in the pervasive developmental spectrum.

All subjects underwent an initial, week-long period of baseline studies and acclimation to the study/laboratory "classroom" setting. Following this, subjects were administered MPH in 0.3- and 0.6-mg/kg doses or placebo for 1 week each. The three conditions were randomly assigned, but because of concern of untoward effects, the 0.3-mg/kg dose always preceded the 0.6-mg/kg dose. Efficacy was measured on the CTRS, the Preschool Behavioral Questionnaire (PBQ), the Side Effects Checklist, and several measures of behavior in the laboratory classroom (waiting task, resistance-to-temptation task, an 8-minute play session, compliance task, and cleanup task). Data were analyzed for the 10 children who completed the study as one child experienced significant increase in social withdrawal, irritability, tearfulness, whining, and anxiety on 0.3 mg/kg and further treatment with MPH was not recommended.

Overall, 8 (73%) of the 11 subjects responded positively to MPH with a minimum of 40% decrease on the Hyperactivity Index of the CTRS and/or the Hyperactive-Distractible subscale of the PBQ. Ratings on MPH, 0.6 mg/kg, compared with placebo on three of the CTRS indices (Hyperactivity [$P < .005$], Inattention-Passivity [$P < .05$], and Hyperactivity Index [$P < .05$]) and the PBQ Hyperactive-Distractible subscale ($P < .005$) all showed significant improvement. In the "laboratory classroom" play intensity and movement during free play decreased significantly, and during the compliance and cleanup tasks, vocalization and disruptive behavior decreased and compliance increased significantly on the omnibus test (but not the pairwise *post hoc* tests) while on MPH. Most children experienced a positive but not significant change on the MPH 0.3-mg/kg dose; the 0.6-mg/kg MPH dose was better for most of the variables, which showed significant improvement. Unfortunately, more clinically important untoward effects (e.g., social withdrawal and irritability) also occurred more frequently at the higher MPH dose. Overall, 45% of the 11 subjects developed untoward effects on MPH. The authors concluded that preschoolers with ADHD and mental retardation responded to MPH similarly to typically developing children with ADHD. They also noted that children with developmental disabilities (e.g., mental retardation) may be at greater risk for developing untoward effects on MPH, especially at higher doses, than children without such disabilities.

Pearson et al. (2003, 2004a, 2004b) reported on the behavioral adjustment, cognitive functioning, and individual variation in treatment response in a 5-week, within-subject, crossover, placebo-controlled, double-blind study of 24 children (18 males, 6 females; mean age 10.9 ± 2.4 years) diagnosed by DSM-III-R (APA, 1987) criteria with ADHD (22, combined type; 2, inattentive type) and mental retardation (17, mild mental retardation; 7, moderate mental retardation; estimated mean IQ of the 24 subjects using the Stanford Binet 4th edition, was 56.5 ± 10.24). Subjects were treated with placebo or MPH in doses of 0.15, 0.30, and 0.60 mg/kg administered twice daily, before breakfast and at lunch time. During the first week, all subjects received placebo; during the following 4 weeks, they were randomly administered each of the four conditions for 1 week. None of the children had other comorbid psychiatric diagnoses.

Behavioral adjustment (Pearson et al., 2003) was assessed by rating scales completed by teachers and parents. Symptoms of inattention, hyperactivity, oppositional behavior, conduct problems, and asocial behavior declined steadily with increasing MPH doses. The most significant findings were reported by teachers for the 0.60-mg/kg dose as follows: attention ($P = .024$), hyperactivity ($P < .001$), and oppositional behavior ($P = .012$) compared with placebo on the ADD-H Comprehensive Teacher Rating Scale and hyperactivity ($P < .001$), conduct problem ($P < .001$), emotional overindulgence ($P = .006$), asocial ($P = .009$), daydream-attention ($P = .022$), and Hyperactivity Index ($P < .001$) on the CTRS. The only parent rating that showed significant improvement was Impulsive-Hyperactive ($P = .018$) on the Conners Parent Rating Scale. The only adverse effects reaching significance were insomnia and loss of appetite, which were dose related. Parents reported that 16.7% (4/24) of the subjects experienced insomnia and that 29.2% (7/24) experienced significantly decreased appetite at the 0.60-mg/kg b.i.d. dose. Subjects did not experience significant increases in staring, social withdrawal, or anxiety. The authors noted that their findings of increasing improvement with increasing dose in the 0.15-to-0.60-mg range were consistent with the MTA study findings (MTA Cooperative Group, 1999a). The authors also noted that their results suggest that, whenever possible, dose regulation should be done when feedback from subjects' teachers is available.

In the same subjects, Pearson et al. (2004b) investigated the effects of MPH on cognitive functioning as assessed by their performance on tasks of sustained attention (using a modified version of the Continuous Performance Test [CPT]), visual sustained attention (using the Speeded Classification Task [SCT]), auditory selective attention (using the Selective Listening Task [SLT]), impulsivity/inhibition (using a Delay of Gratification Task [DGT] and the Matching Familiar Figure Test [MFFT]), and immediate memory (using the Delayed Match to Sample [DMTS]) task. Overall, higher MPH doses were associated with significantly greater gains in cognitive task performance on all the above measures except the DMTS, where no significant MPH effects were found. The 0.15-mg/kg b.i.d. dose was relatively ineffective compared with the 0.60-mg/kg b.i.d. dose. The authors noted that, for subjects who could not tolerate the 0.60-mg/kg b.i.d. dose because of untoward effects such as appetite suppression or insomnia, 0.30 mg/kg b.i.d. also produced significant, but lesser gains.

Pearson et al. (2004a) also looked at their 24 subjects' individual variations in cognitive and behavioral responses to MPH. The authors reported that 57% of subjects on 0.15 mg/kg b.i.d., 63% of subjects on 0.30 mg/kg b.i.d., and 71% of subjects on 0.60 mg/kg b.i.d. showed (any) gains in cognitive task performance. When "significant cognitive gains," defined as >30% improvement relative to placebo on tasks where such a score was possible, were assessed, these percentages decreased to 31%, 37%, and 46%, respectively. The authors also looked at deterioration in cognitive task performance. The authors reported that 35% of subjects on 0.15 mg/kg b.i.d., 29% of subjects on 0.30 mg/kg b.i.d., and 23% of subjects on 0.60 mg/kg b.i.d. showed some deterioration in cognitive task performance. When "significant cognitive deterioration," defined as >30% deterioration relative to placebo, were assessed, these percentages decreased to 14%, 15%, and 9%, respectively. The authors noted that these data suggest that MPH is not causing the deterioration, as fewer children exhibited cognitive deterioration as the MPH dose increased.

Regarding behavioral responses to MPH, Pearson et al. (2004a) reported that 45% of subjects on 0.15 mg/kg b.i.d., 58% of subjects on 0.30 mg/kg b.i.d., and 68% of subjects on 0.60 mg/kg b.i.d. showed (any) behavioral gains. When "significant behavioral gains," defined as >30% improvement, were assessed, these percentages decreased to 25%, 38%, and 55%, respectively. The authors also looked at deterioration in behavior. The authors reported that 38% of subjects on 0.15 mg/kg b.i.d., 24% of subjects on 0.30 mg/kg b.i.d., and 13% of subjects on 0.60 mg/kg b.i.d. showed some degree of deterioration in behavioral functioning. When "significant behavioral deterioration," defined as >30% deterioration relative to placebo, were assessed, these percentages decreased to 22%, 16%, and 9%, respectively.

Importantly, the authors noted that there was substantial independence between the effects of MPH on behavioral and cognitive changes and suggested that the clinician should monitor both responses when treating such children to determine the overall efficacy in a given child. The authors concluded that children with ADHD and MR show substantial improvement in cognitive and behavioral domains when treated with MPH, that the percentage of subjects who improve far outweighs subjects who substantially worsen, and that this favorable ratio improved as the study dose of MPH increased. They reported that at the 0.60-mg/kg b.i.d. dose, five times as many subjects showed substantial cognitive and behavioral gains compared with subjects who showed substantial declines in these domains. The authors concluded that treating children diagnosed with ADHD and mild to moderate MR with MPH results in improvement in both cognitive and behavioral domains and that, on average, higher doses are more effective. The authors also noted that the response rate of children with ADHD and mental retardation to MPH is not as favorable as in children with ADHD who are not retarded (Pearson et al., 2004a).

MPH in Conduct Disorder with and without ADD

Klein et al. (1997) conducted a double-blind, placebo-controlled study in which 84 children (age range, 6 to 15 years; mean, 10.2 ± 2.3 years; 74 males, 10 females) who were diagnosed with conduct disorder by DSM-III criteria were randomly assigned to a 5-week trial of MPH (N = 41) or placebo (N = 42). One subject dropped out before beginning treatment. A comorbid diagnosis of ADHD consistent with DSM-IV criteria was made in 69% of the subjects. Medication was administered twice daily (morning and noon doses) and was gradually raised to a total of 60 mg/day unless untoward effects prevented this. Subjects received no psychosocial therapy, although their parents were given weekly supportive counseling.

Seventy-four subjects completed the study as four taking MPH and five receiving placebo withdrew. The average dose of MPH at the termination of the study was 41.3 mg/day or 1 mg/kg, with the morning and noon doses never varying >5 mg. Untoward effects were reported by 31 (84%) of the subjects receiving MPH; the most common were decreased appetite and delay of sleep, with only a few instances of the latter being severe. Seventeen (46%) of the subjects on placebo reported at least one untoward effect. The authors noted that 72 (97.6%) of the subjects completing the study had at least three symptoms of conduct disorder consistent with DSM-IV criteria and that 51 (69%) had comorbid ADHD.

Compared with subjects receiving placebo, those taking MPH were rated significantly better by teachers and parents on all ratings of ADHD symptoms and all ratings of conduct disorder except socialized aggression, which measures severe delinquent behavior, such as membership in a gang, which was rare in this population. Teachers' ratings specifically noted significant reductions in "obscene language, attacks others, destroys property and deliberately cruel," whereas parents' ratings on "cruel to others, bad companions, and steals outside the home" showed significant decreases. Global improvement ratings of improved or better versus slightly improved or worse were statistically significant (P < .001) for subjects on MPH compared with those on placebo (teachers, 59% vs. 9%; mothers, 78% vs. 27%; and psychiatrists, 68% vs. 11%). Further analysis of the data showed that the significant improvements in symptoms of conduct disorder in subjects treated with MPH were not influenced significantly by the presence, absence, or severity of comorbid ADHD. The authors concluded that MPH had an independent positive influence on provocative, aggressive, mean behaviors and that MPH had a clinically significant effect in the treatment of conduct disorder that was independent of the presence or absence of ADHD.

MPH in the Treatment of Children Diagnosed with Autistic Disorder with Symptoms of ADHD

MPH has been investigated in the treatment of children diagnosed with autistic disorder who also have symptoms of ADHD. Although most of the earlier literature states that stimulants are contraindicated for autistic children and cause a worsening in behavior and/or stereotypies, several recent studies have reported that MPH is effective in treating some children with autistic disorder who also exhibit such symptoms as hyperactivity, impulsivity, short attention spans, and aggression. Strayhorn et al. (1988) reported on two autistic children, a 6-year-old autistic boy given MPH in a randomized trial with either placebo or MPH given each day and a preschool child treated openly with MPH. The former child was reported to show improvement in attention and activity levels, less destructive behavior, and a decrease in stereotyped movements, but sadness and temper tantrums significantly worsened. The preschooler was said to have had similar results.

Birmaher et al. (1988) treated nine hyperactive autistic children aged 4 to 16 years with 10 to 50 mg/day of MPH. Eight of the children improved on all rating scales; the oldest child improved on all scales except the one measuring behavior in school. In contrast, Realmuto et al. (1989), who treated two 9-year-old autistic boys with 10 mg of MPH administered twice daily, found that one became fearful and unable to separate from significant adults, had a worsening of his hyperactivity, and developed a rapid pulse. The second child's baseline behaviors did not change significantly, although he developed mild anorexia.

Quintana et al. (1995) reported a 6-week, double-blind, placebo-controlled crossover study of monotherapy with MPH in the treatment of 10 children (6 males, 4 females; mean age, 8.5 ± 1.3 years; age range, 7 to 11 years) who were diagnosed with autistic disorder by DSM-III-R (APA, 1987) criteria; subjects' mean developmental quotient was 64.3 ± 9.9. Efficacy was determined by ratings on the Childhood Autism Rating Scale (CARS; scores of ≤29 = nonautistic; 30 to 36.5 = mildly to moderately autistic; 37 to 60 = severely autistic) and the 10-item Conners Abbreviated Parent Questionnaire, the hyperactivity factor of the Conners Teacher Questionnaire (CTQ), the Aberrant Behavior Checklist (ABC; scores of 1 to 58 = slight behavioral problem; 59 to 116 = moderate problem; and 117 to 174 = severe problem) and three subscales of the ABC (I = irritability factor; III = stereotypies; and IV = hyperactivity factor). Untoward effects were rated on the Side Effects Checklist.

All subjects had previously been treated with neuroleptics but not with MPH; all were off medication for at least 1 month and completed a 2-week baseline rating period off medication. Subjects were then randomly assigned to 1 week of placebo or of MPH 10 mg twice daily (morning and noontime doses) dose range, 0.17 to 0.33 mg/kg/day, followed by a second week of placebo or MPH 20 mg twice daily or 0.34 to 0.68 mg/kg/day. Subjects then crossed over to receive the treatment they had not received for the final 2 weeks of the study.

Ratings over baseline improved significantly, more when subjects were taking MPH compared with placebo on the hyperactivity factor of the CTQ ($P = .02$), the ABC total score ($P = .04$), ABC irritability factor ($P = .01$), and the ABC hyperactivity factor ($P = .02$). However, all these ratings except the ABC irritability factor also improved significantly over baseline when on placebo, but the improvements were significantly less than when receiving MPH. There were no statistically significant differences in improvement between the two doses of MPH or any correlation with age or developmental quotient. Untoward effects were few and not statistically different from placebo; there was no significant change in ratings on the Abnormal Involuntary Movement Scale (AIMS) or on stereotypy ratings on the ABC stereotypic movement subscale. The authors concluded that MPH produced modest but significant improvement in hyperactivity in these patients without clinically significant untoward effects. They also recommended that hyperactive children diagnosed with autistic disorder be given a trial of MPH before a neuroleptic is administered. In some cases, this may result in sufficient improvement so that a neuroleptic is not required, and in some other cases, a lower dose of neuroleptic may be effective if combined with MPH (Quintana et al., 1995).

Handen et al. (2000) conducted a double-blind, placebo-controlled crossover study of MPH in the treatment of 13 children (10 males, 3 females; mean age,

7.4 years; age range, 5.6 to 11.2 years), 9 of whom were diagnosed by DSM-IV (APA, 1994) criteria with autistic disorder and 4 of whom were diagnosed with pervasive developmental disorder not otherwise specified. In addition, all had co-morbid diagnoses of both ADHD and ODD (ODD [N = 5], ADHD only [N = 6], or ODD only [N = 2]). Intelligence quotients were in the following ranges: average (N = 1), mild mental retardation (N = 4), moderate mental retardation (N = 5), severe/profound mental retardation (N = 3). Seven children were in special education classes and six were inpatients or in an intensive day-treatment program. Subjects were administered MPH in 0.3- or 0.6-mg/kg doses or placebo for 1 week each. The three conditions were randomly assigned, but because of concern about untoward effects, the 0.3-mg/kg dose always preceded the 0.6-mg/kg dose. Doses were given to all subjects at breakfast and lunch times; 11 subjects were given an optional third dose at about 4:00 PM. Efficacy was assessed by ratings on the Conners Teacher Scale 10-item Hyperactivity Index (CTSHI), the IOWA CTRS, the ABC, the Childhood Autism Rating Scale, and the Side Effects Checklist. Responders were a priori defined as having a >50% decrease on the CTSHI on MPH (either dose) versus placebo treatments.

Eight children (61.5%) were rated "responders"; seven of them showed improvement on both doses of MPH, and the eighth only on the higher (0.6 mg/kg dose). Significant improvements occurred on one or both doses of MPH on the CTSHI, the aggression subscale of the IOWA CTRS, and two (hyperactivity and inappropriate speech) of the five factors on the ABC. Significant change occurred on measures on the Stereotype and Inappropriate Speech subscales of the ABC, with the greatest improvements in "odd, bizarre behavior" and "repetitive speech." No significant changes in core features of autism were evident on the Childhood Autism Rating Scale, which is a global assessment of autistic symptoms. There were no significant differences in clinical response between the two doses of MPH and no correlation of response with age or IQ. The authors concluded that clinically significant behavioral gains were obtained on MPH at the lower 0.3-mg/kg dose and that children diagnosed with autism may be at greater risk for untoward effects, especially in the 0.6-mg/kg dose range. One child developed crying, tantrums, aggression, and skin picking on the 0.3-mg/kg dose and was dropped from the study without getting the 0.6-mg dose; two children on the 0.6-mg/kg dose were dropped during the week, one for severe staring spells and one for increased aggression in school. Other children developed increased levels or irritability and/or social withdrawal, especially at the higher dose. At the end of the study, eight children had benefited enough to continue to be prescribed MPH in doses of 0.2 to 0.6 mg/kg.

Single Isomer Dexmethylphenidate Hydrochloride (Focalin; Focalin XR)

Pharmacokinetics of Dexmethylphenidate Hydrochloride

Single Isomer

Dexmethylphenidate hydrochloride (D-MPH) is the D-threo-enantiomer, the more pharmacologically active enantiomer of racemic methylphenidate hydrochloride (D,L-MPH), which is a 50/50 mixture of the D-threo- and the L-threo-enantiomers. Dexmethylphenidate is thought to block the reuptake of norepinephrine and dopamine into the presynaptic neuron and increase the release of these monoamines into the extraneuronal space. The drug is well absorbed orally, and it may be taken with or without food. Peak plasma concentrations are reached in approximately 1 to 1½ hours after ingestion in the fasting state. When taken with a high-fat breakfast, peak plasma levels are about the same but take about twice as long to be reached. The medication is administered twice daily with at least 4 hours between doses. There is evidence that the therapeutic effects of D-MPH are of somewhat longer duration (approximately 5 to 6 hours) compared with a dose of D,L-MPH containing an equivalent amount of the D-isomer (D-MPH) (Wigal et al., 2004).

Dexmethylphenidate is metabolized primarily to ritalinic acid, which has little or no pharmacologic activity and is excreted primarily by the kidneys. The mean plasma elimination half-life of dexmethylphenidate is approximately 2.2 hours.

Contraindications of Dexmethylphenidate Hydrochloride

Dexmethylphenidate is contraindicated in patients with marked anxiety, tension, and agitation as it may worsen such symptoms.

Dexmethylphenidate is contraindicated in patients with hypersensitivity to MPH or other components of the drug. It is contraindicated in patients with glaucoma. Patients with motor tics or with a family history or diagnosis or TS should not be prescribed dexmethylphenidate.

To avoid a potential hypertensive crisis, dexmethylphenidate should not be prescribed to patients who are taking monamine oxidase inhibitors or within a minimum of 14 days of discontinuation of such drugs.

Adverse Effects of Dexmethylphenidate Hydrochloride

In premarketing trials with a total of 684 children, age range 6 to 17 years, the most frequently reported untoward effects were stomach pain, fever, decreased appetite, and nausea. Other, less frequent untoward effects included vomiting, dizziness, sleeplessness, nervousness, tics, allergic reactions, increased blood pressure, and psychosis (abnormal thinking or hallucinations). A total of 50 children (7.3%) experienced untoward effects that resulted in the drug's discontinuation. The untoward effects most frequently responsible for this were twitching (described as motor or vocal tics), anorexia, insomnia, and tachycardia, approximately 1% each.

Indications for Dexmethylphenidate Hydrochloride in Child and Adolescent Psychiatry

FDA approved for treating ADHD.

Dexmethylphenidate Dosage Schedule

Immediate-release dexmethylphenidate should be taken twice daily with at least a 4-hour interval between doses and may be taken with or without food.

- *Children <6 years of age:* not approved for use.
- *Children at least 6 years of age, adolescents, and adults who were not taking racemic MPH or who were on other (non-MPH) stimulants:* Start with 2.5 mg twice daily. Titrate at approximately weekly intervals in increments of 2.5 to 5.0 mg to a maximum of 20 mg daily.

Conversion Strategy

- *Children at least 6 years of age, adolescents, and adults who are currently taking racemic MPH:* Start with one-half the dose of racemic D- and L-methylphenidate to a maximum of 20 mg daily (10-mg doses administered approximately 4 hours apart).

Single Isomer Dexmethylphenidate Hydrochloride Dose Forms Available

- *Tablets:* 2.5, 5, and 10 mg (unscored)
- *Extended-release capsules (Focalin XR):* 5, 10, 15, 20, 25, 30, 35, and 40 mg. The 35- and 40-mg dosages are approved for adults only. This preparation permits once-daily dosing and produces a bimodal plasma concentration-time profile of two distinct peaks—an initial immediate release and the second approximately 4 hours later. Doses >30 mg/day in pediatrics have not been studied and are not recommended. The capsule can be taken whole, or the capsule contents can be sprinkled on applesauce and ingested without chewing the beads.

Reports of Interest

Dexmethylphenidate Hydrochloride in the Treatment of ADHD

Wigal et al. (2004) compared dexmethylphenidate hydrochloride (D-MPH) and D,L-threo-methylphenidate (D,L-MPH) in a 5-week, multicenter, double-blind, placebo-controlled study of 132 subjects (age range, 6 to 17 years; mean 9.8 years; 116 male, 16 female), diagnosed by DSM-IV criteria (APA, 1994) with an ADHD. Following a 1-week, single-blind placebo lead in, subjects received D-MPH ($N = 44$), D,L-MPH ($N = 46$), or placebo ($N = 42$) twice daily (between 7 and 8 AM and between 11:30 AM and 12:30 PM) for 4 weeks; dosage was adjusted on a weekly basis to a maximum of 10 mg twice daily for D-MPH (85% were titrated to the maximum dose) and 20 mg twice daily for D,L-MPH (69% were titrated to the maximum dose). At endpoint, the average daily dose for the D-MPH group was 18.25 mg and that for the D,L-MPH group was 32.14 mg.

Primary efficacy was rated on the Swanson, Nolan, and Pelham (SNAP) Rating Scale completed by the teacher (Teacher SNAP) twice weekly in the afternoon. Secondary efficacy measures included the Parent SNAP (Saturdays and Sundays at 3:00 PM and 6:00 PM), Clinical Global Impressions Scale–Improvement (CGI-I), and a math test; these ratings were obtained at 6:00 PM to test the hypothesis that the duration of action of D-MPH would be longer than that of D,L-MPH.

On the Teacher SNAP, both the D-MPH group ($P = .0004$) and the D,L-MPH group ($P = .0042$) had significantly greater improvement than the placebo group; the effect size was large (1.0) and equal for both drugs. Duration of significant efficacy was longer for the D-MPH group as measured by the Parent SNAP (D-MPH score significance at 3:00 PM, $P < .0001$; at 6:00 PM, $P = .0003$) than that for the D,L-MPH group (D,L-MPH score significance at 3:00 PM was .0073; at 6:00 PM, $P = .0640$). On the CGI-I, 22% of subjects of placebo were rated "much" (16.2%) or "very much improved" (5.4%). Compared with the placebo group, 67% of D-MPH subjects were rated "much" (35.7%) or "very much improved" (31%) with $P = .0010$; 49% of D,L-MPH subjects were rated "much" (26.8%) or "very much improved" (22.0%) with $P = .0130$. The D-MPH group improved significantly more from baseline to endpoint than the placebo group ($P = .0007$); the D,L-MPH group's improvement did not quite reach significance compared with the control group ($P = .0589$).

On the 6:00 PM math test, the D-MPH group scored significantly better that the placebo group; the placebo group worsened from baseline with an average of 3.9 fewer correct answers, whereas the D-MPH group got an average of 12.5 more problems correct ($P = .0236$). The D,L-MPH group scores on the 6:00 PM math test were not significantly different from those of the placebo group.

No patients experienced serious adverse effects (AEs). Headache, abdominal pain, nausea, and diminished appetite were the most frequently reported AEs. Abdominal pain was reported more frequently in the D-MPH group compared with the D,L-MPH group ($P = .0252$). Clinically significant changes occurred in the vital signs of 13 subjects (3 D-MPH, 8 D,L-MPH, and 2 placebo). Significant weight loss, ranging from 5% to 18% of baseline weight, was reported for four subjects in the D-MPH group, six subjects in the D,L-MPH group, and two subjects in the placebo group.

The authors concluded that D-MPH (mean, 18.25 mg) and D,L-MPH (mean, 32.14 mg) have similar efficacy and safety in treating ADHD, similar large effect sizes, and suggest that D-MPH has a longer duration of action that D,L-MPH after twice-daily dosing (Wigal et al., 2004).

As part of a multicenter study, Arnold et al. (2004) administered dexmethyl-phenidate hydrochloride (D-MPH) to 89 subjects (72 males, 17 females; mean age 10.1 ± 2.9 years, age range 6 to 16 years) who were diagnosed with ADHD; 71.9% were treatment naive. The first phase of the study was an open-label, dose-titration study of 6-weeks' duration; this was followed by a 2-week, double-blind, randomized, placebo-controlled withdrawal phase.

Efficacy was measured on the CGI-I Scale, the Swanson, Nolan, and Pelham–ADHD Rating Scale, and a "Math Test," which was used as a measure of "duration-of-effect" of the medication. The CGI-Severity (CGI-S) Scale was used to assess the severity of the subject's illness.

Medication was begun at doses ranging from 2.5 to 10 mg twice daily (morning dose and a noontime dose) depending on subjects' prior medication histories. During the first 4 weeks, medication was titrated upward to a maximum total dose of 20 mg daily or until adverse effects prevented increase or a CGI-I score of 1 ("very much improved") or 2 ("much improved") was achieved. During weeks 5 and 6, the dose was held constant.

Of the 89 subjects, 76 completed the 6-week open-label phase. The 13 dropouts were due to therapeutic failure (4), adverse effects (4), lost to follow-up (3), withdrawn consent (1), and protocol violation (1). Seventy-three completers (82% of the subjects) were rated 1 or 2 on the CGI-I; 89.2% were rated "normal to mildly ill" on the CGI-S Scale versus only 1.1% at baseline ($P < .001$). A total of 77 patients (86.5%) experienced adverse effects. Four subjects were discontinued because of adverse effects (one with rambling speech and tremor, one with labile mood, one with moderate headaches, and one with sleep terrors with somnambulism). Eight subjects had reduction in dosage because of tremor and anergy, gastrointestinal distress (including nausea, emesis, and diarrhea), headache, insomnia, unusual sensory experience, and irritability; except for insomnia, these adverse effects remitted with dose reduction.

Seventy-five of the subjects entered the subsequent 2-week withdrawal phase; 35 were assigned to D-MPH and 40 to placebo; 1 dropped out from each group. At the time of assignment 88.6% of the subjects in the D-MPH group and 87.5% of those in the placebo group were rated as showing only mild to no ADHD symptoms. Similarly, 70.6% of the D-MPH group and 80% of the placebo group were taking 10 mg of dexmethylphenidate twice daily. The placebo group showed significantly more treatment failures than the D-MPH group on the CGI-I: 61.5% had scores of 6 ("much worse") or 7 ("very much worse") versus 17.1% ($P = .001$), deterioration in the 3:00 PM Math Test ($P = .024$) and the 6 PM Math Test ($P < .0001$), Teacher SNAP-ADHD ($P = .028$) and the Parent SNAP-ADHD scores at 3:00 PM ($P = .0026$) and at 6:00 PM ($P = .0381$).

The authors also noted that adverse effects were similar to those of other stimulants and that score on the Math Tests at 3 and 6 hours after the noon dose, confirmed the earlier reported duration of efficacy for dexmethylphenidate to be at least 6 hours after the second daily dose (Arnold et al., 2004).

Silva et al. (2006) reported a multicenter, 2-week, double-blind, placebo-controlled, crossover study in which 54 subjects, age range 6 to 12 years, mean age 9.4 ± 1.6 years, who were diagnosed with ADHD by DSM-IV criteria, were randomly assigned to treatment for a 7-day period, which consisted of a 20-mg dose of D-MPH-ER (extended release) for 5 days, a day off medication, then on the seventh day, ratings in the (period 1) classroom laboratory setting on D-MPH-ER followed by another 7-day period consisting of placebo for 5 days, a day off medication, and then on the seventh day ratings in the (period 2) classroom laboratory setting on placebo (sequence A) or the reverse order (sequence B). All subjects had been stabilized on a total daily dose of 20 to 40 mg of D,L-MPH for a minimum of 1 month before beginning the study. All subjects had four visits: an initial screening visit, a practice day in the classroom, and two evaluation classroom days.

The primary efficacy variable was the Swanson, Kotkin, Agler, M-Flynn, and Pelham (SKAMP)-Combined scores at time 1-hour postdose. Secondary efficacy variables over the 12-hour classroom session were SKAMP-Attention and SKAMP-Deportment scores and the written math test score; these ratings were done at postdose hours 1, 2, 4, 6, 8, 9, 10, 11, and 12. The adjusted mean change in the SKAMP-Combined score from predose to 1-hour postdose was –10.014 for subjects when on D-MPH-ER compared with 0.878 when on placebo ($P < .001$) and the scores on D-MPH-ER were consistently significantly superior to placebo for the 12-hour period of laboratory classroom measurements ($P < .001$). The authors estimated the duration of effect of D-MPH-ER to be from 1 to 12 hours postdose. Scores on the SKAMP-Attention and SKAMP-Deportment Scales were significantly better with D-MPH-ER than with placebo at all time points. Mean changes from predose in the number of math problems attempted and the number of math problems correctly answered indicated that D-MPH-ER was significantly more effective than placebo ($P < .001$).

Because of imbalanced predose scores on the SKAMP-Combined and SKAMP–Attention-Math-Attempted and Math-Completed scores were significantly different between the two treatment weeks, a *post hoc* analysis was performed. In that analysis, for the SKAMP scores, the imbalance was mainly due to higher predose values in subjects given D-MPH-ER during the first week (period 1). The *post hoc* analysis of the 27 subjects who had D-MPH-ER during the first week was no longer significantly different from placebo at times 8, 10, 11, and 12 hours. Similarly, for both Math-Attempted and Math-Correct, scores at time 9, 10, 11, and 12 hours were not significantly different from placebo. The authors noted that this constraint may have contributed to the significant difference between drug and placebo during the later hours and recommended a larger sample without issues of imbalanced predose values to further clarify the duration of action of D-MPH-ER.

AEs were obtained by observation in the laboratory classroom, spontaneous reporting by the subjects, and parental reports of the period preceding each assessment day. One subject, on placebo, dropped out of the study because of nausea. Reported AEs were mild or moderate; no clinically significant cardiovascular AEs or laboratory abnormalities occurred. AEs that occurred more frequently on D-MPH-ER than placebo and possibly related to the drug were decreased appetite (9.4% vs. 0%), anorexia (7.5% vs. 0%), upper abdominal pain (5.7% vs. 1.9%), fatigue (3.8% vs. 0%), and insomnia (3.8% vs. 0%). The authors noted that because subjects had been stabilized on D, L-MPH prior to entering the study, the number and severity of adverse effects reported would tend to be less than would be the case if subjects were treatment naive.

Overall, the authors concluded that in this group of subjects, D-MPH-ER was both safe and effective in treating ADHD. Its duration of action may last for up to 12 hours (Silva et al., 2006).

Amphetamine Stimulant Drugs Approved for Use in Child and Adolescent Psychiatry

Amphetamine Sulfate: Dextroamphetamine Sulfate (Dexedrine, Dexedrine Spansules); Mixed Amphetamine Salts (Adderall)

Pharmacokinetics of Dextroamphetamine Sulfate

Amphetamines are noncatecholamine sympathomimetic amines with CNS activity. Dextroamphetamine sulfate is the dextro isomer of racemic (dextro [D-] levo- [L-]) amphetamine sulfate (Benzedrine), which was historically the first stimulant used in child and adolescent psychopharmacology (Bradley, 1937). The D-isomer is biologically more active than the L-isomer. However, as noted in the preceding text, some individuals respond positively to the L-isomer and not to the D-isomer (Arnold et al., 1976). Maximal dextroamphetamine plasma concentrations occur approximately 3 hours after oral ingestion. Average plasma half-life is approximately 12 hours.

Contraindications for the Administration of Dextroamphetamine Sulfate

The administration of dextroamphetamine sulfate is contraindicated in individuals with symptomatic cardiovascular disease, moderate to severe hypertension, hyperthyroidism, hypersensitivity to the sympathomimetic amines, or glaucoma. Sudden death has been reported in children with structural cardiac abnormalities who were treated with amphetamines at usual therapeutic doses.

Individuals who are in an agitated state or who have a history of drug abuse should also not be prescribed this drug.

Amphetamines should not be prescribed during or within 14 days of the administration of a MAOI to avoid the risk of a hypertensive crisis.

Amphetamines should be used with caution in individuals who have motor or vocal tics, TS, or a family history of such. This is discussed in more detail in the introductory part of this chapter.

Untoward Effects of Dextroamphetamine Sulfate

Dextroamphetamine sulfate elevates the systolic and diastolic blood pressure and has weak bronchodilator and respiratory stimulant action. Tachycardia may occur. The most frequent and troublesome immediate untoward effects include insomnia, anorexia, nausea, abdominal pain or cramps, vomiting, constipation or diarrhea, headache, dry mouth, thirst, lability of mood, irritability, sadness, weepiness, tachycardia, and blood pressure changes. Many of these symptoms diminish over a few weeks, although the cardiovascular changes may persist.

Clinical experience suggests that behavioral symptoms and thought disorder in psychotic children may be worsened by the administration of amphetamines. Amphetamines may cause short-term suppression of growth. Their long-term effects on growth inhibition are not certain, and growth should be monitored during their administration. This is discussed in more detail in the introductory part of this chapter.

Indications for Amphetamine Preparations in Child and Adolescent Psychiatry

Dextroamphetamine sulfate is FDA approved for treating ADDH, narcolepsy, and exogenous obesity. (ADDH is a DSM-III [APA, 1980a] diagnosis that, in large part, corresponds to the DSM-IV [APA, 1994, 2000] diagnosis, ADHD.)

Immediate-Release Amphetamine Sulfate Dosage Schedule for Treating ADHD

The serum half-life for standard-preparation dextroamphetamine sulfate is approximately 6 to 8 hours in children. This half-life makes it possible for some children to take the medication before leaving for school and maintain clinical effectiveness for the duration of the school day without taking a noontime dose, which is required when the standard-preparation MPH is used.

- *Children <3 years of age:* not approved for use.
- *Children 3 through 5 years of age:* begin with 2.5 mg daily; raise by 2.5-mg increments once or twice weekly; titrate for optimal dose.
- *Patients 6 years and older:* begin with 5 mg daily; raise by 5-mg increments once or twice weekly; the usual maximum dose is 40 mg/day or less.

The usual optimal individual dose falls between 0.15 and 0.5 mg/kg for each dose (Duncan, 1990), administered two to three times daily (total daily dose range, 0.30 to 1.5 mg/kg/day).

Mixed amphetamine salts (Adderall), which is a combination of equal parts of dextroamphetamine saccharate, amphetamine aspartate, dextroamphetamine sulfate, and amphetamine sulfate, is also approved for the treatment and narcolepsy. Peak plasma concentration occurs approximately 3 hours after ingestion. The manufacturer states that its plasma half-life is 7 to 8 hours, based on the amphetamine component. Usually, the first dose is given soon after awakening or before leaving for school; this may be followed by an additional one or two doses at 4- to 6-hour intervals. Whether this combination has clinically significant benefits compared with standard- or extended-release dextroamphetamine sulfate is uncertain at present.

Immediate-Release Amphetamine Sulfate Dose Forms Available

- *Tablets (Dexedrine):* 5 mg
- *Tablets (DextroStat):* 5 and 10 mg

Immediate-Release Mixed Amphetamine Salts Preparations Available

- *Tablets (Adderall):* 5, 7.5, 10, 12.5, 15, 20, and 30 mg

(continued)

Indications for Amphetamine Preparations in Child and Adolescent Psychiatry *(continued)*

Extended-Release Amphetamine Preparations Dosage Schedule and Available Dose Forms for Treating ADHD

Extended-Release Dextroamphetamine Sulfate (Dexedrine)

- *Sustained-release capsules (Dexedrine spansules):* 5, 10, and 15 mg

The maximum dextroamphetamine plasma concentrations of Dexedrine spansules occurs approximately 8 hours after oral ingestion of the sustained-release capsule. The plasma half-life is approximately 12 hours, similar to that of the immediate-release form. The manufacturer also noted that this "formulation has not been shown superior in effectiveness over the same dosage of the standard, noncontrolled-release formulation given in divided doses" (*PDR*, 2005, p. 1465).

Extended-Release L-Lysine-Dextroamphetamine Sulfate (Vyvanse)

- *Sustained-release capsules (Vyvanse-lisdexamfetamine dimesylate spansules):* 20, 30, 40, 50, 60, and 70 mg. Originally approved in February 2007. Vyvanse is approved for ADHD in children 6 to 17 years old as well as adults.

Lisdexamfetamine dimesylate or L-lysine-D-amphetamine is the first stimulant prodrug that is therapeutically inactive until it is converted to active D-amphetamine in the body upon cleavage of the lysine portion of the molecule. It was originally developed for the intention of creating a longer-lasting and more difficult to abuse version of dextroamphetamine, as the requirement of conversion into dextroamphetamine via enzymes in red blood cells increases its duration, regardless of the route of ingestion. Release of the active ingredient in Vyvanse does not reportedly rely on gastrointestinal factors such as GI transit time or Gastric pH.

When first released, it was recommended for pediatric patients either beginning treatment or switching from another medication, to initiate treatment at 30 mg once daily in the morning. Later a 20-mg capsule was released to allow another option to initiate treatment at a lower dosage. Dosage may be adjusted in increments of 10 or 20 mg at approximately weekly intervals up to maximum dose of 70 mg/day. Doses >70 mg/day have not been studied. The capsules may be taken whole or may be opened and the entire contents dissolved in a glass of water and consumed immediately.

The plasma half-life is 12 to 13 hours and time to maximum concentration (T_{max}) of Vyvanse is consistent with little interpatient variability at 3.5 hours postdose. After oral administration, lisdexamfetamine is rapidly absorbed from the gastrointestinal tract. Lisdexamfetamine is converted to dextroamphetamine and L-lysine primarily in blood due to the hydrolytic activity of red blood cells. *In vitro* data demonstrated that red blood cells have a high capacity for metabolism of lisdexamfetamine via hydrolysis. Lisdexamfetamine is not metabolized by cytochrome P450 enzymes reportedly.

Vyvanse demonstrated significant improvement in attention for up to 13 hours in a pediatric analog classroom study utilizing SKAMP-A scores (SKAMP = Swanson, Kotkin, Agler, M-Flynn, and Pelham rating scale). Vyvanse provided >70% reduction in ADHD-RS total score in patients who completed 12 months of treatment (Findling et al., 2007a; 2. Data on file, LDX014. Shire US Inc.).

Adverse Effects

The most common AEs reported during the dose-optimization phase of regulatory studies were decreased appetite, insomnia, headache, upper abdominal pain, irritability, and affect lability.

The most common side effects reported in studies of Vyvanse were

- anxiety
- decreased appetite
- diarrhea
- dizziness
- dry mouth
- irritability
- loss of appetite
- nausea
- trouble sleeping
- upper stomach pain
- vomiting
- weight loss

Reports of Interest

Vyvanse demonstrated a significantly lower abuse-related liking effect (DRQ-S Scores) than an equivalent oral dose of D-amphetamine in an abuse liability study. Oral administration of 150 mg/day of Vyvanse produced increases in positive subjective responses that were statistically indistinguishable from the positive subjective responses produced by 40 mg/day of oral IR D-amphetamine (data on file, LDX009. Shire US Inc.; Vyvanse [package insert], 2007).

Studies conducted by Jasinski and Krishnan seem to indicate that lisdexamfetamine dimesylate is less addictive than its counterparts such as Adderall and Concerta due to its unique formulation (Jasinski and Krishnan, 2009a). There is no increased onset of effect as occurs with IV administration of dextroamphetamine compared with oral use of lisdexamfetamine. Intravenously administered lisdexamfetamine produced likability effects similar to placebo, which the authors contend affirmed the drug's ability to reduce abuse potential (Jasinski and Krishnan, 2009b).

Vyvanse is also being investigated for possible treatment of major depressive disorder in adults, cognitive impairment associated with schizophrenia, excessive daytime sleepiness, and binge eating disorder in adults (http://www.shire.com/shireplc/en/rd/pipeline).

Extended-Release Mixed Amphetamine Salts (Adderall XR) and Dose Forms Available

• *Extended-release capsules (Adderall XR):* 5, 10, 15, 20, 25, and 30 mg

The average time to maximum serum levels of Adderall XR is approximately 7 hours. Its duration of action is roughly equivalent to taking two doses of immediate-release Adderall of the same total dose 4 hours apart. The capsule can be opened and sprinkled on applesauce without significantly changing its rate of absorption.

Dextroamphetamine in the Treatment of ADDH/ADHD

Dextroamphetamine sulfate and Adderall, a preparation of four amphetamine salts, are two amphetamines commonly used to treat ADHD in the United States and are the only stimulants currently in use that are approved by the FDA for administration to children as young as 3 years of age. Hence, they are officially the standard treatment for children up to age 6 years; however, many clinicians do prescribe MPH for some patients <6 years of age as there is considerable clinical experience and literature supporting this. Methamphetamine hydrochloride (Desoxyn) is approved for use in children above 6 years of age; however, as in the author's experience, it is infrequently prescribed and is not discussed in this book. Additionally, some clinicians (Wilens) believe it to be neurotoxic. If MPH does not provide satisfactory benefit in controlling symptoms of ADHD, it is recommended that an amphetamine product be tried before moving on to another class of drugs.

Reports of Interest

Amphetamines in Treatment Involving Seizures or ECT

Amphetamines may obtund the maximal electroshock seizure discharge and have been reported to prevent typical three-per-second spike-and-dome petit mal seizures and to abolish the abnormal EEG pattern in some children (Weiner, 1980). Amphetamine preparations may therefore be the stimulants of choice for individuals who have seizures or who are at risk for developing them, although, as noted earlier, MPH does not appear to increase the frequency of seizures or their development *de novo* when administered in usual therapeutic doses.

Amphetamine Sulfate in the Treatment of ADHD

Gillberg et al. (1997) reported a 12-month, randomized, double-blind, placebo-controlled study in which 62 subjects (52 males, 10 females; mean age, 9.0 ± 1.6 years; range, 6 to 11 years), diagnosed by DSM-III-R (APA, 1987) criteria with severe ADHD (26 [42%] of whom had various comorbid disorders) were treated with (racemic) amphetamine sulfate. For 72 subjects, the entire 18-month-long protocol was preceded by a 1-month baseline evaluation. During months 1 through 3, they were administered amphetamine sulfate in a single-blind fashion beginning with initial daily doses of 5 mg at breakfast and 5 mg at lunch times. Subsequent dose regulation permitted a maximum total daily dose of 60 mg. Ten subjects dropped out during this period because of untoward effects or lack of clinical response. The remaining 62 subjects all improved significantly. The 4th through 15th months consisted of the double-blind, placebo-controlled administration of amphetamine sulfate or placebo. The mean amphetamine sulfate dose of the 62 participating subjects at the beginning of this portion was 17 mg/day or 0.52 mg/kg/day, with a range of 5 to 35 mg/day or 0.20 to 1.10 mg/kg/day. During the double-blind portion, dosage was increased for 11 subjects and decreased for 8 subjects. Only 32 subjects (24 of 32 [75%] on active medication and 8 of 30 [27%] receiving placebo) completed the 12-month double-blind, placebo-controlled portion of the protocol. Most of the subjects assigned to the placebo group required switching to open treatment with amphetamine before the completion of the double-blind portion. Months 16 through 18 consisted of administration of single-blind placebo. Efficacy was assessed by ratings on Conners Parent and Teacher Scales and the Wechsler Intelligence Scale for Children–Revised (WISC-R).

During the 12-month placebo period, the group assigned to amphetamine retained the improvements achieved during the 3-month period on amphetamine, but the group assigned to placebo experienced reexacerbation of ADHD symptoms, as shown by comparison of ratings on the Conners Parent Scale, with mean scores declining from 43% to 47% ($P < .001$) and the Conners Teachers Scale with mean scores declining from 27% to 43% ($P < .01$). Comparing baseline WISC-R Scores to those at 15 months, the 35 subjects taking amphetamine for ≥9 months showed FSIQ a mean increase of 4.5 ± 4.7 points versus a mean increase of 0.7 ± 7.2 for the 8 subjects taking placebo for ≥6 months ($P < .05$). With the exception of decreased appetite for the amphetamine group, there were no significant differences in untoward effects for the placebo and amphetamine groups during the double-blind portion of the study. Four males developed hallucinations during the study; three were on active drug and one was on placebo. Upon stopping medication or with dose reduction, the hallucinations rapidly ceased. This study is one of the few long-term studies of amphetamines and suggests that the drug is safe and effective in treating children with ADHD for up to 15 months. Interestingly, when amphetamine was replaced with placebo during the 16th to 18th months of the study, there was no change in parent ratings and only a nonsignificant decline in teachers' ratings, suggesting that behavioral improvements were being maintained without the active drug.

Dextroamphetamine Sulfate in the Treatment of ADHD in Children Diagnosed with Pervasive Developmental Disorder

Geller et al. (1981) reported that dextroamphetamine administered to two children with pervasive developmental disorder and ADDH improved their attention spans with no significant worsening of behavior.

Adderall

Adderall (mixed amphetamine salts [MAS]) is composed of equal proportions of four amphetamine salts (D-amphetamine saccharate, D-amphetamine sulfate, D,L-amphetamine sulfate, and D,L-amphetamine aspartate), resulting in a 3:1 ratio of D-isomer to L-isomer.

Two double-blind placebo-controlled studies, the 4-week, multicenter study of Biederman et al. (2002) in naturalistic home and school settings with an N of 584, and the 6-week analog classroom study of McCracken et al. (2003) with an N of 51 reported that an extended-release formulation of MAS (Adderall XR) was effective and safe in treating children 6 to 12 years of age who were diagnosed with ADHD for at least 12 hours. In 2005, McGough et al. reported on the long-term tolerability and effectiveness of once-daily MAS XR in a 24-month, multicenter, open-label extension of these two studies. A total of 568 subjects who had completed one of the double-blind studies with no significant adverse effects (AEs) or had withdrawn for reasons other than AEs entered the long-term study. MAS XR was initiated in all subjects at a once-daily morning dose of 10 mg; 10-mg increases were permitted at weekly intervals during the first month to a maximum of 30 mg/day. The primary measure of effectiveness was the 10-item Conners Global Index Scale, Parent (CGIS-P) version. A total of 273 subjects (48%) completed the 24-month extension; the major reasons for discontinuing prematurely were as follows: withdrew consent (87, 15.3%), AEs (84, 14.8%), and lost to follow-up (74, 13%). The mean once-daily dose for completers was 22.4 ± 6.9 mg. Improvement of >30% in CGIS-P scores was maintained over the duration of the study ($P < .001$). Most AEs were of mild or moderate severity. The most frequent AEs responsible for withdrawal from the study were weight loss (27, 4.8%), anorexia/decreased appetite (22, 3.9%), insomnia (11, 1.9%), depression (7, 1.2%), and emotional lability (4, 0.7%). Mean systolic and diastolic blood pressure increased by 3.5 and 2.6 mm Hg, respectively; heart rate increased by 3.4 beats per minute. There were no clinically significant changes in laboratory test values. The authors concluded that MAS XR in once-daily doses of between 10 and 30 mg was well tolerated and resulted in significant clinical benefits over the 24-month extension period in children diagnosed with ADHD (McGough et al., 2005).

Adderall Versus MPH

Several studies have compared Adderall and MPH in the treatment of children and adolescents diagnosed with ADHD.

Swanson et al. (1998) conducted a 7-week, double-blind, placebo-controlled, crossover study of placebo, MPH, and Adderall in doses of 5, 10, 15, and 20 mg. All subjects had prior significant clinical responses to MPH (average total daily dose was 31.06 ± 13.59 mg divided into three doses), and each subject received an initial dose of MPH identical to that he or she had been taking (average dose was 12.5 mg) during the week on that condition. Each subject was on one of the six conditions for a week; during the seventh week, one of the conditions was repeated randomly, or if one condition had been missed, the medication appropriate for that week was given.

Findings of particular clinical interest were as follows: peak clinical effects of MPH occurred at an average of 1.88 hours, more rapidly than Adderall at usual doses, where peak clinical effects occurred at 1.5, 2.6, 2.6 [sic], and 3 hours for the 5-, 10-, 15-, and 20-mg doses, respectively.

MPH had a shorter duration of action that ended rather abruptly at an average of 3.98 hours. The duration of action of Adderall was dose dependent, increasing with the dose; duration of action was 3.52, 4.83, 5.44, and 6.40 hours for the 5-, 10-, 15-, and 20-mg doses, respectively.

Adderall was efficacious in the treatment of ADHD, and there were no unexpected or serious untoward effects; those that occurred were typical of stimulants.

Manos et al. (1999) compared the efficacy of MPH given twice daily (breakfast and lunch times) and a single breakfast-time dose of Adderall in a 4-week, double-blind titration, placebo-controlled study of 84 subjects (66 males, 18 females; mean age, 10.1 years; range, 5 to 17 years) diagnosed with ADHD by DSM-IV (APA, 1994) criteria. Each child's physician decided which active drug the child would be prescribed; parents and clinicians were aware of which active drug their child would receive but not of the dose titration or when placebo would be given. All subjects received 7 days of treatment with placebo, and 5-, 10-, and 15-mg doses of either MPH or Adderall. The four conditions were assigned randomly except that the week of the 10-mg dose had to precede the week of the 15-mg/day dose. Seven children on MPH and four on Adderall did not receive the 15-mg/day dose because their physician thought they were too young or weighed too little and had made an assessment that the optimal dose had already been achieved.

Efficacy was determined by the ADHD rating scale, the Conners Abbreviated Symptoms Questionnaire, Composite Ratings, School Situations Questionnaire–Revised, and the Side Effect Behavior Monitoring Scale. The average optimal dose of MPH was 19.5 mg/day and of Adderall was 10.6 mg/day, suggesting that Adderall is clinically about twice as potent as MPH. The optimal dose was significantly better than baseline or placebo conditions. There were no significant differences between parent and teacher ratings of subjects on MPH or Adderall. There were no clinically or statistically significant medication effects at any dose for pulse, blood pressure, or weight. The most commonly reported untoward effects at optimal dose for MPH were "anxious" (7/42, 16.7%), "perseveration" (5/42, 11.9%), "stares a lot" (4/42, 9.6%), "sad/unhappy" (9.6%), and "drowsiness" (3/42, 7.1%). For Adderall, the most common untoward effects at optimal dose were "insomnia" (5/42, 11.9%), "sad/unhappy" (11.9%), "prone to cry" (11.9%), and "irritability" (3/42, 7.1%). These children actually experienced more total untoward effects when not receiving medication, but the differences were not significant. The authors concluded that their data showed that the efficacy of a single morning dose of Adderall was comparable to that of morning and noon doses of MPH and that therefore a single morning dose of Adderall can eliminate the need of a noontime dose in school and simplify the drug management of such children. Of additional clinical interest, all 15 of the Adderall subjects who had previously tried MPH without clinical benefit (7 were nonresponders and 8 had serious untoward effects) showed clinical improvement on Adderall. The only two subjects who showed no clinical improvement in the study were both receiving Adderall. No subjects receiving MPH had previous trials of MPH.

Pliszka et al. (2000) conducted a 3-week, double-blind, placebo-controlled, parallel-group study comparing placebo, Adderall, and MPH in the treatment of 58 children, mean age 8.2 ± 1.4 years diagnosed with ADHD. A flexible dosing algorithm was devised to permit blind titration of the dose at the end of the first and second weeks based on clinical response. At the end of the study, the mean dose of Adderall was 12.5 ± 4.1 mg/day and the mean dose of MPH was 25.2 ± 13.1 mg/day. The most important clinical findings of the study were that both drugs were superior to placebo. The positive effects of Adderall on behavior lasted longer than those of MPH. No subject receiving Adderall required a noon dose; however, 7 of the 13 MPH responders also did not require a noon dose. There was a greater tendency for the children on Adderall to have more stomachaches and to manifest a sad mood than for those receiving MPH.

NONSTIMULANT DRUGS APPROVED FOR ADHD IN CHILD AND ADOLESCENT PSYCHIATRY

Selective Norepinephrine Reuptake Inhibitors

Atomoxetine Hydrochloride (Strattera)

Atomoxetine hydrochloride is a SNRI. This selective inhibition of the presynaptic norepinephrine transporter is the primary mechanism of action by which atomoxetine treats the symptoms of ADHD. In 2002, atomoxetine gained FDA approval for the treatment of ADHD, and it remains one of the few nonstimulant medications with this FDA-approved indication.

While stimulant medications are generally considered to be the first-line agents in the treatment of ADHD, stimulants are not well tolerated by some patients. For these patients, atomoxetine is then often considered as a first-line agent. For instance, stimulant medications may cause clinical worsening of anxiety and tics. Patients with ADHD that is comorbid with either anxiety and/or tics may therefore benefit from a trial of atomoxetine. Most individuals have either no change or an improvement in their anxiety and tic symptoms once treatment with atomoxetine is initiated, although in rare instances tics and anxiety have been worsened by the initiation of atomoxetine. Atomoxetine may also be considered a first-line agent in patients who have a history of illicit substance use. Cases where there is a concern about medication diversion (either by the patient or the patient's family members) are often good candidates for a trial of a nonstimulant such as atomoxetine.

In addition, atomoxetine is often used as either a second-line agent or as an augmentation strategy. For patients who have failed one or more stimulants, a trial of atomoxetine is often considered. In other cases, atomoxetine can be used as an augmenting agent for those patients whose stimulant dose has been maximized. Additionally, if a patient has an unpleasant medication side effect with a stimulant, the stimulant dose can be reduced and atomoxetine can be added to the regimen.

Atomoxetine can have profound effects on the symptoms of ADHD. An additional benefit of atomoxetine is that it can provide 24-hour treatment of ADHD symptoms (which is not feasible with stimulants). Atomoxetine generally does not worsen sleep, tics, or anxiety, and it can be taken at any time of the day. Atomoxetine has less abuse potential than stimulants, and since it is not a Schedule II medication, prescriptions can be written with refills and/or called in to the pharmacy.

While atomoxetine is a SNRI, its only FDA-approved indication is for the treatment of ADHD. Although it does not have FDA approval for other diagnoses, some patients who take it for ADHD have noticed improvements in their symptoms of anxiety, depression, and/or tics.

Although atomoxetine can have a significantly positive impact on ADHD symptoms and on patient's lives, patients must be aware of atomoxetine's black-box warning regarding suicidal ideation (discussed at the end of this section). They should also be aware that since atomoxetine is an NRI, it can take at least 6 weeks for its full effects to be realized. However, some benefits may be noticed after the first dose. Since it takes time to build up in the body, it can also take time to wash out. As a consequence of this, if there is an adverse event with atomoxetine, it could possibly take longer to resolve than an adverse event with a stimulant.

Pharmacokinetics of Atomoxetine Hydrochloride

Taken orally, atomoxetine hydrochloride is rapidly absorbed with maximal plasma concentrations being reached in approximately 1 to 2 hours. Absorption is minimally affected by food but taking it with meals does result in a 9% lower maximum plasma concentration in children and adolescents. Mean elimination half-life is approximately 5.2 hours. At standard doses, 98% of atomoxetine in plasma is protein bound (mostly to albumin). Atomoxetine is metabolized primarily via oxidative metabolism through the CYP2D6 enzymatic pathway followed by glucuronidation. The major metabolite is 4-hydroxyatomoxetine, which is equipotent to atomoxetine but circulates at a much lower plasma concentration. Atomoxetine is excreted primarily as 4-hydroxyatomoxetine-O-glucuronide (about 80% of which is excreted in urine and 17% in feces). Less than 3% of atomoxetine is excreted unchanged.

About 7% of Caucasians and 2% of African Americans are poor metabolizers of atomoxetine because they have reduced ability to metabolize CYP2D6 substrates. Such individuals have a net increase in the maximum plasma concentration of atomoxetine of 500% compared with extensive (normal) metabolizers of the medication. These poor metabolizers therefore have roughly five times as much medication in their system as extensive (normal) metabolizers due to their reduced ability to metabolize atomoxetine. The elimination half-life of atomoxetine for poor metabolizers is approximately 24 hours (nearly five times that of extensive metabolizers). Laboratory testing is available to determine if someone is a poor metabolizer of CYP2D6 medications. Atomoxetine itself neither inhibits nor induces the CYP2D6 pathway (Atomoxetine 2012).

Interactions of Atomoxetine with Other Medications

The current or recent use of nonselective MAOIs is contraindicated with atomoxetine (discussed below). Both nonselective and selective MAOIs should be avoided.

Medications such as quinidine, fluoxetine (Prozac), and paroxetine (Paxil), which inhibit CYP2D6, can result in significant increases in plasma levels of atomoxetine. Fluoxetine and paroxetine may increase the maximum plasma concentration of atomoxetine by up to three or four times in extensive (normal) metabolizers. Co-administration of atomoxetine with these medications will therefore require downward adjustment of the dose of atomoxetine (Michelson et al, 2007).

Patients who are taking blood pressure medications (either pressors or antihypertensives) will need close monitoring with any dosing changes of atomoxetine due to atomoxetine's effects on blood pressure. Co-administration of atomoxetine and beta-2 agonists (e.g., Albuterol) can result in clinically significant increases in blood pressure and heart rate.

Changes in gastric pH do not affect the bioavailability of atomoxetine, so no dosing adjustments need to be made if a patient is also being treated for gastroesophageal reflux (GERD).

Contraindications for Atomoxetine Administration

Atomoxetine is contraindicated in patients with known hypersensitivity to the medication. It should not be taken concomitantly with an MAOI or within 2 weeks of discontinuing an MAOI. Additionally, an MAOI should not be administered within the 2-week period after discontinuing atomoxetine.

Atomoxetine is also contraindicated in individuals with narrow-angle glaucoma since atomoxetine use in clinical trials was associated with an increased risk of mydriasis. Atomoxetine is contraindicated in patients with a history of pheochromocytoma and in people who have severe cardiovascular disorders that may deteriorate with the increases in heart rate and blood pressure that often occur from atomoxetine's effect on norepinephrine. In placebo-controlled registration studies with pediatric patients, the mean heart rate increase with atomoxetine was 5 beats per minute. Overall, 5% to 10% of pediatric patients taking atomoxetine have clinically important changes in blood pressure (≥15 to 20 mm Hg) and/or heart rate (≥20 beats per minute).

It is important to note that the co-administration of MPH and atomoxetine did not increase cardiovascular effects beyond those seen with MPH alone.

Warnings and Precautions

Administration of atomoxetine can cause an increase in suicidal ideation. It is therefore recommended that the patient be monitored closely for suicidality, worsening of symptoms, and unusual behavioral changes (particularly during the initiation phase and during any changes in medication dosing).

Atomoxetine has also been associated with severe liver injury in some cases. The medication should be stopped and not restarted if the patient develops jaundice or has lab values consistent with liver injury. Patients with signs of possible liver dysfunction (e.g., dark urine, pruritis, jaundice, unexplained flu-like symptoms, or right-upper-quadrant pain) should have liver enzyme levels tested. It should be noted that routine labs prior to starting atomoxetine are not required.

Sudden death has been reported in association with atomoxetine treatment (at usual doses) in children and adolescents with structural cardiac abnormalities or other serious heart problems. In adults, sudden death, myocardial infarction, and stroke have been reported in association with atomoxetine treatment (particularly in individuals with preexisting cardiovascular ailments). Atomoxetine should generally not be used in children and adolescents with known serious structural cardiac abnormalities, serious heart rhythm abnormalities, cardiomyopathy, or other serious cardiovascular problems that may worsen with an increase in norepinephrine. Prior to starting atomoxetine, it is therefore important to screen for both a personal and family history of cardiac disease (including a family history of sudden death or ventricular arrhythmia). An EKG and echocardiogram are not considered a part of the routine ADHD workup unless there is a personal or family history of concerning cardiovascular ailments. Blood pressure and heart rate should be monitored routinely, and questions about syncope and orthostasis should be asked. Patients who develop unexplained syncope, exertional chest pain, or other symptoms of possible cardiac disease should have a prompt cardiac evaluation.

With the administration of atomoxetine, it is also important to monitor both height and weight in children since this medication has been shown to have some effects on appetite and growth. In general, gains in both height and weight for patients taking atomoxetine is less than expected (based on population norms) for the first 9 to 12 months of medication use. After about 12 months, gains in height and weight stabilize with them approaching expected norms.

Children and adolescents should also be monitored for increases in aggressive behavior and possible mania/hypomania. Other potential side effects include that some adults have developed urinary hesitancy and retention, priapism, and/or sexual side effects with this medication. Individuals may also develop a rash with atomoxetine.

No fatal overdoses of atomoxetine occurred in clinic trials. There have been several fatalities reported with a mixture of medications, but none involving atomoxetine alone (including overdoses of up to 1,400 mg). In some cases of overdose of atomoxetine, seizures have occurred. Since atomoxetine is mostly protein bound, dialysis is not thought to be useful for atomoxetine overdose. Treatment of an atomoxetine overdose is mostly symptomatic (including monitoring for and treatment of cardiovascular symptoms [changes in blood pressure, heart rate, QTc prolongation]).

Untoward Effects of Atomoxetine

In clinical trials, the most common untoward effects of atomoxetine in children and adolescents (with an incidence of ≥5% and occurring at least twice as frequently as in patients treated with placebo) were nausea, vomiting, fatigue, abdominal pain, decreased appetite, and somnolence.

Indications for Atomoxetine in Child and Adolescent Psychiatry

Note: Review the Black Box Warning at the end of this section or in the package insert before prescribing.
Atomoxetine is FDA approved for the treatment of ADHD in individuals at least 6 years of age.

Atomoxetine Hydrochloride Dosage Schedule

- *Children <6 years of age:* Not recommended. The safety and efficacy of atomoxetine have not been established for this age group.
- *Children and adolescents ≥6 years of age and who weigh <70 kg:* Atomoxetine should be administered as a single morning dose or in two divided doses (in the morning and late afternoon/early evening). The initial total daily dose should be approximately 0.5 mg/kg. After a minimum of 3 days, the dose should be increased to reach a total target daily dose of 1.2 mg/kg. No additional benefit has been demonstrated for doses over 1.2 mg/kg/day, and the maximum recommended total daily dose should not exceed 1.4 mg/kg or 100 mg, whichever is less.
- *Children and adolescents ≥6 years of age and who weigh ≥70 kg and adults:* Atomoxetine should be administered as a single morning dose or in two divided doses (in the morning and late afternoon/early evening). The initial total daily dose should be 40 mg. After a minimum of 3 days, the dose should be increased to reach a total target daily dose of approximately 80 mg. After 2 to 4 additional weeks, the dose may be increased to a maximum of 100 mg.
- Dosing adjustments should be made for individuals who have hepatic impairment, are taking CYP2D6 inhibitors (fluoxetine, paroxetine), or are CYP2D6 poor metabolizers.
- Atomoxetine is considered a Category C medication in pregnancy. It is recommended that pregnant and breastfeeding women not use atomoxetine unless the potential benefit outweighs the potential risk to the fetus/infant.

Atomoxetine Hydrochloride Dose Forms Available and Instructions for Administration

- *Capsules:* 10, 18, 25, 40, 60, 80, 100 mg.
- Capsules should not be opened since the contents of the capsule may be an ocular irritant.
- Capsules can be taken with or without food, but should be taken with at least a glass of water.
- Patients should be instructed to use caution when driving a car or operating heavy machinery until they are reasonably certain that their performance is not adversely affected by atomoxetine.
- Atomoxetine may be discontinued without a taper, although a taper may be recommended.
- Consumption of ethanol with atomoxetine has not been shown to change the intoxicating effects of ethanol.

Reports of Interest

Atomoxetine versus Stimulants in the Treatment of Attention-Deficit/
Hyperactivity Disorder in Children and Adolescents

In head-to-head studies, the stimulants have been more efficacious than atomoxetine in the treatment of ADHD. In a multicenter, randomized, double-blind, forced-dose-escalation laboratory school study, Wigal et al. (2005) compared mixed amphetamine salts extended release (MAS XR; Adderall XR) to atomoxetine in 203 children aged 6 to 12 years who were diagnosed with ADHD (combined or hyperactive/impulsive type). The MAS XR group ($N = 102$) demonstrated significantly greater improvement from baseline than did the atomoxetine group ($N = 101$). The authors noted that AEs were similar in both groups and that their data suggested that with its extended duration of action and greater therapeutic efficacy, MAS XR was more effective than atomoxetine in children diagnosed with ADHD.

Hanwella et al. (2011) published a meta-analysis comparing the efficacy and acceptability of MPH and atomoxetine in the treatment of ADHD in children and adolescents. Nine randomized trials with a total of 2,762 subjects were included. The authors concluded from their analysis that atomoxetine and immediate-release

MPH have comparable efficacy in the treatment of ADHD; however, OROS MPH was considered to be more effective than atomoxetine. Regarding all-cause discontinuation, the authors noted that there was no significant difference between MPH and atomoxetine.

Kemner et al. (2005) reported on the treatment outcomes for African American children who participated in the Formal Observation of Concerta versus Strattera (FOCUS) study (funded by the maker of OROS MPH). Within the study, 183 children (13.8%) were African American. Of the 183, 125 were assigned to OROS MPH and 58 to atomoxetine. The authors noted that both medications were associated with significant improvement in ADHD symptoms from baseline but the group receiving OROS MPH demonstrated significantly greater improvement in total ADHD symptoms, inattentiveness, and CGI-I ratings.

Atomoxetine in the Treatment of ADHD in Children and Adolescents

In 2009, Newcorn et al. published their findings from the IDEA study. In this retrospective analysis of six randomized controlled trials, there were 1,069 subjects (age range from 6 to 18 years of age). The authors reported that (with regard to ADHD symptoms) with atomoxetine: 47% of patients were much improved, 13% had a minimal response, and 40% did not respond. They suggested that there seems to be a bimodal response to atomoxetine (e.g., responders and nonresponders). They noted that most of the responders had at least some improvement in symptoms by week 4 of treatment. They suggested that perhaps any patient who is a nonresponder at week 4 should either have another agent added to the atomoxetine regimen or they should be switched from atomoxetine to another medication.

Wehmeier et al. (2010) published the results of a meta-analysis of five atomoxetine trials. In all, there were 794 subjects (611 children and 183 adolescents). Atomoxetine was shown to be effective in improving some aspects of health-related quality of life (HR-QoL) in both children and adolescents (including in the achievement domain [academic performance and peer relations] and the risk avoidance domain).

Michelson et al. (2001) showed in a randomized, placebo-controlled, dose-response study, that atomoxetine was effective and safe in treating ADHD in children and adolescents when administered twice daily. In 2002, Michelson et al. conducted a study showing that (for most patients) atomoxetine could also be administered once daily with good clinical results. They reported a 6-week, double-blind, placebo-controlled study of once-daily treatment with atomoxetine in 171 children and adolescents (age range 6 to 16 years) who were diagnosed with ADHD. The treatment effect size (0.71) was noted to be similar to those observed in studies that used twice-daily atomoxetine dosing. The authors noted that this study suggested that once-daily dosing with atomoxetine is an effective treatment for ADHD. Despite its relatively short half-life, beneficial effects of one morning dose lasted into the evening for many subjects.

Weiss et al. (2005) also studied once-daily dosing of atomoxetine. In this multicenter, randomized, placebo-controlled, 7-week study in the school setting, 153 subjects (123 male, 30 female) were enrolled (age range 8 to 12 years). At its conclusion, 69% of the atomoxetine group versus 43% of the placebo group were rated as responders. Safety and tolerability was examined, and the authors concluded that once-daily dosing of atomoxetine is safe and effective in the treatment of ADHD.

Two studies by Wehmeier et al. examined possible gender differences in atomoxetine treatment of ADHD. This 2011 study was a pooled analysis of gender differences in five atomoxetine trials. Data from 136 girls and 658 boys were pooled. It was concluded that atomoextine was effective in improving some aspects of the HR-QoL in both genders without any significant difference across genders.

Atomoxetine in the Treatment of ADHD with Comorbid ODD or Conduct Disorder in Children and Adolescents

ADHD and ODD are frequent comorbidities. Newcorn et al. (2005) reported on the effects of atomoxetine on 293 subjects (8 to 18 years old) who were diagnosed with either ADHD-only ($N = 178$, 61%) or ADHD comorbid with ODD ($N = 115$, 39%). This was a 13-site, outpatient-only, approximately 8-week, randomized, double-blind, placebo-controlled study. At the conclusion of the study, in the ADHD/ODD group, atomoxetine was superior to placebo in reducing ADHD symptoms only for the 1.8 mg/kg/day dose (and not for the lower doses that were studied). The authors concluded that atomoxetine resulted in statistically and clinically significant improvements. They also stated that their results suggested that higher doses are required when ODD is comorbid with ADHD.

Wehmeier et al. (2010) conducted a study on the effects of atomoxetine on patients with ADHD and comorbid ODD or conduct disorder. The 9-week study of 180 patients showed that atomoxetine improved quality of life as measured by the KINDL-R scores on emotional well-being, self-esteem, friends, and family. However, there were no significant effects on family burden in these children and adolescents with ADHD and either ODD or conduct disorder.

Atomoxetine in the Treatment of Children and Adolescents Diagnosed with Comorbid Anxiety Disorder

Geller et al. (2007) reported that 25% to 35% of children with ADHD have comorbid anxiety disorders. Their 12-week, double-blind study of patients (age 8 to 17 years old) with ADHD and comorbid generalized anxiety disorder, separation anxiety disorder, and/or social phobia showed that atomoxetine was efficacious in reducing both ADHD symptoms and anxiety symptoms. The medication was reported to be well tolerated in this population.

Atomoxetine in the Treatment of Children and Adolescents Diagnosed with Pervasive Developmental Disorders

Harfterkamp et al. (2012) published a study which included 97 patients between the ages of 6 and 17 with an autism spectrum disorder and ADHD-like symptoms. This 8-week, double-blind study showed that hyperactivity improved significantly with atomoxetine compared with placebo. AEs (mostly nausea, decreased appetite, fatigue, and early morning awakening) were reported in 81.3% of patients receiving atomoxetine and 65.3% of patients receiving placebo. The authors concluded that atomoxetine moderately improved ADHD symptoms and was generally well tolerated. It has generally been noted that the effects of medications on the treatment of ADHD-like symptoms associated with an autism spectrum disorder are less robust than their effects on ADHD-only.

Atomoxetine in the Treatment of Children and Adolescents Diagnosed with ADHD and Lower IQ

Two studies (one by Mazzone et al. {2011} and another by Fernández-Jaén et al. {2010}) examined the use of atomoxetine in patients with ADHD and lower-than-average IQ. Mazzone's study included children whose IQs ranged from 43 to 117. The authors' conclusion at the completion of the study was that children and adolescents with IQs < 85 were less likely to respond to atomoxetine than children and were adolescents with IQs ≥ 85. Fernández-Jaén reported that patients with mental retardation and ADHD-like symptoms did show clinically significant improvements in their ADHD-like symptoms with the use of atomoxetine.

Review of Atomoxetine's Black Box Warning

Atomoxetine increased the risk of suicidal ideation in short-term studies in children or adolescents with ADHD. Anyone considering the use of atomoxetine in a child or adolescent must balance this risk with the clinical need. Comorbidities occurring with ADHD may be associated with an increase in the risk of suicidal ideation and/or behavior. Patients who are started on therapy should be monitored closely for suicidality (suicidal thinking and behavior), clinical worsening, or unusual changes in behavior. Families and caregivers should be advised of the need for close observation and communication with the prescriber.

Pooled analyses of short-term (6 to 18 weeks), placebo-controlled trials of Strattera (atomoxetine) in children and adolescents (a total of 12 trials involving more than 2,200 patients, including 11 trials in ADHD and 1 trial in enuresis) have revealed a greater risk of suicidal ideation early during treatment in those receiving Strattera compared with placebo. The average risk of suicidal ideation in patients receiving Strattera was 0.4% (5/1,357 patients), compared with none in placebo-treated patients (851 patients). There was 1 suicide attempt among the 2,200 patients. No suicides occurred in these trials (Bangs et al, 2008).

All reactions were reported to have occurred in children 12 years of age and younger. All reactions occurred in the first month of treatment.

A similar analysis in adult patients treated with Strattera for either ADHD or major depressive disorder (MDD) did not reveal an increased risk of suicidal ideation or behavior in association with the use of Strattera.

ALPHA-ADRENERGIC AGONISTS

While the dopamine system is believed to be innately involved in frontal lobe executive functioning and manifests in the syndrome of ADHD when impaired, the norepinephrine system also appears to be important in causing behavioral and cognitive abnormalities, in at least some children with ADHD.

Clonidine Hydrochloride Extended Release (KAPVAY), Clonidine Hydrochloride (Catapres), Clonidine (Catapres-Transdermal Therapeutic System)

Clonidine is a centrally acting antihypertensive agent. The only formulation that has a pediatric indication for ADHD is clonidine hydrochloride extended release (CXR), which is indicated for the treatment of ADHD as monotherapy and as adjunctive therapy to stimulant medications. The only therapeutic indication that immediate-release clonidine has been approved for by the FDA is the treatment of hypertension in older adolescents and adults; its safety and efficacy in children have not been established.

Clonidine is an alpha-2-adrenergic receptor agonist whose binding is independent of norepinephrine levels. There are three different subtypes of alpha-2 adrenoceptors in humans: the 2A, 2B, and 2C. The 2A and 2C subtypes have wide distributions in the brain, most importantly for ADHD in the prefrontal cortex (PFC), whereas the 2B receptors are most concentrated in the thalamus. Both the A and C subtypes are localized in the PFC, with the A subtype being more prevalent. Differential binding of alpha-2 receptors in these varying brain areas may account for their effects on cognitive as well as emotional functioning. It is theorized that alpha-2 agonists exhibit their therapeutic effects by strengthening (PFC) regulation of attention and behavior through direct stimulation of postsynaptic alpha-2A adrenoceptors (Arnsten et al., 2007). Alpha-2 agonists have been shown to bind to the alpha-2B and alpha-2C receptors as well. All three alpha-2-adrenoceptors subtypes are associated with sedative effects; in addition, hypotensive effects have been associated with subtype 2C (Arnsten et al., 2007; Franowicz and Arnsten, 2002). Clonidine appears to bind to all three alpha-2-receptor subtypes fairly equally, whereas guanfacine appears to be 15× to 20× more selective for the alpha-2A-receptor subtype.

Pharmacokinetics of CXR

The pharmacokinetic profile of KAPVAY administration was evaluated in an open-label, three-period, randomized, crossover study of 15 healthy adult subjects who received three single-dose regimens of clonidine: 0.1 mg of KAPVAY under fasted conditions, 0.1 mg of KAPVAY following a high-fat meal, and 0.1 mg of clonidine immediate-release (Catapres) under fasted conditions. Treatments were separated by 1-week washout periods.

After administration of KAPVAY, maximum clonidine concentrations (C_{max} pg/mL) were approximately 50% of the Catapres maximum concentration means (443 pg/mL) and T_{max} occurred approximately 5 hours later (6.8 hours) relative to Catapres (2.07 hours). Similar elimination half-lives (T_{max} hour) were observed at 12 hours and total systemic bioavailability (AUC) following KAPVAY was approximately 89% of that following Catapres.

Food had no effect on plasma concentrations, bioavailability, or elimination half-life.

Pharmacokinetics of Clonidine Hydrochloride Immediate Release

Peak plasma levels of clonidine occur between 3 and 5 hours after ingestion, and plasma half-life is between 12 and 16 hours (package insert). Leckman et al. (1985), however, give different pharmacokinetic values for children and adolescents, stating that clonidine's half-life is approximately 8 to 12 hours in adolescents and adults, whereas in prepubertal children it is considerably shorter at approximately 4 to 6 hours. Between 40% and 60% of the drug is excreted unchanged by the kidneys within 24 hours after oral ingestion, and approximately 50% is metabolized by the liver (package insert).

Contraindications for Clonidine Hydrochloride Administration

Known hypersensitivity to clonidine hydrochloride is a contraindication. Significant cardiovascular disease is a relative contraindication; if clonidine is used in patients with such conditions, careful and frequent monitoring is required.

Children and adolescents with depressive symptomatology, past history of depression, or family history of mood disorder should not be given clonidine (Hunt et al., 1990).

Interactions of Clonidine Hydrochloride with Other Drugs

Tricyclic antidepressants may decrease the effects of clonidine, necessitating higher doses.

The CNS depressive effects of alcohol, barbiturates, and other drugs may be enhanced by simultaneous administration with clonidine. Due to a potential for additive effects such as bradycardia and AV block, caution is warranted in patients receiving clonidine concomitantly with agents known to affect sinus node function or AV nodal conduction (e.g., digitalis, calcium channel blockers, and beta-blockers). Interactions with additional drugs have been reported.

Clonidine and MPH

In the summer of 1995 (July 13th), a National Public Radio broadcast reported that sudden deaths had occurred in three children taking a combination of MPH and clonidine, which caused alarm among parents and physicians of patients taking this combination of medications. Popper's editorial concerning this noted that the Food and Drug Administration (FDA) had not publicized the data or informed clinicians, as it considered the "link between the deaths and the medications highly dubious." Detailed reviews of the medications and the three cases by Popper (1995) and Fenichel (1995) concluded that there was no convincing evidence of an adverse MPH–clonidine interaction in any of the cases. Popper (1995) and Swanson et al. (1995) concluded that combined clonidine–MPH treatment of ADHD is usually safe and that the available evidence did not support discontinuation of such therapy in patients experiencing significant clinical benefit. All authors also noted the lack of systematic studies of the efficacy and safety of combined MPH–clonidine treatment.

Swanson et al. (1995) noted in their review of untoward effects that when the combination of clonidine and a stimulant was given, sedation–hypotension–bradycardia would be most expected when the clonidine effect was at its peak and the stimulant's effect is decreasing and, conversely, that hypertension–tachycardia would be most expected when the stimulant is at its peak and clonidine's effect is waning.

In 1999, in a "Debate Forum" on "Combining Methylphenidate and Clonidine" published in the *Journal of the American Academy of Child and Adolescent Psychiatry,* Wilens and Spencer argued the affirmative ("A Clinically Sound Medication Option") and Swanson, Connor, and Cantwell argued the negative ("Ill-Advised"). Before prescribing this combination, it is recommended that the clinician reviews this literature and thoroughly discusses the risks and benefits with the parents/legal guardian and patient.

Untoward Effects of CXR

The most common side effects of KAPVAY include

- sleepiness
- tiredness
- irritability
- sore throat
- trouble sleeping (insomnia)
- nightmares
- change in mood
- constipation
- stuffy nose
- increased body temperature
- dry mouth
- low blood pressure and low heart rate

It is advised that the treating practitioner should check heart rate and blood pressure before starting treatment and regularly during treatment with KAPVAY.

Sleepiness may be an early and bothersome side effect.

Somnolence and sedation were commonly reported adverse reactions in clinical studies. In patients who completed 5 weeks of therapy in a controlled fixed-dose pediatric monotherapy study, 31% of patients treated with 0.4 mg/day and 38% treated with 0.2 mg/day versus 7% of placebo-treated patients reported somnolence as an adverse event. In patients who completed 5 weeks of therapy in a controlled flexible-dose pediatric adjunctive to stimulants study, 19% of patients treated with KAPVAY+stimulant versus 8% treated with placebo+stimulant reported somnolence.

The incidence of "sedation-like" AEs (somnolence and fatigue) appeared to be independent of clonidine dose or concentration within the studied dose range in the titration study.

Withdrawal Symptoms

Suddenly stopping KAPVAY may cause withdrawal symptoms, including increased blood pressure, headache, increased heart rate, lightheadedness, "tightness" in the chest, and nervousness.

Interestingly, the incidence of "sedation-like" AEs (somnolence and fatigue) appeared to be independent of clonidine dose or concentration within the studied dose range in the titration study.

Results from the add-on study showed that clonidine body weight normalized clearance (CL/F) was 11% higher in patients who were receiving MPH and 44% lower in those receiving amphetamine compared with subjects not on adjunctive therapy.

Untoward Effects of Clonidine Hydrochloride Immediate Release

Hunt et al. (1991) reported that sedation is the most frequent and troublesome untoward effect of clonidine in treating children. Cardiovascular untoward effects, including hypotension, were not usually clinically significant.

Clonidine worsened or induced depressive symptomatology in approximately 5% of children (Hunt et al., 1991). McCracken and Martin (1997) reported the case of an 8-year-old boy with autistic disorder who developed an apparent severe depressive reaction on a total daily dose of 0.2 mg of clonidine; there was rapid improvement following discontinuation of clonidine. They cautioned clinicians to monitor for depressive reactions secondary to clonidine that could be mistaken for worsening of the primary disorder.

Levin et al. (1993) reported the onset of precocious puberty in two 7-year-old girls with mild mental retardation who were being treated with clonidine for aggressivity; of note, discontinuation of clonidine halted the progression of puberty in both cases. Many other untoward effects have been reported in patients on clonidine (*PDR*, 1995).

Swanson et al. (1995) reviewed briefly 20 MedWatch adverse-event reports concerning subjects <19 years of age who were taking clonidine and added three additional cases, one of which was fatal. Of the 23 cases, 4 were fatalities. Eleven cases were treated with clonidine only, 11 with combined clonidine–MPH therapy, and 1 with combined clonidine–dexedrine therapy. In 12 cases, the untoward effect occurred after a change in medication protocol (e.g., prescribed dose change, accidental change, or noncompliance). In 10 of the 19 nonfatal cases, hypotension and/or bradycardia was reported, and in 5 cases hypertension and/or tachycardia was reported. (See also the preceding discussion on clonidine–MPH under drug interactions.)

Effects of CXR and Clonidine Hydrochloride Immediate Release on the Electrocardiograms of Children and Adolescents

In the CXR studies, there were no changes on ECGs to suggest a drug-related effect.

Several studies have looked at cardiac issues when using immediate-release clonidine hydrochloride. Kofoed et al. (1999) reviewed relevant literature and conducted a retrospective study of the effects of clonidine alone ($N = 12$) and clonidine combined with stimulants (MPH [$N = 14$], dextroamphetamine [$N = 13$], or magnesium pemoline [$N = 3$]) on 12-lead, electrocardiograms (ECGs) of 42 children and adolescents (36 males and 6 females; age range, 4 to 16 years). The mean clonidine dose was 0.16 ± 0.075 mg/day (dose range, 0.05 to 0.30 mg/day). The mean daily MPH dose was 60 mg; the mean daily dextroamphetamine dose was 40 mg; and the mean daily magnesium pemoline dose was 112 mg. The authors stated that their data should be able to detect a difference of 0.012 second between baseline and postclonidine treatment PR intervals and of 0.015 second between pretreatment and postclonidine treatment for the QTc interval. Their data should also detect differences between clonidine only and clonidine plus a stimulant of 0.020 second for the PR interval and 0.024 second for the QTc interval. Two pediatric cardiologists, blinded to treatment condition, evaluated all ECGs.

The mean PR interval for all 42 subjects before clonidine was 0.140 ± 0.020 second versus 0.140 ± 0.022 second after clonidine treatment. The mean QTc interval calculated by cardiologist A before clonidine was 0.407 ± 0.025 second versus 0.407 ± 0.021 second after clonidine; for cardiologist B, the QTc interval before clonidine was 0.402 ± 0.027 second and after clonidine, 0.399 ± 0.023 second.

For the 12 subjects in the clonidine-only group, the mean pretreatment PR interval was 0.137 second and the posttreatment PR interval was also 0.137 second. There was also no pretreatment to posttreatment change in the mean PR interval for the 30 subjects receiving a combination of clonidine and a stimulant (PR = 0.142 second for both); there was no statistically significant effect of treatment, drug group, or treatment–drug group interaction term on PR intervals.

For the 12 subjects in the clonidine-only group, cardiologist A calculated the mean QTc pretreatment interval to be 0.409 versus 0.405 second posttreatment. For the 30 subjects receiving a combination of clonidine and a stimulant, the mean QTc pretreatment interval was calculated to be 0.406 versus 0.408 second post-treatment; there was no statistically significant effect of treatment, drug group, or treatment–drug group interaction term on the QTc interval.

For the 12 subjects in the clonidine-only group, cardiologist B calculated the mean QTc pretreatment interval to be 0.412 versus 0.398 second posttreatment. For the 30 subjects receiving a combination of clonidine and a stimulant, the mean QTc pretreatment interval was calculated to be 0.398 versus 0.400 second post-treatment; there was no statistically significant effect of treatment or drug group. However, treatment–drug group interaction term on the QTc interval showed a significant difference (0.014 increase for clonidine only versus 0.002 increase for clonidine and stimulant, $P = .034$). The authors noted that the 0.014-second shortening calculated for the clonidine-only group was not consistent with known effects of clonidine and thought this value resulted from the combination of a small N with other confounding errors.

Six (14%) of the 42 subjects had ECG abnormalities before medication treatment (3 sinus bradycardia, 2 ectopic atrial rhythm, and 1 short PR interval), and 7 (17%) had ECG abnormalities after medication. The abnormal ECGs of two subjects normalized on medication and three subjects with normal pretreatment ECGs developed abnormal ECGs on medication ($P = .50$, not significant), suggesting spontaneous variability rather than drug effect. Except for a 10-year-old boy with a short PR interval that later required ablation of an accessory atrial pathway, all subjects had normal PR, QRS, and QTc intervals, suggesting that clonidine alone or in combination with stimulants has no significant effect on these ECG parameters.

The authors emphasized the importance of pretreatment ECGs, as 14% of their subjects had abnormalities on their ECGs, some of which could have been attributed to clonidine if baseline data were not available. They also noted that spontaneous variations in ECGs over time occurred that were not caused by medication. Such variations in QTc occur randomly with changes in the balance of sympathetic/parasympathetic input to the heart and possibly due to diurnal variations that have been reported in adults. The authors made the valuable suggestion that each subject's pre- and posttreatment ECGs should be recorded at the same time of day to minimize some of these possible confounding spontaneous variations. The authors concluded that clonidine alone or in combination with stimulants had no systematic cardiac effects on these behaviorally disturbed children but that rare idiosyncratic responses could occur.

Guidelines for the Administration of CXR to Children and Adolescents

The dose of KAPVAY, administered either as monotherapy or as adjunctive therapy to a psychostimulant, is the same. Dosing should be initiated with one 0.1-mg tablet at bedtime, and the daily dosage should be adjusted in increments of 0.1 mg/day at weekly intervals until the desired response is achieved. Doses should be taken twice a day, with either an equal or higher split dosage being given at bedtime. Note that immediate-release clonidine hydrochloride and CXR have different pharmacokinetic characteristics; dose substitution on a milligram-for-milligram basis will result in differences in exposure. A comparison across studies suggests that the C_{max} is 50% lower for CXR compared with immediate-release clonidine hydrochloride.

■ *Guidelines for the Administration of Clonidine Hydrochloride*
Immediate Release to Children and Adolescents

Hunt et al. (1990) recommend beginning clonidine administration with bedtime doses to utilize the usual initial sedative effect to facilitate sleep. Sedation is most severe during the first 2 to 4 weeks, after which tolerance usually develops (Hunt et al., 1991). Because of its short serum half-life, clonidine is usually administered three to four times daily and at bedtime. Hunt et al. (1990) have reported that some children have shown a loss of therapeutic effect or withdrawal symptoms when it is administered less frequently; CXR or transdermal patches eliminate this difficulty.

Cantwell et al. (1997) expressed additional concern about untoward effects and the lack of methodologically sound studies on using combined clonidine/stimulant treatment for behavioral disturbances in children. The following is a summary only of their suggested guidelines for clonidine.

- *Screening*: Preexisting cardiac or vascular disease is a contraindication for clonidine therapy for behavioral reasons. Sinus node and atrioventricular node disease and renal disease are relative contraindications.
- *Pulse and blood pressure*: Pulse rate and blood pressure should be obtained to provide a baseline, should be done weekly during titration, and should be repeated every 4 to 6 weeks on maintenance dosage. A thorough evaluation of "new-onset treatment-emergent" symptoms, especially if exercise related, is essential.
- *ECG*: Baseline bradycardia or impaired atrioventricular conduction indicating first-degree, second-degree, or complete heart block or QRS interval >120 milliseconds necessitates cardiac consultation for medical clearance. Baseline ECG should be compared with an ECG recorded on full dose of clonidine.
- *Dose titration*: Clonidine should be titrated gradually and not exceed a 0.05-mg increment every 3 days. Drug termination should be by gradual tapering of dose to minimize withdrawal effects.

■ *Clonidine Administration with the Transdermal Therapeutic System*

When transdermal patches were used in treating subjects diagnosed with ADHD, Hunt (1987) found that their efficacy wore off and that they had to be replaced in 50% of subjects after 5 days rather than the 7 days stated by the manufacturer. He also noted that, to achieve the same degree of symptom control, three of his eight subjects whose daily oral dose was 0.2 mg/day had to have their doses increased to 0.3 mg/day when clonidine was administered transdermally. Comings (1990), who has extensive clinical experience with patients with TS, stated that he found that clonidine administered using a patch may work when oral clonidine is ineffective. Comings also found it convenient and useful to adjust the dose of clonidine by using scissors to cut the patch to the necessary size.

Indications for Clonidine Hydrochloride in Child and Adolescent Psychiatry

CXR (KAPVAY) released in 2011 was the second alpha-2A-receptor agonist FDA indicated for the treatment of ADHD in children and adolescents ages 6 to 17 as monotherapy and as adjunctive therapy to stimulant medications. The efficacy of CXR in the treatment of ADHD is based on two controlled trials (one monotherapy and one adjunctive to stimulant medication) in children and adolescents ages 6 to 17 who met DSM-IV criteria for ADHD hyperactive or combined hyperactive/inattentive subtypes. In the adjunctive study, CXR was administered to patients who had been on a stable regimen of either MPH or amphetamine (or their derivatives) and who had not achieved an optimal response. The effectiveness of CXR for longer-term use (more than 5 weeks) has not been systematically evaluated in controlled trials.

(continued)

Indications for Clonidine Hydrochloride in Child and Adolescent Psychiatry *(continued)*

Previously, clonidine immediate release (CIR) had been investigated in many clinical studies for the treatment of children and adolescents diagnosed with ADHD and/or TS who have not responded to standard treatments for these disorders. Studies of these uses and the doses employed by the researchers are summarized later for each of these conditions.

CXR and Clonidine Discontinuation/Treatment Withdrawal

When discontinuing CXR, the total daily dose should be tapered in decrements of no more than 0.1 mg every 3 to 7 days.

CIR should be gradually reduced over a period of 2 to 4 days to avoid a possible hypertensive reaction and other withdrawal symptomatology such as nervousness, agitation, and headache (package insert).

Clonidine Hydrochloride Dose Forms Available

- *CXR tabs:* 0.1, 0.2 mg (available in starter packs)—tablets must be swallowed whole and never crushed, cut, or chewed.
- *CIR tablets (single scored):* 0.1, 0.2, and 0.3 mg
- *Transdermal therapeutic system (TTS):* Programmed delivery by skin patch of 0.1 mg (Catapres-TTS 1), 0.2 mg (Catapres-TTS 2), or 0.3 mg daily (Catapres-TTS 3) for 1 week.

Safety and Efficacy Studies Involved in FDA Approval of CXR

Two CXR ADHD clinical studies evaluated 256 patients who received active therapy, in one of the two placebo-controlled studies (Studies 1 and 2) with primary efficacy endpoints at 5 weeks.

Study 1: Fixed-Dose CXR Monotherapy

Study 1 was an 8-week, multicenter, randomized, double-blind, fixed-dose, placebo-controlled study with primary efficacy endpoint at 5 weeks, of two fixed doses (0.2 or 0.4 mg/day) of CXR in children and adolescents aged 6 to 17 ($N = 236$) with a 5-week primary efficacy endpoint who met DSM-IV criteria for ADHD hyperactive or combined inattentive/hyperactive subtypes. Patients were randomly assigned to one of the following three treatment groups: CXR 0.2 mg/day ($N = 78$), CXR 0.4 mg/day ($N = 80$), or placebo ($N = 78$).

Dosing for the CXR groups started at 0.1 mg/day and was titrated in increments of 0.1 mg/week to their respective dose (as divided doses). Patients were maintained at their dose for a minimum of 2 weeks before being gradually tapered down to 0.1 mg/day at the last week of treatment. At both doses, improvements in ADHD symptoms were statistically significantly superior in CXR-treated patients compared with placebo-treated patients at the end of 5 weeks as measured by the ADHDRS-IV total score.

Study 2: Flexible-Dose CXR as Adjunctive Therapy to a Psychostimulant

Study 2 was an 8-week, multicenter, randomized, double-blind, placebo-controlled study, with primary efficacy endpoint at 5 weeks, of a flexible dose of CXR as adjunctive therapy to a psychostimulant in children and adolescents 6 to 17 ($N = 198$) with a 5-week primary efficacy endpoint who met DSM-IV criteria for ADHD hyperactive or combined inattentive/hyperactive subtypes. Patients had been treated with a psychostimulant (MPH or amphetamine) for 4 weeks with inadequate response. Patients were randomly assigned to one of two treatment groups: CXR adjunct to a psychostimulant ($N = 102$) or psychostimulant alone ($N = 96$). The CXR dose was initiated at 0.1 mg/day, and doses were titrated in increments of 0.1 mg/week up to 0.4 mg/day, as divided doses, over a 3-week period based on tolerability and clinical response. The dose was maintained for a minimum of 2 weeks before being gradually tapered to 0.1 mg/day at the last week of treatment. ADHD symptoms were statistically significantly improved in CXR plus stimulant group compared with the stimulant-alone group at the end of 5 weeks as measured by the ADHDRS-IV total score.

Thirteen percent of patients receiving KAPVAY discontinued from the pediatric monotherapy study due to AEs, compared with 1% in the placebo group. The most common adverse reactions leading to discontinuation of KAPVAY monotherapy-treated patients were somnolence/sedation (5%) and fatigue (4%).

KAPVAY treatment was not associated with any clinically important effects on any laboratory parameters in either of the placebo-controlled studies. Mean decreases in blood pressure and heart rate were seen (see "Warnings and Precautions"). There were no changes on ECGs to suggest a drug-related effect.

In Study 2, the adjunctive therapy study, the most common adverse reactions, defined as events that were reported in at least 5% of drug-treated patients and at least twice the rate as in placebo patients, during the treatment period were somnolence, fatigue, upper respiratory tract infection, irritability, throat pain, insomnia, nightmares, emotional disorder, constipation, nasal congestion, increased body temperature, dry mouth, and ear pain. The most common adverse reactions that were reported during the taper phase were upper abdominal pain and gastrointestinal virus.

Reports of Interest

CIR in the Treatment of ADHD

Hunt et al. (1982) reported on an open pilot study in which clonidine 3 to 4 µg/kg/day was administered orally for 2 to 5 months to four children between 9 and 14 years of age diagnosed with ADDH. Improvement was noted by parents and teachers. The authors noted that distractibility often persisted but that the children were nevertheless more able to return to and complete tasks.

Hunt et al. (1985) conducted a double-blind, placebo-controlled crossover study of 12 children (mean age, 11.6 ± 0.54 years) who were diagnosed with ADDH. Ten children completed the study. Seven subjects had previously received stimulant medication; in four cases, stimulants had been discontinued because of significant untoward effects. Clonidine was begun at 0.05 mg and increased every other day until a dose of 4 to 5 µg/kg/day (approximately 0.05 mg four times daily) was attained. Parents, teachers, and clinicians all noted statistically significant improvements on clonidine for the group as a whole. The best responders were children who had been overactive and who were uninhibited and impulsive, which, in turn, had impaired their opportunities to use their basically intact capacities for social relatedness and purposeful activity. During the placebo period, parents, teachers, and clinicians noted significant deterioration in overall behavior for the group, with symptoms usually returning between 2 and 4 days after discontinuing the medication (Hunt et al., 1985).

The most frequent untoward effect seen in this study was sedation, occurring approximately 1 hour after ingestion and lasting 30 to 60 minutes. In all but one case, tolerance to this effect developed within 3 weeks. Mean blood pressure also decreased approximately 10%.

Hunt et al. (1990, 1991) have reported that children diagnosed with ADHD and treated with clonidine have been maintained on the same dose for up to 5 years without diminution of clinical efficacy. However, approximately 20% of such children require an increase in dose after several months of treatment, probably secondary to autoinduction of hepatic enzymes (Hunt et al., 1990).

Hunt (1987) compared the efficacies of clonidine (administered both orally and transdermally) and MPH in an open study of 10 children diagnosed with ADDH, all of whom had ratings by both parents and teachers of >1.5 SD above normal on

Conners Behavioral Rating Scales. Eight subjects (seven males, one female; mean age, 11.4 ± 0.6 years; range, 6.7 to 14.4 years) completed the protocol. Subjects received placebo, low-dose (0.3 mg/kg) MPH, or high-dose (0.6 mg/kg) MPH. Each of these conditions was randomized for a period of 1 week. All subjects then received an open trial of clonidine 5 µg/kg/day administered orally for 8 weeks. Eight subjects completed the open trial with positive results and were then switched from tablets to transdermal clonidine skin patch. Both clonidine and MPH were significantly more effective than placebo, and clonidine in both dosage forms was as effective as MPH (Hunt, 1987). Children reported that they felt more "normal" on clonidine than on MPH. Transdermal administration was preferred to oral administration by 75% of the children and their families, not only because the embarrassment of taking pills at school was avoided but also because it was more convenient. Skin patches caused localized contact dermatitis, usually presenting with itching and erythema, in approximately 40% of children and at times limited their usefulness (Hunt et al., 1990).

Hunt (1987) noted that in contrast to the stimulants, clonidine appears to increase frustration tolerance but does not decrease distractibility. He noted that an additional small dose of MPH may be safely added to help focus attention and that this combination frequently permits a much lower dose of MPH than would be required if it were the only drug used (Hunt, 1987).

In a review of clonidine use in child and adolescent psychiatry, Hunt et al. (1990) explained more specifically the differences between clonidine and MPH in treating ADHD and their possible synergistic use in treating ADHD and suggested the subgroups of ADHD children for whom each treatment would be most useful. Stimulants (MPH) improve attentional focusing and decrease distractibility, whereas clonidine decreases hyperarousal and increases frustration tolerance and task orientation.

The authors found that children with ADHD who respond best to clonidine often have an early onset of symptoms, are extremely energetic or hyperactive (hyperaroused), and have a concomitant diagnosis of conduct disorder or oppositional disorder. Such children often respond to clonidine treatment with increased frustration tolerance and consequent improvement in task-orientated behavior; more effort, compliance, and cooperativeness; and better learning capacity and achievement. Clonidine was also efficacious in nonpsychotic inpatient adolescents with ADHD who were aggressive and hyperaroused (Hunt et al., 1990).

Unlike stimulants, clonidine in the original studies did not seem to directly improve distractibility; hence, stimulants were recommended preferable to immediate-release clonidine for mildly to moderately hyperactive children with significant deficits in distractibility and attentional focus. The combination of clonidine and MPH was found to be helpful for children who were diagnosed with coexisting conduct or oppositional disorder and ADHD and who were both highly aroused and very distractible (Hunt et al., 1990). The combined use of these drugs may permit the effective dose of MPH to be reduced by approximately 40%, making it potentially useful for ADHD patients in whom significant motor hyperactivity persists, or in whom rebound symptoms or dose-limiting side effects such as aggression, irritability, insomnia, or decrements in weight or height gain have occurred with stimulant treatment (Hunt et al., 1990).

Steingard et al. (1993) published a retrospective chart review of 54 patients (age range, 3 to 18 years; mean, 10.0 ± 0.5 years) who were diagnosed with ADHD only ($N = 30$) or ADHD and comorbid tic disorder ($N = 24$) and treated with clonidine. Of note, 17 subjects in the ADHD-only group had prior unsatisfactory responses to stimulant or tricyclic antidepressant medication. In the comorbid group, 9 had developed tics when treated with stimulants and 10 had unsuccessful prior trials of tricyclic antidepressants. Clonidine was initiated at a low dose and titrated upward until a positive clinical result occurred or untoward effects prevented further increase. Mean optimal daily dose for all subjects was 0.19 ± 0.02 mg/day (range, 0.025 to 0.6 mg/day). There was no significant difference in mean daily dose between subjects with and without tics, responders and nonresponders, or subjects less and more than 12 years of age. Although 72% (39) of 54 subjects were rated as improved on the Clinical Global Improvement Scale subset of items for ADHD symptoms, a significantly greater proportion ($P = .0005$) of subjects with a comorbid tic disorder (23 [96%] of 24) improved than did subjects with ADHD only (16 [53%] of 30). On Clinical Global Improvement Scale items pertinent to tics, 75% (18 of 24) showed improvement. Sedation, the most frequent untoward effect, was reported in 22 (41%) patients. All seven patients whose untoward effects resulted in discontinuation of medication were in the ADHD-only group. Five were discontinued because of sedation, one because of increased anxiety, and one because of a depressive episode.

At present, CIR may be regarded as a possible alternative treatment for ADHD. It may eventually prove useful in treating, in particular, a subgroup of ADHD children who do not respond well to stimulants. Clonidine may also be a useful alternative treatment for some ADHD children who have chronic tics or who develop side effects of sufficient severity as to preclude the use of stimulants (Hunt et al., 1985; Steingard et al., 1993).

Conner et al. (1999) reviewed the literature from 1980 to 1999 on the use of clonidine in the treatment of ADHD with and without comorbid diagnoses of conduct disorder, tic disorder, or developmental delay. Eleven of the 39 reports provided data sufficient to be used in a meta-analysis. The authors reported the overall effect size of clonidine for symptoms of ADHD to be moderate. It was similar to the effect size for tricyclic antidepressants but less than the large effect size for stimulants. The authors concluded that clonidine in doses of 0.1 to 0.3 mg/day was moderately effective in ameliorating common symptoms of ADHD and should be considered as a second-tier treatment. They also noted that clonidine's use is associated with many untoward effects, in particular sedation, irritability, and, when administered by transdermal patch, skin irritation and rash.

Clonidine in the Treatment of Sleep Disturbances in Children and Adolescents Diagnosed with ADHD

Wilens et al. (1994) reported their experience in using the sedation that clonidine often produces to treat more than 100 patients diagnosed with ADHD who also had spontaneous or drug-induced sleep difficulties. The effect has allowed some children who responded very well to stimulants, but could not tolerate them because of significant insomnia to be treated successfully with them. Typically, an initial dose of 0.05 mg of clonidine for patients between 4 and 17 years of age was given about half an hour before bedtime and was increased by 0.05-mg increments to a maximum of 0.4 mg. A few very young or underweight children required only 0.025 mg, whereas a few other children required >0.4 mg. Patients and parents reported better sleep, and there were decreased familial conflicts around sleep activities and fewer ADHD-like symptoms after treatment. Some of the latter improvement is likely to result from the fact that clonidine is also effective in treating ADHD independent of its sleep-enhancing qualities. Clonidine should be tapered gradually when it is discontinued, even if used only at night for insomnia.

Clonidine in the Treatment of Chronic Severe Aggressiveness

Kemph et al. (1993) treated openly with clonidine 17 outpatients (14 males and 3 females; age range, 5 to 15 years old; mean age, 10.1 years) diagnosed with conduct or ODD. All subjects had a history of chronic and violent aggressiveness in multiple settings that had not responded to behavioral management. Clonidine was begun at an initial dose of 0.05 mg/day. After 2 days, it was increased to 0.05 mg twice daily, and on day 5 it was increased to 0.05 mg three times daily, following which it was titrated as clinically indicated on an individual basis. The maximum effective dose was 0.4 mg daily administered in divided doses. A comparison of mean baseline and follow-up scores on the Rating of Aggression against People and/or Property Scale (RAAPP) showed significant improvement on drug ($P < .0001$). Drowsiness was the major untoward effect most frequently reported; it usually occurred during the first weeks of treatment, and most patients developed tolerance to it. There were no significant changes in blood pressure or cardiovascular parameters. The authors noted that plasma gamma-aminobutyric acid (GABA) levels increased significantly ($P < .01$) in five of the six children for whom it was available at follow-up, suggesting that GABA plasma levels may be correlated with childhood aggressiveness and may also be useful to verify compliance. Clonidine may be a useful agent in the control of aggression in children and adolescents and merits further study.

Clonidine in the Treatment of Autistic Disorder Accompanied by Inattention, Impulsivity, and Hyperactivity

Jaselskis et al. (1992) treated eight males (age range, 5.0 to 13.4 years; mean, 8.1 ± 2.8 years) diagnosed with autistic disorder who also had significant inattention, impulsivity, and hyperactivity that had not responded to prior psychopharmacotherapy (e.g., MPH or desipramine); they received clonidine in a double-blind, placebo-controlled, crossover protocol. Clonidine or placebo was titrated over the initial 2 weeks to a daily total of 4 to 10 µg/kg/day (0.15 to 0.20 mg/day) divided into three doses; this regimen was maintained for the next 4 weeks. During the seventh week, subjects were tapered off clonidine or placebo. At week 8, subjects were crossed over to the other condition for 6 weeks. Parents' ratings on the Conners Abbreviated Parent–Teacher Questionnaire showed significant improvement while their children were on clonidine. Teachers' ratings on the Aberrant Behavior Checklist were significantly better during clonidine treatment for irritability ($P = .03$), hyperactivity ($P = .03$), stereotypy ($P = .05$), and inappropriate speech ($P = .05$). ADDH: Comprehensive Teacher's Rating Scale scores improved significantly only for oppositional behavior ($P = .05$). Although significant, improvement was modest. Clinician ratings at the end of each 6-week period showed no significant differences between clonidine and placebo. Untoward effects included significant drowsiness and hypotension requiring reduction of dosage in three subjects.

Clonidine in the Treatment of Tourette Syndrome

Cohen et al. (1980) reported that clonidine was clinically effective in at least 70% of 25 patients between 9 and 50 years of age diagnosed with TS who either did not benefit from haloperidol or could not tolerate the untoward effects of that medication. Dosage was begun at 1 to 2 µg/kg/day (usually 0.05 mg/day) and gradually titrated up to a maximum of 0.60 mg/day. Most patients did best with small doses three to four times daily. Comings (1990) recommends a starting dose of 0.025 mg/day (one-fourth of a tablet) and sometimes found it necessary to administer as many as five divided doses daily for best results. He found it to be an excellent drug for the approximately 60% of his patients who responded and noted that it ameliorated oppositional, confrontational, and obsessive-compulsive behaviors and symptoms of ADHD when these were also present. In contrast, Shapiro and Shapiro (1989) noted that, in their experience, clonidine was only rarely effective in treating unselected patients with tics and TS.

Cohen et al. (1980) delineated five phases of treatment response to clonidine:

Phase I: Within hours or days, patients felt calmer, less angry, and more in control.

Phase II: Approximately 3 to 4 weeks after initiation of clonidine (usually coinciding with a therapeutic dose of 3 to 4 µg/kg/day [0.15 mg/day]), the patient recognized progressive benefits characterized by decreased compulsive behavior, further behavioral control, and decreased phonic and motor tics.

Phase III: A plateauing of improvement started at about the third month.

Phase IV: Five or more months after beginning, an increase in dosage up to 4 to 6 µg/kg/day (0.30 mg/day) of clonidine was needed to maintain clinical improvement.

Phase V: Further tolerance to clonidine may occur at a dose considered too high to increase further.

A review of the use of clonidine in TS (Leckman et al., 1982) noted discrepant results among studies. The reviewers estimated that approximately 50% of subjects improved meaningfully. Behavioral symptoms showed the most improvement and maximum benefit could take from 4 to 6 months. A minority of patients did not respond, and a few worsened.

Leckman et al. (1985) reported a 20-week, single-blind, placebo-controlled trial of clonidine in 13 patients, aged 9 to 16 years, diagnosed with TS. This was followed by a 1-year open clinical trial. The mean dose of clonidine was 5.5 µg/kg/day (range, 3 to 8 µg/kg/day) (0.125 to 0.3 mg/day). There was significant improvement in motor and phonic tics and associated behavioral problems. Forty-six percent of subjects were unequivocal responders, and 46% responded equivocally. Of interest is the fact that 9 of the 13 patients reported by Leckman et al. also had an additional diagnosis of ADDH. As noted earlier, some children with ADHD have symptoms that respond to clonidine.

Leckman et al. (1991) reported a 12-week, double-blind, placebo-controlled trial of clonidine completed by 40 subjects (age range, 7 to 48 years; mean, 15.6 ± 10.4 years; 31 of the subjects were younger than 18 years old) diagnosed with TS. Clonidine was titrated gradually during the first 2 weeks to a total daily dose of 4 to 5 µg/kg/day (maximum, 0.25 mg/day) and administered in two to four divided doses per day, depending on the total dose. Mean clonidine dose at the end of the 12 weeks for the 21 subjects randomly assigned to clonidine was 4.4 ± 0.7 µg/kg/day (range, 3.2 to 5.7 µg/kg/day); clonidine serum levels, available for 19 subjects, ranged from 0.24 to 1.0 ng/mL, with a mean of 0.48 ± 0.23 ng/mL. Subjects receiving clonidine were rated as significantly more improved than those receiving placebo on the Tourette Syndrome Global Scale for motor tics ($P = .008$) and total score ($P = .05$); on the anchored Clinical Global Impressions Scale for TS (TS-CGI); on the Shapiro Tourette Severity Symptom Scale for decrease in "tics noticeable to others"; and on the Conners Parent Questionnaire for total score ($P = .02$) and the impulsive/hyperactive factor ($P = .01$). Untoward effects most frequently reported were sedation/fatigue (90%), dry mouth (57%), faintness/dizziness (43%), and irritability (33%). Although clonidine is not as effective in controlling tic behavior as the D_2-dopamine receptor-blocking agents haloperidol and pimozide, its more favorable untoward effect profile should prompt the clinician to consider a trial of clonidine before using antipsychotic drugs in milder cases (Leckman et al., 1991).

Bruun (1983) has provided useful guidelines for prescribing clonidine for TS. She suggests initiating daily dosage at 0.025 mg twice daily for small children and at 0.05 mg twice daily for older children and adolescents. Medication is titrated upward gradually with increases of no >0.05 mg/week; this slow pace often prevents untoward effects from interfering with the treatment. The usual optimal daily dose is between 0.25 and 0.45 mg. Doses above 0.5 mg/day may be required, but untoward effects (e.g., drowsiness, fatigue, dizziness, headache, insomnia, and increased irritability) become more troublesome. Bruun (1983) notes that drowsiness may occur at very low doses and suggests that no further increases in dosage be made until drowsiness subsides. Some patients note a decrease in beneficial effects 4 to 5 hours after their last dose, and treatment is usually more effective for all patients with total daily dosage administered in three or four smaller doses (Bruun, 1983).

Although presently not an approved treatment, there is evidence that some children and adolescents with TS respond favorably with significant symptom reduction when treated with clonidine. Clonidine may be regarded as a possible treatment for those youngsters with TS who have not responded satisfactorily or who have intolerable untoward effects to standard treatments.

Clonidine in the Treatment of Children Who Stutter

Althaus et al. (1995) reported that clonidine was *not effective* in the treatment of 25 children 6 to 13 years of age diagnosed with stuttering by DSM-III-R (APA, 1987) criteria. In a 28-week, double-blind, placebo-controlled crossover study. Medication or placebo was gradually increased for 1 week, followed by maintenance for 8 weeks; dosage was then tapered for 4 days followed by 4.5 weeks of washout before beginning the other condition or at the end of the study before the final ratings. Clonidine was given in a total dose of 4 µg/kg/day divided into three equal portions over the day. Efficacy was determined by ratings of repetitions, prolongations, blockades, and interjections at baseline, before first dose reduction, after first washout period, before second dose reduction, and after the final washout. There was no significant improvement in any of the measures used. Parents and teachers also rated no significant difference between placebo and clonidine and improvement of children's stuttering, but they did notice significant behavioral improvements in hyperactivity, task orientation, and greater approachability. The authors concluded that clonidine was not a useful drug for treating children diagnosed with stuttering.

Guanfacine Hydrochloride (Tenex)

INTUNIV (Guanfacine) Extended-Release Tablets

Generic guanfacine hydrochloride is a centrally acting antihypertensive agent with alpha-2-adrenoreceptor agonist properties. Guanfacine is not a CNS stimulant.

Guanfacine is a selective alpha-2A-adrenergic receptor agonist in that it has a 15 to 20 times higher affinity for this receptor subtype than for the alpha-2B or alpha-2C subtypes (compared with clonidine affinities). Guanfacine has no known potential for abuse. INTUNIV is a once-daily, extended-release formulation of guanfacine hydrochloride (HCl) in a matrix tablet formulation for oral administration only. INTUNIV, released in 2009, was the first alpha-2A-receptor agonist FDA indicated for the treatment of ADHD in children and adolescents ages 6 to 17. The efficacy of INTUNIV or guanfacine extended-release (GXR) tablets as a monotherapy treatment for ADHD is based on results of two 8 to 9 week studies in children and adolescents aged 6 to 17. In 2011, GXR tablets received additional FDA approval as Adjunctive Therapy to Stimulant Medications in 6- to 17-year-olds with ADHD who had a suboptimal response to stimulant monotherapy based on a 9-week trial.

The only other FDA-approved indication for guanfacine hydrochloride is the treatment of hypertension. As INTUNIV (guanfacine) tablets are the only FDA-approved formulation of guanfacine for pediatric ADHD, it will be highlighted and preferentially discussed versus the guanfacine immediate-release (GIR) formulation which is not FDA approved.

Pharmacokinetics of GXR Tablets

GXR tablets were developed with rate-limiting excipients in its matrix to slow guanfacine absorption, thereby reducing the peak-to-trough fluctuations (Shojaei et al., 2006). Peak plasma levels occur from 4 to 8 hours (mean, 6 hours) after ingestion. Average plasma half-life is approximately 18 ± 4 hours. Although younger subjects tend to metabolize GIR more rapidly, this has not been studied in GXR tablets. The long-acting formulation of guanfacine results in a much lower (60%) C_{max} (ng/mL) of 1.0 versus 2.5 for GIR and thus provides a slower rise to maximum concentration compared with GIR. Steady-state blood levels usually occur within 4 days. GXR is a unique formulation of guanfacine; therefore, one cannot substitute for GIR tablets on a milligram-for-milligram basis because of the differing pharmacokinetic profiles. Guanfacine and its metabolites are excreted primarily by the kidneys.

Contraindications for Guanfacine Hydrochloride Administration

GXR tablets should not be used in patients with a history of hypersensitivity to guanfacine or any of its inactive ingredients or by patients taking other products containing guanfacine.

Interactions of Guanfacine Hydrochloride with Other Drugs

The depressive effects of alcohol, barbiturates, and other drugs on the CNS may be enhanced by simultaneous administration of guanfacine. Interactions with additional drugs have been reported.

Untoward Effects of Guanfacine Hydrochloride

Untoward effects include those typical of the central alpha-2-adrenoreceptor agonists such as dry mouth, sedation, fatigue, dizziness, low blood pressure, constipation, weakness/asthenia, irritability, and upper abdominal pain. Most are mild and transient if treatment is continued. Adverse reactions in GXR studies 301 and 304 that were dose related include somnolence, abdominal pain, dizziness, hypotension/decreased blood pressure, dry mouth, and constipation.

Horrigan and Barnhill (1998) reported five cases in which intense activation with a cluster of signs and symptoms resembling an acute-onset manic episode occurred within 3 days following the administration of guanfacine (GIR). These cases were from a series of 95 outpatients who were treated with guanfacine (GIR) during a 12-month period. All five patients were reported to have personal and family risk factors for bipolar disorder.

Indications for Guanfacine Hydrochloride in Child and Adolescent Psychiatry

INTUNIV, released in 2009, was the first alpha-2A-receptor agonist FDA indicated for the treatment of ADHD in children and adolescents ages 6 to 17.

GXR Tablets Dosage Schedule

GXR is an extended-release tablet and should be dosed once daily. Tablets should not be rushed, chewed, or broken before swallowing because this will increase the rate of guanfacine release. Prescribing instructions advise to not administer with high-fat meals, due to increased exposure (C_{max} approximately 75% and AUC approximately 40%). One cannot substitute GXR for GIR tablets on a milligram-for-milligram basis because of differing pharmacokinetic profiles. It is recommended to begin at a dose of 1 mg/day and adjust in increments of no more than 1 mg/week. The dose is recommended to be kept within the studied range of 1 to 4 mg once daily, depending on clinical response and tolerability. In the initial clinical trials, patients were randomized to doses of 1, 2, 3, or 4 mg and received GXR once daily in the morning when used as monotherapy. Later adjunctive therapy studies demonstrated the efficacy of GXR when dosed either in the morning or evening when combined with stimulant therapy dosed in the morning.

In the monotherapy studies, clinically relevant improvements were observed beginning at doses in the range of 0.05 to 0.08 mg/kg once daily. Efficacy increased with increasing weight-adjusted dose (mg/kg). If well tolerated, doses up to 0.12 mg/kg once daily seemed to provide additional benefit. Unfortunately, dosages above 4 mg/day have not been studied which may allow more efficacious treatment in larger individuals but safety data are available on dosages up to 0.17 mg/kg/day.

(continued)

Indications for Guanfacine Hydrochloride in Child and Adolescent Psychiatry *(continued)*

GIR Dosage Schedule

- *Children up to 11 years of age:* Not recommended. Efficacy and safety have not been established in this age group. Hunt et al. (1995) begin guanfacine at a dose of 0.5 mg/day and, on the basis of clinical response, individually titrate guanfacine in 0.5-mg increments every 3 days to a maximum of 4 mg/day, which appears to be appropriate in the treatment of ADHD in this age group.
- *Adolescents >12 years of age and adults:* For the treatment of hypertension, an initial dose of 1 mg at bedtime is recommended to minimize the impact of any initial sedation that may occur. If clinically indicated, higher doses may be administered.

GXR Tablets Discontinuation/Treatment Withdrawal

In vitro studies with human liver microsomes and recombinant CYP's demonstrated that guanfacine was primarily metabolized by CYP3A4. In pooled human hepatic microsomes, guanfacine did not inhibit the activities of the major cytochrome P450 isoenzymes (CYP1A2, CYP2C8, CYP2C9, CYP2C19, CYP2D6, or CYP3A4/5). Guanfacine is a substrate of CYP3A4/5 and exposure is affected by CYP3A4/5 inducers/inhibitors.

Drug Interactions

It is recommended to use caution when guanfacine is administered to patients taking ketoconazole and other strong CYP3A4/5 inhibitors, since elevation of plasma guanfacine concentrations increases the risk of AEs such as hypotension, bradycardia, and sedation.

When patients are taking guanfacine concomitantly with a CYP3A4 inducer such as rifampin, an increase in the dose of guanfacine within the recommended dose range may be indicated and considered.

There was a significant decrease in the rate and extent of guanfacine exposure when co-administered with rifampin, a CYP3A4 inducer. The exposure to guanfacine decreased by 70% (AUC).

Valproic Acid

Co-administration of guanfacine and valproic acid can result in increased concentrations of valproic acid. The mechanism of this interaction is unknown, although both guanfacine (via a Phase I metabolite, 3-hydroxy guanfacine) and valproic acid are metabolized by glucuronidation, possibly resulting in competitive inhibition. In such cases, patients should be monitored for potential additive CNS effects and consideration given to monitoring serum valproic acid concentrations. Adjustments in the dose of valproic acid may be indicated when co-administered with guanfacine.

Guanfacine Discontinuation/Treatment Withdrawal

Because of possible rebound phenomena, including nervousness and anxiety (from relative increases in catecholamines) and increases in blood pressure to over baseline, GIR should be tapered gradually when discontinued. When discontinuing GXR formulations, it is recommended to taper the dose in decrements of no more than 1 mg every 3 to 7 days. Because of guanfacine's relatively long half-life, if rebound is to occur, it usually does so 2 to 4 days after abrupt withdrawal. Although rebound hypertension can occur, it is infrequent and blood pressure usually returns to pretreatment levels over 2 to 4 days.

GXR Dose Forms Available

- *Extended-release tablets:* 1, 2, 3, and 4 mg

Guanfacine Hydrochloride (GIR) Dose Forms Available

- *Tablets:* 1 and 2 mg

CLINICAL STUDIES

Safety and Efficacy Studies Involved in FDA Approval of GXR

Studies 1 and 2: Fixed-Dose GXR Monotherapy

The efficacy of GXR in the treatment of ADHD was established in two placebo-controlled trials in children and adolescents ages 6 to 17. Study 1 evaluated 2, 3, and 4 mg of GXR dosed once daily in an 8-week, double-blind, placebo-controlled, parallel-group, fixed-dose design ($N = 345$). Study 2 evaluated 1, 2, 3, and 4 mg of GXR dosed once daily in a 9-week, double-blind, placebo-controlled, parallel-group, fixed-dose design ($N = 324$). In Studies 1 and 2, patients were randomized to a fixed dose of GXR. Doses were titrated in increments of up to 1 mg/week. The lowest dose of 1 mg used in Study 2 was assigned only to patients <50 kg (110 lb). Patients who weighed <25 kg (55 lb) were not included in either study.

Guanfacine Extended Release

Signs and symptoms of ADHD were evaluated on a once weekly basis using the clinician-administered and scored ADHD Rating Scale–IV (ADHD-RS), which includes both hyperactive/impulsive and inattentive subscales. In both studies, the primary outcome was the change from baseline to endpoint in mean ADHD-RS scores.

The mean reductions in ADHD-RS scores at endpoint were statistically significantly greater for GXR compared with placebo for Studies 1 and 2. Placebo-adjusted changes from baseline were statistically significant for each of the 2-, 3-, and 4-mg GXR randomized treatment groups in both studies, as well as the 1-mg GXR treatment group (for patients 55 to 110 lb) that was included only in Study 2.

Interestingly, dose-responsive efficacy was evident, particularly when data were examined on a weight-adjusted (mg/kg) basis. When evaluated over the dose range of 0.01 to 0.17 mg/kg/day, clinically relevant improvements were observed beginning at doses in the range 0.05 to 0.08 mg/kg/day. Doses up to 0.12 mg/kg/day were shown to provide additional benefit and some clinicians consider this to be a "sweet spot" for dosing but each patient must be individualized on a risk/benefit ratio.

GXR

Controlled, long-term efficacy studies (>9 weeks) have not been conducted for GXR. Subgroup analyses were performed to identify any differences in response based on gender or age (6 to 12 vs. 13 to 17). Analyses of the primary outcome did not suggest any differential responsiveness on the basis of gender. Analyses by age subgroup revealed a statistically significant treatment effect only in the age 6 to 12 subgroup. Due to the relatively small proportion of adolescent patients (ages 13 to 17) enrolled into these studies (approximately 25%), these data may not be sufficient to demonstrate efficacy in the adolescent subgroup. In these studies, patients were randomized to a fixed dose of INTUNIV™ rather than optimized by body weight. Therefore, it is likely that some adolescent patients were randomized to a dose that resulted in relatively low plasma guanfacine concentrations compared with the younger subgroup. More than half (55%) of the adolescent patients received doses of 0.01 to 0.04 mg/kg. In studies in which systematic pharmacokinetic data were obtained, there was a strong inverse correlation between body weight and plasma guanfacine concentrations.

Study 3: Flexible-Dose GXR as Adjunctive Therapy to Psychostimulants

Study 3 evaluated 1, 2, 3, and 4 mg of INTUNIV dosed once daily in a 9-week, double-blind, placebo-controlled, dose-optimization study. This study evaluated the safety and efficacy of GXR, dosed either in the morning or in the evening, compared with placebo, when given in combination with a psychostimulant, in children and adolescents aged 6 to 17 years with a diagnosis of ADHD, with a suboptimal response to stimulants ($N = 455$). Subjects were started at the 1-mg GXR dose level and were titrated weekly over a 5-week dose-optimization period to an optimal GXR dose not to exceed 4 mg/day based on tolerability and clinical response. The dose was then maintained for a 3-week dose-maintenance period before entry to 1 week of dose tapering. Subjects took GXR either in the morning or in the evening while maintaining their current dose of psychostimulant treatment given each morning. Allowable psychostimulants in the study were ADDERALL XR, VYVANSE, CONCERTA, FOCALIN XR, RITALIN LA, METADATE CD, or FDA-approved generic equivalents.

Symptoms of ADHD were evaluated on a weekly basis by clinicians using the ADHD Rating Scale (ADHD-RS-IV), which includes both hyperactive/impulsive and inattentive subscales. The primary efficacy outcome was the change from baseline to endpoint in ADHD-RS-IV total scores. Endpoint was defined as the last postrandomization treatment week prior to dose tapering for which a valid score was obtained (up to Week 8).

Mean reductions in ADHD-RS-IV total scores at endpoint were significantly greater for GXR given in combination with a psychostimulant compared with placebo given with a psychostimulant for Study 3, for both morning and evening GXR dosing. Nearly two-thirds (64.2%) of subjects reached optimal doses in the 0.05 to 0.12 mg/kg/day range.

Controlled adjunctive long-term efficacy studies (>9 weeks) have not been conducted.

Pearls

Study 3 was a dose-optimization study and thus theoretically more clinically relevant to actual prescribing practices. While previous experience with short-acting alpha-2 agonists led many clinicians to perceive guanfacine and clonidine as primarily useful for hyperactive and emotional impulsivity/anger features of ADHD, Study 3 seemed to demonstrate that GXR was beneficial for both hyperactive and inattentive symptoms of ADHD. This adjunctive medication study also indicated that the combination of stimulant and GXR was more efficacious than each agent given alone. GXR appeared to have very similar efficacy whether dosed in the morning or in the evening. The fact that evening dosing is effective is useful as one of the more common dose-related side effects of GXR is sedation, which may allow sleep onset complaints by patients to be addressed successfully utilizing evening administration of GXR. Although GXR is only FDA approved for once-a-day dosing, clinicians sometimes utilize bid dosing to address efficacy issues or side effect issues such as daytime sedation.

Reports of Interest Using GIR Tablets

Guanfacine in the Treatment of ADHD

Guanfacine appears to have potential advantages over clonidine in the treatment of ADHD because it has a longer plasma half-life and appears to be less sedating (Hunt et al., 1995).

Hunt et al. (1995) treated, with guanfacine, 13 subjects (11 males, 2 females; age range, 4 to 20 years; mean, 11.1 years) who were diagnosed with ADHD. Guanfacine was begun at a dose of 0.5 mg/day and individually titrated by 0.5-mg increments every 3 days to achieve optimal clinical response to a maximum of 4 mg/day. Mean therapeutic dose was 3.2 mg/day (0.091 mg/kg/day). Medication was usually administered in four divided doses with the morning, noon, and approximately 4:00 PM doses being somewhat less than the bedtime dose. Parental ratings on the Conners 31-item Parent Questionnaire at baseline and after 1 month of treatment with guanfacine showed a significant improvement on guanfacine in total average score ($P < .015$), Factor I (hyperactivity) ($P < .002$), Factor II (inattention) ($P < .004$), and Factor V (immaturity) ($P < .002$). In addition, scores on the following individual behavioral items of the Conners questionnaire were significantly improved while on guanfacine: less fidgety ($P < .002$), less restless ($P < .01$), making fewer disruptive sounds ($P < .01$), less easily frustrated ($P < .005$), less anxious ($P < .005$), less excessive energy ($P < .01$), better able to finish projects

($P < .005$), more attentive ($P < .01$), functional with less supervision ($P < .025$), less rejected and unpopular in social groups ($P < .01$), less uncooperative ($P < .05$), and less constricted or rigid ($P < .01$). Untoward effects included significant initial tiredness on guanfacine compared with baseline ($P < .01$), which resolved within 2 weeks. Headaches and stomachaches were reported by approximately 25% of subjects but resolved within 2 weeks except in one patient. Decreased appetite occurred initially in 16% of the subjects but stabilized within 2 weeks. No subject had clinically significant changes in blood pressure.

Guanfacine in the Treatment of ADHD and Tics and/or Tourette Syndrome

Chappell et al. (1995) reported an open study of 10 subjects, aged 8 to 16 years, who were diagnosed with ADHD and TS and treated with guanfacine. Two subjects received other psychoactive medications concurrently. An initial bedtime dose of 0.5 mg of guanfacine was titrated upward in 0.5-mg increments every 3 to 4 days and was given in two or three divided doses. Daily doses ranged from 0.75 to 3 mg; optimal daily dose was 1.5 mg for seven of the subjects. Although analysis of the group data did not show significant improvement in ADHD symptoms, three subjects had moderate and one had marked improvement based on ratings on the 48-item Conners Parent Rating Scale. Group means measuring the severity of motor and phonic tics decreased in ratings by clinicians and patients themselves. The most common untoward effects were lethargy or fatigue (60%), headache (40%), insomnia (30%), and dizziness or lightheadedness (20%); these symptoms usually remitted over 3 to 4 days. No child experienced clinically significant exacerbation of tics. Guanfacine may be a useful drug for some children and adolescents who have comorbid ADHD and a chronic tic disorder.

Horrigan and Barnhill (1995) administered guanfacine to 15 treatment-resistant boys (age range, 7 to 17 years; mean, 13.3 years) diagnosed with ADHD. Most subjects also were diagnosed with comorbid psychiatric disorders, including TS ($N = 8$) and specific developmental disorders ($N = 11$). Overall, the subjects had a mean of 3.46 Axis I and Axis II diagnoses. Subjects failed to respond satisfactorily to a mean of 2.0 prior medications, including dextroamphetamine, MPH, clonidine, imipramine, fluoxetine, carbamazepine, lithium, haloperidol, thyroid hormone, tryptophan, and biotin. Guanfacine was initiated with a 0.5-mg dose at bedtime and increased every 5 to 7 days by 0.25-to-0.5-mg increments as clinically indicated. Because the pediatric population metabolizes guanfacine more rapidly than adults, it was administered in two divided doses. After 10 weeks, the range of optimal doses was from 0.5 mg to 3 mg/day, with 0.5 mg twice daily being the most frequent optimal dose. Thirteen subjects received guanfacine only; one subject additionally received lithium carbonate 1,800 mg/day, and another received fluoxetine 10 mg/day.

Overall, guanfacine produced a significant clinical response. Parental ratings, made 4 to 8 weeks after the dose was stabilized on the 13 subjects who completed the study, showed decreases on the Conners Parent–Teacher Scale (short form) of 11.1 points (from 19.9 to 8.8); on the Edelbrock CAP Inattention Subscale of 4.85 points; and on the Edelbrock CAP Overactivity Subscale of 3.23. The authors noted that the greater improvement in inattention compared with overactivity is the opposite of the pattern often seen with clonidine; they thought that this reversal might be explained by guanfacine's having a greater affinity for alpha-2 adrenoreceptors in the prefrontal areas compared with clonidine's having a greater affinity for the alpha-2 adrenoreceptors in more basal regions (Horrigan and Barnhill, 1995). One subject did not complete the trial because his mother discontinued the medication because of lack of improvement and another because he developed symptoms of overactivation/overarousal. The only other untoward effects noted were initial mild sedation in five boys. No patient experienced a significant change in blood pressure or pulse.

Scahill et al. (2000) conducted an 8-week, randomized, double-blind, placebo-controlled trial of guanfacine in the treatment of 34 subjects (31 males, 3 females; mean age, 10.4 ± 2.01 years; age range, 7 to 14 years) diagnosed with ADHD and comorbid TS ($N = 20$), chronic motor tic disorder ($N = 12$), or stimulant-induced tic disorder ($N = 2$). Eleven subjects (32%) were medication naive; 19 of the other 23 subjects who had previous trials on at least one stimulant medication had experienced worsening of tics on stimulants. Subjects were assigned randomly to guanfacine ($N = 14$) or placebo ($N = 14$). Efficacy was determined by ratings on the DuPaul ADHD Rating Scale (Teacher) and the CGI-I Scale (CGI-I), the Total Tic Score of the Yale Global Tic Severity Scale (YGTSS), and the Hyperactivity Index (HI) of the Parent Conners. On the CGI-I, nine subjects receiving guanfacine were rated 1 ("very much improved") or 2 ("much improved") at endpoint compared with no such ratings on placebo ($P < .001$). Subjects on guanfacine improved by 38% on the ADHD Rating Scale versus only 8% improvement for subjects on placebo ($P < .001$). Total Tic Score on the YGTSS for subjects on guanfacine decreased by 30% versus no change in the placebo group ($P < .05$). There was no significant difference between placebo and guanfacine on HI Index scores. There were no clinically significant changes in pulse or blood pressure; one subject on guanfacine discontinued the study after 4 weeks because of sedation.

Other Nonapproved FDA Drugs Used for Enhancement of Frontal Lobe Executive Function in Child and Adolescent Psychiatry

Caffeine

Caffeine is a mild stimulant with some clinical suggestions that it may be useful in treating some aspects of Frontal Lobe Functioning. Two reviews of the relevant literature concluded that caffeine is not a therapeutically useful drug in the treatment of ADHD (Klein, 1987; Klein et al., 1980).

Bernstein et al. (1994) investigated the effects of caffeine on learning, performance, and anxiety in 21 prepubescent normal children, 12 males and 9 females, 8 through 12 years old (mean age, 10.6 ± 1.3 years) who ingested a minimum of 20 mg/day of caffeine in their usual diets (average daily caffeine consumption by subjects was 50.9 ± 52.2 mg/day or 1.3 mg/kg/day). Children with significant medical conditions or those ever diagnosed with ADHD were excluded. Subjects were enrolled in a double-blind, placebo-controlled, crossover study in which they were seen for four 2-hour sessions spaced approximately 1 week apart. The four rated conditions were baseline, placebo, low-dose (2.5 mg/kg) caffeine, and high-dose (5 mg/kg) caffeine. Caffeine intake was restricted for 12 to 15 hours before the sessions. Children reported feeling less "sluggish" after receiving caffeine, and their performances improved significantly on two of four measures of attention and a test of manual dexterity for the dominant hand. Self-reported anxiety level showed a trend to increase.

Magnesium Pemoline (Cylert)

Between the second (1995) and third (2001) editions of this book, the situation regarding magnesium pemoline changed significantly. The manufacturer noted in the package insert that Cylert was associated with life-threatening hepatic failure and that 15 cases of acute hepatic failure had been reported to the FDA since it was first marketed in 1975. This was 4 to 17 times the rate expected in the general population. Twelve of the cases resulted in death or liver transplantation, usually within 4 weeks of onset of signs of liver failure.

Pemoline was withdrawn from the market (in 2005) after it was determined by the FDA that the overall risk of liver toxicity from pemoline magnesium outweighed its potential benefits. The interested reader may consult the prior editions if he/she requires further information.

Amantadine Hydrochloride (SYMMETREL)

Gualtieri (2002) in his book *Brain Injury and Mental Retardation*, based primarily on his clinical experience alone, promotes that AMT is an "excellent drug for agitation during coma recovery and disinhibition, behavioral instability, abulia, and hypoarousal after severe TBI" (p. 317). It is thought that most drugs that have therapuetic value in the treatment of traumatic brain injury (TBI) do so by some direct or indirect effect on the dopamine system.

This issue of TBI is not of small significance in the field of child and adolescent psychiatry. Child and adolescent psychiatrists have always assumed a major role in the treatment of children with primary prominent cognitive delays or outright clear mental retardation from known and more commonly unknown causes. The advances in prenatal and neonatal medicine have also made it possible for infants with marked prematurity, or profound medical illness such as severe strokes to now live after birth in numbers never before realized. Unfortunately, many of these early "premies," multiple birth cohorts or infants with profound fetal alcohol syndrome for example, are markedly brain damaged and cognitively impaired. Although many of these children demonstrate frontal lobe executive function deficits and may receive a diagnosis of ADHD, this is not classic or mainstream ADHD. Neuropsychologists may diagnose such children or adults with "Cognitive Disorder NOS secondary to static encephalopathy due to frontal lobe impairment from fetal alcohol effects" for instance. This lengthy but descriptive diagnosis is useful in capturing the true etiology of the underlying brain damage but does not aid the treating clinician in being able to call upon a wealth of clinical data to guide treatment especially in the psychopharmacology realm. This is where the clinical experience of pediatric neurologists and psychiatrists and a few case studies are the only sources of direction available to guide treatment. It is with this background that AMT is included.

AMT is a water-soluble acid salt that is FDA approved only as an antiviral agent for the prophylactic treatment of influenza A and for Parkinson disease (PD). It also can be used for neuroleptic induced side effects such as EPS, pseudoparkinsonism, akathisia, and neuroleptic malignant syndrome. It is comparable to anticholinergic agents or benztropine for EPS but with fewer side effects such as memory impairment. Clinical experience indicates AMT may have utility for a number of other neuropsychiatric conditions. It was originally thought that AMT acted as a pure dopamine agonist, that is, effecting dopamine (DA) neurotransmission by presynaptically enhancing DA release and inhibiting DA reuptake and/or postsynaptically directly effecting DA receptors in some fashion such as facilitating the effects of endogenous DA agonists. However, as Gualtieri explains, it now believed that AMT acts as a weak antagonist of the N-methyl-D-aspartate (NMDA) type glutamate receptor-ion channel which may mitigate the excitotoxic damage of glutamatergic hyperactivity. Its actions on the dopamine system are indirect and appear to be involved more as a modulator of dysfunction in the dopamine system. It also may function as an anticholinergic and is specifically a nicotinic alpha-7 antagonist like the similar pharmaceutical agent memantine which is approved for the treatment of moderate to severe Alzheimer disease.

Pharmacokinetics of Amantadine Hydrochloride

Plasma half-life is 16 ± 6 hours with negligible metabolism before it is renally excreted basically unchanged in the urine. Across studies, the time to C_{max} (T_{max}) averaged about 2 to 4 hours after a 100-mg dose.

Contraindications for AMT

SYMMETREL is contraindicated in patients with known hypersensitivity to amantadine hydrochloride or to any of the other ingredients in SYMMETREL.

Untoward Effects of AMT

CNS side effects include nervousness, anxiety, agitation, insomnia, difficulty in concentrating, and exacerbations of preexisting seizure disorders and psychiatric symptoms in patients with schizophrenia or PD. Clinically, it exhibits anticholinergic-like side effects such as dry mouth, urinary retention, and constipation. A small number of suicidal attempts, some of which have been fatal, have been reported in adult patients treated with SYMMETREL. Patients with a history of epilepsy or other "seizures" should be observed closely for possible increased seizure activity. Behavioral toxicities have been the most important side effect (p. 314).

Overdosage

Deaths have been reported from overdose with SYMMETREL. The lowest reported acute lethal dose was 1 g. Acute toxicity may be attributable to the anticholinergic effects of AMT.

Indications for AMT in Child and Adolescent Psychiatry

There are no approved uses of AMT in psychiatrically disturbed children and adolescents. The safety and efficacy of SYMMETREL in newborn infants and infants below the age of 1 year have not been established.

Amantadine Hydrochloride Dosage Schedule

Dosing Schedule Adopted from Prophylactic Influenza Treatment in Pediatric Patients

1 to 9 years of age: The total daily dose should be calculated on the basis of 2 to 4 mg/lb/day (4.4 to 8.8 mg/kg/day), but not to exceed 150 mg/day.

9 to 12 years of age: The total daily dose is 200 mg given as one tablet of 100 mg (or two teaspoonfuls of syrup) twice a day. The 100 mg daily dose has not been studied in this pediatric population.

Amantadine Hydrochloride Dosage Forms Available

SYMMETREL is available in 100-mg tablets and a syrup containing 50 mg of amantadine hydrochloride per 5 mL and has the following inactive ingredients: artificial raspberry flavor, citric acid, methylparaben, propylparaben, and sorbitol solution.

Reports of Interest

There have been anecdotal reports that low-dose AMT has been successfully used to treat ADHD (Hallowell and Ratey, 2005).

Limited data have shown that AMT may help to relieve SSRI-induced sexual dysfunction (Balogh et al., 1992).

In a 2012 study, 184 patients with severe traumatic brain injury were treated with AMT or placebo for 4 weeks. In this study, the drug accelerated functional brain recovery (Giacino et al., 2012).

For patients with symptoms of agitation and aggression during coma-recovery treatment or problems with disinhibition, behavioral instability, abulia, and hypoarousal after severe TBI, treatment with AMT for several months can be very efficacious. For an indirect dopamine agonist such as AMT to work it requires an intact presynaptic neuron which is not the case in patients with brain stem injuries who may benefit from a direct agonist agent such as bromocriptine. AMT can be used in combination with low to moderate dosages of MPH or amphetamine stimulant agents as well. True stimulants appear to be better for patients with normal IQs, milder brain injuries such as postconcussion syndromes, or in later stages of TBI recovery. AMT seems to have the greatest response for individuals with moderate to severe mental retardation. The adult dosing strategy can be modified for use in pediatrics by using AMT syrup to initiate treatment at 25 to 50 mg and increase the dosage every 4 days to effect in a range of 50 mg b.i.d. to 400 mg/day. AMT is not typically sedating and has a favorable side effect profile, but if behavioral toxicity develops it can be readily addressed by discontinuation of AMT. It should be noted that AMT should not be discontinued abruptly if co-administered with neuroleptics as toxicity in the form of neuroleptic malignant syndrome and catatonia can ensue. For a much more in-depth discussion of this area, one may read Gualtieri's chapter on these agents.

First-Generation/Typical Antipsychotic Drugs

WILLIAM KLYKYLO

INTRODUCTION

Although antipsychotic drugs, also commonly known as *neuroleptics* or *major tranquilizers*, are used in adults primarily to treat psychoses, in children they have also been used to treat other common nonpsychotic psychiatric disorders. At present, antipsychotics are the drugs of first choice in childhood for schizophrenia and autistic disorder. There is, however, some evidence that antipsychotics are not as effective clinically in schizophrenia with childhood onset as in schizophrenia occurring in later adolescence and adulthood (Green et al., 1984). Meyers et al. (1980) noted that serum neuroleptic levels of 50 ng/mL of chlorpromazine equivalents correspond to the threshold for clinical response in adult patients with schizophrenia and suggest that similar therapeutic serum levels are necessary in children. Because children may metabolize and excrete antipsychotics more efficiently than do adults, determination of serum neuroleptic levels, if they are available, is recommended before a trial of an antipsychotic is deemed a failure.

The use of first-generation (FGA) versus second-generation antipsychotics (SGA) in early-onset psychotic disorders remains controversial. The TEOSS (Treatment of Early-Onset Schizophrenia Spectrum Disorders; Sikich et al., 2008) noted that molindone appeared to have similar efficacy to second-generation drugs, with more benign metabolic effects. As the potential adverse effects and cost of second-generation agents in some patients are recognized, familiarity with first-generation/typical agent remains a necessary part of clinical practice.

Shapiro and Shapiro (1989) concluded that antipsychotics were also the drugs of choice for treating chronic motor or vocal tic disorder and Tourette disorder when psychosocial, educational, or occupational functioning was so impaired that medication was required. SGAs are now often used for tic disorders, but FGAs, including haloperidol and pimozide, remain common agents (Roessner et al., 2012; Singer, 2010). Both FGAs and SGAs can lead to increases in body mass index in patients with tic disorders, with resultant metabolic effects.

Antipsychotic drugs are also clinically effective in children with severely aggressive conduct disorders, and some are approved for use in such children. Lithium is also effective in some such children, perhaps more so when an explosive affect is present, and lithium has fewer clinically significant untoward effects than neuroleptics. Because lithium is still not approved for use either in children younger than 12 years or for this indication, and because of the necessity of monitoring serum lithium levels, many clinicians prefer to use antipsychotic drugs.

The use of antipsychotics in the mentally retarded continues to be controversial, but they are prescribed frequently, especially for institutionalized patients. In optimal doses, antipsychotics are effective in decreasing irritability, sleep disturbances, hostility, agitation, and combativeness and may improve concentration and social behavior in agitated individuals with severe intellectual disabilities (American Medical Association, 1986). Aman and Singh (1988) cautioned that the influential studies of the mentally retarded by Breuning, which showed significant detrimental effects on cognition resulting from antipsychotic use, appear to have been fabricated. However, concerns over overuse and misuse of these medications in this population continue, especially as psychosocial resources are threatened.

ANTIPSYCHOTIC DRUGS IN THE TREATMENT OF ATTENTION-DEFICIT/HYPERACTIVITY DISORDERS

Some antipsychotic agents (e.g., haloperidol) have been approved for treating children with symptoms such as excessive motor activity, impulsivity, difficulty sustaining attention, and poor frustration tolerance, which would be found in most children diagnosed with attention-deficit/hyperactivity disorder (ADHD). Double-blind, controlled studies have shown antipsychotic drugs to be effective in treating children who would meet the criteria for ADHD. However, studies comparing antipsychotic drugs with stimulants almost always show that, overall, stimulants are statistically more effective clinically than antipsychotics (Green, 1995; Gittelman-Klein et al., 1976). In addition, many clinicians are reluctant to use antipsychotics to treat patients with ADHD because of the risk that an irreversible tardive dyskinesia (TD) might develop, the possibility of adverse metabolic effects, and the worry that the sedative effects of antipsychotics may interfere significantly with cognition and learning. Because of such factors, antipsychotics should be thought of as third-rank drugs to be used primarily in the treatment of ADHD, which is severely disabling and which has not responded to stimulants and other drugs with untoward effects of more acceptable risk.

Although these caveats in using antipsychotics are not to be dismissed, data moderating these dictums should be cited: (a) the influential studies of Breuning and his colleagues, which showed significant detrimental effects on cognition in mentally retarded patients treated with antipsychotic drugs, appear to have been fabricated (Aman and Singh, 1988); (b) other studies have reported minimal impairment of cognition in subjects diagnosed with ADHD who were treated with appropriate doses of antipsychotics (Klein, 1990/1991); (c) Sallee et al. (1994) examined the effects of haloperidol and pimozide in patients with Tourette syndrome, including subjects with ADHD and found no decrement in cognition associated with FGA use.

In a randomized, crossover, double-blind study, Weizman et al. (1984) noted that the combination of a stimulant and neuroleptics may be useful in some children who do not respond adequately to stimulants alone. Clinically, this may be a potentially useful option for a small subgroup of children who do not respond adequately to stimulants or to other drugs alone. The combination of stimulant and neuroleptic would presumably achieve a satisfactory result that would either not be achieved by the neuroleptic alone or would require higher doses of neuroleptics, which would carry an increased risk of untoward effects, such as TD and cognitive dulling.

PHARMACOKINETICS OF ANTIPSYCHOTIC DRUGS

Rivera-Calimlim et al. (1979) reported plasma chlorpromazine levels in a total of 24 children aged 8 to 16 years who were treated with chlorpromazine for psychiatric disorders, including various psychoses, mental retardation with aggression, hyperactivity, self-injurious behavior, and mood disorders with anxiety. The authors reported wide interpatient variations in chlorpromazine plasma levels for a given dose; for example, nine children receiving 0.8 to 2.9 mg/kg/day achieved mean plasma levels of 6.6 ng/mL, with a range from undetectable to 18 ng/mL. One child receiving 9.8 mg/kg/day showed only trace levels of plasma chlorpromazine. Children and adolescents had chlorpromazine plasma levels that were two to three-and-a-half times lower than those for adults, for a given dose per kilogram of body weight. Clinical improvement in these children usually began when plasma chlorpromazine concentration was at least 30 ng/mL and optimal levels ranged between 40 and 80 ng/mL; suggested optimal plasma levels for adults treated with chlorpromazine were higher, between 50 and 300 ng/mL. A final, clinically important observation was that plasma chlorpromazine levels declined over time in most patients who were on fixed doses (Rivera-Calimlim et al., 1979). It was suggested that one possible reason might be autoinduction of enzymes that metabolize chlorpromazine.

CONTRAINDICATIONS FOR THE ADMINISTRATION OF ANTIPSYCHOTIC DRUGS

Known hypersensitivity to the drug and toxic central nervous system depression or comatose states are absolute contraindications. If a severe adverse event develops (e.g., agranulocytosis, neuroleptic malignant syndrome TD, or a withdrawal dyskinesia), children and adolescents should be managed without antipsychotics, if at all possible.

Neuroleptics may lower the seizure threshold; they should be used cautiously in patients with seizure disorders, and chlorpromazine probably should not be used in such patients.

INTERACTIONS OF ANTIPSYCHOTIC DRUGS WITH OTHER MEDICATIONS

The most frequent clinically important reactions are with other central nervous system depressants such as alcohol, sedatives and hypnotics, benzodiazepines, antihistamines, opiates, and barbiturates, in which an additive central nervous system depressive effect occurs.

Antipsychotic drugs also have varying degrees of anticholinergic effects. When combined with another anticholinergic (antiparkinsonian) agent, such as when one is used prophylactically to prevent acute dyskinesia, pseudoparkinsonism, or akathisia, central nervous system symptoms of cholinergic blockade may result. These symptoms may include confusion, disorientation, delirium, hallucinations, and worsening of preexisting psychotic symptoms. Of clinical importance, this picture may be mistaken for inadequate treatment or worsening of the psychosis, rather than an untoward effect.

The combination of antipsychotic drugs and lithium carbonate, particularly if high doses are used, may lead to an increased incidence of central nervous system toxicity, including neuroleptic malignant syndrome.

Combined use of antipsychotic drugs with tricyclic antidepressants or monoamine oxidase inhibitors may increase plasma levels of antidepressants.

Neuroleptics may also have noteworthy interactions with many other medications. Given today's easy access to databases of drug interactions, a review of all possible interactions in every patient receiving these drugs should be standard clinical practice.

UNTOWARD EFFECTS OF ANTIPSYCHOTIC DRUGS

Although antipsychotic drugs may have numerous serious untoward effects, those of greatest concern in children and adolescents are the effects of sedation on cognition and the extrapyramidal syndromes, in particular the possible development of irreversible TD with the standard antipsychotics. We note that even older references documenting these effects remain current and unchallenged.

Agranulocytosis

Agranulocytosis is a major concern in patients treated with clozapine; it is discussed in more detail later. Agranulocytosis has also been reported with other antipsychotics. It usually occurs relatively early in treatment (e.g., for chlorpromazine, usually between the 4th and 10th weeks). Parents and older patients should be warned to report indications of sudden infections, such as fever and sore throat, to the physician. White blood cell count should be determined immediately, and if it is significantly depressed, medication should be stopped and therapy instituted.

Untoward Cognitive Effects

Both high-potency and low-potency antipsychotic agents are effective when given in equivalent doses, but they differ in the frequency and severity of their untoward effects. Usually, the higher-potency antipsychotic drugs cause less sedation, fewer autonomic side effects, and more extrapyramidal untoward effects; the lower-potency antipsychotic drugs cause greater sedation, more autonomic side effects, and fewer extrapyramidal effects (Baldessarini, 1990). Because of the great importance of minimizing any cognitive dulling in schoolchildren and in the mentally retarded, whose cognition is already compromised, high-potency, less-sedative antipsychotic drugs are often preferred. Over a period of days to weeks, however, considerable tolerance often develops to the sedative effects of high-dose, low-potency antipsychotic drugs, and thus they are still useful when untoward effects are carefully monitored (Green, 1989).

Extrapyramidal Syndromes

Significant numbers of children and adolescents receiving antipsychotic medication develop extrapyramidal syndromes. Baldessarini (1990) has enumerated six types of extrapyramidal syndromes associated with the use of antipsychotic drugs. The risk of extrapyramidal syndromes with clozapine and other atypical antipsychotics appears to be considerably reduced compared with that of standard antipsychotics.

Effects Usually Appearing During Drug Administration

Acute Dystonic Reactions

The period of maximum risk is within hours to 5 days of initiation of neuroleptic therapy. There may also be increased risk following increments in dose. High-potency, low-dose antipsychotic drugs are more likely to precipitate an acute dystonic reaction than are low-potency, high-dose antipsychotic drugs, and young males, both children and adolescents, may be at increased risk (APA, 1980b). Untreated acute dystonic reactions may last from a few minutes to several hours, and they may recur. Symptoms, which may be painful and frightening, particularly if the patient does not understand what is happening, include muscular hypertonicity; tonic contractions (spasms) of the neck (torticollis), mouth, and tongue, which may make speaking difficult; oculogyric crisis (eyes rolling upward and remaining in that position); and opisthotonos (spasm in which the spine and extremities are bent with an anterior convexity). Acute dystonic reactions respond rapidly to anticholinergic and antiparkinsonian drugs, such as 25 to 50 mg diphenhydramine (Benadryl) orally or intramuscularly, or 1 to 2 mg benztropine (Cogentin) intramuscularly. (The manufacturer of benztropine cautions that, because of its atropine-like untoward effects, its use is contraindicated in children younger than 3 years and that it should be used with caution in older children [*Physicians' Desk Reference* (PDR), 1995].) If the dystonia is very severe, administering either 25 mg of diphenhydramine or 1 to 2 mg of benztropine intramuscularly will reverse the dystonia within a few minutes. The prophylactic use of anticholinergic and antiparkinsonian agents to prevent acute dystonic reactions is discussed following the section on "Akathisia."

Parkinsonism (Pseudoparkinsonism)

Symptoms of parkinsonism include tremor, cogwheel rigidity, drooling, and decrease in facial expressive movements (mask-like or expressionless facies), and akinesia (slowness in initiating movements). These symptoms respond to antiparkinsonian medications; for example, benztropine (Cogentin), 1 to 2 mg given two or three times daily, usually provides relief within a day or two. Antiparkinsonian medication may be withdrawn gradually after 1 or 2 weeks to see if it is still necessary for symptomatic relief.

The period of maximum risk for developing parkinsonism is 5 to 30 days after initiation of neuroleptic therapy. The risk for development of parkinsonism appears to be greater for females and to increase with age. It is rarely seen in preschool children treated with therapeutic doses of neuroleptics; it occurs commonly in school-aged children and adolescents (Campbell et al., 1985). Richardson et al. (1991) reported that 21 (34%) of 61 hospitalized children and adolescents, of whom only 7 were diagnosed with psychotic or affective disorders, who were taking neuroleptics at the time of evaluation exhibited symptoms of parkinsonism when rated on several movement disorder scales. Three (14.3%) of the 21 children were rated as having parkinsonism despite the fact that they were concurrently receiving antiparkinsonian drugs. Development of parkinsonism was significantly ($P = .05$) associated with a longer duration on medication at the time of evaluation (mean of 117 days for patients with parkinsonism and mean of 34 days for patients without parkinsonism).

Akinesia, perhaps the most severe form of parkinsonism, is defined by Rifkin et al. (1975) as a "behavioral state of diminished spontaneity characterized by few gestures, unspontaneous speech and, particularly, apathy and difficulty with initiating usual activities" (p. 672). It may be particularly difficult to differentiate from the negative symptoms of schizophrenia, such as apathy and blunting. Van Putten and Marder (1987) suggested that akinesia might be the most toxic behavioral side effect of antipsychotic drugs. The authors noted that a subjective sense of sedation or drowsiness, excessive sleeping, and a lack of any leg-crossing during an interview of approximately 20 minutes correlated with the presence of akinesia. Akinesia also interferes with social adjustment, and the patient may appear to have a "postpsychotic depression." Patients with akinesia are often less concerned with any psychotic symptoms and report that everything is fine; they may experience an absence of emotion and appear emotionally dead (Van Putten and Marder, 1987). Although antiparkinsonian drugs may be helpful, in some cases they do not adequately control symptoms of akinesia. There is some evidence that antiparkinsonian drugs become less effective at higher daily dosages of antipsychotics (Van Putten and Marder, 1987).

The prophylactic use of anticholinergic and antiparkinsonian agents to prevent pseudoparkinsonism is discussed following the section on "Akathisia."

Akathisia (Motor Restlessness)

The period of maximum risk for developing this condition is 5 to 60 days after initiation of neuroleptic therapy, but it has been reported to occur in as few as 6 hours after an oral dose of a neuroleptic (Van Putten et al., 1984). Symptoms include constant uncomfortable restlessness, a feeling of tension in the lower extremities often accompanied by a strong or irresistible urge to move them, inability to sit still, and foot-tapping or pacing. Clinically, blunted affect, emotional withdrawal, and motor retardation may also be observed (Van Putten and Marder, 1987).

Akathisia may or may not respond to antiparkinsonian drugs such as trihexyphenidyl (Artane). Van Putten and Marder (1987) noted the dual nature of akathisia: a subjective experience of restlessness and observable motor restlessness. In their clinical experience, all patients with moderate or severe akathisia exhibited either rocking from foot to foot or walking on the spot. Akathisia was also strongly associated with depression, dysphoria, and, at times in severe and treatment-resistant cases, exacerbation of psychotic symptoms and homicidal and suicidal ideation and behavior (Van Putten and Marder, 1987). Of particular clinical importance, patients who have unpleasant untoward effects, especially akathisia, with antipsychotics, are more likely to be noncompliant and to unilaterally discontinue medication early in treatment (Van Putten and Marder, 1987).

Fleischhacker et al. (1989) have published a rating scale for akathisia that includes two subjective items: "a sensation of inner restlessness" and "the urge to move," and three items that characterize the frequency and magnitude of observed akathisia phenomena.

Propranolol may be helpful in ameliorating akathisia (Adler et al., 1986); benzodiazepines and clonidine have also been reported to be effective in some cases.

Clonazepam was administered to 10 first-onset psychotic adolescents (8 of whom were diagnosed with schizophrenia, paranoid subtype) between 16 and 19 years of age who experienced distressing akathisia following treatment with antipsychotics (Kutcher et al., 1987). Nine of the patients had also been receiving benztropine concomitantly with their antipsychotic medication. All patients reported subjective improvement, and scores on an akathisia subscale decreased significantly after 1 week's treatment with 0.5 mg/day of clonazepam.

In some cases, reduction in dose of the antipsychotic may be necessary. Neppe and Ward (1989) recommend that if only akathisia develops (i.e., without accompanying parkinsonism), a beta-blocker be used rather than an anticholinergic agent.

Prophylactic Use of Antiparkinsonian Agents for Acute Dystonic Reaction, Parkinsonism, and Akathisia

The use of antiparkinsonian (anticholinergic) agents prophylactically to minimize the likelihood of the patient's developing an acute dystonic reaction, parkinsonism, or akathisia from antipsychotic drug use is controversial. Some of the reasons relate to the effects caused by the anticholinergic agents themselves. Anticholinergic agents may adversely affect cognition and may aggravate psychotic symptomatology. In addition, there is some suggestion that at least part of the effectiveness of these agents is that they may lower the serum concentration of the antipsychotic drug (Rivera-Calimlim et al., 1976). Because of their reluctance to give an additional medication that itself may have untoward effects, many clinicians choose to minimize the risk of these extrapyramidal effects by beginning with a low dose and titrating the medication slowly. If an acute dystonic reaction should occur, it may be treated with diphenhydramine and the dosage of antipsychotic lowered temporarily if necessary. Conversely, some clinicians routinely prescribe an agent such as benztropine for approximately 1 month to 6 weeks, covering the period of maximal risk for the development of both acute dystonic reactions and parkinsonian untoward effects. Another option for outpatients is to prescribe a small amount of an anticholinergic (e.g., diphenhydramine) with an explanation of how it is to be administered should a dystonic reaction occur (e.g., to take one capsule should such a reaction begin, to take another dose in 20 to 30 minutes if there is no improvement, and to go to an emergency room if the reaction is severe and alert the physician to the medication being taken).

In their review of the management of acute extrapyramidal syndromes induced by neuroleptics, Neppe and Ward (1989) note that anticholinergics can significantly reduce the rate of acute dystonias especially in the highest-risk group, males younger than 30 years of age treated with high-potency antipsychotic agents. However, as acute dystonic reactions tend to be transient, prophylactic treatment for more than 2 weeks is not usually indicated. These authors recommend no prophylaxis for parkinsonism and akathisia because they rarely present as dramatically emergent a picture as acute dystonia. The parents and/or patient, as appropriate, may be carefully informed about the possibility of these conditions arising, to aid in their early detection. The clinician can then decide how best to treat the particular symptom in the particular patient (Neppe and Ward, 1989).

Van Putten and Marder (1987) point out that prophylactic use of antiparkinsonian drugs may not fully prevent symptoms of akinesia from developing and that some schizophrenic patients who have been stabilized using antiparkinsonian medication may experience increased anxiety, depression, general dysphoria, and suffering when the anticholinergics are withdrawn.

The clinician should decide on a case-by-case basis which of the preceding possibilities is best for a given patient. This decision will be based on such factors as whether a high- or low-potency neuroleptic is given, how rapidly the dose is increased, previous experience of the patient, whether it is administered to an outpatient or an inpatient (who has ready access to clinical staff), how such a reaction might affect the relationship with the patient and/or the parents and subsequent compliance, and the patient's environment. For example, it can be particularly difficult for a patient and family if the patient develops an acute dystonic reaction while attending school.

Neuroleptic Malignant Syndrome

Neuroleptic malignant syndrome is life-threatening and can occur after a single dose, but occurs most frequently within 2 weeks of initiation of neuroleptic therapy or an increase in dosage; males and younger individuals appear to be most often affected (for review see Kaufmann and Wyatt, 1987). Symptoms include severe muscular rigidity, altered consciousness, stupor, catatonia, hyperpyrexia, labile pulse and blood pressure, and occasionally myoglobinemia. Most patients have elevated creatine phosphokinase (CPK) levels. Neuroleptic malignant syndrome can persist for up to 2 weeks or longer after medication is discontinued and can be fatal. Treatment consists of immediate cessation of medication and hospitalization, under intensive care, with supportive treatment. Dopaminergic agonists (e.g., bromocriptine and amantadine) and/or dantrolene have also been reported to reduce the mortality rate significantly (Sakkas et al., 1991). Antiparkinsonian drugs are not useful.

Latz and McCracken (1992) conducted an extensive literature search and reported a total of 49 cases of neuroleptic malignant syndrome (NMS) in patients 18 years or younger. The youngest reported case was that of an 11-month-old. Five (83%) of the six preschoolers developed NMS after a single dose of neuroleptic that either was an accidental overdose or was prescribed for a nonpsychiatric illness. Overall lethality for all cases reviewed was 16.3% (8 of 49). However, the death rate for patients 12 years of age or younger was 27% (3 of 11), more than twice the death rate of 13% (5 of 38) for adolescents 13 to 18 years old.

Steingard et al. (1992) also published a review with detailed summaries of 35 cases of neuroleptic malignant syndrome in patients younger than 19 years of age. Fever, rigidity, altered mental status, and tachycardia were present in >70% of the cases. Five (14%) of the patients died; however, only one of these died within the past two decades, and that was a 2-year-old who had ingested chlorpromazine accidentally. Croarkin et al. (2008) reported on 16 cases in subjects 18 years old and younger from 1991 through 2007, mostly male, all of whom survived. These data suggest that the standard of care for these patients has improved, but do not address reporting bias.

Late-Appearing Syndromes (After Months or Years of Treatment)

Tardive Dyskinesia

Definitions and descriptions of TD and related dyskinesias (withdrawal, masked dyskinesias) vary. Perhaps the most influential definition at present is the research diagnostic criteria proposed in 1982 by Schooler and Kane. They note that, if possible, the absence of abnormal involuntary movements before beginning pharmacotherapy should be documented. Schooler and Kane's (1982) research diagnostic criteria for TD proposed three prerequisites for making the diagnosis:

1. Exposure to neuroleptic drugs for a minimum total cumulative exposure of 3 months.
2. The presence of at least "moderate" abnormal involuntary movements in one or more body areas (face, lips, jaw, tongue, upper extremities, lower extremities, trunk) or at least "mild" movements in two or more body areas.
3. Absence of other conditions that might produce abnormal movements.

   Once these prerequisites have been met by a patient, Schooler and Kane (1982) proposed six diagnostic categories of TD:

   a. (i) Probable TD "concurrent neuroleptics" if the patient is currently receiving neuroleptic therapy or (ii) probable TD "neuroleptic-free" if no longer receiving neuroleptic medication. (Only one of these two diagnoses would be possible the first time the patient is examined.)
   b. Masked probable TD: within 2 weeks of an increase in dose in a patient diagnosed with 1a or resumption of neuroleptic drug treatment in a patient diagnosed with 1b, prerequisite 2 is no longer met.
   c. Transient TD: within 3 months of a patient being diagnosed with 1a and with no increase in dose of neuroleptic (a dose reduction is permissible), prerequisite 2 is no longer met; or, within 3 months of a patient being diagnosed with 1b, prerequisite 2 is no longer met and the patient has remained neuroleptic-free.
   d. Withdrawal TD: while receiving neuroleptics the patient does not meet prerequisite 2, but within 2 weeks of cessation of neuroleptics with usual serum half-lives or 5 weeks after stopping a long-acting neuroleptic (e.g., a depot dosage form), the patient develops abnormal movements consistent with prerequisite 2. If the movements cease or no longer satisfy prerequisite 2 within 3 months, this diagnosis stands.
   e. (i) Persistent TD "concurrent neuroleptics" if the patient was diagnosed with 1a and has continuously received neuroleptics over the subsequent 3 months and continues to satisfy prerequisite 2. (ii) Persistent TD "neuroleptic-free" if the patient was diagnosed with 1a (and neuroleptic drug was immediately stopped), with 1b, or with 4 (withdrawal TD) and no neuroleptic was administered during the subsequent 3 months and the patient continues to fulfill prerequisite 2. (iii) Persistent TD "unspecified" if the patient was diagnosed 1a, 1b, or 4, and the patient received neuroleptics for part of the subsequent 3-month period and still meets prerequisite 2.
   f. Masked persistent TD if a patient diagnosed with 5a or 5c no longer meets prerequisite 2 within 3 weeks of an increase in dosage of the neuroleptic agent or if a patient diagnosed with 5b no longer meets prerequisite 2 within 3 weeks of resumption of a neuroleptic.

Four additional diagnostic criteria were suggested by the American Psychiatric Association Task Force on TD (American Psychiatric Association [APA], 1992):

1. The abnormal movements are exacerbated or may be provoked by a decrease or withdrawal of an antipsychotic drug. Increasing the dose of antipsychotic will suppress (or dampen) the movements at least temporarily.
2. Anticholinergic medication does not ameliorate and may worsen the movements.
3. Emotional stress may worsen the movements.
4. The movements decrease or disappear during sleep.

TD develops while actively receiving a neuroleptic drug, as opposed to a withdrawal dyskinesia that occurs when a neuroleptic is withdrawn or its dose is decreased. TD, which may be both severely disabling and irreversible, is the most clinically significant common long-term untoward effect of antipsychotic use. Baldessarini (1990) notes that in some cases, especially in younger patients, TD will disappear over the course of weeks to as much as 3 years. It is believed that the risk of developing irreversible TD increases with both total cumulative dose and duration of treatment. Older females appear to be at increased risk. It has been reported that fine, worm-like (vermicular) movements of the tongue may be an early sign of TD and that discontinuation of the medication when this occurs may prevent further development of the syndrome (PDR, 1995). Symptoms of TD most typically include involuntary choreoathetotic movements that affect the face; tongue; perioral, buccal, and masticatory musculature; and neck but may also involve the torso and extremities.

Atypical and less common forms of TD, such as tardive akathisia, a persisting restlessness, and tardive dystonia, also occur. Burke et al. (1982) reported 42 cases of tardive dystonia that they diagnosed by the following criteria:

1. The presence of chronic dystonia.
2. History of antipsychotic drug treatment preceding or concurrent with the onset of dystonia.
3. Exclusion of known causes of secondary dystonia by appropriate clinical and laboratory evaluation.
4. A negative family history for dystonia.

Symptoms of tardive dystonia began after as few as 3 days and up to 11 years after initiation of antipsychotic medication. The incidence of tardive dystonia was more frequent in younger male patients than in older patients; was characterized by sustained abnormal postures accompanied by torticollis, torsion of the trunk and extremities, blepharospasm, and grimacing; and was incapacitating in severe cases. Spontaneous remission occurred in a few patients, but dystonia persisted for years in most. Of the many medications used to ameliorate the tardive dystonia, the most helpful were tetrabenzine, which improved symptoms in 68% of patients, and anticholinergics, which were helpful in 39% of patients (Burke et al., 1982).

In TD and other choreoathetotic syndromes, emotional stress typically causes worsening of the movements, drowsiness or sedation causes them to diminish, and sleep causes them to disappear (APA, 1980b). There is no adequate treatment; antiparkinsonian drugs may worsen the condition (for review, see APA, 1980b, 1992). There is evidence, however, that the atypical antipsychotic drug clozapine not only produces little or no TD when it is the only neuroleptic ever used, but also significantly decreases or eliminates existing symptoms of TD during the period it is prescribed (Birmaher et al., 1992; Mozes et al., 1994; Small et al., 1987). Upon its discontinuation, however, the dyskinetic movements that were suppressed by clozapine rapidly returned in 18 of 19 patients (Small et al., 1987).

Vitamin E and TD

Vitamin E has also been reported to be helpful in treating TD in adults. Adler et al. (1999) note that although several short-term, controlled studies found vitamin E to be helpful, they were from a single site, had relatively small numbers, and treatment duration was short. To further investigate the effectiveness of vitamin E, the authors conducted a prospective, randomized, nine-site, double-blind, placebo-controlled study. They found no significant differences between vitamin E and placebo on any of the rating scales at the end of the study and concluded that vitamin E is not effective in treating TD in patients who are actively being treated with neuroleptics.

In addition, a withdrawal dyskinesia may emerge when neuroleptic medication is withdrawn or the dose is reduced. Withdrawal-emergent dyskinesias can occur for two different reasons. First, antidopaminergic drugs, including antipsychotics, can suppress TD; thus, decreasing their serum levels can "unmask" ongoing TD. Second, Baldessarini (1990) points out that a "disuse supersensitivity" to dopamine agonists may also occur following withdrawal of antidopaminergic drugs; he suggests that this phenomenon may explain withdrawal dyskinesias that resolve within a few weeks.

The reported prevalence of neuroleptic-induced TD and withdrawal TD in children and adolescents has ranged from 0% to 51% (Wolf and Wagner, 1993). It is thought that the risk of developing TD that will become irreversible increases with both total cumulative dose and duration of treatment. No cases of irreversible TD developing in children or adolescents have been reported; the longest neuroleptic-free persistent TD was reported to last 4.5 years. Usually, withdrawal dyskinesias resolve within a few weeks to a few months of discontinuation of the neuroleptic (Wolf and Wagner, 1993).

Richardson et al. (1991) reported that 5 (12%) of 41 hospitalized children and adolescents (mean age, 15.5 years), of whom only 10 were diagnosed with psychotic or affective disorders, who had taken neuroleptics for at least one period of 90 continuous days before the time of evaluation exhibited symptoms of treatment-emergent TD (occurring while receiving neuroleptics) when rated on the Simpson Abbreviated Dyskinesia Scale. The five patients who developed TD were significantly more likely to have had a history of assaultive behavior ($P = .003$) and a first-degree relative who had been hospitalized for a psychiatric disorder ($P = .009$) than patients who did not develop TD. Using the more stringent research criteria of Schooler and Kane (1982), three (7%) were diagnosed with TD. McDonagh et al. (2010) reported a Cochrane review that disclosed that risperidone resulted in an increased risk of new-onset TD (3% compared with 1% to 2% for others).

If TD develops, every effort should be made to discontinue or at least reduce the dose of antipsychotic drug as much as possible. The dyskinesia should be monitored with serial ratings on the Abnormal Involuntary Movement Scale (AIMS). If the severity of the psychiatric disorder precludes discontinuation of antipsychotic medication (e.g., in a patient diagnosed with autistic disorder who exhibits severe self-injurious behavior [SIB] and aggressiveness and who has not responded adequately to other medications such as lithium or propranolol), the clinician must carefully document the rationale for reinstituting antipsychotic medication and verify that the legal guardians (and patient when appropriate) have given their informed consent. Reinstating or increasing the dose of antipsychotic may suppress or mask TD.

Because of such risks, antipsychotic agents should be given only to children and adolescents for whom no other potentially less harmful treatment is available; for example, although effective in some children diagnosed with ADHD, antipsychotic drugs should not be used unless stimulant medications and other nonstimulant drugs with safer untoward-effect profiles have been treatment failures (Green, 1995).

Although antipsychotics are the only drugs that result in persistent TD in a significant proportion of patients, a number of different drugs may cause dyskinesias after short- or long-term treatment. Jeste and Wyatt (1982) note that the dyskinesia produced by L-dopa most closely resembles the TD resulting from antipsychotics and that, typically, the dyskinesias caused by most other drugs are usually acute, sometimes toxic, effects and almost always remit when the drug is discontinued. Among the drugs used in child and adolescent psychopharmacotherapy for which dyskinesias have been reported are amphetamines, methylphenidate, monoamine oxidase inhibitors, tricyclic antidepressants, lithium, antihistamines, benzodiazepines, and antiepileptic drugs (Jeste and Wyatt, 1982).

Rabbit Syndrome (Perioral Tremor)

Rabbit syndrome (perioral tremor), which may be a late-onset variant of parkinsonism, is uncommon. Its name derives from the fact that patients so afflicted make rapid chewing movements similar to those of rabbits (Villeneuve, 1972). It may respond to antiparkinsonian medication.

Other Untoward Effects of Antipsychotic Drugs

Table 5.1 is a compilation of most of the reported untoward effects of chlorpromazine, the prototype antipsychotic drug. Most of these untoward effects have also been reported to occur to a greater or lesser degree with other antipsychotic drugs.

TABLE 5.1 » Untoward Effects of Chlorpromazine

Allergic
    Mild urticaria
    Photosensitivity, exfoliative dermatitis
    Asthma
    Anaphylactoid reactions
    Laryngeal edema
    Angioneurotic edema
Autonomic nervous system
    Antiadrenergic effects
        Orthostatic hypotension
        Ejaculatory disturbances
    Anticholinergic effects
        Decreased secretion, resulting in dry mouth, dry eyes, nasal congestion
        Blurred vision, mydriasis
        Glaucoma attack in patients with narrow-angle closure
        Constipation, paralytic ileus
        Urinary retention
        Impotence
Cardiovascular
    Postural (orthostatic) hypotension
    Tachycardia
    ECG changes
    Sudden death due to cardiac arrest
Central nervous system
    Neuromuscular effects
        Dystonias
        Akasthisia (motor restlessness)
        Pseudoparkinsonism
        Tardive dyskinesia
    Seizures, lowering of seizure threshold
    Drowsiness, sedation
    Behavioral effects
        Increased psychotic symptoms
        Catatonic-like states
Dermatological
    Photosensitivity
        Skin pigmentation changes in exposed areas
        Rashes

(continued)

TABLE 5.1 » Untoward Effects of Chlorpromazine (Continued)	

Endocrinological
  Elevated prolactin levels
  Gynecomastia
  Amenorrhea
  Hyperglycemia, glycosuria, and hypoglycemia
Hematological
  Agranulocytosis
  Eosinophilia
  Leukopenia
  Hemolytic anemia
  Aplastic anemia
  Thrombocytopenic purpura
  Pancytopenia
Hepatological
  Jaundice
Metabolic
  Weight gain, increased appetite
Ophthalmologic
  Blurred vision
  Precipitation of acute glaucoma attack in persons with narrow-angle glaucoma
  Deposition of pigmented material and star-shaped opacities in lens
  Deposition of pigmented material in cornea
  Pigmentary retinopathy
  Epithelial keratopathy
Teratogenic effects possible (seen in animal studies)
Other
  Neuroleptic malignant syndrome
  Sudden death, which may be related to cardiac failure or suppression of cough reflex

REPRESENTATIVE FIRST-GENERATION/TYPICAL ANTIPSYCHOTIC DRUGS

Table 5.2 summarizes representative first-generation/typical antipsychotic drugs commonly used in child and adolescent psychiatry, as well as clozapine. It compares their relative potencies and expected potential sedative, autonomic, and extrapyramidal untoward effects with chlorpromazine, the prototype of the antipsychotics. FDA age limitations and recommended dosages for approved use in children and adolescents are also given when available. We note the deletion of thioridazine from this table because of its well-documented adverse effects including cardiac conductivity disturbance related to QT-interval elongation and retinal pigmentation leading to blindness.

Considerations about Dosage

The antipsychotic effects of neuroleptic agents evolve gradually. The depolarization inactivation of dopaminergic neurons, which is necessary for antipsychotic efficacy, takes approximately 3 to 6 weeks to develop. Hence, it is important to have a trial of adequate duration of an antipsychotic drug at usual therapeutic doses rather than rapidly increasing the dose, which can lead to the erroneous clinical impression that a much higher dose than necessary was responsible for the patient's clinical improvement. Studies have also suggested that there is a therapeutic window of approximately 300 to 1,000 mg of chlorpromazine or its equivalent for most psychotic adult patients. Patients receiving <300 mg tend to improve less, and

TABLE 5.2 » Representative First-Generation/Typical Antipsychotic Drugs and Clozapine

Antipsychotic Drug/Trade Name	Chemical Classification	Therapeutically Equivalent Oral Dose in Milligrams	Effects			Approved Age for Use	Usual Optimal Dose/ Maintenance Dose Range
			Sedation	Autonomic[a]	Extrapyramidal Reaction[b]		
Chlorpromazine/Thorazine	Phenothiazine: aliphatic compound	100	+++	+++	++	Over 6 mo	See text
Clozapine/Clozaril	Dibenzodiazepine	75	+++	+++	0?	16 y	As per adults; see text
Mesoridazine/Serentil	Phenothiazine: piperidine compound	50	+++	++	+	12 y	No specific doses for children
Loxapine/Loxitane	Dibenzoxazepine	15	++	+/++	++/+++	16 y	As per adults
Molindone/Moban	Dihydroindolone	10	++	+	+	12 y	No specific doses for children
Perphenazine/Trilafon	Phenothiazine: piperazine compound	10	++	+	++/+++	12 y	No specific doses for children
Trifluoperazine/Stelazine	Phenothiazine: piperazine compound	5	++	+	+++	6 y	See text
Thiothixene/Navane	Thioxanthene	5	+	+	+++	12 y	No specific doses for children
Fluphenazine/Permitil, Prolixin	Phenothiazine: piperazine compound	2	+	+	+++	16 y	See text
Haloperidol/Haldol	Butyrophenone	2	+	+	+++	3 y	See text
Pimozide[c]/Orap	Diphenyl-butylpiperidine	10	+	+	+++	Over 12 y	0.2 mg/kg/d or maximum, 10 mg/d

[a]Alpha-antiadrenergic and anticholinergic effects.

[b]Excluding tardive dyskinesia, which appears to be produced to the same degree and frequency by all agents except clozapine with equieffective antipsychotic doses. Clozapine has produced agranulocytosis; therefore, recommendations for its use are limited (see text).

[c]Only indicated for Tourette disorder that has not responded to other standard treatments; not approved for use in psychoses.

Adapted from American Medical Association. *Drug Evaluations Annual 1994*. Chicago, IL: American Medical Association; 1994.

those receiving >1,000 mg of chlorpromazine or its equivalent show no increased benefit (for review, see Levy, 1993). It is usually recommended that antipsychotic agents initially be administered in divided doses, most frequently three or four times daily. Once the optimal dose is established, however, their relatively long serum half-lives usually permit either once-daily dosage (e.g., before bedtime) or twice-daily dosage (in the morning and before bedtime).

FIRST-GENERATION/TYPICAL ANTIPSYCHOTIC DRUGS

Chlorpromazine Hydrochloride (Thorazine)

Indications for Chlorpromazine Hydrochloride in Child and Adolescent Psychiatry

In addition to being approved for uses similar to those for adults, including psychotic disorders, chlorpromazine is approved for the treatment of severe behavioral problems in children, marked by combativeness and/or explosive hyperexcitable behavior. It is also noted that dosages >500 mg/day are unlikely to further enhance behavioral improvement in severely disturbed mentally retarded patients.

Chlorpromazine may lower the threshold to seizures; another antipsychotic should be chosen for seizure-prone individuals.

Chlorpromazine Dosage Schedule for Children and Adolescents

* *Infants younger than 6 months of age:* not recommended.
* *Children aged 6 months to 12 years with severe behavioral problems or psychotic conditions:*

  Oral: 0.25 mg/kg every 4 to 6 hours as needed. Titrate upward gradually. In severe cases, daily doses of 200 mg or higher may be required.
  Rectal: 1 mg/kg every 6 to 8 hours as needed.
  Intramuscular: 0.5 mg/kg every 6 to 8 hours as needed. Maximum daily intramuscular dose for a child younger than 5 years or below 22 kg is 40 mg; for a child 5 to 12 years of age or 22 to 45 kg, maximum daily dose is 75 mg.

* *Adolescents:* depending on severity of symptoms, begin with 10 mg three times to 25 mg four times daily. Titrate upward with increases of 20 to 50 mg twice weekly. For severely agitated patients, 25 mg may be given intramuscularly and repeated if necessary in 1 hour. Any subsequent intramuscular medication should be at 4- to 6-hour intervals.

Chlorpromazine Hydrochloride Dose Forms Available

* *Tablets:* 10, 25, 50, 100, and 200 mg
* *Spansules (extended release, not recommended for children):* 30, 75, and 150 mg
* *Syrup:* 10 mg/5 mL
* *Oral concentrate:* 30 and 100 mg/mL
* *Suppositories:* 25 and 100 mg
* *Injection (intramuscular):* 25 mg/mL

Reports of Interest

Chlorpromazine in the Treatment of Children and Adolescents Diagnosed with ADHD

Werry et al. (1966) reported that chlorpromazine was significantly superior to placebo ($P = .005$) in reducing hyperactivity in a double-blind, placebo-controlled, 8-week study of 39 hyperactive children (mean age, 8.5 years; IQ, 85 or greater), a large number of whom had additional symptoms of distractibility, irritability, and specific cognitive defects. Intellectual functioning and symptoms of distractibility, aggressivity, and excitability did not appear to have been significantly affected by the drug. The authors concluded that chlorpromazine could be used for behavioral symptoms in therapeutic doses (mean dose was 106 mg/day with a maximum daily dose of 5 mg/kg or 150 to 200 mg) without fear of significantly impairing learning.

The most frequent untoward effects were mild sedation and mild photosensitization of the skin (Werry et al., 1966).

Weiss and her colleagues (1975) reported that 5 years after initial diagnosis, there were no differences on measures of emotional adjustment, antisocial behavior, and academic performance among a group of hyperactive children treated with chlorpromazine for 1.5 to 5 years, a similar group treated for 3 to 5 years with methylphenidate, and a group whose medication was discontinued after 4 months because of poor response.

Thioridazine Hydrochloride (Mellaril)

In July of 2000, Novartis, the manufacturer of Mellaril (thioridazine hydrochloride), issued major changes in their labeling. This included a boxed warning indicating that thioridazine has been shown to prolong the QTc interval in a dose-related manner and that drugs with this potential, including thioridazine, have been associated with torsade de pointes and sudden death.

The current FDA Black Box Warning (PDR, 2006) states, "Thioridazine has been shown to prolong the QTc interval in a dose-related manner, and drugs with this potential, including thioridazine, have been associated with torsade de pointes–type arrhythmias and sudden death. Because of its potential for significant, possibly life-threatening proarrhythmic effects, thioridazine should be reserved for use in the treatment of schizophrenic patients who fail to show an acceptable response to adequate courses of treatment with other antipsychotic drugs, either because of insufficient effectiveness or the inability to achieve an effective dose due to intolerable adverse effects from those drugs."

Currently, thioridazine no longer has FDA approval for treating severe behavioral problems marked by combativeness and/or explosive hyperexcitable behavior, or for the short-term treatment of hyperactive children who show excessive motor activity with accompanying conduct disorders consisting of some or all of the following symptoms: impulsivity, difficulty sustaining attention, aggressivity, mood lability, and poor frustration tolerance. Use of thioridazine in child and adolescent psychiatry would not only be "off-label" but also would ignore the new recommendations and warnings, and cannot be recommended. Further information about the history of the use of this agent is contained in the Appendix.

Trifluoperazine Hydrochloride (Stelazine, Vesprin)

Indications for Trifluoperazine Hydrochloride in Child and Adolescent Psychiatry

One manufacturer has a specific disclaimer that trifluoperazine has not been proved effective in the management of behavioral complications in patients with mental retardation and recommends it only for the treatment of psychotic individuals and for the short-term treatment of nonpsychotic anxiety in individuals with generalized anxiety disorder who have not responded to other medications.

Trifluoperazine Dosage Schedule

- *Children younger than 6 years of age:* not recommended.
- *Children aged 6 to 12 years of age:* a starting dose of 1 mg once or twice daily with gradual upward titration is recommended. Dosages in excess of 15 mg/day are usually required only by older children with severe symptoms.
- *Adolescents:* 1 to 5 mg twice daily. Usually the optimal dose will be 15 to 20 mg/day or less; occasionally, up to 40 mg/day will be required. Titration to optimal dose can usually be accomplished within 2 to 3 weeks.

(continued)

Indications for Trifluoperazine Hydrochloride in Child and Adolescent Psychiatry *(continued)*

Trifluoperazine Hydrochloride Dose Forms Available

- *Tablets:* 1, 2, 5, and 10 mg
- *Oral concentrate:* 10 mg/mL
- *Injection (intramuscular):* 2 mg/mL (One manufacturer notes that there is little experience using intramuscular trifluoperazine with children and recommends 1 mg intramuscularly once, or maximally twice, daily if necessary for rapid control of severe symptoms.)

Haloperidol (Haldol)

Pharmacokinetics of Haloperidol

Morselli et al. (1983) noted that steady-state haloperidol plasma levels in children may vary up to 15-fold at a given mg/kg daily dosage, but for a given individual the relationship between dosage and plasma level is fairly consistent. Most children had haloperidol plasma half-lives that were shorter than those of adolescents and adults. However, the authors also emphasized that despite their more rapid metabolism of haloperidol, children did not require proportionally higher daily doses because they also appear to be more sensitive to both the therapeutic and the untoward effects of haloperidol at lower plasma concentrations than were older adolescents and adults (Morselli et al., 1983).

Indications for Haloperidol in Child and Adolescent Psychiatry

Haloperidol is indicated for the treatment of acute and chronic psychotic disorders and for the control of tics and vocal utterances in Tourette disorder. Only after the failure of treatment with psychotherapy and nonantipsychotic medications has haloperidol been approved for treating children with severe behavioral disorders (e.g., "combative, explosive hyperexcitability [which cannot be accounted for by immediate provocation]" [package insert]) and for the short-term treatment of hyperactive children with coexisting conduct disorders, who exhibit such symptoms as "impulsivity, difficulty sustaining attention, aggressivity, mood liability, and poor frustration tolerance."

Haloperidol Dosage Schedule for Children and Adolescents with Psychotic Disorders, Tourette Disorder, or Severe Nonpsychotic Behavioral Disorders

- *Children younger than 3 years of age:* not recommended.
- *Children 3 to 12 years of age (weight: 15 to 40 kg):* begin with 0.5 mg daily; titrate upward by 0.5-mg increments at 5- to 7-day intervals. Therapeutic dose ranges are usually from 0.05 to 0.075 mg/kg/day for nonpsychotic behavioral disorders and Tourette disorder; for psychotic children, the upper range is usually 0.15 mg/kg/day, but may be higher in severe cases. Morselli et al. (1983) reported good therapeutic results in children with tics and Tourette disorder associated with haloperidol plasma levels in the range of 1 to 3 ng/mL. Higher haloperidol plasma levels, usually between 6 and 10 ng/mL, were necessary for significant improvement in psychotic conditions.
- *Adolescents:* depending on severity, 0.5 to 5 mg two or three times daily. Higher doses may be necessary for more rapid control in some severe cases.

Haloperidol Dose Forms Available

- *Tablets:* 0.5, 1, 2, 5, 10, and 20 mg
- *Oral concentrate:* 2 mg/mL
- *Injectable immediate release (intramuscular):* Haloperidol lactate (Haldol IR injection): 5.0 mg/mL. Safety has not been established for children and younger adolescents. If necessary, in acutely agitated older adolescents, an initial dose of 2 to 5 mg may be given intramuscularly. Additional medication may be given every 1 to 8 hours as determined by ongoing evaluation of the patient.

(continued)

Indications for Haloperidol in Child and Adolescent Psychiatry *(continued)*

- *Injection, long-acting (intramuscular), Haloperidol Decanoate 50 and 100 mg:* Haldol Decanoate Injection 50 and Haldol Decanoate Injection 100 contain 50 and 100 mg of haloperidol (present as 70.52 and 141.04 mg of haloperidol decanoate), respectively. The safety and efficacy of haloperidol decanoate has not been established for children and younger adolescents, and it is currently used primarily for treating adults diagnosed with chronic schizophrenia. However, in some severely disturbed adolescents, particularly when compliance is a major therapeutic issue, haloperidol decanoate may be indicated. Peak plasma concentration is reached approximately 6 days after injection and plasma half-life is approximately 3 weeks. The usual interval between doses is 4 weeks, but this may need to be adjusted for some patients.

◼ *Reports of Interest*

Haloperidol in the Treatment of Schizophrenia with Childhood Onset

Green et al. (1992) administered haloperidol on an open basis to 15 hospitalized children younger than 12 years of age diagnosed with schizophrenia. They reported the optimal dose to range between 1 and 6 mg/day. Acute dystonic reactions occurred in approximately 25% of the children despite low initial doses and gradual increments of the drug.

Spencer et al. (1992) administered haloperidol to 12 patients (9 males, 3 females; ages 5.5 to 11.75 years) in an ongoing, double-blind, placebo-controlled study of hospitalized children diagnosed with schizophrenia. Optimal haloperidol dose ranged from 0.5 to 3.5 mg/day (range, 0.02 to 0.12 mg/kg/day; mean, 2.02 mg/day). Haloperidol was significantly better than placebo on staff Global Clinical Judgments ($P = .003$) and on four of the eight Children's Psychiatric Rating Scale (CPRS) items selected for their pertinence to schizophrenia: ideas of reference ($P = .04$), persecutory ($P = .01$), other thinking disorders ($P = .04$), and hallucinations ($P = .04$). Two children (16.7%) experienced acute dystonic reactions. All 12 improved on haloperidol and were discharged on that medication.

In a double-blind, head-to-head comparison of haloperidol and clozapine, Kumra et al. (1996) reported that clozapine was significantly superior to haloperidol in treating treatment-resistant adolescents with childhood-onset schizophrenia. Because of its severe untoward-effect profile, however, clozapine is not a first-line therapeutic drug for schizophrenia. This study is reviewed in detail later under clozapine.

Haloperidol in the Treatment of Tourette Disorder

Shapiro and Shapiro (1989) concluded that the most effective neuroleptics in the treatment of tics and Tourette disorder were pimozide (Orap), haloperidol, fluphenazine (Prolixin, Permitil), and penfluridol (Semap, an investigational drug). Studies by Shapiro and Shapiro (1984), Shapiro et al. (1983), and Sallee et al. (1997) comparing haloperidol and pimozide found pimozide to be more efficacious and to have significantly less severe untoward effects in treating Tourette disorder. These studies are reviewed later under pimozide. Dysphoria upon withdrawal of haloperidol in treatment of Tourette disorder has been reported (Braña-Berríos et al., 2011).

Haloperidol in the Treatment of Autistic Disorder and Atypical Pervasive Developmental Disorders

Haloperidol is the most well-studied first-generation antipsychotic used in the treatment of autistic disorder. In a study of 40 autistic children 2.33 to 6.92 years of age, haloperidol in optimal doses of 0.5 to 3 mg/day yielded global clinical improvement and significantly decreased the symptoms of withdrawal, stereotypies, abnormal object relationships, hyperactivity, fidgetiness, negativism, and angry and labile affect (Anderson et al., 1984). However, a high rate of dyskinesias remains a problem. Significant numbers of autistic children (22%, or 8 of 36) developed TD or withdrawal dyskinesia in a prospective study in which 0.5 to 3 mg/day of haloperidol was administered for periods ranging from 3.5 to 42.5 months; thus, close monitoring is necessary (Perry et al., 1985).

In autistic disorder, stereotypies existing at baseline may be suppressed by administration of haloperidol. When the drug is withdrawn, there is potential for confusion between the reappearance of stereotypies and a withdrawal dyskinesia; this is of special concern if a physician unfamiliar with the child at baseline assumes treatment responsibilities for the child while he or she is on maintenance medication.

Joshi et al. (1988) administered fluphenazine or haloperidol to 12 children aged 7 to 11 years who were hospitalized and diagnosed with childhood onset or atypical pervasive developmental disorders (PDDs) (i.e., approximately equivalent to the DSM-III-R [APA, 1987] diagnoses of autistic disorder with childhood onset and PDD not otherwise specified [PDDNOS]). The children responded with remarkable improvement in peer interactions and reality testing and decreases in autistic-like behavior, aggressiveness, impulsivity, and hyperactivity. Seven of the 12 children were able to return home rather than be admitted for residential treatment as had been planned. Haloperidol was begun at a dose of 0.02 mg/kg/day and titrated based on behavioral response, with increases at 3- to 5-day intervals. Mean optimal dose of haloperidol was 0.04 ± 0.01 mg/kg/day. Untoward effects were remarkably infrequent. Drowsiness occurred initially in some children, but it was transient and did not interfere with their later cognitive performance. Two children receiving haloperidol developed some rigidity and cogwheeling that responded to oral diphenhydramine during the first few days of treatment; the extrapyramidal symptoms did not recur when the diphenhydramine was discontinued.

Haloperidol in the Treatment of Aggressive Conduct Disorder

In a double-blind, placebo-controlled study of 61 treatment-resistant hospitalized children, aged 5.2 to 12.9 years, with undersocialized aggressive conduct disorder, both haloperidol and lithium were found to be superior to placebo in ameliorating behavioral symptoms (Campbell et al., 1984b). Optimal doses of haloperidol ranged from 1 to 6 mg/day. The authors reported that, at optimal doses, the untoward effects of haloperidol appeared to interfere more significantly with the children's daily routines than did those of lithium.

Haloperidol in the Treatment of ADHD

Werry and Aman (1975) investigated the effects of methylphenidate and haloperidol on attention, memory, and activity in 24 children (ages 4.11 to 12.4 years), more than half of whom were diagnosed with hyperkinetic reaction and the remainder with unsocialized aggressive reaction. Each child received one of four drug conditions—placebo, methylphenidate (0.3 mg/kg), low-dose haloperidol (0.025 mg/kg), or high-dose haloperidol (0.05 mg/kg)—in a double-blind, placebo-controlled, crossover (within-subject) design. For all statistically significant measures of cognitive functions of vigilance and short-term memory, the rank order of the means was methylphenidate, haloperidol (low dose), placebo, and haloperidol (high dose). The data suggested that methylphenidate and low-dose haloperidol, although to a lesser degree, improved these cognitive functions, whereas high-dose haloperidol appeared to cause them to deteriorate (Werry and Aman, 1975). The clinical importance of observing this biphasic effect is that it is the dose of haloperidol, not the drug itself, that may cause cognitive impairment. Based on this study, most children and adolescents treated for ADHD with haloperidol should receive doses between 0.5 and 2.0 mg/day (i.e., 0.025 mg/kg for a weight range of 20 to 80 kg).

Thiothixene (Navane)

Indications for Thiothixene in Child and Adolescent Psychiatry

Thiothixene is an antipsychotic drug of the thioxanthene series. It is indicated in the management of symptoms of psychotic disorders. It has not been evaluated in the management of behavioral disturbances in individuals with intellectual disabilities nor is its use recommended in children younger than 12 years of age because safe conditions for its use in that age group have not been established (PDR, 2000). Information concerning its use appears in the Appendix.

 ## Loxapine Succinate (Loxitane)

Indications for Loxapine Succinate in Child and Adolescent Psychiatry

Loxapine is a dibenzoxazepine compound with antipsychotic properties used in treating psychotic disorders. The manufacturer does not recommend its use in persons younger than 16 years of age. Information concerning its use appears in the Appendix.

Molindone Hydrochloride (Moban)

Molindone hydrochloride is a dihydroindolone compound with antipsychotic properties; it is structurally unrelated to the phenothiazine, butyrophenone, and thioxanthene antipsychotics. Its clinical action resembles that of the piperazine phenothiazines (e.g., perphenazine [Trilafon]) (*Drug Facts and Comparisons*, 1995). Moban is rapidly absorbed from the gastrointestinal tract, and peak blood levels of unmetabolized drug are achieved approximately 1.5 hours after ingestion. Moban has many metabolites, and pharmacologic effects from a single dose may last up to 36 hours (PDR, 2000). Although molindone has been associated with sinus tachycardia, it is one of the few antipsychotics that have no warning of increased QTc intervals in the package insert (Gutgesell et al., 1999).

Indications for Molindone Hydrochloride in Child and Adolescent Psychiatry

Molindone hydrochloride is approved for the treatment of psychotic disorders. Its use in children younger than 12 years of age is not recommended as its efficacy and safety have not been established for use in that age group (PDR, 2000). However, its use in the TEOSS study (Sikich et al., 2008) suggests that it may have utility in the treatment of early-onset schizophrenia. It was found to have equal efficacy to risperidone and olanzapine, while conveying a lower metabolic risk.

Molindone Dosage Schedule

- *Children younger than 12 years of age:* not recommended.
- *Adolescents and adults:* the usual starting dose for treatment of psychotic symptoms is 50 to 75 mg/day, with an increase to 100 mg/day in 3 to 4 days. The medication should be titrated according to symptom response; up to 225 mg/day may be required in severely disturbed patients.

Molindone Hydrochloride Dose Forms Available

- *Tablets:* 5, 10, 25, 50, and 100 mg
- *Oral concentrate:* 20 mg/mL

Reports of Interest

Molindone Hydrochloride in the Treatment of Children Diagnosed with Conduct Disorder

Greenhill et al. (1985) compared molindone and thioridazine in treating 31 hospitalized boys, ages 6 to 11 years, who were diagnosed with undersocialized conduct disorder, aggressive type. Children were assigned randomly to either medication in an 8-week, double-blind, parallel-design study. Subjects were drug-free for the baseline week and were on placebo the second week of the study. During week 3, medication was raised until it produced sedation; this was followed by a fixed dose of drug during weeks 4 through 6. The final 2 weeks of the study were again with placebo. The mean dose of thioridazine over the 4-week treatment period was 169.9 mg/day (4.64 mg/kg/day), and the mean dose of molindone was 26.8 mg/day (1.3 mg/kg/day).

The groups were similar on baseline ratings, which showed them to be severely aggressive. In fact, the initial or terminal placebo periods had to be shortened for 11 subjects and drug begun because of their severe symptomatology. Symptoms improved significantly during the 4 weeks on either drug compared with the placebo periods. On Clinical Global Impressions (CGI), nurses rated the severity of illness at the end of the study as less in the molindone group ($P < .08$) and the degree of improvement as significantly greater ($P < .035$). Untoward effects differed, although not significantly, between the drugs; acute dystonic reactions occurred more frequently in the molindone group (23.5% vs. 6.1%), whereas sedation and gastrointestinal symptoms were more frequent among subjects treated with thioridazine. The authors concluded that molindone is relatively safe for inpatient children and adolescents and thought its efficacy in this population was similar to the more commonly used neuroleptics. Thioridazine is no longer to be used with children.

Fluphenazine Hydrochloride (Prolixin, Permitil)

Indications for Fluphenazine Hydrochloride in Child and Adolescent Psychiatry

Fluphenazine hydrochloride is approved for the treatment of psychotic disorders. It is not approved for administration to children younger than 12 years of age, however, because of lack of studies proving its efficacy and safety in this age group. A manufacturer notes that it has not been shown to be effective in treating behaviorally disturbed patients with intellectual disabilities.

Fluphenazine Dosage Schedule

- *Children younger than 12 years of age:* safety and efficacy have not been established; however, United States Pharmacopeial Dispensing Information (USPDI, 2005) recommends 0.25 to 0.75 mg one to four times daily for psychotic disorders in children.
- *Adolescents and adults:* the manufacturer recommends an initial daily total dose of 2.5 to 10 mg for adults, divided and administered every 6 to 8 hours. One should be at least this conservative in adolescents (see also Joshi et al., 1988).

Fluphenazine Hydrochloride Dose Forms Available

- *Tablets:* 1, 2.5, 5, and 10 mg
- *Elixir:* 0.5 mg/mL (2.5 mg/5 mL)
- *Oral concentrate:* 5 mg/1 mL
- *Injectable preparation (intramuscular):* 2.5 mg/mL
- *Long-acting preparations for parenteral administration:* fluphenazine enanthate, 25 mg/mL, and fluphenazine decanoate, 25 mg/mL, are available. (They are used primarily in treating adults diagnosed with chronic schizophrenia. However, USPDI [2005] suggests an intramuscular or subcutaneous dose of between 3.125 and 12.5 mg every 1 to 3 weeks as needed and tolerated in children aged 5 to 11 years. In children aged 12 years and older, an initial dose of 6.25 to 18.75 mg is suggested with a subsequent increase to 12.5 to 25 mg, with injections every 1 to 3 weeks.)

Report of Interest

Fluphenazine Hydrochloride in the Treatment of Children
Diagnosed with Pervasive Developmental Disorders

As discussed earlier for haloperidol, Joshi et al. (1988) found fluphenazine to be efficacious in treating children diagnosed with childhood-onset PDD or atypical PDD. Fluphenazine was begun at 0.02 mg/kg/day and increased at 3- to 5-day intervals based on behavioral responses. Mean optimal dose of fluphenazine was 1.3 ± 0.7 mg/day. Untoward effects of fluphenazine were remarkably infrequent. Initial drowsiness occurred in some children, but it was transient.

Pimozide (Orap)

Pimozide is an antipsychotic of the diphenyl-butylpiperidine series. It is indicated for the suppression of motor and phonic tics in patients with Tourette disorder who have failed to respond to standard treatment (e.g., haloperidol). It is not intended as a treatment of first choice, and it is seldom used as a psychotropic medication. However, it remains in use and some studies suggest that it may be more efficacious that other FGAs (Roessner et al., 2012). A "Dear Health Care Provider" letter dated September 1999, from the manufacturer warned that sudden, unexpected deaths have occurred in patients taking pimozide at doses >10 mg/day.

Indications for Pimozide in Child and Adolescent Psychiatry

Pimozide is indicated only in the treatment of patients diagnosed with Tourette disorder whose development and/or daily life function is severely compromised by the presence of motor and phonic tics and who have not responded satisfactorily to or cannot tolerate standard treatments, such as haloperidol. Pimozide should not be considered a drug of first choice.

Unexplained deaths, perhaps cardiac related, and grand mal seizures have occurred in patients taking high doses of pimozide (>20 mg/day) (PDR, 1995). In September 1999, the manufacturer reported that sudden, unexplained deaths had occurred with doses >10 mg/day. Information concerning the use of pimozide appears in the Appendix.

6 CHAPTER

Second-Generation/Atypical and Other Antipsychotic Drugs

RICK BOWERS

"ATYPICAL" ANTIPSYCHOTIC DRUGS

The FDA has directed manufacturers of all atypical antipsychotic drugs to add a black box warning that elderly patients with dementia-related psychosis treated with atypical antipsychotic drugs are at increased risk of death of 1.6 to 1.7 times that seen in placebo-treated patients. Atypical antipsychotic drugs are not approved for treatment of patients with dementia-related psychoses.

In addition, despite the early hopes that atypical antipsychotic drugs would be entirely free of the serious adverse effects associated with first-generation antipsychotics (FGAs), the possibility of these adverse effects has not disappeared. Clinicians using these medications must remain alert for the possibility of adverse effects, including neuroleptic malignant syndrome and tardive dyskinesia (TD), associated with any of these agents.

Atypical antipsychotic drugs, including clozapine, risperidone, olanzapine, quetiapine, ariprazole, and ziprasidone differ from the traditional antipsychotic drugs in that in addition to being dopamine receptor (D_2) blockers, they are significant serotonin receptor (S_2) blockers. The simultaneous blocking of D_2 and S_2 receptors in the brain is thought to account for the increased efficacy of these drugs in improving "negative" symptoms of schizophrenia as well as the decreased incidence of extrapyramidal untoward effects that occur with the atypical antipsychotic drugs compared with standard antipsychotic drugs (Borison et al., 1992; *PDR*, 2000). These drugs may also have a positive therapeutic effect when administered to some patients with preexisting TD (Birmaher et al., 1992; Chouinard et al., 1993; Mozes et al., 1994).

Because prepubertal children diagnosed with schizophrenia differ from their adolescent and adult counterpart on some significant parameters and frequently respond less satisfactorily to treatment with standard antipsychotics, specific investigations of the various atypical antipsychotics will be necessary to determine their efficacy in this age group (Green and Deutsch, 1990).

Neuroprotection and Neurogenesis

It is now apparent that several psychiatric disorders such as schizophrenia, bipolar disorder, and recurrent major depression demonstrate atrophic brain changes. The recent discovery that some psychotropic medications used in treating those disorders are neuroprotective and induce new nerve growth or neurogenesis has brought about a new understanding of the causes and healing of neuropsychiatric diseases. The concept of *neuroprotection* now needs to be considered in the risk–benefit analysis when considering medication therapy in the treatment of these chronic psychiatric conditions.

A series of brain neuroimaging studies by Thompson et al. (2001) led clinicians to associate the clinical and functional deterioration in schizophrenia with the progressive neurodegeneration that was found in this brain disorder. Neuroimaging studies in childhood-onset schizophrenia revealed a subcortical gray matter and cortical volume loss estimated at 1% to 3% per year during the first 5 years. This is a very significant finding when one compares this with Alzheimer disorder, which has a 5% cortical loss per year.

Researchers began to explore the pathogenesis of brain tissue loss in schizophrenia and discovered several interrelated causes. These include

- dopaminergic overstimulation which can lead to cell death
- glutamate excitotoxicity and oxidative stress (similar to Alzheimer disorder)
- a decline in protective growth factors or neurotropins such as nerve growth factor (NGF), which stimulate brain-derived neurotropic factor (BDNF) production. These neurotropins, which are critical in brain development, neuroplasticity, and synaptic connectivity, are reduced in treatment-naive schizophrenia.

FGAs and second-generation antipsychotics (SGAs) have different effects on neurotropins in schizophrenia.

The FGAs never gave a promising neurogenesis signal in atrophic brain regions in schizophrenia such as the cerebral cortex or the hippocampus (Chakos et al., 1995). Several studies indicate that not only does haloperidol fail to stimulate neurogenesis in rats, but it also appears to be neurotoxic by inducing apoptotic cell death (Wang et al., 2004).

This appears to occur in part due to the decline of neurotropins, such as brain-derived neurotropic factor. Nasrallah et al. (2004) found via neuroimaging that geriatric patients on FGA's long term experienced greater progressive brain loss and higher mortality rates, with haloperidol being the worst offender. Haloperidol causes pronounced reductions in NGF and brain-derived neurotropic factor, which is reversed by SGAs. FGAs induce caudate nucleus hyperplasia, which may be related to development of TD. The SGAs do not induce caudate hyperplasia (Corson et al., 1999) and in fact may reverse it (Chakos et al., 1995). The SGAs reduce whole-brain gray matter volume loss compared with FGAs. SGAs stimulate the genesis of glial cells, which create the myelin covering that pervades brain white matter. White matter deficits have been widely documented in schizophrenia. SGAs and mood stabilizers are known to have neuroprotective properties such as promotion of new nerve cell development and regeneration of cortical gray matter.

The role of neurotransmitters in neurogenesis is important, and the SGAs seem to have an advantage in this area as well. All the leading neurotransmitters that have been implicated in schizophrenia play a role in neurogenesis:

- Dopamine: D_3 receptor stimulation has been shown to promote neurogenesis; however, the role of the D_2 receptor is unclear.
- Serotonin: The $5\text{-}HT_{1A}$ receptor has been implicated in selective serotonin reuptake inhibitor-induced adult neurogenesis, and the $5\text{-}HT_{2A}$ and $5\text{-}HT_{2C}$ receptors have been definitely linked to neurogenesis.

- GABA: GABA plays a pivotal role in adult neurogenesis, which is evidenced by the fact that GABA precedes all other neurotransmitters in innervating newborn neurons.
- Glutamate: Group I metabotropic glutamate receptors promote adult neurogenesis; however, stimulation of the NMDA or AMPA receptors leads to a reduction in neurogenesis.

Clozapine (Clozaril)

The FDA has directed manufacturers of atypical antipsychotic drugs to add a black box warning that elderly patients with dementia-related psychosis treated with atypical antipsychotic drugs are at increased risk of death of 1.6 to 1.7 times that seen in placebo-treated patients. Clozapine is not approved for treatment of patients with dementia-related psychosis.

Clozapine, a dibenzodiazepine, was approved by the U.S. Food and Drug Administration (FDA) for marketing in the United States in late 1989. It differs from typical antipsychotic drugs in its dopaminergic effects. It functions as a dopamine blocker at both D_1 and D_2 receptors, but does not induce catalepsy or inhibit apomorphine-induced stereotypy. Clozapine also appears to block limbic dopamine receptors more than striatal dopamine receptors. This may account for the fact that no confirmed cases of TD have been reported in more than 20 years of worldwide experience in patients who have received only clozapine (*PDR*, 2000).

Volavka (1999) suggested that clozapine's antiaggressive effect in patients diagnosed with schizophrenia may result from its unique pharmacologic properties of preferentially blocking the D_1-mediated function and its serotonergic actions.

Clozapine has significantly greater efficacy in treating the "negative" symptoms of schizophrenia and a lower incidence of extrapyramidal symptoms (EPS) than do traditional antipsychotics. There is also evidence that clozapine has a positive therapeutic effect on some patients with preexisting TD. Like traditional antipsychotic drugs, clozapine initially suppresses the involuntary movements, but, unlike traditional antipsychotics, the abnormal movements do not worsen over time with clozapine, sometimes even with dose reduction. There is a suggestion that, although it may not be curative, clozapine may alleviate TD over time in some patients (Jann, 1991).

Because of the increased risk for serious and potentially life-threatening untoward effects that has been reported in patients receiving clozapine, its administration was previously deemed appropriate only for severely dysfunctional patients with schizophrenia who had not responded satisfactorily to adequate trials of at least two other antipsychotic drugs or who could not tolerate the untoward effects present at therapeutic dose levels. Given the realization that neurodegeneration begins to occur with the first psychotic episode in the adolescent brain and continues each year, some clinicians now advocate the implementation of clozapine sooner than later. The logic of using clearly the most efficacious antipsychotic agent currently available is sound and acceptable to many clinicians given the blood monitoring requirements have made the risk of serious injury or death exceedingly rare.

In their comparison of clozapine and olanzapine in the treatment of treatment-resistant schizophrenia with childhood onset, Kumra et al. (1998) reported that clozapine was superior to olanzapine and remains the "gold standard" treatment for schizophrenia. They also concluded that all children and adolescents with treatment-refractory schizophrenia should be given a trial of clozapine despite the increased risk of serious untoward effects (agranulocytosis/neutropenia and seizures) and the inconvenience of mandatory and necessary monitoring.

Pharmacokinetics of Clozapine

Peak plasma concentrations during steady-state maintenance at 100 mg twice daily occurred on an average of 2.5 hours (range, 1 to 6 hours) after dosing; mean peak plasma concentration was 319 ng/mL (range, 102 to 771 ng/mL). Clozapine is almost completely metabolized to demethylated, hydroxylated, and N-oxide derivatives, of which approximately 50% are secreted in the urine and 30% in the feces. Serum half-life after a single 75-mg dose averages 8 hours (range, 4 to 12 hours); at steady state on 100 mg twice daily, serum half-life averaged 12 hours (range, 4 to 66 hours). Food does not affect the absorption/bioavailability of clozapine; it may be taken with or without food.

Contraindications for Clozapine Administration

Hypersensitivity to clozapine is a contraindication. Also, patients with myeloproliferative disorders, uncontrolled epilepsy, or a history of clozapine-induced agranulocytosis or severe granulocytopenia should not take clozapine. Clozapine should not be administered together with another drug known to cause agranulocytosis or to suppress bone marrow function.

Adverse Effects of Clozapine

Agranulocytosis is reported to occur in association with administration of clozapine in 1% to 2% of patients. Because of this, weekly monitoring of white blood cell (WBC) counts is mandatory, with discontinuation of treatment if the WBC decreases significantly. It has been recommended that if the WBC falls below 3,500, monitoring should be increased to twice weekly, and if the WBC falls below 3,000, clozapine should be discontinued. Alvir et al. (1993) reported that 73 of 11,555 patients who received clozapine during a 15-month period developed agranulocytosis; of these, 2 died from complications of infection. The cumulative incidence of agranulocytosis was 0.80% after 1 year and 0.91% after 18 months. Agranulocytosis occurred during the first 3 months of treatment in the large majority of cases (61 [83.6%] of 73). In general, older patients and females appear to be at higher risk for developing agranulocytosis. However, an exception appeared to be that patients younger than 21 years of age were at somewhat higher risk than patients between 21 and 40 years of age. The authors also noted that subsequent to the period of their study, an additional five patients between 40 and 72 years of age died from complications resulting from agranulocytosis within 3 months of taking clozapine (Alvir et al., 1993). The manufacturer reports that more than 68,000 patients in the United States had been prescribed clozapine as of January 1, 1994. Of these, 317 developed agranulocytosis; despite weekly monitoring, 11 cases were fatal (PDR, 1995). As of August 21, 1997, the number of patients who were prescribed clozapine had increased to 150,409, with 585 cases of agranulocytosis and 19 fatalities (PDR, 2000).

Kumra et al. (1996) reported that 5 (24%) of 21 adolescent patients enrolled for up to 30 ± 15 months in their study had mild to moderate neutropenia, compared with an estimated cumulative risk of 1.5% to 2.0% in adults. They suggested that this might occur because, in metabolizing clozapine, children produce relatively higher concentrations of N-desmethyl-clozapine, which is associated with hematopoietic toxicity, than do adults.

Administration of clozapine is also associated with an increased incidence of seizures that is apparently dose-dependent. At doses below 300 mg/day, approximately 1% to 2% of patients develop seizures; at moderate doses of 300 to 599 mg/day, approximately 3% to 4% develop seizures; at high doses of 600 to 900 mg/day, approximately 5% of patients develop seizures. Baseline EEG and periodic monitoring should be mandatory for children and adolescents receiving clozapine.

Gerbino-Rosen et al. (2005) reported a retrospective chart review of the hematologic adverse events (HAE) in 172 children and adolescents admitted over a 12-year period to a long-term chronic care facility for treatment-resistant disorders, defined as having failed treatment (i.e., continued need for hospitalization secondary to potential for self-harm, harm to others, or inability to care for self) with at least two antipsychotics in at least two chemical classes in clinically appropriate doses; the large majority of patients were diagnosed with schizophrenia spectrum disorders (N = 139) or bipolar disorder (N = 25). Patients, none of whom had previously received clozapine, were administered clozapine (mean age at clozapine initiation was 15.03 ± 2.13 years) on an open-label basis following a standard drug-monitoring program, with weekly assessments of WBC counts with differential, including absolute neutrophil counts (ANCs). The median observation period was 8 months. Neutropenia (an ANC $< 1,500/mm^3$) occurred in 29 (16.9%) patients; 5 of these patients continued clozapine as a repeated blood sample had a safe ANC and were not included among the patients who developed clozapine-induced HAE ($N = 24$). One of the 24 (0.6%) developed agranulocytosis (ANC $< 500/mm^3$). The cumulative probability of developing an HAE over a 1-year period was 16.1% (95% CI, 9.7% to 22.5%); for developing agranulocytosis, the cumulative probability over a 1-year period was 0.99% (95% CI, 0.98% to 1.0%). Twenty of the 24 patients with an HAE were rechallenged with clozapine; of these, 11 did not develop another episode of HAE and remained on clozapine. The nine patients who developed a second episode were administered a third trial of clozapine, with five being successfully maintained on clozapine without subsequent HAE and four patients eventually stopping because of HAEs. Overall only eight (5%) patients stopped clozapine because of HAEs. The authors noted that the risk for agranulocytosis in children and adolescents treated with clozapine is similar to that reported for adults and that with careful monitoring and prompt discontinuation of clozapine at the first sign of an HAE, there were no long-term negative sequelae in these patients (Gerbino-Rosen et al., 2005).

BOXED WARNING [Summary]: Because of significant risk of developing potentially fatal agranulocytosis, only severely ill patients who have failed to respond adequately to (or could not tolerate) at least two other antipsychotics should be considered for treatment with clozapine. If given, mandatory monitoring protocols must be followed. READ PACKAGE INSERT COMPLETELY BEFORE PRESCRIBING.

Indications for Clozapine in Child and Adolescent Psychiatry

Clozapine is indicated for the management of severely ill, treatment-resistant, schizophrenic patients, and to reduce the risk of recurrent suicidal behavior in patients with schizophrenia or schizoaffective disorder who are judged to be at risk of reexperiencing suicidal behavior. The manufacturer noted that safety and efficacy of clozapine have not been established in children younger than 16 years of age.

Clozapine Dosage Schedule

- *Children and adolescents 15 years of age and less:* not recommended.
- *Adolescents 16 years of age and adults:* initially, a dose of 12.5 mg once or twice daily is recommended. The dose can be increased daily by 25 to 50 mg, if tolerated, to reach a target dose of 300 to 450 mg by 2 weeks' time. Subsequent dose increases of a maximum of 100 mg may be made once or twice weekly. Total daily dosage should not exceed 900 mg.

Clozapine Dose Forms Available

- *Scored tablets:* 25 and 100 mg
- FazaClo (clozapine, USP) is available as yellow, orally disintegrating tablets of 12.5, 25, 100, 150, and 200 mg for oral administration without water and may be chewed

Mandatory Monitoring

Baseline WBC count must be $\geq 3,500/mm^3$, with the differential having an ANC of $\geq 1,500/mm^3$. Weekly monitoring of these parameters is required, with WBC counts $\geq 3,000/mm^3$ and ANCs $\geq 1,500/mm^3$ necessary to continue on medication. If lower counts occur, clozapine must be interrupted and the patient monitored daily. If both blood counts for the first 6 months are always within the acceptable range, biweekly monitoring may be initiated after 6 months. If both counts for the second 6 months are always within the acceptable range, monthly monitoring may be initiated after 12 months. Read the complete monitoring instructions in package insert or *PDR* before prescribing.

Other untoward effects include adverse cardiovascular effects such as orthostatic hypotension, tachycardia, and ECG changes.

Clozapine in the Treatment of Children and Adolescents Diagnosed with Schizophrenia

Siefen and Remschmidt (1986) administered clozapine to 21 inpatients, 12 of whom were younger than 18 years (average age, 18.1 years). Their patients had an average of 2.4 inpatient hospitalizations and had been tried on an average of 2.8 different antipsychotics without adequate therapeutic response or with severe extrapyramidal effects. In addition, the authors considered it a risk that their patients' psychotic symptoms would become chronic if clozapine was not administered.

Clozapine was administered over an average of 133 days. The average maximum dose was 415 mg/day (range, 225 to 800 mg/day) and the average maintenance dose was 363 mg/day (range, 150 to 800 mg/day). In addition, 11 of the 21 subjects were administered one or more other unidentified drugs for about half of the time they were receiving clozapine.

Approximately 67% of symptoms that had been relatively resistant to previous treatment with antipsychotics disappeared or improved markedly in 11 (52%) of the patients, and an additional 6 (29%) patients showed at least slight improvement in the same number of symptoms. Four patients, however, had no changes or worsening of more than half of their psychopathologic symptoms during clozapine therapy. Positive symptoms of schizophrenia improved more than negative symptoms. Specifically, improvements in incoherent/dissociative thinking, aggressiveness, hallucinations, agitation, ideas of reference, anxiety, inability to make decisions, psychomotor agitation, motivation toward achievement, impoverished and restricted thinking, and ambivalent behavior were reported. Symptoms such as lack of self-confidence, fear of failure, psychomotor retardation, irritability, slowed thinking, blunted affect, and unhappiness showed no improvement or deteriorated during treatment with clozapine (Siefen and Remschmidt, 1986).

The most frequent untoward effects observed early in treatment with clozapine were daytime sedation, dizziness, tachycardia, orthostatic hypotension, sleepiness, and increased salivation. No patients developed agranulocytosis, and the hematologic changes that occurred in approximately 25% of patients were clinically insignificant and normalized during continued maintenance on clozapine (Siefen and Remschmidt, 1986).

Schmidt et al. (1990) reported a total of 57 cases of children and adolescents (age range, 9.8 to 21.3 years; mean, 16.8 years; 30 males and 27 females) who were treated with clozapine. Forty-eight patients were diagnosed with a schizophrenic disorder, five with schizoaffective disorder, two with monopolar manic disorder, and two with pervasive developmental disorders (PDDs). These patients had a mean duration of illness of 19.4 months (range, 0 to 74 months) before this hospitalization, which was the first for 16 patients, the second for 16 patients, and the third or more for the remaining 25 patients. Clozapine was begun on an average approximately 3 months after hospitalization following treatment failures with other antipsychotic drugs and concern about chronicity, intolerable untoward effects, or uncontrolled excitation. Average dose during the length of hospitalization was 318 mg/day (range, 50 to 800 mg/day); average dose at discharge was somewhat lower, 290 mg/day (range, 75 to 800 mg/day). Thirty-five patients received only clozapine. In 22 cases, one or more additional other neuroleptics, primarily phenothiazines, were administered simultaneously, but in about one-half of these cases the additional drugs were tapered off and discontinued so that eventually 80% of the patients were on clozapine only. Mean duration on clozapine during hospitalization was 78 days (range, 7 to 355 days), and 17 (31%) patients were discharged on clozapine.

Clozapine was discontinued in 15 (28%) of the patients between the 8th and 132nd days of treatment (average, 50th day) when they were taking a mean dose of 143 mg/day (range, 25 to 350 mg/day) for the following reasons: insufficient antipsychotic effect in 7 cases; poor compliance and a change to depot medication in 5 cases; and severe untoward effects in 3 cases (cholinergic delirium, seizure, and questionable clinically significant decrease of erythrocytes to 2.3 million).

The authors reported that two-thirds of the patients significantly improved in the whole range of symptoms. Paranoid-hallucinatory symptoms and excitation responded best, followed by a reduction in aggressivity. Clozapine was less effective in decreasing agitation and improving negative symptoms, and these symptoms sometimes worsened. Untoward effects were noted in all subjects. These included increased heart rates (during the first 8 weeks only) from 94 to 109 beats per minute in 37 (65%) patients, daytime sedation in 29 (51%) patients, hypersalivation in 20 (35%) patients, orthostatic hypotension in 20 (35%) patients, and an unspecified rise in temperature in 15 (26%) patients. Abnormal movements were observed in nine patients, including tremor (six cases), akathisia (one case), and unspecified EPS in two cases. During the first 16 weeks of clozapine therapy, a significant decrease of various hematologic parameters, including number of erythrocytes, was observed, but did not reach pathologic values; a relative shift from lymphocytes to neutrophils was seen in the differential during the first 2 weeks. There was a reversible increase in liver enzymes, which peaked during the third and fourth weeks. On EEGs, there was evidence that clozapine induced increased neuronal disinhibition (e.g., spike discharges) and a shift in background activity to lower frequencies. Pathologic EEG changes were present in 30 (55%) patients on clozapine compared with 17 (30%) patients before its administration ($P < .01$). One patient developed a seizure (Schmidt et al., 1990). The authors later noted that they considered EEG monitoring before and during treatment with clozapine to be mandatory (Blanz and Schmidt, 1993).

Birmaher et al. (1992) treated three inpatient adolescents (an 18-year-old female and two 17-year-old males) with clozapine; they were diagnosed with schizophrenia that was chronic and resistant to treatment with standard antipsychotics. Clozapine was titrated upward, resulting in markedly better symptom control than was achieved in previous drug trials. Doses at discharge were 100 mg/day for the female and 300 mg/day for the two males. The female patient experienced a reexacerbation of symptoms after approximately 1 year despite good compliance, and rehospitalization was required. She was discharged in 2 weeks, but it was necessary to increase clozapine to 400 mg/day; her functioning was described as satisfactory, but some auditory hallucinations remained.

The only untoward effects that these three patients complained about were sedation and increased salivation, and these gradually remitted. The buccolingual dyskinesia, which one of the males had developed during treatment with standard antipsychotics, disappeared while on clozapine (Birmaher et al., 1992).

Mandoki (1993) administered clozapine to two hospitalized males of age 14 and 16 years, diagnosed with schizophrenia, who had unsatisfactory responses to trials of many medications, including antipsychotics. The younger patient had predominantly severe negative symptoms and the older one predominantly severe positive symptoms. Clozapine in doses of 300 to 400 mg/day resulted in significant improvements. The 14-year-old was discharged on 300 mg/day of clozapine 11 weeks after clozapine treatment began. At follow-up, he was attending school. Clozapine had been increased to 200 mg every morning and 400 mg at bedtime. Untoward effects were significant weight gain, mild hypersalivation, and severe drowsiness. The 16-year-old was discharged on 300 mg/day of clozapine 2 months after beginning clozapine. Dose was increased to 400 mg/day after 2 months because inappropriate touching behaviors recurred. No untoward effects were reported. At follow-up, both adolescents were continuing to experience gradual clinical improvement.

Remschmidt et al. (1994) reported a retrospective study of 36 adolescent inpatients aged 14 to 22 years, diagnosed with schizophrenia, who were treated on an open basis with clozapine following treatment failures with at least two other antipsychotic drugs. Doses ranged from 50 to 800 mg/day (mean, 330 mg/day), and the mean duration of clozapine administration was 154 ± 93 days. Twenty-seven patients (75%) had clinically significant improvement; four (11%) had complete remissions. Three patients (8%) showed no improvement. Six (17%) developed untoward effects necessitating the discontinuation of clozapine: leuko-penia without agranulocytosis (two patients); hypertension, tachycardia, and ECG abnormalities (two); elevations in liver transaminases to 10 times normal values without other signs of hepatitis (one); and worsening of symptoms and develop-ment of stupor when given in combination with carbamazepine 400 mg/day (one). Five patients developed EPS over a period of several months: Four (11%) devel-oped akathisia and one developed a course tremor. Overall, positive symptoms improved significantly more than negative symptoms. For example, delusions, hallucinations, and excitation improved in approximately 65% of patients. Some negative symptoms (e.g., flat affect and autistic behavior) showed little improve-ment, but other negative symptoms (e.g., anergy, muteness, bizarre behavior, and thought blocking) showed improvement in 11% to 22% of the patients. Nine (90%) of 10 patients who had predominantly negative symptoms did not improve clinically.

Levkovitch et al. (1994) treated 13 adolescents (7 males and 6 females; mean age, 16.6 years; range, 14 to 17 years) who were diagnosed with adolescent-onset schizophrenia with clozapine. All had experienced treatment failures, with an aver-age of three traditional antipsychotics. Patients received an average daily dose of 240 mg of clozapine for a mean of 245 days. After 2 months, 10 patients (76.9%) showed significant improvement of at least a 50% decrease in scores on the Brief Psychiatric Rating Scale (BPRS); 2 patients showed more modest improvements. Clozapine was discontinued after 2 days in one patient because of significant orthostatic hypotension. Other untoward effects were tiredness in four (30.8%) patients, hypersalivation in one (7.7%), and temperature elevation in one (7.7%). No leukopenia occurred during weekly monitoring.

Frazier et al. (1994) treated 11 hospitalized adolescents (age range, 12 to 17 years; mean, 14.0 ± 1.5 years) diagnosed with childhood-onset schizophrenia with a 6-week open trial of clozapine. Subjects were chronically and severely ill and had received at least two previous neuroleptic medications without significant clinical benefit or experienced intolerable untoward effects. Following a 4-week washout/observation period, clozapine was begun at 12.5 or 25 mg/day. Dose was titrated individually based on symptom response versus untoward effects and in-creased by one to two times the initial dose every 4 days to a potential maximum of 900 mg/day. The main untoward effects responsible for limiting dose increases were tachycardia (three patients) and sedation (seven patients). Other untoward effects reported included hypersalivation (eight patients), weight gain (seven), en-uresis (four), constipation (four), orthostatic hypotension (two), nausea (one), and dizziness (one).

Extrapyramidal untoward effects also occurred: Four adolescents developed akathisia after several months and one developed a coarse tremor. The mean dose of clozapine at the end of the 6-week period was 370.5 mg/day (range, 125 to 825 mg/day). Six (55%) of the patients improved over 30% on the BPRS on opti-mal dose of clozapine, compared with admission ratings when nine of the patients were receiving other drugs; nine (82%) of the patients improved on clozapine over 30% on the BPRS compared with ratings during the washout period. Nine of the 11 patients also received 6-week courses of haloperidol following 4-week wash-out/observation periods during their hospitalizations; of these, 5 (56%) showed more than a 30% improvement on the BPRS while on clozapine, compared with earlier ratings while on haloperidol. Both positive and negative symptoms of schizophrenia improved (Frazier et al., 1994).

Mozes et al. (1994) treated four children with clozapine; the three males and one female, 10 to 12 years of age, were diagnosed with schizophrenia and had not responded satisfactorily to other neuroleptics. Clozapine was begun in doses of 25 to 100 mg/day and titrated upward. Three patients had significantly reduced symptomatology in <2 weeks. Further decreases in both positive and negative symptoms occurred during the next 10 to 15 weeks of treatment. All four children improved significantly on the BPRS, with a mean reduction of 41 within 15 weeks. At the time of the report, patients had been in treatment between 23 and 70 weeks, and maintenance dosage ranged from 150 to 300 mg/day. The most frequent untoward effect was drooling, which spontaneously decreased over time; drowsiness, experienced by three patients, peaked during the first week and then gradually faded away. Excitatory EEG changes occurred in three patients, and dosage was not increased to decrease the likelihood of seizures. Of note, two cases of TD caused by previous neuroleptic drugs disappeared on clozapine.

Kumra et al. (1996) reported a double-blind study comparing clozapine and haloperidol in 21 hospitalized patients (11 males, 10 females; mean age, 14.0 ± 2.3 years) who had been diagnosed with schizophrenia by DSM-III-R (American Psychiatric Association [APA], 1987) criteria by age 12 and who were treatment refractory. All patients had failed to respond to at least two standard neuroleptics, often at high doses, and augmented with mood stabilizers or antidepressants; most patients also had failed to respond to risperidone. Medications were discontinued over a 2-week period, which was followed by a 4-week washout before active medication whenever this could be tolerated. Patients were randomly assigned to a 6-week parallel treatment with clozapine ($N = 10$) or haloperidol ($N = 11$); the two groups did not differ significantly on any demographic variables. To maintain the blind and to minimize any extrapyramidal effects secondary to haloperidol, all patients receiving that drug were prescribed up to 6 mg/day of benztropine, whereas subjects on clozapine received identical placebo tablets. Initial doses were based on patients' weights and ranged from 6.25 to 25 mg/day for clozapine and from 0.25 to 1.0 mg/day for haloperidol. Increases in the dose by one or two times the initial dose were permitted every 3 to 4 days if clinically indicated. Three patients receiving clozapine and one patient on haloperidol were unable to complete the 6-week trial because of severe untoward effects and were dropped during the fourth and fifth weeks, and the ratings of the final week were carried forward in data analysis. The mean dose of haloperidol during the last treatment week was 16.0 ± 8 mg/day (range, 7 to 27 mg/day) or 0.29 ± 0.19 mg/kg/day (range, 0.08 to 0.69 mg/kg/day). The mean dose of clozapine during the last treatment week was 176 ± 149 mg/day (range, 25 to 525 mg/day) or 3.07 ± 2.59 mg/kg/day (range, 0.34 to 7.53 mg/kg/day); the mean dose of clozapine for the seven subjects who completed the entire 6-week trial was higher: 239 ± 134 mg/day. Clozapine was statistically superior to haloperidol on ratings at the 6-week endpoint on the BPRS ($P = .04$), the Bunney-Hamburg Psychosis Rating Scale ($P = .02$), the Scale for the Assessment of Positive Symptoms ($P = .01$), and the Scale for the Assessment of Negative Symptoms ($P = .002$). Clozapine was also superior to haloperidol on the depression ($P = .02$), thinking disturbance ($P = .05$), withdrawal ($P = .03$), and total ($P = .03$) rating scores on the BPRS. After the double-blind study was completed, the 11 patients who received haloperidol were administered clozapine openly for 6 weeks. The combined sample of 21 subjects was rated on the Clinical Global Impressions (CGI) Scale as follows: very much improved, 2 (9.5%); much improved, 11 (52.4%); minimally improved, 7 (33%); and worsened, 1 (4.8%). The authors also noted that for some patients, clinical improvement continued and peaked only after 6 to 9 months of treatment, as has been reported for adults.

Despite the superiority of clozapine over haloperidol, Kumra et al. (1996) noted serious untoward effects secondary to clozapine. Five of the 10 patients in the double-blind portion developed toxic hematopoietic effects with an ANC of <1,500. In three patients, the WBC normalized spontaneously and they were successfully restarted on clozapine; the other two patients, however, had recurrences of neutropenia when rechallenged with clozapine and were dropped from the study. One patient developed myoclonus and had a tonic-clonic seizure the next day; epileptiform spikes continued on the EEG despite lowering the dose of clozapine and antiepileptic medication, and clozapine was discontinued. Another patient who had bifrontal and posterior delta wave slowing during the study had tonic-clonic seizures as an outpatient on 275 mg/day of clozapine and continued to have petit mal seizures despite a reduction in dosage and treatment with valproate sodium, necessitating discontinuation of clozapine. Three of the 11 patients treated openly with clozapine also developed significant EEG changes associated with worsening behavior, such as increased aggression, psychosis, or irritability. Two of these individuals improved with a reduction of the dose of clozapine and addition of valproate sodium; however, the third experienced further clinical deterioration and facial myoclonus with associated EEG spikes, which required the discontinuation of clozapine. Children and adolescents appear to be at greater risk than adults to develop clinically significant EEG changes. One patient on clozapine had clinically significant increases in liver enzymes and two had tachycardias of more than 100 beats per minute. The authors also felt that excessive weight gain occurred secondary to clozapine; the two best responders during the double-blind protocol gained the most weight. Only one patient was dropped from the haloperidol group, and that was for signs of incipient neuromalignant syndrome; the discontinuing of haloperidol and initiation of supportive measures resulted in normalization of laboratory abnormalities and vital signs within a few days. The extrapyramidal tract untoward effects expected from haloperidol were minimized by the prophylactic benztropine. This study provides significant support for the importance of clozapine in treatment-resistant schizophrenia in children and adolescents but underscores the importance of monitoring the WBC for untoward effects, such as neutropenia/agranulocytosis, and to monitor EEGs for epileptiform changes, to observe for myoclonic movements that may progress to tonic-clonic seizures, and for seizures as the pediatric age group may be at greater risk for all of these than are adults.

In a naturalistic treatment study, Kranzler et al. (2005) administered open-label clozapine, using a flexible titration schedule, to 20 treatment-refractory adolescents (14 males, 6 females; median age 14.19 years; age range 8.5 to 18 years) diagnosed with schizophrenia and hospitalized in a long-term treatment facility (Bronx Children's Psychiatric Center) to evaluate its effectiveness in the treatment of aggression. Subjects were judged to be acutely ill and required a change of medication because of the severity of their psychosis and aggression when clozapine was introduced. The current medication regime was continued and there was a slow cross taper with clozapine. Using a mirror-image study design, effectiveness was measured by comparing the number of emergency oral and injected medications and frequency of seclusion or restraint events in the 12 weeks immediately preceding the trial of clozapine and during a similar period (from week 12 through 24 of clozapine treatment) when optimal clozapine levels had been reached. The mean dose at week 24 was 476 ± 119 mg/day, and 11 of the 20 subjects were on clozapine monotherapy. Comparison of preclozapine and optimal clozapine measures implemented for aggressive behavior showed significant decreases in emergency oral medication ($P = .000$), injectable medication ($P = .007$), and seclusion events ($P = .003$). Another significant finding was that patients who had been hospitalized for a shorter length of time when started on clozapine showed a significantly greater reduction in seclusion events than subjects who had been hospitalized for longer periods when the switch to clozapine was made ($P = .033$). These data suggested that, in such a patient population, clozapine reduces the incidence and severity of violence and aggression and may hasten discharge to a less restrictive setting. The authors think that clozapine treatment may be underutilized because of concerns about its untoward effects and the necessary frequent monitoring with blood tests.

Risperidone (Risperdal)

The FDA has directed manufacturers of atypical antipsychotic drugs to add a black box warning that elderly patients with dementia-related psychosis treated with atypical antipsychotic drugs are at increased risk of death of 1.6 to 1.7 times that seen in placebo-treated patients. Risperidone is not approved for treatment of patients with dementia-related psychosis.

Risperidone belongs to the new chemical class of benzisoxazole derivatives. It was approved by the FDA for marketing in the United States in 1993. The manufacturer suggests that its antipsychotic properties may be mediated through its antagonism of dopamine type 2 (D_2) and serotonin type 2 (5-HT_2) receptors; it also has a high affinity for alpha-1 and alpha-2 adrenergic and H_1 histaminergic receptors Risperdal [package insert] (2010).

Risperidone appears to have significantly greater efficacy in improving "negative" symptoms of schizophrenia than the traditional antipsychotics (Chouinard et al., 1993).

Risperidone has significantly fewer EPS than typical antipsychotics. However, the appearance of EPS is dose related and becomes increasingly greater than that for placebo in the upper approved dosage ranges.

Although the manufacturer notes that there have been isolated reports of TD associated with risperidone, it is likely that the incidence of TD occurring with risperidone only will be significantly less than that with typical antipsychotic agents. Nonetheless, TD has been reported with risperidone since soon after its adoption (Klykylo and Feeney, 1997), and clinicians using this and all antipsychotic agents must be alert for its occurrence.

Pharmacokinetics of Risperidone

Food does not affect the rate or extent of the absorption of risperidone. Peak serum levels of risperidone occur at a mean of 1 hour after ingestion. Risperidone is metabolized in the liver by cytochrome P450IID6 to 9-hydroxyrisperidone, which is the major active metabolite and similar to risperidone in its receptor binding activity. The 9-hydroxyrisperidone active metabolite, developed by Jansen Pharmaceuticals and marketed as Invega, will be described later. Because of genetic polymorphism, approximately 7% of Caucasians and a very low percentage of Asians are slow metabolizers. Peak 9-hydroxyrisperidone levels occur in approximately 3 hours in extensive metabolizers and 17 hours in poor metabolizers. Half-life ($T_{1/2}$) of risperidone is approximately 3 hours in extensive metabolizers and 20 hours in poor metabolizers; $T_{1/2}$ of 9-hydroxyrisperidone is approximately 21 hours in extensive metabolizers and 30 hours in poor metabolizers.

Contraindications for Risperidone Administration

Risperidone is contraindicated in patients with a known hypersensitivity to it.

Risperidone should be administered with caution to patients with hepatic impairment, which may increase free risperidone by up to 35%, and/or renal impairment, which may decrease clearance of risperidone and its active metabolite by up to 60%.

Interactions of Risperidone with Other Drugs

Carbamazepine

Plasma concentrations of risperidone and 9-hydroxyrisperidone were decreased by approximately 50% with coadministration of carbamazepine over a 3-week period. Plasma levels of carbamazepine did not appear to be affected.

Valproate

Oral doses (4 mg/day) of risperidone did not affect the predose or average plasma concentrations and exposure area under the curve (AUC) of valproate (a total of 1,000 mg administered in three divided doses), but there was a 20% increase in valproate peak plasma concentration after concomitant administration of risperidone.

Lithium

Risperidone (6 mg/day in two divided doses) did not affect the exposure (AUC) or lithium's peak plasma concentration.

Fluoxetine

Fluoxetine in doses of 20 mg/day increased risperidone's plasma concentration from 2.5 to 2.8 times, but did not affect the plasma concentration of 9-hydroxyrisperidone.

Paroxetine

Paroxetine in doses of 20 mg twice daily increased risperidone's plasma concentration by three to nine times and lowered the concentration of 9-hydroxyrisperidone by approximately 13%.

Adverse Effects of Risperidone

Black Box Warning

There is a "Black Box Warning" that there is increased mortality in elderly patients with dementia-related psychosis who are treated with atypical antipsychotic drugs including risperidone.

Extrapyramidal Symptoms

The incidence of EPS in patients treated with risperidone appears to be dose related, and clinicians often opt to maintain the dosage below the 6 mg/day dosage.

Hepatotoxicity

Kumra et al. (1997) reviewed the medical records of the 13 children and adolescents (3 males and 10 females) diagnosed with schizophrenia who were admitted to the NIMH over a period of 28 months and treated with risperidone. Two of the three males, but none of the females, showed evidence of steatohepatitis with obesity, elevated liver enzyme values, and evidence of fatty liver on ultrasound, which was confirmed by biopsy in one case. Following discontinuation of risperidone, liver function tests returned to normal within 2 weeks to 3 months. The authors noted that two additional males who were subsequently admitted developed hepatotoxicity during long-term treatment with risperidone. The authors strongly recommended determining baseline liver function tests, obtaining liver aminotransferases, cholesterol, and triglycerides every 3 months, and monitoring weight frequently in pediatric patients who are being maintained on risperidol. Males in this age range may be particularly at risk for hepatotoxicity.

Szigethy et al. (1999) retrospectively reviewed the charts of 38 children and adolescents (32 males, 6 females; mean age, 10.6 ± 3.7; age range, 4 to 17 years) who had been treated with a mean dose of 2.5 mg/day (range, 0.5 to 10.0 mg/day) or 0.05 mg/kg/day (range, 0.01 to 0.11 mg/kg/day) of risperidone for a mean of 15.2 ± 10.0 months (range, 1 to 35 months) to assess hepatic function during risperidone treatment and to identify any clinical factors associated with hepatic dysfunction. Diagnoses of the subjects were autistic disorder ($N = 12$), other PDDs ($N = 8$), mood disorders ($N = 6$), disruptive behavior disorders (DBDs) ($N = 7$), and psychotic disorders ($N = 5$). Thirty-seven (97.4%) of the subjects had normal values for aspartate aminotransferase (AST), alanine aminotransferase (ALT), and total bilirubin after treatment with risperidone for a mean duration of 12.2 ± 9.8 months (range, 1 to 30 months). The thirty-eighth subject, who had received 24 months of risperidone and a peak dose of 4 mg/day, had an ALT of 46 U/L, 7 U/L above the upper limit of normal, which was not considered clinically significant. Baseline liver function tests were available for 14 subjects; comparison of these values with those obtained after an average of 5.47 ± 4.9 months (range, 1 to 19 months) showed no clinically meaningful increases. All subjects for whom baseline weights were available gained weight during treatment (see following text). The authors noted that obesity itself is associated with both steatohepatitis and elevated transaminases and that weight gain alone may have caused the elevated ATL in their patients. Overall, the authors concluded from their review that the risk for risperidone-induced hepatotoxicity is probably low in relatively short-term therapy in this age group.

Weight Gain

Weight gain is often a problem in patients treated with risperidone, usually secondary to a marked increase in appetite. Horrigan and Barnhill (1997) noted a positive correlation between the degree of clinical improvement, increased appetite, and weight gain. They noted that serotonin plays a role in signaling satiety and that, by blocking 5-HT$_2$ receptors, risperidone may cause dysregulation of the "satiety switch."

In their chart review of 38 patients who received risperidone, Szigethy et al. (1999) reported that weight gain occurred in all 23 subjects for whom baseline weights were available; mean baseline weight was 37.92 ± 16.0 kg (range, 15.0 to 73.6 kg), and mean end-of-study weight was 48.28 ± 18.97 kg (range, 19.10 to 82.95 kg). The mean weight gain was 1.01 ± 0.73 kg/month (range, 0.18 to 3.1 kg/month). The mean duration of risperidone therapy for all 38 subjects was 15.2 ± 10.0 months (range, 1 to 35 months), demonstrating that risk of weight gain with risperidone therapy is an important therapeutic issue.

Martin et al. (2000) conducted a retrospective chart review comparing 37 child and adolescent inpatients treated for a minimum of 6 continuous months with risperidone, with 33 inpatients having no exposure to atypical antipsychotics with regard to baseline weight, standardized z scores of weight for age and gender, and percentage of subjects whose weight increased ≥7% (chosen a priori as the standard cutoff for extreme weight gain in clinical trials). After 6 months of risperidone, significantly more subjects on risperidone (78%) versus 24% of controls gained ≥7% of their baseline weight ($P = .001$). A significant difference was evident within 2 months of treatment ($P = .001$). Risperidone-treated subjects gained an average of 1.2 kg/month over the 6-month study, and their weight gain showed no tendency to plateau during that period. There was no correlation between dose of risperidone and demographic or clinical characteristics such as discharge diagnosis or concomitant medication. Weight gain is an important consideration in the treatment of children and adolescents with risperidone and must be considered in the risks and benefits discussed as part of the informed consent process.

Hyperprolactinemia

Risperidone may cause elevations of prolactin that are significantly above normal values and may persist during chronic administration. This is discussed in detail and relevant literature reviewed under the section "Prolactin Levels" in Chapter 2.

Hyperglycemia and Type 2 Diabetes

Epidemiologic studies suggest an increased risk of treatment-emergent hyperglycemia-related adverse events (AEs) in patients treated with atypical antipsychotic drugs, including risperidone (*PDR*, 2006).

Other Untoward Effects

Orthostatic hypotension, dizziness, tachycardia, increase of QTc interval on ECG to >450 msec, insomnia or somnolence, constipation, rhinitis, and many other untoward effects have been reported.

Indications for Risperidone in Child and Adolescent Psychiatry

Risperidone is indicated for the management of the manifestations of schizophrenia in adolescents aged 13 to 17 years, the short-term (3-week) treatment of bipolar mania of acute manic or mixed episodes associated with Bipolar I disorder in children and adolescents aged 10 to 17 years, and the treatment of irritability associated with autistic disorder in children and adolescents aged 5 to 16 years.

Risperidone Dosage Schedule for Schizophrenia

- *Children 12 years of age or less:* not recommended. The safety and effectiveness of risperidone in this pediatric age group have not been established.
- *Adolescents:* an initial dose of 0.5 mg once daily in AM or PM is recommended, with increases of 0.5 to 1.0 mg occurring in intervals of no less than 24 hours as tolerated to a recommended dose of 3 mg/day. It is recommended that any subsequent adjustments of dosage be made at weekly intervals to allow adequate time for steady-state serum levels to be achieved. The manufacturer indicates that although efficacy has been demonstrated in studies of adolescent patients with schizophrenia at doses between 1 and 6 mg/day, no additional benefit was seen above 3 mg/day, and higher doses were associated with more AEs. Doses higher than 6 mg/day have not been studied in adolescents. It is recommended that patients experiencing persistent somnolence may benefit from administering half the daily dose twice daily.

Risperidone Dosage Schedule for Bipolar

- *Children 9 years of age or less:* not recommended. The safety and effectiveness of risperidone in this pediatric age group have not been established.
- *Children and adolescents:* an initial dose of 0.5 mg once daily in am or pm is recommended, with increases of 0.5 to 1.0 mg occurring in intervals of no less than 24 hours as tolerated to a recommended dose of 2.5 mg/day. The manufacturer indicates that although efficacy has been demonstrated in studies of adolescent patients with bipolar mania at doses between 0.5 and 6 mg/day, no additional benefit was seen above 2.5 mg/day, and higher doses were associated with more AEs. Doses higher than 6 mg/day have not been studied in children and adolescents.

Risperidone Dosage Schedule for Autism

- *Children 4 years of age or less:* not recommended. The safety and effectiveness of risperidone in this pediatric age group have not been established.
- *Children and adolescents:* Dosing should be initiated at 0.25 mg/day for patients <20 kg and 0.5 mg/day for patients ≥20 kg. After a minimum of 4 days from treatment initiation, the dose may be increased to the recommended dose of 0.5 mg/day for patients <20 kg and 1 mg/day for patients ≥20 kg. This dose should be maintained for a minimum of 14 days. In patients not achieving sufficient clinical response, dose increases may be considered at ≥2-week intervals in increments of 0.25 mg/day for patients <20 kg or 0.5 mg/day for patients ≥20 kg. Caution should be exercised with dosage for smaller children who weigh <15 kg. In clinical trials, 90% of patients who showed a response (based on at least 25% improvement on Aberrant Behavior Checklist Irritability subscale [ABC-I]), received dosages between 0.5 and 2.5 mg/day. The maximum daily dose of risperidone in one of the pivotal trials, when the therapeutic effect reached plateau, was 1 mg in patients <20 kg, 2.5 mg in patients ≥20 kg, or 3 mg in patients >45 kg. No dosing data are available for children who weighed <15 kg. The manufacturer recommends consideration be given to gradually lowering the dose to achieve the optimal balance of efficacy and safety once sufficient clinical response has been achieved and maintained.

Risperidone Dose Forms Available

- *Tablets:* 0.25, 0.5, 1, 2, 3, and 4 mg
- *Orally disintegrating tablets (Risperdal M-TAB):* 0.5, 1, and 2 mg
- *Oral solution:* 1 mg/mL
- *Long-acting injection (Risperal Consta):* 25, 37.5, and 50 mg vials. This dosage form is indicated for the treatment of schizophrenia and is designed to provide 2 weeks of medication coverage. Its use is not recommended in patients younger than 18 years of age as its safety and efficacy has not been studied in this age group.

Schizophrenia

FDA Registry Trials

The efficacy and safety of risperidone in the short-term treatment of schizophrenia in adolescents aged 13 to 17 years was demonstrated in two short-term (6 and 8 weeks), double-blind controlled trials. All patients met DSM-IV diagnostic criteria for schizophrenia and were experiencing an acute episode at time of enrollment.

In the first trial (study 1), patients were randomized into one of three treatment groups: Risperdal 1 to 3 mg/day ($N = 55$, mean modal dose = 2.6 mg), Risperdal 4 to 6 mg/day ($N = 51$, mean modal dose = 5.3 mg), or placebo ($N = 54$). In the second trial (study 2), patients were randomized to either Risperdal 0.15 to 0.6 mg/day ($N = 132$, mean modal dose = 0.5 mg) or Risperdal 1.5 to 6 mg/day ($N = 125$, mean modal dose = 4 mg).

In all cases, study medication was initiated at 0.5 mg/day (with the exception of the 0.15 to 0.6 mg/day group in study 2, where the initial dose was 0.05 mg/day) and titrated to the target dosage range by approximately Day 7. Subsequently, dosage was increased to the maximum tolerated dose within the target dose range by Day 14. The primary efficacy variable in all studies was the mean change from baseline in total Positive and Negative Syndrome Scale (PANSS) score. Results of the studies demonstrated efficacy of Risperdal in all dose groups from 1 to 6 mg/day compared with placebo, as measured by significant reduction of total PANSS score. The efficacy on the primary parameter in the 1-to-3-mg/day group was comparable to the 4-to-6-mg/day group in study 1, and similar to the efficacy demonstrated in the 1.5-to-6-mg/day group in study 2. In study 2, the efficacy in the 1.5-to-6-mg/day group was statistically significantly greater than that in the 0.15-to-0.6-mg/day group.

Doses higher than 3 mg/day did not reveal any trend toward greater efficacy (Risperdal [package insert], 2010).

Autism

FDA Registry Trials

The efficacy and safety of risperidone in the treatment of irritability associated with autistic disorder were established in two 8-week, double-blind, placebo-controlled trials in 156 children and adolescents (aged 5 to 16 years) who met the DSM-IV criteria for autistic disorder. The Research Units on Pediatric Psychopharmacology (RUPP) Autism Network Study Part 1 was a randomized 8-week, multisite, randomized, double-blind, placebo-controlled, parallel-group, flexible-dose study. This study was to compare the safety and efficacy of risperidone and placebo in the treatment of severe tantrums, aggression, and/or self-injurious behavior (SIB) in 101 children (82 males, 19 females; age range 5 to 17 years, mean age 8.8 + 2.7 years) who were diagnosed with autistic disorder by DSM-IV (APA, 1994) criteria (McCracken et al., 2002). The primary outcome measures were the Irritability subscale of the Aberrant Behavior Checklist (ABC) and the Clinical Global Impressions–Improvement (CGI-I) Scale; a positive response required a minimum 25% reduction on the Irritability score and a rating of 1 or 2 (much improved or very much improved) on the CGI-I Scale at time 8 weeks. Forty-nine subjects were assigned to risperidone and 52 to placebo.

The initial dose of risperidone was determined by subjects' weights. More than 90% of these subjects were below 12 years of age and most weighed more than 20 kg (16 to 104.3 kg). Children weighing ≤20 kg received 0.25 mg daily; those weighing 20 to 45 kg received 0.5 mg daily at bedtime for the first 3 days and then increased to 0.5 mg twice daily on Day 4 followed by titration in 0.5-mg increments to a maximum of 1 mg in the morning and 1.5 mg at bedtime by Day 29. Children weighing ≥45 kg were prescribed medication at a somewhat accelerated rate to achieve a maximum permitted dose of 1.5 mg in the morning and 2.0 mg at bedtime. The final mean dose of risperidone was 1.8 + 0.7 mg/day, with a range of 0.5 to 3.5 mg.

At time 8 weeks, subjects on risperidone had a 56.9% decrease on the Irritability subscale of the ABC versus 14.1% decrease for subjects receiving placebo ($P < .001$). On the CBI-I Scale, 75.5% of subjects on risperidone were rated 1 or 2 (very much improved or much improved) versus only 11.5% of subjects on placebo. Positive responders included 69% of the risperidone group versus only 12% of the group on placebo ($P < .001$). The authors also noted that, compared with the group receiving placebo, the risperidone group improved significantly on the Stereotypy and Hyperactivity Scales, but there were no significant differences on the Social Withdrawal and Inappropriate Speech Scales of the ABC. The authors also noted that 23 of the 34 subjects who were "responders" continued to show benefit after 6 months on medication.

No child dropped out of the study because of AEs; no serious AEs occurred in the risperidone group and most were mild and self-limited (e.g., fatigue/drowsiness subsided in most subjects within 4 to 6 weeks). Increased appetite ("mild" 49% vs. 25%, $P = .03$; "moderate" 24% vs. 4%, $P = .01$), fatigue 59% versus 27%, drowsiness 49% versus 12% ($P < .001$), dizziness 16% versus 4% ($P = .05$), and drooling 27% versus 6% ($P = .02$) were each significantly more frequent in the risperidone group than in the placebo group. Over the 8-week study, subjects on risperidone gained significantly more weight—an average of 2.7 + 2.9 kg versus 0.8 + 2.2 kg for subjects in the placebo group ($P < .001$). Three (6%) of the subjects in the risperidone group withdrew from the study because of lack of clinical efficacy versus 18 (35%) of the subjects in the placebo group, of whom 12 withdrew because of lack of clinical efficacy ($P = .001$).

The authors concluded that risperidone was safe and effective with a favorable risk-benefit ratio in the short-term treatment of children diagnosed with autistic disorder. Significant improvements were noted in tantrums, aggression, SIB, stereotypic behavior, and hyperactivity.

Aman et al. (2005) reported further on the long-term safety and efficacy of risperidone for up to 6 months in the subjects in an 8-week double-blind, placebo-controlled trial reported by McCracken et al. (2002). Upon completion of this 8-week study, 37 placebo nonresponders were treated with risperidone on an open basis for an additional 8 weeks; of these subjects, 30 who responded to risperidone then entered a 16-week open extension phase of treatment with risperidone (Scahill et al., 2001). Of the 34 risperidone responders in the initial 8-week double-blind, placebo-controlled trial, 30 entered the 16-week open extension phase of treatment with risperidone. An additional 3 subjects who were in the risperidone group during the initial 8-week placebo-controlled double-blind study but did not meet all criteria to be "responders" were also enrolled in the 16-week extension phase for a total of 63 subjects; the authors noted that including these 3 subjects in the analyses did not alter clinical results for any outcome. Finally, upon completing the 16-week open extension, 32 of the 63 subjects were rerandomized in an additional 8-week, double-blind phase to either continue therapy with risperidone ($N = 16$) or to enter a placebo substitution phase ($N = 16$) during the first 4 weeks of which risperidone was reduced by 25% of the dose each week with only placebo being given for the last 4 weeks. The authors noted that only 32 subjects participated in this final phase as interim analysis showed that significantly more subjects relapsed on placebo compared with those maintained on risperidone (62.5% vs. 12.5%, $P = .01$), and they then stopped this portion of the study.

Regarding AEs, subjects on risperidone experienced the following significantly more frequently than those on placebo: daytime tiredness (94% vs. 54% "at all" and 37% vs. 12% moderate/severe; $P < .0001$), difficulty waking ($P = .05$), excessive saliva/drooling (29% vs. 16%; $P = .04$), and dizziness/loss of balance (22% vs. 8%; $P = .04$). On the other hand, difficulty falling asleep (65% vs. 47%; $P = .02$)

and anxiety (48% vs. 32%; $P = .05$) were significantly more frequent in the placebo group than in the risperidone group. Excessive appetite was reported in 82% of the risperidone group versus 38% in the placebo group. There was significantly greater weight gain in the risperidone group; however, the authors noted that weight gain decelerated over time with ongoing risperidone treatment. There were no significant changes in height. As noted in the preceding text, only three (6.1%) of the subjects who were treated with risperidone dropped out of the study during the initial 8-week period (McCracken et al., 2002).

During the 16-week extension, six (9.5%) of the subjects treated with risperidone dropped out because of AEs and two of these were because of seizures, which did not appear to be related to risperidone (Aman et al., 2005). The authors concluded that safety and tolerability remained favorable in treating these subjects. They cautioned that the number of patients in the study was too small to identify infrequent/rare AEs and likewise too short in duration to determine rates of TD, obesity, and diabetes.

Pandina et al. (2007) conducted a secondary analysis of data from an earlier study by Shea et al. (2004) of children with autism and other PDDs who were treated with risperidone. This subgroup analysis of the children with autism evaluated the same behavior and clinical assessment measures included in the RUPP autism study by McCracken et al. (2002). The investigators concluded risperidone was well tolerated and significantly improved behavioral problems associated with autism.

In the Shea et al. study, the subjects who were taking risperidone (mean dosage: 0.04 mg/kg/day; 1.17 mg/day) experienced a significantly greater mean decrease on the irritability subscale of the ABC (primary endpoint) compared with those who were taking placebo. By study endpoint, risperidone-treated subjects exhibited a 64% improvement over baseline in the irritability score almost double that of placebo-treated subjects (31%). Risperidone-treated subjects also exhibited significantly greater decreases on the other four subscales of the ABC; on the Conduct Problem, Insecure/Anxious, Hyperactive, and Overly Sensitive subscales of the Nisonger Child Behavior Rating Form (N-CBRF) (parent version); and on the Visual Analog Scale of the most troublesome symptom. More Risperidone-treated subjects (87%) showed global improvement in their condition compared with the placebo group (40%). Somnolence, the most frequently reported AE, was noted in 72.5% versus 7.7% of subjects (risperidone vs. placebo) and seemed manageable with dose/dose-schedule modification. Risperidone-treated subjects experienced statistically significantly greater increases in weight (2.7 vs. 1.0 kg), pulse rate, and systolic blood pressure. EPS scores were comparable between groups.

Long-Term Trials

Additional safety information was also assessed in a long-term study in patients with autistic disorder, or in short- and long-term studies involving 1,885 pediatric patients with psychiatric disorders other than autistic disorder, schizophrenia, or bipolar mania who were of similar age and weight and who received similar dosages of risperidone as patients treated for irritability associated with autistic disorder (Risperdal [prescribing information], 2007).

Weight Changes

In longer-term pediatric studies, the majority of weight gain occurred during the first 6 months. At 12 months, expected normal growth (7 to 8 lb) accounted for approximately half of the 17 lb weight gain observed with risperidone.

Tardive Dyskinesia

Of the 1,885 patients with autistic disorder and other psychiatric disorders, 2 patients were reported to have TD (0.1%). In both cases, TD resolved upon discontinuation.

Reports of Interest

Horrigan and Barnhill (1997) reported treating 11 males ranging from children to adults with risperidone (mean age, 18.3 years; age range, 6 to 34 years); 10 of these subjects were diagnosed with autistic disorder with comorbid moderate to severe mental retardation. All 11 exhibited explosive aggressive behavior, including SIB of such a magnitude that their present caretakers were considering placing them elsewhere; eight of them had poor sleep patterns, which additionally aggravated the situation. On average, the 11 patients had prior trials on 5.45 psychotropic drugs with no, or only partial, improvement. After appropriate washout, five subjects were begun on risperidone only and six had risperidone added to partially efficacious medications, which were continued. Risperidone was initiated with a bedtime dose of 0.5 mg daily and titrated upward in 0.25- to 0.5-mg increments every 5 to 7 days. All patients improved, with the most significant clinical gains apparent within 24 hours. Aggression, self-injury, explosivity, overactivity, and poor sleep patterns improved the most, and caregivers reported that many of the patients tolerated frustration and transitions better and appeared calmer and focused. Optimal daily dose after 4 weeks ranged from 0.5 to 2.0 mg, with a modal dose of 0.5 mg b.i.d. ($N = 10$); after 4 months, the modal dose remained unchanged for the eight patients who continued on the study. Untoward effects reported included three patients with initial mild sedation that ceased by the third week. One patient developed possible chemical hepatitis, with gamma-glutamyltranspeptidase (GGT) increasing from a baseline of 32 to 295 at week 10, necessitating discontinuation. Possible precipitation of a new complex partial seizure disorder and a weight loss of 3.5 kg occurred in one patient, and significant weight gain was reported in eight patients, with gains of 1.6 to 3.6 kg within 4 weeks. None of the patients developed any extrapyramidal tract symptoms or significant changes in blood pressure or heart rate.

Bipolar Disorder

FDA Registry Trials

The efficacy and safety of risperidone in the short-term treatment of acute manic or mixed episodes associated with bipolar I disorder in 169 children and adolescent patients, aged 10 to 17 years, were demonstrated in one double-blind, placebo-controlled, 3-week trial.

See section "FDA-Approved SDA Antipsychotics as Mood Stabilizers in Pediatrics" at the end of chapter for summary description of these agents.

Reports of Interest

Risperidone in the Treatment of Children and Adolescents Diagnosed with Bipolar Disorder

Frazier et al. (1999) conducted a retrospective chart review of outpatients at a university center who were diagnosed by DSM-IV criteria (APA, 1994) with bipolar disorder and treated with risperidone. Twenty-eight such subjects, mean age 10.4 ± 3.8 (range, 4 to 17 years; 27 males, 1 female), were identified. Twenty-five subjects were diagnosed with bipolar I disorder, most recent episode mixed, and three with bipolar I disorder, most recent episode hypomanic. In addition, there was an average of 2.6 ± 0.8 comorbid diagnoses, including attention-deficit/hyperactivity disorder (ADHD) in 25 (89%) and PDD in 8 (29%), and 13 subjects had psychotic symptoms. Subjects had been previously medicated with an average of 3.6 ± 1.7 drugs. Outcome was measured using the NIMH CGI Scale, including CGI-S (illness severity) and CGI-I (global improvement).

Risperidone was begun at a low dose and titrated to reach the lowest dose, achieving acceptable clinical improvement. Mean optimal daily dose of risperidone was 1.7 ± 1.3 mg. Mean length of treatment was 6.1 ± 8.5 months (range,

1 week to 34 months). A mean of 1.8 ± 1.1 drugs was administered concurrently to 27 (96%) of the subjects. Optimal clinical response to risperidone was 1.9 ± 1.0 months; 16 (57%) responded within the first month. CGI-S scores stratified for syndromes of mania, psychosis, and aggression all showed significant improvement, with decreases from marked severity to within the mild severity range. Such scores for ADHD declined significantly but still remained in the moderately severe range. Using a CGI-I rating of 2 or less ("much" or "very much improved") to define robust improvement, 82% of subjects improved for mania, 82% for aggression, 69% for psychosis, and 8% for ADHD. No serious untoward effects were reported; common untoward effects were weight gain (18%), mild sedation (18%), and drooling (7%). There were no cases of extrapyramidal side effects. Prolactin levels were available for 11 subjects; mean prolactin level was 32.8 ± 12.05 ng/mL (normal range, 0 to 15 ng/mL) and was above normal in 9 (82%) of these subjects.

The authors concluded that risperidone treatment resulted in rapid and sustained improvement of manic, psychotic, and aggressive symptoms in these 28 children diagnosed with bipolar I disorder, all but 1 of whom had been previously medicated with limited success. They noted that the efficacy of risperidone was in contrast to similar subjects treated with mood stabilizers, which, although efficacious, took many months to reach maximum clinical improvement and were associated with a high percentage of relapse.

Biederman et al. (2005b) conducted an 8-week, open-label, prospective study of risperidone monotherapy in 30 subjects, mean age 10.1 ± 2.5 years, 22 (73%) males, 8 (27%) females, diagnosed by DSM-IV criteria with bipolar I or bipolar disorder NOS. All subjects had clinically significant mania and a Young Mania Rating Scale (YMRS) score >15; at entry, the overall mean YMRS score was 27.9 ± 9.1, which is in the severe range. Risperidone was begun at a daily dose of 0.25 mg for subjects 12 years of age or younger and 0.50 mg/day for subjects 13 years of age or older. Based on clinical response, dose was titrated at weekly intervals to a maximum of 2.0 mg/day in the younger subjects and a maximum of 4.0 mg/day in the older group. Subjects taking stimulants as treatment of comorbid ADHD were permitted to continue if the dose had remained constant for a minimum of 30 days prior to the study.

Subjects were rated on the YMRS, the Children's Depression Rating Scale–Revised (CDRS-R), the BPRS, and the Clinical Global Impressions–Severity (CGI-S) and CGI-I Scales. A positive response was defined as a ≥30% reduction in YMRS or a score of ≤2 (much or very much improved) on the CGI-I Scale. Euthymia was defined as a score of <10 on the YMRS and a CDRS-R score of ≤28.

Twenty-two subjects completed the entire 8-week study. Analyses were intention to treat (ITT) with the last observation carried forward (LOCF) for noncompleters. At endpoint, there was significant improvement in manic symptoms (P < .0001) on the YMRS (baseline 27.9 ± 9.2 vs. endpoint 13.5 ± 9.7) although subjects remained with residual manic symptoms; 21 (70%) of subjects had at least a 30% reduction in baseline YMRS scores and 15 (50%) had reductions of at least 50%. The reduction in depressive symptoms as measured on the CDRS-R (baseline rating of 40.9 ± 11.5 vs. endpoint rating of 30.7 ± 11.0) was also significant (P = .0001), but indicated that symptoms of depression continued. Overall, euthymia was achieved in 7 (23%) subjects and remitted mania with residual depression in 5 (16%) subjects. Of note, 5 (55%) of subjects with a codiagnosis of conduct disorder, 10 (46%) of the subjects with a codiagnoses of depression, and 9 (35%) of the subjects with a codiagnosis of ADHD were rated ≤2 (much or very much improved) on the CGI-I.

Regarding AEs, the most commonly reported were gastrointestinal complaints (20%), increased appetite (16%), and sedation (13%). Prolactin levels increased significantly from a baseline of 7.9 ± 5.3 ng/dL to 34.4 ± 21.9 ng/dL at endpoint ($P < .001$). Subjects also had a significant increase in weight, 2.1 ± 2.0 kg ($P < .001$), and pulse rate from a baseline of 90.6 ± 13.3 beats per minute to 98.0 ± 14.0 beats per minute ($P = .006$) (Biederman et al., 2005b).

Risperidone in the Treatment of Children and Adolescents Diagnosed with Conduct Disorder (and Various Intelligence Quotients)

Findling et al. (2000) conducted a small 10-week, randomized, double-blind, placebo-controlled-study at an inner-city, academic medical center to address if risperidone was superior to placebo in ameliorating aggression in children and adolescents. More specifically, the study attempted to examine the safety, tolerability, and efficacy of risperidone in children and adolescents suffering from a primary diagnosis conduct disorder with prominent aggressive behavior. Notably, exclusion criteria included moderate or severe ADHD and significant psychiatric comorbidity including mood disorders.

Twenty youths (19 males and 1 female) were selected as subjects. Ten were randomly assigned to receive placebo and 10 youths were randomly assigned to receive risperidone. Half of the youths assigned to each treatment arm were White. The ages of the patients ranged from 6 to 14 years. Nine of the youths (six in the risperidone group and three in the placebo group) had not improved with community-based treatments with other psychotropic medications. These nine youths had all previously received methylphenidate. Other medications that had been previously prescribed to these youths included dextroamphetamine ($N = 4$), clonidine ($N = 3$), an antidepressant ($N = 5$), divalproex sodium ($N = 2$), and thioridazine ($N = 1$).

Patients were seen weekly throughout the trial. The starting dose of medication was one 0.25 or 0.50 mg tablet per day, depending on patient weight, given in the morning. Medications could be increased at weekly intervals during the first 6 weeks of the study. Patients weighing <50 kg had a maximum total daily dose of risperidone of 1.5 mg. Patients weighing 50 kg or greater had a maximum total daily dose of risperidone of 3.0 mg.

Of the 10 youths assigned to risperidone, 6 completed the entire study. Only 3 youths who received placebo finished the trial. The average estimated end-of-study dose for those youths assigned to risperidone was 0.028 ± 0.004 mg/kg/day (range, 0.75 to 1.50 mg/day). Although investigators were permitted to use their discretion to alter dosing to bedtime or in divided dosages, all but one subject received their medication as a once-daily dose in the morning.

The primary outcome measure was the Rating of Aggression Against People and/or Property Scale (RAAPPS). The authors concluded that risperidone was clearly superior to placebo in ameliorating aggression on this primary outcome measure during the last 4 weeks of the study. Statistically significant differences were not found for all measures of aggression in the secondary outcome measures but there were positive trends on many measures and this finding may have been the result of the small sample size. The once-a-day dosages used in this study were fairly modest and larger dosages or the utilization of multiple dosages over the course of a day may have been more beneficial for some patients. Risperidone was reasonably well tolerated, with none of the risperidone-treated patients developing extrapyramidal side effects or requiring treatment with oral benztropine, which the study allowed. There were no clinically significant changes in any laboratory values such as elevations of serum transaminases or electrocardiogram. The predicted weight gain for the risperidone group was 4.2 ± 0.7 kg and for the placebo group 0.74 ± 0.9 kg suggesting that treatment with risperidone was associated with weight gain. The modest side-effect rates found in the study were likely due to the low dosing ranges and slow titration utilized in the study as well as the short duration of the study. The authors concluded that these data provide preliminary evidence that risperidone may have efficacy in the treatment of youths with conduct disorder. Because of the small sample size and the brief length of this study, further research is necessary to confirm these findings.

Findling et al. (2000) noted that, despite the small sample size, clinical improvement on almost all measures of aggressive behavior were highly significant in patients receiving risperidone compared with those on placebo. Risperidone, in low daily doses, appears to be a promising short-term treatment for at least some youngsters diagnosed with conduct disorder and exhibiting prominent aggressive behavior (Findling et al., 2000).

Aman et al. (2000) conducted a 6-week, randomized, double-blind, placebo-controlled study of risperidone in the treatment of 118 children (age range, 5 to 12 years) exhibiting severe conduct problems and who had intelligence quotients ranging from 35 (moderate retardation) to 84 (borderline intelligence). Efficacy was determined by ratings on the N-CBRF, the ABC, the Behavior Problems Inventory, and the CGI Scale. Risperidone dosage was titrated to be within a range of 0.02 to 0.06 mg/kg/day. The mean treatment dose was 1.23 mg/day. Patients on risperidone improved significantly more on the N-CBRF than patients on placebo, beginning within the first week and continuing for the duration of the study. At endpoint, risperidone was also significantly better than placebo, as evidenced by ratings on the other scales. No serious untoward effects were reported.

Croonenberghs et al. (2005) conducted an international multisite (16 European, 11 North American, and 5 South African) 1-year open-label trial of risperidone with 504 patients (419 males, 85 females; mean age 9.7 ± 2.5 years, range 4 to 14 years; 375 [74.4%] were older than 12 years of age and 425 [84.3%] were White) diagnosed with DBDs and subaverage intelligence to determine risperidone's long-term safety and effectiveness in the treatment of such disorders. Subjects had DSM-IV Axis Diagnoses of conduct disorder (23.8%), conduct disorder and ADHD (20.8%), oppositional defiant disorder (ODD, 17.9%), ODD and ADHD (18.8%), DBD NOS (6.5%), DBDNOS and ADHD (10.1%), and ADHD only (2.0%) and Axis II diagnoses of borderline intelligence (37.6%), or mild (43.1%) or moderate (19.3%) mental retardation (mean IQ was 64.2 ± 13.4; range 36 to 84).

The primary rating scales employed in measuring results were the N-CBRF Conduct Problem Subscale and the Vineland Adaptive Behavior Scale for conduct problems; a modified children's version of the California Verbal Learning Test (MCVLT-CV) and the Continuous Performance Task (CPT) for cognitive functioning; and the Extrapyramidal Symptom Rating Scale and Adverse Effects "Query" were also recorded. The ABC and the CGI Scale were used to assess overall effectiveness. After an initial 3-day screening, eligible subjects were treated with a weeklong, single-blind, placebo period. At the end of this period, they were administered the N-CBRF Conduct Problem Subscale and the Vineland Adaptive Behavior Scale; those scoring <24 on the former or >84 on the latter were excluded. Subjects were administered 0.01 mg/kg of an oral risperidone solution once daily for the first 2 days of the study; this was increased to 0.02 mg/kg beginning the third day. Thereafter, doses could be adjusted at weekly intervals, but increases could not be >0.02 mg/kg/day and the maximum permitted dose was 0.06 mg/kg/day.

Of the 504 subjects, 367 (73%) completed the 1-year study. The primary reasons for noncompletion were adverse effects (43; 8.5%), lost to follow-up (26; 5.2%), withdrawal of consent (18; 3.6%), and noncompliance (17; 3.4%). The most frequent reason for discontinuing was weight gain (9 subjects). The median dose was 1.5 mg/day (range, 0.1 to 4.3 mg/day).

Subjects' scores improved significantly on both measures of cognitive functioning ($P < .001$). On the conduct problem subscale of the N-CBRF, the mean score decreased from 32.9 ± 7.5 at baseline to 17.0 ± 11.0 at endpoint, a 48% decrease ($P < .001$). On the positive social behavior subscale of the N-CBRF compliant/ calm and adaptive/social behavior, both improved significantly ($P < .001$) from baseline, and on the problem behavior subscale, insecure/anxious, hyperactive, self-injury/stereotypic, self-isolated/ritualistic, and overly sensitive behaviors decreased significantly ($P < .001$). On the CGI Scale, at baseline 72% were rated as having marked to extremely severe symptoms; at the end of the study, only 12% were so rated and 66% had mild symptoms or were rated as not ill. Scores on the ABC decreased from 64.3 ± 25.0 at baseline to 37.4 ± 27.4 at endpoint ($P < .001$).

At least one adverse effect was reported by 462 (91.7%) of the subjects, and most were mild or moderate in intensity. The most common adverse effects that appeared to be related to the medication were somnolence (149, 29.6%), weight gain (87, 17.3%), fatigue (69; 13.7%), hyperprolactinemia (56, 11.1%), and increased appetite (53, 10.5%). There was a low baseline incidence of EPS, and ratings decreased over time throughout the study. However, five subjects required antiparkinsonian medication during the study and six patients discontinued the study because of EPS. Two subjects developed TD, which remitted after medication was discontinued and one subject possibly experienced a withdrawal dyskinesia within 12 hours of discontinuing risperidone.

The authors concluded that risperidone is generally safe and well tolerated by children and adolescents over a period of up to 1 year.

Snyder et al. (2002) conducted a double-blind, placebo-controlled 6-week study of 110 children (age range, 5 to 12 years) with subaverage IQs (15 were moderately retarded [IQ = 35–49], 42 were mildly retarded [IQ = 50–69] and 53 had borderline IQs [IQs = 70–85]) to determine the efficacy of risperidone in reducing the severe disruptive behaviors they exhibited, including aggression, destruction of property, impulsivity, and defiance of authority. The children were diagnosed with conduct disorder, ODD, or DBD NOS; 80% of subjects were also diagnosed with ADHD, and 45 of these continued treatment with the stimulant medication they were already receiving at time of entry to this study. Subjects had to have a score of 24 or greater on Conduct Problem subtest of the N-CBRF at baseline and at the end of a weeklong single-blind placebo run-in period that preceded the 6-week study to enter the double-blind phase. Of the 133 children beginning the study, 23 (17.3%) were placebo responders who dropped out of the study before the double-blind phase.

Subjects were randomly assigned to placebo ($N = 57$) or risperidone ($N = 53$). Twenty-five subjects dropped out of the double-blind portion; the most common reason being insufficient response. All 19 dropouts from the placebo group were for insufficient response whereas only 2 of the 6 dropouts from the risperidone group were for this reason ($P < .001$).

Risperidone or placebo was administered as an oral solution, beginning at 0.01 mg/kg/day and titrated upward with a maximum permitted weekly increase of 0.02 mg/kg to a total maximum dose of 0.06 mg/kg/day. The mean dose of risperidone at the endpoint was 0.98 ± 0.06 mg/day (range 0.40 to 3.80 mg/day) or 0.033 ± 0.001 mg/kg/day. The risperidone group showed a significantly greater reduction in ratings on the primary outcome variable, the N-CBRF Conduct Problem subtest, than the placebo group (47.3% vs. 20.9% reduction, $P < .001$). In addition, significant improvements for subjects on risperidone were reported on several other subscales of the N-CBRF (conduct problem scale) and on various subscales of the Behavior Problems Inventory (aggressive behavior), the ABC (irritability), and the Visual Analog Scale (VAS) (symptom) compared with the placebo group. Ratings on the CGI-I Scale for subjects who completed the 6-week double-blind phase were significantly better for the risperidone group ($N = 42$), which improved significantly more than the placebo group ($N = 37$). No clinically significant ECG changes occurred. There were no significant cognitive changes on the CPT or on the MCVLT-CV.

The most common adverse effects reported in the risperidone group were somnolence (41.5%), headache (17%), appetite increase (15.1%), and dyspepsia (15.1%). At endpoint, the risperidone group gained significantly more weight than the placebo group, 2.2 versus 0.2 kg ($P < .001$). Prolactin levels increased significantly in both males (from 6.96 at baseline to 27.08 at endpoint) and females (from 11.30 at baseline to 30.38 at endpoint) taking risperidone; the authors attributed this increase in the group to a minority of subjects whose increased prolactin levels fell within the 35 to 105 ng/mL range (normal range is 2 to 18 ng/mL for males and 3 to 30 ng/mL for females).

The authors concluded that risperidone was effective in reducing aggression, hyperactivity, and self-injury associated with DBDs and that it was adequately tolerated.

Risperidone in the Treatment of an Adolescent Diagnosed with Obsessive-Compulsive Disorder

Simeon et al. (1995) reported that a 16-year-old male diagnosed with severe obsessive-compulsive disorder, symptoms of anxiety, and aggressive and oppositional behavior and who had failed prior trials of clomipramine alone and in combination with standard neuroleptics and fluvoxamine showed minimal improvement and remained severely dysfunctional when risperidone was used in combination with clomipramine and fluvoxamine.

Risperidone in the Treatment of Children and Adolescents Diagnosed with Tic Disorders

Gilbert et al. (2004) conducted a randomized, double-blind crossover trial comparing risperidone and pimozide in 19 children and adolescents (15 males, 4 females; age range, 7 to 17 years, mean 11 ± 2.5 years) who were diagnosed with Tourette disorder ($N = 16$) or chronic motor tic disorder ($N = 3$). Subjects were randomized to active treatment for a 4-week period; this was followed by a 2-week washout and administration of the other drug for 4 additional weeks. All subjects received placebo for an initial 2-week period, at the completion of which baseline tic severity was determined. The active drugs were titrated for the first 2 weeks and then held constant for the final 2 weeks of each period. Doses were increased if there was minimal or no improvement and held constant if untoward effects developed. Both treatments were administered twice daily; however, the morning dose of pimozide was a placebo. Pimozide was begun at a dose of 1 mg at bedtime and could be titrated up to a maximum of 4 mg/day. Risperidone was begun at a dose of 0.5 mg twice daily (morning and bedtime) and could be titrated up to a maximum of 2mg twice daily. Two subjects taking risperidone and one subject taking pimozide discontinued the study because of worsening tics. Thirteen subjects completed the study. The final daily doses of risperidone ranged from 1 to 4 mg (mean 2.5 mg/day); final daily doses of pimozide ranged from 1 to 4 mg (mean 2.4 mg/day). Changes in tic severity were rated on the Yale Global Tic Severity Scale (YGTSS; baseline rating = 43.3 ± 17.5). For the first 4-week period, subjects on risperidone had significantly lower tic severity scores on the YGTSS than subjects on pimozide (25.2 ± 13.6 vs. 34.2 ± 14.2; $P = .05$). The mean 18 point (42%) decrease on the YGTSS in the subjects receiving risperidone is clinically meaningful. Subjects on both drugs experienced weight gain; during the 4-week treatment periods, subjects on risperidone gained a mean of 1.9 kg whereas those on pimozide gained about half as much, 1.0 kg. Untoward effects were rated as mild. The authors conclude that their study supports the idea that risperidone and other atypical dopamine blocking agents are effective in treating Tourette disorder, but caution that excessive weight gain and high dropout rates in this and other studies suggest that, when such drugs are used as monotherapy, the efficacy–to–adverse-effect ratio is unfavorable for some patients.

Olanzapine (Zyprexa)

Olanzapine belongs to the thienobenzodiazepine class. It was approved by the FDA for marketing in the United States in 1997. The manufacturer suggests that its antipsychotic properties may be mediated through a combination of dopamine and serotonin type 2 (5-HT$_2$) antagonism. Olanzapine also antagonizes muscarinic M$_{1-5}$ receptors, which may explain its anticholinergic effects; histamine H$_1$ receptors, which may explain the somnolence that may occur; and adrenergic alpha-1 receptors, which may explain the orthostatic hypotension sometimes observed.

Pharmacokinetics of Olanzapine

Food does not affect the rate or extent of absorption of olanzapine. Peak serum concentrations occur approximately 6 hours after oral administration. The half-life of olanzapine ranges from 21 to 54 hours in 90% of the population, with a mean half-life of 30 hours. With once-daily dosing, steady-state serum concentrations occur in approximately 7 days.

Olanzapine is metabolized primarily by direct glucuronidation and cytochrome P450 (CYP)-mediated oxidation. The major circulating metabolites during steady state, 10-N-glucuronide and 4′-N-desmethyl olanzapine, are clinically inactive at usual doses. The drug is highly metabolized, with only approximately 7% being recovered unchanged in the urine. Approximately 60% of the drug is excreted through the kidneys, and approximately 30% is recovered in the feces.

Tobacco smoking induces cytochrome CYP1A2, a principal enzyme mediating the metabolism of olanzapine; hence, adult smokers have lower plasma olanzapine levels than nonsmokers.

It is noted that olanzapine clearance is approximately 30% greater in males than in females and approximately 40% greater in smokers than in nonsmokers; however, dosage modifications are not usually necessary.

Olanzapine Pharmacokinetics in Child and Adolescent Inpatients Diagnosed with Schizophrenia

Grothe et al. (2000) studied the pharmacokinetics of olanzapine in an 8-week, open-label treatment of eight inpatients (four males, four females; age range, 10 to 18 years) diagnosed with schizophrenia who were subjects in the NIMH study investigating the efficacy and safety of atypical antipsychotic drugs in treatment-refractory schizophrenia with childhood onset. As all eight were nonsmokers, their olanzapine pharmacokinetics were compared with those reported for adult nonsmokers. Olanzapine was begun at a dose of 2.5 mg/day, with an increase to 5.0 mg/day on Day 3. Subsequently, olanzapine was titrated upward in 2.5- to 5.0-mg increments every 5 to 9 days based on clinical response up to a maximum of 20 mg/day. Blood samples were drawn weekly; at the end of treatment, plasma level determinations were made for 0, 1, 2, 4, 8, 12, 24, and 36 hours after the final dose. At the end of the 8-week study, seven subjects were receiving olanzapine 20 mg/day and one was receiving 15 mg/day. Plasma olanzapine levels increased linearly in this dose range, making dose adjustments relatively predictable. At a fixed-dose, steady-state levels developed in approximately 7 days, with olanzapine's concentration approximately doubling over that period. The seven subjects receiving 20 mg/day had an average steady-state plasma olanzapine concentration of 92.6 ± 27.0 ng/mL; average trough concentration (measured 24 hours after the last dose) was 75.6 ± 27.2 ng/mL. The seven subjects' mean maximum plasma concentration (C_{max}) was 115.6 ± 26.7 ng/mL, which occurred at a mean time (T_{max}) of 4.7 ± 3.7 hours after the dose was given. Mean elimination half-life ($T_{1/2}$) was 37.2 ± 5.1 hours. Olanzapine plasma levels of these seven mostly adolescent subjects were comparable to those reported for adult nonsmokers.

Interactions of Olanzapine with Other Drugs

Of particular note, carbamazepine, a potent inducer of CYP1A2 activity, in doses of 200 mg b.i.d. causes an increase of approximately 50% in the clearance of olanzapine; higher doses may cause an even greater increase, necessitating upward adjustment of the dose of olanzapine.

Contraindications for Olanzapine Administration

Olanzapine is contraindicated in patients with known hypersensitivity to the drug.

Adverse Effects of Olanzapine

Extrapyramidal Symptoms

At doses up to 15 ± 2.5 mg, there were no statistically significant differences in treatment-emergent EPS assessed by rating scales between placebo and olanzapine. This was also true for adverse effects spontaneously reported by patients, except that akathisia was reported significantly more frequently at doses of 10 ± 2.5 mg or more for olanzapine than for placebo.

Other Adverse Effects

Orthostatic hypotension, tachycardia, weight gain, liver transaminase elevations, somnolence, insomnia, constipation, dizziness, agitation, and dry mouth have been reported to occur in patients treated with olanzapine.

Indications for Olanzapine in Child and Adolescent Psychiatry

The PI states that the increased potential (in adolescents compared with adults) for weight gain and hyperlipidemia may lead clinicians to consider prescribing other drugs first in adolescents.

Olanzapine is indicated in adolescents 13 to 17 years of age for the treatment of schizophrenia and the treatment of acute mixed or manic episodes associated with bipolar I disorder.

Olanzapine Dosage Schedule

- *Children and adolescents 12 years of age and less:* not recommended. The safety and effectiveness of olanzapine have not been established for pediatric populations <13 years of age.

Treatment of Schizophrenia

Adolescents 13 to 17 years of age: An initial dose of 2.5 to 5 mg without regard to meals is recommended, with dose increases in increments of 2.5 to 5.0 mg over several days as tolerated to a target dose of 10 mg/day. Although a flexible dose range of 2.5 to 20 mg was used in clinical trials and was shown to be efficacious, doses above 10 mg/day have not been demonstrated to clearly increase efficacy. The safety of doses above 20 mg/day has not been evaluated in clinical trials.

Treatment of Acute Mixed or Manic Episodes Associated with Bipolar I Disorder

Adolescents 13 to 17 years of age: An initial dose of 2.5 to 5 mg without regard to meals is recommended, with dose increases in increments of 2.5 to 5.0 mg over several days as tolerated to the dose range of 2.5 to 20 mg/day which demonstrated efficacy in clinical trials. The safety of doses above 20 mg/day has not been evaluated in clinical trials.

Olanzapine Dose Forms Available

- *Tablets:* 2.5, 5, 7.5, 10, 15, and 20 mg
- *Orally disintegrating tablets (Zyprexa Zydis):* 5, 10, 15, and 20 mg
- *Injection, intramuscular:* 10 mg vial

Schizophrenia

FDA Registry Trials

Adolescents (ages 13 to 17): Efficacy was established in one 6-week trial in patients with schizophrenia. PI indicates the increased potential (in adolescents compared with adults) for weight gain and hyperlipidemia may lead clinicians to consider prescribing other drugs first in adolescents. Compared with patients from adult clinical trials, adolescents were likely to gain more weight, experience increased sedation, and have greater increases in total cholesterol, triglycerides, LDL cholesterol, prolactin, and hepatic aminotransferase levels.

Commonly Observed Adverse Reactions

Commonly observed treatment-emergent adverse reactions of ≥5% incidence among adolescents (13 to 17 years old) (combined incidence from short-term, placebo-controlled clinical trials of schizophrenia or bipolar I disorder [Manic or Mixed Episodes]) were sedation, weight increase, increased appetite, headache, fatigue, dizziness, and dry mouth in decreasing order of incidence (Zyprexa [package insert], 2011).

Reports of Interest

Olanzapine in the Treatment of Children and Adolescents Diagnosed with Schizophrenia

Sholevar et al. (2000) treated with olanzapine 15 hospitalized subjects (9 males, 6 females; age range, 6 to 13 years; mean age, 9.4 ± 1.99 years) who were diagnosed with childhood-onset acute schizophrenia by DSM-IV criteria before age 12. Medication was begun between 24 and 48 hours after admission. Because the first 3 subjects experienced morning sedation and lethargy on initial doses of 5 mg of olanzapine daily, the subsequent 12 patients were begun on 2.5 mg daily. Medication was increased to 5 mg daily after 5 days if no untoward effects were apparent. Average hospitalization during which this study took place was 11.3 days. At the end of hospitalization, 14 (93%) of the subjects were maintained on 5 mg olanzapine daily. Psychiatric improvement was rated on a four-point scale: 0 = no improvement, 1 = slight improvement, 2 = moderate improvement, and 3 = great improvement. Five subjects (33.3%) were greatly improved, five (33.3%) were moderately improved, three (20%) were slightly improved, and two (13.3%) showed no improvement. Sedation was the most common untoward effect and lasted from 0 to 4 days. There were no clinically significant changes in laboratory values or vital signs. The authors reported that longer duration of initial sedation was significantly positively correlated with increased clinical improvement ($P = .004$). Younger age was significantly correlated with increased clinical improvement ($P < .05$). The 11 subjects who were being treated for the first time with an antipsychotic showed greater clinical improvement than the 4 subjects who had failed prior treatments with antipsychotics.

Kumra et al. (1998) compared the efficacy of olanzapine in an 8-week, open-label trial in 8 patients (mean age, 15.3 ± 2.3 years) with that of clozapine in a 6-week, open-label trial in 15 patients (mean age, 13.6 ± 1.5 years) in the treatment of subjects diagnosed with schizophrenia by DSM-III-R (APA, 1987) criteria. Subjects receiving olanzapine in this study had treatment-resistant schizophrenia (all had failed prior treatment with at least two other neuroleptics) with childhood onset, which comprises an even rarer subgroup than schizophrenia with childhood onset. In addition, four of the subjects on olanzapine had experienced good clinical response to clozapine but developed significant untoward effects requiring its discontinuation. In addition, most clinicians would now administer a trial of an atypical antipsychotic rather than a standard neuroleptic as a first-line medication.

Mean dose of olanzapine at the sixth week of treatment was 17.5 ± 2.3 mg/day (range, 12.5 to 20 mg/day) or 0.27 ± 0.11 mg/kg/day (range, 0.15 to 0.41 mg/kg/day). The mean dose of clozapine at the sixth week of treatment was 317 ± 147mg/day (range, 100 to 600 mg/day) or 5.42 ± 2.84 mg/kg/day (range, 1.28 to 8.88 mg/kg/day). Efficacy was rated using scores of the BPRS and the CGI Scale.

The most clinically important findings of this study were that 8 (53%) of the 15 subjects on clozapine and none of the 8 subjects on olanzapine met "responder" criteria by week 6. At week 8, two (25%) of the subjects receiving olanzapine met "responder" criteria and one (12.5%) was a partial responder. Clinical improvement of subjects on clozapine at 6 weeks was rated better than that of subjects on olanzapine at 8 weeks for all clinical ratings. Even the four subjects who could not tolerate clozapine because of untoward effects had shown greater clinical improvement on clozapine than on olanzapine. Of the eight patients on olanzapine, three were rated "much improved"; two, "minimally improved"; one, "no change"; one, "minimally worse"; one, "much worse." Four subjects, who improved on olanzapine at 8 weeks and continued to take the drug, showed further clinical improvement. Untoward effects of olanzapine were moderate but frequent; the most common were insomnia (seven, 87.5%), transient liver transaminase elevation (seven, 87.5%), increased appetite (six, 75%), nausea/vomiting (six, 75%), headache (six, 75%), sustained tachycardia (six, 75%), increased agitation (six, 75%), difficulty concentrating (five, 62.5%), and constipation (five, 62.5%). During the 8-week trial, seven (87.5%) of the patients on olanzapine were treated with lorazepam, 2 to 8 mg/day, for agitation or insomnia. No patient on olanzapine required prophylactic anticonvulsant treatment for developing an abnormal EEG or convulsions, but four of the patients on clozapine required such medication (Kumra et al., 1998). The authors concluded that clozapine remains the "gold standard" for the treatment of schizophrenia but that, because of olanzapine's much more favorable untoward-effect profile and indication of therapeutic efficacy in some of their subjects, it is a good first-line choice for treating schizophrenia with childhood onset.

Olanzapine in the Treatment of Children and Adolescents Diagnosed with PDDs

Potenza et al. (1999) reported a 12-week, open-label, pilot study in which olanzapine monotherapy was prescribed to eight patients (mean age, 20.9 ± 11.7 years; range, 5 to 42 years), of whom four were children or adolescents, diagnosed by DSM-IV (APA, 1994) criteria with autistic disorder ($N = 5$) or with PDD not otherwise specified (PDDNOS) of at least moderate severity. Four subjects had full-scale intelligence quotients (FSIQs) in the mildly retarded range, and three subjects had FSIQs in the moderately retarded range. Seven of the subjects had prior drug trials, including at least one typical antipsychotic that was clinically ineffective or produced unacceptable untoward effects. Efficacy was assessed using the Yale-Brown Obsessive-Compulsive Scale Compulsion subscale (Y-BOCS-CS), the Self-Injurious Behavior Questionnaire (SIB-Q), the Vineland Adaptive Behavior Scale Maladaptive Behavior subscales (VMBS), the Ritvo-Freeman Real-Life Rating Scale (RFRLRS), the CGI-I Scale, and the Clinician-Rated Visual Analog Scale (VAS).

All subjects had a 4-week, drug-free period before beginning the 12-week protocol. An initial daily dose of 2.5 mg of olanzapine was prescribed for the first 2 weeks. Olanzapine was then titrated upward in 2.5- to 5.0-mg increments to a maximum of 20 mg/day, usually given at bedtime. Seven subjects completed the study and the eighth dropped out after 9 weeks because of failure to improve, the last observation of that case was carried forward, intent-to-treat methodology was used in the data analysis. The mean dose of olanzapine at week 12 was 7.8 ± 4.7 mg/day (range, 5 to 20 mg/day). Six patients were considered responders, and the response was not correlated with dose, age, IQ, SIB or repetitive behaviors, or baseline severity of illness. By the end of week 4, subjects showed a significant mean improvement over baseline on the CGI-I ($P = .015$) with further improvement at the end of the 8th and 12th weeks ($P < .001$). There was also significant improvement on items of the VAS, such as temper tantrums, impulsivity, anxiety, social withdrawal, rocking, destruction of property, and inappropriate sexual behavior; and the RFRLRS behavioral constellations for sensory motor behaviors, social relationship to people, affectual reactions, sensory responses, and language use and response, and the SIB-Q showed a significant reduction in aggressive behavior over time. Repetitive behaviors rated on the Y-BOCS-CS showed no significant improvement. The most clinically significant untoward effects were sedation in three subjects and significant weight gain in six subjects. The group mean weight at the end of the 12-week period was 70.88 ± 25.06 kg, compared with 62.50 ± 25.37 kg at baseline ($P = .008$). The guardians of two children who were responders discontinued their olanzapine 2 and 8 weeks after the initial period because they felt the clinical benefit was not sufficient to tolerate the significant weight gain.

Bipolar Disorder

FDA Registry Trials

Adolescents (ages 13 to 17): Efficacy was established in one 3-week trial in patients with manic or mixed episodes associated with bipolar I disorder. The increased potential (in adolescents compared with adults) for weight gain and hyperlipidemia may lead clinicians to consider prescribing other drugs first in adolescents. Compared with patients from adult clinical trials, adolescents were likely to gain more weight, experience increased sedation, and have greater increases in total cholesterol, triglycerides, LDL cholesterol, prolactin, and hepatic aminotransferase levels.

Reports of Interest

Olanzapine in the Treatment of Children and Adolescents Diagnosed with Bipolar Disorder

Frazier et al. (2000) treated 23 subjects (age range, 5 to 14 years), diagnosed with bipolar disorder and currently manic or mixed, with olanzapine on an open-label basis for up to 8 weeks. The dose ranged from 2.5 to 20 mg/day. Efficacy was evaluated by ratings on the YMRS with responders defined a priori as having $\geq 30\%$ improvement in total score from baseline to endpoint and by ratings of ≤ 3 ("very much improved," "much improved," or "improved") on the Clinical Global Impressions–Bipolar Mania (CGI-BP) Improvement Scale. Twenty-two (95.7%) completed the study, the 23rd developed depressive symptoms and dropped out. Mean ratings on the YMRS decreased by 19.04 ± 9.21 ($P < .001$), and 60.9% were rated as responders. No significant EPS were noted; however, subjects' weights increased significantly (4.98 ± 2.32 kg over the course of the treatment).

Quetiapine Fumarate (Seroquel)

Quetiapine fumarate (Seroquel) belongs to a new chemical class, the dibenzothiazepine derivatives. The drug antagonizes 5-HT_{1a}, 5-HT_3, dopamine D_1, dopamine D_2, histamine H_1, adrenergic alpha-1, and adrenergic alpha-2 neurotransmitter receptors in the brain. It has no appreciable affinity at cholinergic muscarinic and benzodiazepine receptors. It is suggested that its antipsychotic properties may be mediated through its antagonism of dopamine type 2 (D_2) and serotonin type 2 (5-HT_2) receptors. Quetiapine's antagonism of H_1 and adrenergic alpha-1 receptors may explain the sedation and hypotension, respectively, sometimes observed with the drug. It was approved by the FDA in 1997 for adult patients.

Pharmacokinetics of Quetiapine Fumarate

Food affects the bioavailability of quetiapine fumarate only marginally. Peak serum levels occur at a mean of 1.5 hours after ingestion. Quetiapine fumarate is extensively metabolized, primarily in the liver, by sulfoxidation by cytochrome P450 3A4 isoenzyme, to its major, sulfoxide metabolite, and by oxidation; both metabolites are pharmacologically inactive.

Steady-state serum concentrations occur after approximately 2 days on a given dose regimen. Terminal serum half-life is approximately 6 hours.

Gender, race, and smoking have no clinically significant effects on the metabolism of quetiapine fumarate.

Contraindications for Quetiapine Fumarate Administration

Quetiapine fumarate is contraindicated in patients with a known hypersensitivity to it.

Quetiapine fumarate should be administered with caution to patients with hepatic impairment, which may increase plasma levels.

▌ Advantages of Quetiapine Fumarate

Quetiapine fumarate does not cause statistically significant changes in the QT, QTc, and PR intervals of the ECG.

▌ Adverse Effects of Quetiapine Fumarate

Extrapyramidal Symptoms

The incidence of treatment-emergent EPS in patients treated with quetiapine fumarate is not significantly different from that in patients treated with placebo over a daily dose range of 75 to 750 mg.

Other Adverse Effects

Orthostatic hypotension, dizziness, tachycardia, weight gain, somnolence, constipation, dry mouth, dyspepsia, and many other untoward effects have been reported in patients taking quetiapine.

Indications for Quetiapine Fumarate in Child and Adolescent Psychiatry

The PI states because of the increased potential (in adolescents compared with adults) for weight gain and hyperlipidemia may lead clinicians to consider prescribing other drugs first in adolescents.

Quetiapine is indicated in adolescents 13 to 17 years of age for the treatment of schizophrenia and in children and adolescents 10 to 17 years of age for the treatment of manic episodes associated with bipolar I disorder.

Quetiapine Dosage Schedule

Quetiapine can be taken without regard to food.

- *Children and adolescents 12 years of age and less:* not recommended in schizophrenia.
- *Children and adolescents 9 years of age and less:* not recommended in bipolar I disorder. The safety and effectiveness of quetiapine have not been established for pediatric populations <10 years of age.

Treatment of Schizophrenia

Adolescents 13 to 17 years of age: Day 1: 25 mg twice daily. Day 2: twice-daily dosing totaling 100 mg. Day 3: twice-daily dosing totaling 200 mg. Day 4: twice-daily dosing totaling 300 mg. Day 5: twice-daily dosing totaling 400 mg. A flexible dose range of 400 to 800 mg was used in clinical trials based on response and tolerability and shown to be efficacious. However, no additional benefit was seen in the 800-mg group. The safety of doses over 800 mg/day has not been evaluated in clinical trials. Based on tolerability issues, quetiapine may be administered three times daily when indicated.

Treatment of Acute Manic Episodes Associated with Bipolar I Disorder

Children and adolescents 10 to 17 years of age: Day 1: 25 mg twice daily. Day 2: twice-daily dosing totaling 100 mg. Day 3: twice-daily dosing totaling 200 mg. Day 4: twice-daily dosing totaling 300 mg. Day 5: twice-daily dosing totaling 400 mg. Dosage adjustments should be in increments of no greater than 100 mg/day. A flexible dose range of 400 to 600 mg was used in clinical trials based on response and tolerability and shown to be efficacious. However, no additional benefit was seen in the 600-mg group. The safety of doses over 600 mg/day has not been evaluated in clinical trials. Based on tolerability issues, quetiapine may be administered three times daily when indicated.

Quetiapine Fumarate Dose Forms Available

- *Tablets:* 25, 50, 100, 200, 300, and 400 mg

Quetiapine Fumarate XR (Extended-Release) Dose Forms Available

- *Tablets:* 50, 150, 200, 300, and 400 mg

Schizophrenia

FDA Registry Trials

Adolescents (ages 10 to 17): Efficacy was established in one 3-week, double-blind, placebo-controlled trial in patients with schizophrenia.

Bipolar Disorder

FDA Registry Trials

Adolescents (ages 13 to 17): Efficacy was established in one 3-week double-blind, placebo-controlled, multicenter trial in patients with manic episodes associated with bipolar I disorder.

The increased potential (in adolescents compared with adults) for weight gain and hyperlipidemia may lead clinicians to consider prescribing other drugs first in adolescents. Compared with patients from adult clinical trials, adolescents were likely to gain more weight, experience increased sedation, and have greater increases in total cholesterol, triglycerides, LDL cholesterol, prolactin, and hepatic aminotransferase levels.

Reports of Interest

Quetiapine Fumarate in the Treatment of Children and Adolescents Diagnosed with Autistic Disorder

Martin et al. (1999) treated six male outpatients (mean age, 10.9 ± 3.3 years; age range, 6.2 to 15.3 years) diagnosed with autistic disorder by DSM-IV (APA, 1994) criteria with quetiapine in a 16-week, open-label study. All were mentally retarded (two mild, three moderate, one severe). Target symptoms for five patients were aggression, self-injury, and poor impulse control, and for the sixth interfering stereotypies and repetitive behaviors. Quetiapine was begun with a nighttime dose of 25 mg and titrated on the basis of clinical response, with increases up to 100 mg/ week permitted. Efficacy was assessed by ratings on the ABC, the CGI-I Scale, with subjects rated "much improved" or "very much improved" considered responders, the Ritvo-Freeman Real-Life Rating Scale (RFRLRS), and the Children's Yale-Brown Obsessive-Compulsive Scale (CY-BOCS). Only two subjects completed the 16-week study. Three (50%) dropped out (two after 4 weeks and one after 8 weeks) because sedation and the lack of clinical improvement were so problematic that the dose of quetiapine could not be increased (one of the three also had an apparent seizure), and the fourth dropped out after 4 weeks because of behavioral activation and apparent akathisia. Mean dose of quetiapine at endpoint or at dropout was 225 ± 108 mg/day (range, 100 to 350 mg/day). Based on the CGI-I, only the two subjects who completed the 16 weeks were responders, one "very much improved" and the other "much improved"; of the four nonresponders, one was "much worse," two were "minimally worse," and one was "no change." Four subjects experienced increased appetite and a mean weight gain of 2.9 ± 3.6 kg. Overall, quetiapine was poorly tolerated and/or ineffective for two-thirds of the subjects, and only one of the two responders continued to benefit from long-term treatment with quetiapine.

Findling et al. (2004) reported a 12-week, open-label study in nine subjects (age range 12.0 to 17.3 years; eight males, one female) diagnosed with autistic disorder and having a score of >30 on the Childhood Autism Rating Scale (CARS), and a rating on the CGI-S of at least moderately ill. Target symptoms included aggression, SIB, tantrums, irritability, overactivity, and social withdrawal. Quetiapine was begun at 25 mg twice daily for 3 days and then increased to 50 mg twice daily for the next 11 days. At the beginning of week 3, the dose was increased by 50 mg twice daily every other week to reach a target dose of 150 mg twice daily (300 mg/ day). Following this, the dose could be increased by a total of 25 to 75 mg/week, based on tolerability and clinical response, to a maximum of 750 mg/day.

Mean total quetiapine daily dose was 291.7, dose range 100 to 450 mg. Responders were defined as having ratings of 1 (very much improved) or 2 (much improved) on the CGI-I rating at endpoint. Six patients completed the study; one dropped out because of increased aggression/agitation and one dropped out because of drowsiness, whereas the final patient was lost to follow-up after 1 week. Only two of the eight patients (25%) who received medication were responders. The most frequent side effects reported by parents were sedation ($N = 7$), weight gain ($N = 5$), agitation ($N = 4$), and aggression ($N = 2$). The authors noted that quetiapine was not particularly effective clinically in these treatment-resistant adolescents with autistic disorder (Findling et al., 2004).

Quetiapine in Children and Adolescents with Conduct Disorder

Findling et al. (2006a) conducted an 8-week, open-label outpatient trial of quetiapine in patients aged 6 to 12 years with a primary diagnosis of CD to address if quetiapine was superior to placebo in ameliorating aggression in children. Notably, exclusion criteria included any other psychiatric comorbidity with the exception of ADHD, nor could they participate if they had any other clinically significant general medical condition or any organic mental syndrome including mental retardation. Of the 17 subjects enrolled, 16 were boys with a mean age of 8.9 years and all subjects met diagnostic symptom criteria for comorbid ADHD/combined type. The study also collected pharmacokinetic (PK) data in children via intensive blood sampling to complement a study by McConville et al. (2000), which found that the PK properties of quetiapine in a group of 10 adolescents aged 12 to 15 years were similar to those previously described in adults.

During the acute trial phase, patients were seen at a predose baseline visit, 12 to 24 hours following the first dose of medication, and then at the end of study week 1. Patients were then seen weekly for the next 3 weeks and at study weeks 6 and 8.

Initial dosing was weight based with patients weighing <35 kg administered a single morning dose of 25 mg quetiapine. Patients weighing >35 kg began treatment with 25 mg quetiapine in the morning and 25 mg quetiapine 1 hour before bedtime. Each subject's study medication was increased until a total daily dose of approximately 3 mg/kg/day was reached by the end of week 1. This dose was then maintained until the end of week 2 when blood was drawn for PK sampling. Patients treated with >25 mg quetiapine per day were dosed twice daily. After completion of the end of week 2 when the first PK sampling occurred, patients could then have their medication increased to either a total daily dose of 6 mg/kg/day or 750 mg/day (whichever was lower). Dose increases from 25 to 50 mg/week were permitted at any time up to the end of week 7 at the discretion of the patient's treating psychiatrist. Dose decreases were also permitted. No concomitant psychotropic or general medical medications were allowed during this study. After blood was drawn for PK analysis at the end of week 2, an additional blood drawn for PK analysis occurred at the end of week 8 of treatment.

The primary outcome measure was the RAAPPS score (Kemph et al., 1993). The clinician-rated RAAPPS records severity of aggressive behaviors with lower scores representing more modest degrees of aggressive behavior. This single-item scale has a possible score ranging from 1 (no aggression) to 5 (intolerable). Multiple secondary measures were utilized to assess various behaviors and emotions, overall psychosocial functioning, and the severity of a patient's psychiatric condition.

At the patient's final study visit, those attaining a CGI-I Scale score of 1 or 2, indicative of being "very much" or "much improved," respectively, were considered responders.

Twelve of the 17 patients enrolled completed all 8 weeks of the study. The median study dose of quetiapine at week 8 was 150 mg (range 75 to 300 mg) with a mean dose of 4.4 mg/kg. RAAPPS and CGI-S scores at weeks 4 and 8 evidenced significant differences reflecting improvement for several domains, including aggression and conduct problems. At week 8, 6 of the 12 patients who completed treatment were given CGI-I scores of 1 or 2 and were considered responders.

Regarding AEs, 15 (88.2%) of the 17 dosed patients experienced an AE during the course of the study. The most frequently reported side effects included the following: fatigue ($N = 11$), nasal congestion ($N = 8$), headache ($N = 7$), nausea ($N = 4$), sedation ($N = 4$), increased appetite ($N = 4$), vomiting ($N = 3$), stomach pain ($N = 3$), irritability ($N = 2$), and fever ($N = 2$). No patient withdrew from the study because of an AE, however.

A significant change in patient body weight from baseline to week 8 LOCF was observed in the 12 patients who completed the study. Overall median increase in weight in these 12 patients was 2.3 kg at week 8 ($P < .001$). Fasting morning blood chemistry evaluations showed no clinically significant changes between baseline and week 8 LOCF visits. Prolactin levels were obtained in 16 patients at the screening visit and in 10 patients at week 8. No elevation of prolactin levels was found. No neurological symptoms were observed during the course of the study as measured by the Neurological Rating Scale, Barnes Akathisia Scale, and the Abnormal Involuntary Movement Scale. In addition, no significant changes on physical examination were noted during the course of this study.

A statistical analysis of quetiapine PK data was conducted. Comprehensive blood sampling for the determination of timed quetiapine plasma concentrations was possible in 12 patients at study week 2 and in 10 patients at study week 8. Calculated quetiapine PK parameter estimates for both study periods indicate that the drug was rapidly absorbed from the intestinal tract, reflected by the average T_{max} of 1.2 and 1 hour at study weeks 2 and 8, respectively. Quetiapine $T_{1/2}$ averaged 3.9 and 2.9 hours and total body clearance (Cl) averaged 3.5 and 3.0 L/hr/kg at weeks 2 and 8, respectively. Furthermore, the disposition of quetiapine was linear over the dose range studied. No statistically significant relationships or differences were observed for quetiapine C_{max}, T_{max}, or Cl relative to age, study period, or dose. In general, it appears that the PK profile of quetiapine, including the critical assessment of drug body elimination, is similar across studies of adults (DeVane and Nemeroff, 2001), adolescents (McConville et al., 2000), and children based on this study. Week 8 concentration data were used to examine graphically the possibility that overall concentrations, or concentration at a single time point could differentiate between responder and nonresponder status. No relationships were observed. In contrast, for the 10 patients with plasma quetiapine concentration determinations at week 8, statistical analysis revealed patients with 1-hour postdose quetiapine plasma concentrations >300 ng/mL were significantly more likely to be considered responders than those patients with plasma quetiapine concentrations <300 ng/mL (Fisher exact test, $P = .048$). Despite these observed trends, caution should be used in considering this preliminary finding because of the small number of patients that were studied and the limited age range (6 to 12 years) of these patients.

As approximately 99% of quetiapine is metabolized in the liver predominantly via cytochrome P450 3A4 (CYP 3A4) and a small contribution by CYP 2D6 (DeVane and Nemeroff, 2001), concurrent drug administration and/or hepatic dysfunction affecting these pathways may markedly affect PK parameters.

Given the limitations of a short, open-label design study with a small sample size the authors proposed quetiapine was found to be beneficial and generally well tolerated in the acute treatment of aggressive behavior in a small number of children with CD. Some of the author's concerns about the long-term safety of quetiapine in the pediatric population have been better delineated since this study was published. Quetiapine continues to be considered an agent with a mild risk of EPS or other neurological side-effects but its potential for significant weight gain and metabolic syndrome are clearly relative to a risk–benefit analysis when considering quetiapine in this pediatric population.

Aripiprazole (ABILIFY)

Aripiprazole belongs to the chemical class of quinolinone derivatives. It was approved by the FDA for marketing in the United States in 2002 for adults. The manufacturer suggests that its antipsychotic properties may be mediated through its partial agonism of dopamine type 2 (D_2) and serotonin type 1 (5-HT_{1A}) receptors and antagonism of serotonin type 2 (5-HT_{2A}) receptors.

Pharmacokinetics of Aripiprazole

Taken orally, aripiprazole is well absorbed and peak plasma concentrations occur within 3 to 5 hours. Taking it with food does not significantly alter peak plasma concentrations; however, it may delay them for several hours. Activity is due to aripiprazole (approximately 60%) and its major metabolite dehydro-aripiprazole (approximately 40%) at steady-state plasma levels, which are achieved for both within 14 days. Mean elimination half-lives are approximately 75 hours for aripiprazole and approximately 94 hours for dehydro-aripiprazole. The major metabolism is through the hepatic P450 isomers CYP2D6 and CYP3A4. Most of the metabolites and some unchanged drug are excreted in the feces; a lesser but significant amount is excreted by the kidneys.

Approximately 8% of Caucasians are poor metabolizers of aripiprazole because they have decreased ability to metabolize CYP2D6 substrates. Such individuals have a net increase of approximately 60% on exposure to the drug, compared with extensive (normal) metabolizers of the drug. The elimination half-life of aripiprazole for poor metabolizers is approximately 146 hours, nearly twice that of extensive metabolizers.

Interactions of Aripiprazole with Other Drugs

Drugs such as quinine, which inhibit CYP2D6, can result in more than a doubling of plasma levels and require downward adjustment of the dose of aripiprazole. If fluoxetine or paroxetine, both potential CYP2D6 inhibitors, is given concomitantly, the aripiprazole dose should be reduced by at least one-half of the usual dose.

Contraindications for Aripiprazole Administration

Aripiprazole is contraindicated in patients with known hypersensitivity to the drug.

Adverse Effects of Aripiprazole

Commonly observed adverse reactions (>5% incidence and at least twice the rate of placebo for ABILIFY vs. placebo, respectively):

- *Pediatric patients (13 to 17 years) with schizophrenia:* extrapyramidal disorder (17% vs. 5%), somnolence (16% vs. 6%), and tremor (7% vs. 2%)
- *Pediatric patients (10 to 17 years) with bipolar mania:* somnolence (23% vs. 3%), extrapyramidal disorder (20% vs. 3%), fatigue (11% vs. 4%), nausea (11% vs. 4%), akathisia (10% vs. 2%), blurred vision (8% vs. 0%), salivary hypersecretion (6% vs. 0%), and dizziness (5% vs. 1%)

ECG Changes

No significant ECG differences were found between subjects administered placebo and aripiprazole in the pooled data of the premarketing trials; within the dose range of 10 to 30 mg, aripiprazole tended to slightly shorten the QTc interval. There was a median increase in heart rate of 4 beats per minute in subjects treated with aripiprazole.

Weight

In premarketing studies of 4 to 6 weeks duration, subjects receiving aripiprazole gained a mean of 0.7 kg compared with subjects on placebo who lost a mean of 0.05 kg. In a 52-week study, weight gain or loss was related to initial BMI. Subjects with a BMI of <23 gained a mean of 2.6 kg and 30% had an increase in weight of >7% over baseline measures. The data for subjects with baseline BMIs of 23 to 27 were a mean weight gain of 1.4 kg with 19% experiencing a weight gain of >7%. Subjects with a BMI >27 lost a mean weight of 1.2 kg, but 8% of them still gained >7% of their baseline body weight.

Indications for Aripiprazole in Child and Adolescent Psychiatry

Aripiprazole is indicated in adolescents 13 to 17 years of age for the treatment of schizophrenia, in children and adolescents 10 to 17 years of age for the treatment of manic or mixed episodes associated with bipolar I disorder, both as monotherapy and as an adjunct to lithium or valproate and in children and adolescents 10 to 17 years of age for the treatment of irritability associated with autistic disorder.

Aripiprazole Dosage Schedule

- *Children 9 years of age and less:* not recommended. The safety and effectiveness of olanzapine have not been established for pediatric populations <12 years of age.

Treatment of Schizophrenia

Adolescents 13 to 17 years of age: The recommended starting daily dose of the tablet formulation is 2 mg, which in the studies was titrated to 5 mg after 2 days and to the target dose of 10 mg after 2 additional days. Subsequent dose increases should be administered in 5 mg increments. The 30-mg/day dose was not shown to be more efficacious than the 10-mg/day dose. ABILIFY can be administered without regard to meals. Maintenance efficacy was demonstrated in one trial in adults and can be extrapolated to adolescents.

Treatment of Acute Manic Episodes Associated with Bipolar I Disorder

Children and adolescents 10 to 17 years of age: The recommended starting dose as monotherapy is 2 mg/day, with titration to 5 mg/day after 2 days, and a target dose of 10 mg/day after 2 additional days. Recommended dosing as adjunctive therapy to lithium orvalproate is the same. Subsequent dose increases, if needed, should be administered in 5-mg/day increments. ABILIFY can be given without regard to meals. The recommended dose for maintenance treatment, whether as monotherapy or as adjunctive therapy, is the same dose needed to stabilize patients during acute treatment, both for adult and pediatric patients. Patients should be periodically reassessed to determine the continued need for maintenance treatment.

Treatment of Irritability Associated with Autistic Disorder

Children and adolescents 6 to 17 years of age: The recommended starting dose is 2 mg/day. The dose should be increased to 5 mg/day, with subsequent increases to 10 or 15 mg/day if needed. Dose adjustments of up to 5 mg/day should occur gradually, at intervals of no less than 1 week. The efficacy of ABILIFY for the maintenance treatment of irritability associated with autistic disorder has not been evaluated. Although there is no body of evidence available to answer the question of how long the patient treated with ABILIFY should be maintained, patients should be periodically reassessed to determine the continued need for maintenance treatment.

Aripiprazole Dose Forms Available

- *Tablets:* 2, 5, 10, 15, 20, and 30 mg
- *DISCMELT Orally Disintegrating Tablets:* 10 and 15 mg
- *Oral solution:* 1 mg/mg
- Injection for intramuscular use is a clear, colorless solution available as a ready-to-use, 9.75 mg/1.3 mL (7.5 mg/mL)

Schizophrenia

FDA Registry Trials

Adolescents (ages 13 to 17): The efficacy of ABILIFY (aripiprazole) in the treatment of schizophrenia in pediatric patients (13 to 17 years of age) was evaluated in one 6-week, placebo-controlled trial of outpatients who met DSM-IV criteria for schizophrenia and had a PANSS score ≥70 at baseline. In this trial ($N = 302$) comparing two fixed doses of ABILIFY (10 or 30 mg/day) to placebo, ABILIFY was titrated starting from 2 mg/day to the target dose in 5 days in the 10-mg/day treatment arm and in 11 days in the 30-mg/day treatment arm. Both doses of ABILIFY were superior to placebo in the PANSS total score, the primary outcome measure of the study. The 30-mg/day dosage was not shown to be more efficacious than the 10-mg/day dose.

Commonly Observed Adverse Reactions

Commonly observed adverse reactions associated with the use of aripiprazole in adolescent patients with schizophrenia (incidence of 5% or greater and aripiprazole incidence at least twice that for placebo) were extrapyramidal disorder, somnolence, and tremor.

Bipolar Disorder

FDA Registry Trials

Children and adolescents (ages 10 to 17): The efficacy of ABILIFY in the treatment of bipolar I disorder in pediatric patients (10 to 17 years of age) was evaluated in one 4-week, placebo-controlled trial ($N = 296$) of outpatients who met DSM-IV criteria for bipolar I disorder manic or mixed episodes with or without psychotic features and had a YMRS score ≥20 at baseline. This double-blind, placebo-controlled trial compared two fixed doses of ABILIFY (10 or 30mg/day) with placebo. The ABILIFY dose was started at 2 mg/day, which was titrated to 5 mg/day after 2 days, and to the target dose in 5 days in the 10-mg/day treatment arm and in 13 days in the 30-mg/day treatment arm. Both doses of ABILIFY were superior to placebo in change from baseline to week 4 on the YMRS total score.

Commonly Observed Adverse Reactions

Commonly observed adverse reactions associated with the use of aripiprazole in adolescent patients with schizophrenia (incidence of 5% or greater and aripiprazole incidence at least twice that for placebo) were somnolence, extrapyramidal disorder, fatigue, and nausea.

Autistic Disorder

FDA Registry Trials

Children and adolescents (ages 6 to 17): The efficacy of ABILIFY in the treatment of irritability associated with autistic disorder was established in two 8-week, placebo-controlled trials in pediatric patients (6 to 17 years of age) who met the DSM-IV criteria for autistic disorder and demonstrated behaviors such as tantrums, aggression, SIB, or a combination of these problems. More than 75% of these subjects were below 13 years of age.

Efficacy was evaluated using two assessment scales: the ABC and the CGI-I Scale. The primary outcome measure in both trials was the change from baseline to endpoint in the Irritability subscale of the ABC (ABC-I). The ABC-I subscale measured the emotional and behavioral symptoms of irritability in autistic disorder, including aggression toward others, deliberate self-injuriousness, temper tantrums, and quickly changing moods. The results of these trials are as follows:

In one of the 8-week, placebo-controlled trials, children and adolescents with autistic disorder ($N = 98$), aged 6 to 17 years, received daily doses of placebo or

ABILIFY 2 to 15 mg/day. ABILIFY, starting at 2 mg/day with increases allowed up to 15 mg/day based on clinical response, significantly improved scores on the ABC-I subscale and on the CGI-I Scale compared with placebo. The mean daily dose of ABILIFY at the end of 8-week treatment was 8.6 mg/day.

In the other 8-week, placebo-controlled trial in children and adolescents with autistic disorder ($N = 218$), aged 6 to 17 years, three fixed doses of ABILIFY (5, 10, or 15 mg/day) were compared with placebo. ABILIFY dosing started at 2 mg/day and was increased to 5 mg/day after 1 week. After the second week, it was increased to 10 mg/day for patients in the 10- and 15-mg dose arms, and after the third week, it was increased to 15 mg/day in the 15-mg/day treatment arm. All three doses of ABILIFY significantly improved scores on the ABC-I subscale compared with placebo (ABILIFY [package insert], 2012).

Commonly Observed Adverse Reactions

Commonly observed adverse reactions associated with the use of aripiprazole in adolescent patients with autism in decreasing order (incidence of 5% or greater and aripiprazole incidence at least twice that for placebo) were sedation, fatigue, vomiting, somnolence, tremor, pyrexia, drooling, decreased appetite, salivary hypersecretion, extrapyramidal disorder, and lethargy (ABILIFY [package insert], 2012).

Reports of Interest

Aripiprazole in Children and Adolescents with Conduct Disorder

Findling et al. (2009) conducted an open-label, 15-day, three-center study with an optional 36-month extension that enrolled a total of 23 patients: 12 children (6 to 12 years) and 11 adolescents (13 to 17 years) with CD and a score of 2 to 3 on the RAAPP. This study consisted of an initial 15-day, outpatient pharmacokinetic study (Phase A) at the end of which subjects were permitted to enter the open-label extension treatment period (Phase B) of 36 months during which frequent reassessment for safety and efficacy occurred. Throughout Phase B, the dose could be adjusted at the discretion of the investigator up to a maximum of 15 mg/day. Notably stimulants were allowed from months 2 through 36. All 23 subjects completed the initial 14 days of treatment (Phase A) and continued into the 36-month continuation phase (Phase B). Of these, only five patients (21.7%, two children and three adolescents) completed 36 months of treatment and 18 (78.3%) discontinued prior to the 36-month time point. The aripiprazole dose was adjusted upward in Phase B for most patients ($N = 14/23$, 60.9%), with 6 of these 14 patients eventually receiving the maximum dose. Overall, RAAPP scores improved during the course of the study. Treatment effect appeared early as both children and adolescents showed a median score of 2 at Day 14 and remained at this level at month 36. By Day 14, 63.6% of children and 45.5% of adolescents were rated as much or very much improved on the CGI-I score. At month 36, 66.7% of children and 100% of adolescents showed this level of CGI-I score (much or very much improved) (observed cases, OC). A neuropsychological battery consisting of the Wisconsin Card Sort Test, pediatric version (WCST), Conners' Continuous Performance Test II (CPT II), and the Verbal Fluency Test (VFT) showed, on average, minor improvements per the authors.

Treatment with aripiprazole was generally well tolerated after the initial dose adjustment was revised following vomiting in four and somnolence in three children. Throughout the study, there were five reports of EPS, three of them being in Phase A. All EPS reports were considered to be of mild intensity by the investigator and did not lead to discontinuation. There were no serious AEs and no subjects discontinued due to AEs. Only two laboratory findings of potential clinical significance were observed; an elevated creatine phosphokinase on Day 737 that lasted for 3 days in one subject and a mild elevation of hepatic enzymes on Day 169 that lasted for 15 days in another subject. Both investigators considered these to be not clinically significant and it was not reported as an AE. An elevated prolactin level was not reported for any subject. No subjects were discontinued from the study because of vital-sign abnormalities.

Mean weight change (LOCF) in patients ≤12 years old from baseline to week 72 was 9.0 ± 11.0 kg. In patients ≤13 years old, the mean change in weight was 3.3 ± 15.5 kg. Mean BMI change in patients ≤12 years old from baseline to week 72 was 1.8 kg/m². In patients ≤13 years old, the mean change in BMI from baseline was 3.4 kg/m². The authors proposed that although weight and BMI increased in children and adolescents over the study duration, weight gain in this population is normal and the findings were therefore not unexpected. No patients discontinued due to weight gain. Total cholesterol and glucose levels did not appear to be affected negatively by treatment.

In regard to the pharmacokinetics studies, it appears the steady state was attained within 14 days of once-daily aripiprazole dosing. The authors concluded the mean apparent oral clearance of aripiprazole, when normalized for body weight, was similar across age groups.

The authors proposed that the preliminary data from this study (which was done before aripiprazole was FDA approved for treatment of schizophrenia and bipolar disorder in adolescent patients) suggest that aripiprazole may improve symptoms of CD with modest impact on cognitive function in both children and adolescents; however, the sample size was too small to draw any firm conclusions. It also supported the learned clinical practice enacted by early clinicians of starting aripiprazole at low doses initially and titrating gradually over the first 10 to 14 days to reduce the incidence of nausea and vomiting which was unfortunately too frequent when more aggressive dosing was utilized.

Ziprasidone Hydrochloride (Geodon)

The manufacturer suggests that ziprasidone's antipsychotic properties may be mediated through its antagonism of dopamine type 2 (D_2) and serotonin type 2 (5-HT_{2A}) receptors.

It was approved by the FDA for marketing in the United States in 2001.

Pharmacokinetics of Ziprasidone Hydrochloride

Taken orally, ziprasidone is well absorbed and peak plasma concentrations occur within 6 to 8 hours. Absorption is increased up to twofold when taken with food. Elimination is mainly through hepatic metabolism; about one-third of the excretory metabolites are oxidized by P450 CYP3A4, and about two-thirds result from reduction by aldehyde oxidase. Approximately 20% is excreted in the urine and 66% in the feces. Mean terminal half-life is approximately 7 hours for doses in the recommended clinical range. Steady-state plasma levels are achieved within 1 to 3 days at a constant dose.

Interactions of Ziprasidone with Other Drugs

Carbamazepine, an inducer of CYP3A4, resulted in a decrease of approximately 35% in ziprasidone AUC ("the total amount of drug absorbed into the systemic circulation and available for distribution to the target organ and site of action"; Ayd, 2000).

Contraindications for Ziprasidone Administration

Ziprasidone is contraindicated in patients with known hypersensitivity to the drug or in patients who have familial long QT syndrome or a history of cardiac arrhythmias or other significant cardiovascular illnesses.

Ziprasidone should not be prescribed concomitantly with other drugs that are known to prolong the QTc interval.

Adverse Effects of Ziprasidone

ECG changes: Ziprasidone is associated with increases in the QTc interval. In placebo-controlled trials, ziprasidone increased the QTc interval by approximately 10 msec at a dose of 160 mg/day compared with placebo. In direct comparisons with five other antipsychotic medications, the mean increase in QTc over baseline in subjects receiving ziprasidone ranged from 9 to 14 msec greater than for subjects receiving risperidone, olanzapine, quetiapine, and haloperidol but was approximately 14 msec less than for subjects receiving thioridazine.

Indications for Ziprasidone Hydrochloride in Child and Adolescent Psychiatry

Ziprasidone is indicated for the treatment of schizophrenia and the treatment of acute mania episodes or mixed episodes associated with bipolar disorder. Ziprasidone intramuscular is indicated for the treatment of acute agitation in patients with schizophrenia and patients who need intramuscular antipsychotic medication for rapid control of the agitation.

Because of ziprasidone's greater capacity to increase the QT/QTc interval compared with several other antipsychotics, careful clinical consideration should be given to prescribing one or more trials of such alternative antipsychotics before undertaking a trial with ziprasidone.

Ziprasidone Dosage Schedule

- *Children and adolescents 17 years of age and less:* not recommended. The safety and efficacy of ziprasidone have not been established for pediatric populations.
- *Adolescents 18 years of age and older and adults:* an initial dose of 20 mg twice daily is recommended. Maximum total daily doses over 160 mg are not usually recommended. As it takes 1 to 3 days to achieve steady-state plasma levels, adjustments in dose should not be made at intervals of <2 days. In long-term studies (52 weeks) of subjects maintained on ziprasidone doses ranging from 20 to 80 mg b.i.d., no clinical advantage was demonstrated for doses over 20 mg b.i.d.

Ziprasidone Hydrochloride Dose Forms Available

- *Capsules:* 20, 40, 60, and 80 mg
- *Injection:* (ziprasidone mesylate) single-use vials 20 mg/mL for intramuscular injection. Doses are different from the oral doses; read package insert before use (Geodon [package insert], 2012).

Reports of Interest

Ziprasidone in the Treatment of Children and Adolescents Diagnosed with Autistic Disorder

McDougle et al. (2002) conducted an open-label trial to evaluate the safety and effectiveness of ziprasidone in treating 12 subjects (mean age 11.62 ± 4.38 years; age range 8 to 20 years) who were diagnosed with autistic disorder ($N = 9$) or PDD not otherwise specified (PDDNOS); ($N = 3$) by DSM-IV criteria; 11 subjects had codiagnoses of mental retardation (mild = 4, moderate = 6, and severe = 1). Target symptoms were aggression, self-injury, property destruction, agitation, irritability, and mood instability. Most subjects were treatment resistant, and 11 were previously treated with one or more other atypical antipsychotic drugs, with significant weight gain often causing their discontinuation. At the beginning of the study, five subjects were receiving an atypical antipsychotic, which was discontinued over a 4-week taper. Four subjects were permitted to continue on their usual dose of other medications during the study.

The initial dose of ziprasidone was 20 mg at bedtime and titrated upward according to clinical response and AEs, in increments of 10 to 20 mg/week, and divided into two daily doses. All subjects completed a minimum of 6 weeks of the study; mean duration was 14.15 ± 8.29 weeks, range 6 to 30 weeks. The final mean ziprasidone dose was 59.23 ± 34.76 mg/day, dose range 20 to 120 mg/day. Responders were defined as subjects with a CGI-I rating of 1 (very much improved) or 2 (much improved). Six (50%) subjects were responders; two subjects with comorbid bipolar disorder were rated much worse. AEs were evaluated using a checklist used by the RUPP Autism Network. Four subjects reported no AEs. Sedation ($N = 5$), usually transient, was the most frequent AE, three experienced increased appetite and two had insomnia. Both the subjects with comorbid bipolar disorder experienced agitation and insomnia. One subject who had a history of TD of the hands developed an oral dyskinesia that resolved when ziprasidone was discontinued. The mean weight change was -5.83 ± 12.52 pounds, range -35 to $+6$ pounds. No cardiovascular AEs were reported; however, only a baseline ECG was performed. The authors suggested that ziprasidone is a potentially useful treatment for aggression, agitation, and irritability in children, adolescents, and young adults diagnosed with autistic disorder or PDDNOS and that further studies should be undertaken (McDougle et al., 2002).

Ziprasidone (Intramuscular) in the Treatment of Children and Adolescents Exhibiting Acute Agitation, Aggression, or Anxiety

Staller (2004) conducted a retrospective chart review of 49 children and adolescents (17 males, 32 females; age range 8 to 16 years), who were administered intramuscular ziprasidone for acute agitation and agitation/anxiety/threat ($N = 47$) or psychosis ($N = 2$) during hospitalization in an acute care private psychiatric hospital in central upstate New York. Most subjects (87%) were administered 20-mg injections; however, six subjects (two males and four females), all 13 years of age or younger, received 10-mg injections. Nursing notes indicated that only two patients continued to exhibit agitation and aggression during the subsequent shift and that only one of these was given a repeat 20-mg dose. There were no adverse reactions reported.

Ziprasidone Treatment of Children and Adolescents With Tourette Syndrome: A Pilot Study

Sallee et al. (2000a) conducted a study to evaluate the efficacy and tolerability of ziprasidone in children and adolescents with Tourette syndrome and chronic tic disorders. Twenty-eight patients aged 7 to 17 years were randomly assigned to ziprasidone or placebo for 56 days. Ziprasidone was initiated at a dose of 5 mg/day and flexibly titrated to a maximum of 40 mg/day. Ziprasidone was significantly more effective than placebo in reducing the Global Severity ($P = .016$) and Total Tic ($P = .008$) scores on the YGTSS. Compared with placebo, ziprasidone significantly reduced tic frequencies as determined by blind videotape tic counts ($P = .039$). The mean ($\pm$SD) daily dose of ziprasidone during the last 4 weeks of the trial was 28.2 ± 9.6 mg. Ziprasidone in a dosage from 5 to 40 mg/day appeared to be effective in the treatment of Tourette syndrome and was well tolerated with mild transient somnolence as the most common AE. No clinically significant effects were observed on specific ratings of EPS, akathisia, or TD.

Paliperidone Extended-Release Tablets (Invega)

Like risperidone, paliperidone is a psychotropic agent belonging to the chemical class of benzisoxazole derivatives. In fact, paliperidone is 9-hydroxyrisperidone, the chief active metabolite of risperidone, an established antipsychotic agent. Paliperidone, which is available in extended-release tablets (paliperidone ER; Invega), is an oral atypical antipsychotic medication that was first approved in December 2006 for the acute and maintenance treatment of schizophrenia in adults. It was the seventh SGA to be introduced to the U.S. market. In April 2011, the FDA approved Invega (paliperidone) extended-release tablets for the treatment of schizophrenia in children and adolescents 12 to 17 years of age.

In vivo studies suggest that the cytochrome P450 enzyme system plays a minimal role in paliperidone metabolism, with none of the metabolites accounting for >10% of a dose. Because of this limited hepatic metabolism, paliperidone should have minimal risks for hepatic drug–drug and drug–disease interactions. The majority (59%) of paliperidone is eliminated through the kidneys as unchanged drug.

Paliperidone demonstrates high affinity for central dopamine 2 and serotonin 2a receptors. In addition, it has affinity for both alpha-adrenergic 1 and 2 and histaminic 1 receptors. Paliperidone does not possess affinity for muscarinic-cholinergic and beta-adrenergic receptors.

Although the manufacturer notes that there have been isolated reports of TD associated with paliperidone, it is likely that the incidence of TD occurring with paliperidone only will be significantly less than that with typical antipsychotic agents.

Pharmacokinetics of Paliperidone

Paliperidone ER utilizes the OROS delivery system, which allows for once-daily dosing and a resulting pharmacokinetic profile, which exhibits a more stable serum concentration. OROS formulation delivers paliperidone at a controlled rate over a 24-hour period. This is the same delivery system as was developed for the stimulant Concerta. Rossenu et al. (2007) found that the OROS technology results in reduced fluctuations between drug peak and trough serum concentrations (e.g., 38% paliperidone ER vs. 125% risperidone immediate release [IR]). To preserve the integrity of the OROS delivery system, the tablet should be swallowed whole and not chewed, split, or crushed (Invega [package insert], 2012). Since the shell of the tablet is nonabsorbable, prescribers should inform patients that the undissolved residue may be observed in their stool.

Administration of this agent after a high-fat or high-calorie meal increased the maximum serum concentration and AUC values by 60% and 54%, respectively. While paliperidone ER can be taken without regard to meals, the presence of food may increase its exposure. Patients in the clinical efficacy trials, however, were dosed without regard to meal timing. The terminal half-life of paliperidone ER is about 23 hours in extensive metabolizers and 30 hours in poor metabolizers with steady-state concentration attained in 4 to 5 days.

Vermeir et al. (2005) reported that paliperidone ER undergoes very limited hepatic metabolism, with approximately 60% of the unchanged drug eliminated renally and 11% eliminated unchanged in the feces. Paliperidone is not expected to cause clinically important pharmacokinetic interactions with drugs that are metabolized by cytochrome P450 isozymes. *In vitro* studies in human liver microsomes showed that paliperidone does not substantially inhibit the metabolism of drugs metabolized by cytochrome P450 isozymes, including CYP1A2, CYP2A6, CYP2C8/9/10, CYP2D6, CYP2E1, CYP3A4, and CYP3A5 (Invega [package insert], 2012), which should translate into less hepatic drug–drug or drug–disease interactions. Rossenu et al. (2006) ascertained that in general the paliperidone ER pharmacokinetic profile demonstrates dose proportionality within the recommended clinical range of 3 to 12 mg/day.

Contraindications for Paliperidone Administration

Paliperidone is contraindicated in patients with a known hypersensitivity to it.

Interactions of Paliperidone with Other Drugs

Carbamazepine. Plasma concentrations of 9-hydroxyrisperidone were decreased by approximately 37% with coadministration of carbamazepine although plasma levels of carbamazepine did not appear to be affected.

Divalproex sodium. Plasma concentrations (C_{max}) and AUC of 9-hydroxyrisperidone were increased by approximately 50% with coadministration of divalproex sodium. In a clinical study, subjects on stable doses of valproate had comparable valproate average plasma concentrations when paliperidone ER 3 to 15 mg/day was added to their existing valproate treatment (Invega [package insert], 2012).

Pharmacokinetic interaction between lithium and paliperidone ER is unlikely.

In an interaction study in healthy subjects in which a single 3-mg dose of paliperidone ER was administered concomitantly with 20 mg/day of paroxetine (a potent CYP2D6 inhibitor), paliperidone exposures were on average 16% higher in CYP2D6 extensive metabolizers.

Adverse Effects of Paliperidone

Black Box Warning. As with all atypical antipsychotics, there is a "Black Box Warning" that there is increased mortality in elderly patients with dementia-related psychosis who are treated with atypical antipsychotic drugs including risperidone.

Extrapyramidal Symptoms. In the adolescents with schizophrenia trial akathisia, tremor, dystonia, and cogwheel rigidity were observed adverse reactions with an incidence ≥5% and at least twice that for placebo.

Hepatotoxicity. Paliperidone should have less hepatic issues than risperidone.

Weight Gain. Weight gain in adolescent subjects (12 to 17 years of age) with schizophrenia was assessed in a 6-week, double-blind, placebo-controlled study and an open-label extension with a median duration of exposure to paliperidone ER of 182 days.

In the open-label long-term study, the proportion of total subjects treated with paliperidone ER with an increase in body weight of ≥7% from baseline was 33%. However, this weight gain should be assessed against that expected increase in weight that occurs with normal growth over the 182-day length of the study to achieve a more clinically relevant measure of changes in weight. The mean change from open-label baseline to endpoint in standardized score for weight was 0.1 (4% above the median for normative data). Based on comparison to the normative data, these changes are not considered to be clinically significant. Although paliperidone ER appears to be well tolerated in short-term studies, long-term follow-up investigations of 1 to 2 years with ongoing clinical monitoring are necessary to confirm their safety in this age group.

Hyperprolactinemia. Paliperidone has a prolactin-elevating effect similar to that seen with risperidone, a drug that is associated with higher levels of prolactin than other antipsychotic drugs.

Hyperglycemia and Dyslipidemia. Previous epidemiologic studies suggested an increased risk of treatment-emergent hyperglycemia-related AEs in patients treated with atypical antipsychotic drugs, including risperidone (*PDR*, 2006). As well, undesirable alterations in lipids have been observed in patients treated with atypical antipsychotics, but as paliperidone was not marketed at the time these studies were performed, it is not known if paliperidone is associated with these increased risks. There were only limited changes in these parameters in the adolescent schizophrenia studies, but these trials were only 6 weeks in duration and of limited benefit in determining the true metabolic risk of paliperidone.

Other Untoward Effects. Paliperidone can induce orthostatic hypotension, tachycardia, dizziness, and syncope in some patients because of its alpha-blocking activity and thus tiration of dosages is indicated. Paliperidone causes a modest increase in the corrected QT (QTc) interval. The use of paliperidone should be avoided in combination with other drugs that are known to prolong QTc. In an adult QTc study, a 4-mg dose of the immediate-release oral formulation of paliperidone, showed an increased placebo-subtracted QTcLD of 6.8 msec on Day 2 at 1.5 hours post dose.

None of the subjects had a change exceeding 60 msec or a QTcLD exceeding 500 msec at any time during this study (Invega [package insert], 2012).

Indications for Paliperidone in Child and Adolescent Psychiatry

Paliperidone is indicated for the management of the manifestations of schizophrenia in adolescents aged 12 to 17 years.

Paliperidone ER Dosage Schedule for Schizophrenia

- *Children 11 years of age or less:* not recommended. The safety and effectiveness of paliperidone in this young pediatric age group have not been established.
- *Adolescents <51 kg:* an initial dose of 3 mg once daily, with a recommended dosing range of 3 to 6 mg and a maximum dosage of 6 mg.
- *Adolescents >51 kg:* an initial dose of 3 mg once daily, with a recommended dosing range of 3 to 12 mg and a maximum dosage of 12 mg.

Initial dose titration is not required. Dose increases, if considered necessary, should be made only after clinical reassessment and should occur at increments of 3 mg/day at intervals of more than 5 days. The manufacturer indicates that there was no clear enhancement to efficacy at the higher doses, that is, 6 mg for subjects weighing <51 and 12 mg for subjects weighing ≥51 kg, while AEs were dose related.

Clinical Pearl: To compare dosages of paliperidone to risperidone, a virtual comparison of the two drugs was conducted by Schooler et al. (2006). The authors combined data from all available randomized placebo-controlled studies of risperidone and paliperidone in adults with schizophrenia. Paliperidone 6 to 12 mg/day was found to be similarly efficacious to risperidone 4 to 6 mg/day, with some tolerability benefits. In addition, paliperidone 6 to 12 mg/day was found to be more efficacious than risperidone 2 to 4 mg/day, but was associated with increased tachycardia.

Paliperidone ER Dose Forms Available

- *Tablets:* 1.5, 3, 6, and 9 mg

Paliperidone Dosage Schedule for Bipolar

Paliperidone is not approved for bipolar disorder in children, adolescents, or adults.

Schizophrenia

FDA Registry Trials

The efficacy of paliperidone ER in adolescents with schizophrenia was established in a single, 6-week randomized, double-blind, placebo-controlled study using a fixed-dose weight-based treatment group design over a dose range of 1.5 to 12 mg/day.

The study was conducted in several countries, including the United States, and involved adolescents ranging in age from 12 to 17 years, all of whom met DSM-IV criteria for schizophrenia, with diagnosis confirmation using the Kiddie Schedule for Affective Disorders and Schizophrenia–Present and Lifetime Version (K-SADS-PL). Efficacy was evaluated using the PANSS, a validated multi-item inventory composed of 30 individual items to evaluate positive symptoms, negative symptoms, disorganized thoughts, uncontrolled hostility/excitement, and anxiety/depression.

The study used a weight-based dosing regimen with a low (1.5 mg), medium (3 mg), and high (9 mg) dose groups. Dosing was in the morning without regard to meals. Overall, this study demonstrated efficacy of paliperidone ER in adolescents within the dose range of 3 to 12 mg a day; however, there was no clear indication of enhanced efficacy at the higher doses, and AEs were dose related.

In the treatment group, the most commonly reported AEs in this study were somnolence (13%), akathisia (9%), headache (9%), and insomnia (9%). Like most atypical antipsychotic medications, significant weight gain can be a side effect as well.

Reports of Interest

Paliperidone ER for Irritability in Autistic Disorder

Stigler et al. (2010) reported on two case reports of autistic patients who manifested treatment-resistant aggression that benefited markedly when treated with paliperidone ER. The authors noted that, given the efficacy of risperidone in youths and adults with autism, paliperidone ER may be of benefit as well and have the advantages of once daily dosing, much less pharmacokinetic interactions and a lower incidence of EPS and weight gain as the latter was of considerable concern in the Risperdal registry trials. During the trial, the two patients received repeated health assessment via EKGs, vitals (including height and weight), and labwork (complete blood count (CBC), liver function tests, fasting glucose, and fasting lipid panel). Symptom improvement with the focus on the target symptom domain of irritability (aggression, SIBs, tantrums) was measured by utilizing the Clinical Global Impressions -Improvement (CGI-I) scale (Guy 1976b). Rated 1 to 7 (1 = very much improved; 2 = much improved; 3 = minimally improved; 4 = no change; 5 = minimally worse; 6 = much worse; 7 = very much worse). In this report, patients were judged treatment responders if assigned a posttrial CGI-I rating of 1 (very much improved) or 2 (much improved).

One patient was female and 16 years of age with verbal autism, comorbid mild mental retardation and intermittent explosive disorder, which was representative of her severe irritability, impulsive aggression toward others, as well as SIB. The patient also had a seizure disorder that was diagnosed in early childhood. Due to the severity of her irritability, physical aggression, SIB, and tantrums, she had received several prior adequate medication trials that were reported as ineffective. These trials included quetiapine, risperidone, aripiprazole, and valproic acid.

At the time of initial assessment, the patient was taking a medication regimen of ziprasidone 80 mg twice daily, naltrexone 75 mg daily, diazepam 10 mg three times daily, and oxcarbazepine 300 mg daily for her seizure disorder, which was well controlled. Her baseline labwork was notable for elevated liver function tests (AST, 74 [reference range, 15–41] and ALT, 108 [reference range, 0–45]). Fasting lipid panel revealed an elevated total cholesterol of 268 (reference range, <200) and LDL of 191 (reference range, 118–142). The investigators tapered off the ziprasidone over a period of 1 month. Paliperidone ER was subsequently initiated at a dosage of 3 mg daily. When the patient was continued at this dosage for 4 weeks with only modest improvement in her symptoms, overall it was elected to increase her dosage to 6 mg daily to target her residual symptoms. The patient responded to such a degree that she was judged to be "very much improved," in relation to her target symptoms of irritability (aggression, SIB, and tantrums). Due to her markedly improved functioning, naltrexone and diazepam were successfully tapered and discontinued over a period of 2 and 4 months, respectively. Repeat labwork obtained at 44 weeks continued to demonstrate a normal CBC and fasting glucose level with a normalizing of her liver function tests. Her fasting lipid panel measures improved as well, with a decrease in total cholesterol to 230 and LDL of 160. An ECG was normal. The investigators reported the patient was maintained at this 6-mg dosage of paliperidone for 50 weeks. No additional adverse effects were observed or recorded including EPS or changes in vital signs. Over the 50 weeks of treatment, the patient recorded a loss of 10 lb (from 162 to 152 lb).

The second patient was a 20-year-old male with minimal language classic autism and moderate mental retardation. He had a history of severe irritability that included multiple daily episodes of aggression, SIB (head banging), and tantrums. Prior adequate medication trials included fluvoxamine, mirtazapine, olanzapine, chlorpromazine, haloperidol, quetiapine, and lithium. At the time of assessment, the patient had been on an ineffective 7-month trial of risperidone 4 mg twice daily, guanfacine 1 mg twice daily, and valproic acid extended-release 1,500 mg nightly. His baseline bloodwork was notable for an elevated total cholesterol of 232 (reference range, <200); triglycerides of 317 (reference range, <150); and a low HDL of 35 (reference range, >40). Due to the health risk of his SIB, it was elected to replace the risperidal with paliperidone ER without a taper period, which he tolerated without incident. The patient was reported to have had a marked reduction in his irritability, aggression, SIB, and tantrums across multiple settings, which warranted a classification of "much improved," with a CGI-I score of 2. The baseline fasting lipid panel measures that were out of normal range improved with a total cholesterol of 212, triglycerides of 192, and HDL of 42. An ECG was normal. He maintained satisfactorily on this dosage of paliperidone ER for 42 weeks. Over this treatment duration, his weight decreased by 2 lb (from 204 to 202 lb).

Albeit a small case study series, the authors proposed that their preliminary experience suggested that paliperidone may be an effective and well-tolerated treatment for severe irritability in adolescent and adult patients with autism and worthy of future study.

FDA-Approved SDA Antipsychotics as Mood Stabilizers in Pediatrics

Beginning in late 2009, several of the atypical antipsychotics received FDA approval for the treatment of bipolar disorder in youth. Lithium was the first medication to be approved for pediatric bipolar disorder many years ago. These agents will be discussed in this section focusing on clinical relevance. Table 6.1 summarizes their specific indications and dosing ranges.

Although FDA approval was given to these four atypical antipsychotic mood stabilizers for the treatment of pediatric bipolar disorder, the FDA panel expressed concerns about side-effects of these medications, especially the propensity for weight gain and metabolic issues such as diabetes or lipid disorders. A study by Correll et al. (2009) found that teens are more prone to weight gain when taking atypical antipsychtic drugs than are adults. Some have speculated that the higher density of histamine receptors in the pediatric versus adult brain may account for this greater propensity for weight gain. The study found children and teens can gain nearly 20 lb and become obese within just 11 weeks. Reviewing the weight

---

TABLE 6.1 » FDA-Approved Mood Stabilizers in Pediatrics

Agent	Pediatric Indication	Dosage (mg/d)
Risperidone	Acute treatment of manic and mixed episodes associated with bipolar I disorder in children and adolescents (10–17 y of age)	0.5–6.0
Aripiprazole	Acute and maintenance treatment of manic or mixed episodes associated with bipolar I disorder in children and adolescents (10–17 y of age), both as monotherapy and as an adjunct to lithium or divalproex	10–30
Quetiapine	Acute treatment of manic episodes associated with bipolar I disorder in children and adolescents (10–17 y of age), both as monotherapy and as an adjunct to lithium or divalproex	400–600
Olanzapine	Acute treatment of manic and mixed episodes associated with bipolar I disorder in adolescents (13–17 y of age)	2.5–20
Lithium	Approved for the treatment of bipolar disorder in adolescents aged 12 y and above	Therapeutic levels 0.8–1.2 mEq/L

gain reported in the randomized controlled trials (RTC), one could rank the weight gain from most to least as olanzapine > risperidone > quetiapine >> aripiprazole > ziprasodone = 0.

Ziprasidone was initially voted to be "acceptably safe" and effective for the treatment of bipolar disorder in teenagers and children by an FDA panel of outside medical experts that reviewed trial data for the FDA in 2009. However, there were comparatively more concerns about its efficacy compared with the other agents in the subgroups of younger patients aged 10 to 14 and patients weighing <45 kg, where ziprasidone did not achieve statistically significant difference versus placebo, given the small numbers of patients in these subgroups, which precluded any meaningful conclusion. Possibly due to these clinical efficacy issues, other safety issues, and concerns about data collection at certain sites, ziprasidone's final formal FDA approval never materialized.

Now that clinicians have several FDA-approved medications for pediatric bipolar, initiating treatment with one of these agents as first-line treatment seems appropriate. The studies indicate some variance in the number needed to treat (NNT), which is the number of how many patients need to be treated for one to benefit. The NNTs were predominantly in the 3-to-4 range, which indicates a clinically significant treatment effect. It is not always possible to accurately compare efficacy data across different studies, and as such many clinicians are apt to select an initial medication based on its side-effect profile and how that relates to the patient or his/her family medical history. These patient variables considered could entail current issues such as BMI, health history, and family history as it relates to obesity, diabetes, lipidemias, or cholesterol problems (Bowers et al., 2012).

For children <10 years old requiring treatment for bipolar disorder, there is very limited data to guide a clinician. Biederman et al. (2005a) evaluated short-term safety and efficacy in 31 preschoolers (4 to 6 years) in an open-label prospective study and found both risperidone (at 1 week) and olanzapine (at 2 weeks) resulted in a rapid reduction of symptoms of mania in children with BPD; however, there were substantial adverse effects and the benefit may not outweigh the risk in this population.

Non–FDA-Pediatric-Approved Antipsychotic Medications of Interest

In 2010, three new antipsychotics, namely, lurasidone (Latuda), iloperidone (Fanapt), and asenapine (Saphris), were approved for schizophrenia. Only asenapine has been approved for the additional condition of bipolar disorder. None of these agents have been FDA approved in children for any psychiatric condition at the time of this printing. These medications may never be FDA approved for pediatric use but because of their seemingly preferable metabolic and weight-gain side-effect profiles, they are of interest to pediatric clinicians, given the current medication options available to them. Because antipsychotics are a basic part of the psychopharmacology of schizophrenia and bipolar disorder, the tolerability relative to other available antipsychotics is very important. All the typical antipsychotic class warnings such as the mortality signal for use in elderly patients for behavioral manifestations of dementia, neuroleptic malignant syndrome, TD, and metabolic changes apply to these most recent antipsychotics and mood stabilizers in the case of asenapine.

Lurasidone (Latuda)

In October 2010, the FDA approved lurasidone for the acute treatment of schizophrenia at a dose of 40 or 80 mg, administered once daily with food. Subsequent dosing revisions now support an upper dosing range of 160 mg/day. Similar to most other atypical antipsychotics, lurasidone has high binding affinity and antagonism at serotonin 2A ($5\text{-}HT_{2A}$) and dopamine D_2 receptors. High binding affinity at $5\text{-}HT_7$, as well as moderate binding affinity at $5\text{-}HT_{1A}$, and alpha-2C-adrenergic receptors is believed to possibly enhance cognition, and $5\text{-}HT_7$ is being studied for a potential role in mood regulation and sensory processing. Lurasidone's low activity on alpha-1, H_1, and M_1 receptors suggests a low risk of orthostatic hypotension, H_1-mediated sedation and weight gain, and H_1- and M_1-mediated cognitive blunting.

Lurasidone is absorbed in the gastrointestinal tract, but its concentration (C_{max}) doubles when lurasidone is administered with food (≥350 cal). Absorption, however, is independent of the meal's fat content. The elimination half-life is approximately 18 hours, and steady-state concentration is reached within 7 days. Lurasidone is eliminated predominantly through cytochrome P450 (CYP) 3A4 metabolism in the liver. The PI indicates that the starting and maintenance does of lurasidone should be reduced by 50% for patients who are taking moderate CYP3A4 inhibitors such as diltiazem. Lurasidone should be avoided if used in combination with a strong CYP3A4 inhibitor (e.g., ketoconazole) or a strong CYP3A4 inducer (e.g., rifampin).

In clinical studies in adults, tolerability was quite good and the rate of discontinuation from clinical trials because of adverse effects was 9.4% for lurasidone versus 5.9% for placebo. Somnolence, akathisia, nausea, parkinsonism, and agitation were the most commonly reported adverse reactions; somnolence and akathisia appear dose related. Of note, orthostatic hypotension associated with dizziness, tachycardia or bradycardia, and syncope may occur, especially early in treatment. Other adverse effects associated with lurasidone were nausea, vomiting, dyspepsia, dystonia, dizziness, insomnia, agitation, and anxiety.

Metabolic changes (hyperlipidemia, hyperglycemia, and increased body weight) were quite favorable and lurasidone is considered to have insignificant effects on serum lipids or glucose while being weight-neutral in 52 week open-label extension studies in adults.

As is the case with other D_2 antagonists, lurasidone is associated with increased prolactin in a small subset of patients, which appears to be greater in females and is dose dependent. However, in the longer-term studies, there was no signal of any prolactin increase, suggesting much as with Zyprexa and others, and unlike Risperdal, any significant elevation in prolactin levels is not sustained.

Lurasidone is not associated with significant QTc prolongation, seizures, transaminases increase, or changes in serum chemistry, hematology, or urinalysis.

Lurasidone does not require initial dose titration in adults and should be given with food that provides ≥350 cal to improve medication absorption. Lurasidone is manufactured as 20-, 40-, 80-, and 120-mg tablets. The tablets are not a long-acting formulation.

The recommended starting dose in adults is 40 mg/day, and the maximum recommended dose is 160 mg/day (a starting dose of 20 mg and a maximum dose of 80 mg is recommended in those on a moderate CYP3A4 inhibitor such as diltiazem) (Latuda{package insert}2012).

Pending Pediatric Clinical Trials (clinicaltrials.gov)

A. Lurasidone Pediatric Pharmacokinetics Study
   (a) Phase 1: Open-label, multicenter, single and multiple ascending-dose study to evaluate pharmacokinetics, safety, and tolerability of lurasidone in subjects 6 to 17 years old with schizophrenia spectrum, bipolar spectrum, autistic spectrum disorder, or other psychiatric disorders. Data from this study will be used to recommend pediatric doses that result in comparable exposures with those observed in currently

approved adult doses of Latuda (40, 80, 120, and 160 mg/day) in subsequent efficacy and safety studies.

B. Study of Lurasidone in Treating Antipsychotic Naive or Quasi-Naive Children and Adolescents

   (b) The overarching purpose of this pilot study is to collect preliminary data regarding the variability of weight gain associated with lurasidone (Latuda) treatment of antipsychotic naive children and adolescents in order to inform decisions about including a lurasidone arm in a future large-scale trial of different approaches to minimize antipsychotic-associated weight gain in the pediatric population. The participants will be 6 to 19 years old with psychotic spectrum, mood spectrum, or autism spectrum disorders. They will have 4 weeks or less of lifetime antipsychotic exposure.

Some pediatric clinicians will be enticed to select lurasidone for its generally favorable tolerability profile to reduce the overall long-term side-effect burden. Until the current pediatric studies in progress are completed, lurasidone should be used cautiously and not used without compelling reason in children because of the lack of clinical and safety data.

Iloperidone (Fanapt)

In May 2009, the FDA approved iloperidone for the acute treatment of schizophrenia in adults at a daily dose of 12 to 24 mg administered with or without food in b.i.d. fashion, initially due to its alpha-2 effects, which can cause hypotension and dizziness. Similar to most other atypical antipsychotics, iloperidone has high binding affinity and antagonism at serotonin 2A ($5-HT_{2A}$) and dopamine D_2/D_3 receptors; in addition, it evidences moderate affinity for dopamine D_4, serotonin $5-HT_7$, and noradrenalin alpha-1 receptors. Moderate binding affinity at $5-HT_6$, $5-HT_7$ receptors is believed to possibly enhance cognition, and $5-HT_7$ is being studied for a potential role in mood regulation and sensory processing. Iloperidone's low activity on histamine H_1 and muscarinic M_1 receptors suggests a low risk of H_1-mediated sedation and weight gain, and M_1-mediated memory/cognitive blunting, blurry vision, and urinary difficulties. Less predictable from its pharmacodynamic profile is that iloperidone has a more favorable EPS and akathisia profile than other $D_2/5-HT_{2A}$ antagonists and would be considered comparable to quetiapine in this regard. This in part may be due to the required titration to avoid orthostasis, and, if started at higher doses, one may precipitate some mild EPS.

Iloperidone is labeled for twice-a-day dosing not because of its half-life, which is 18 to 33 hours, but to minimize the potential for orthostatic hypotension during the titration phase due its peripheral alpha-1 receptor antagonism. This early hypotensive effect seems to only last during the first few weeks of treatment, and thus the long half-life suggests that later conversion to once-a-day dosing is reasonable. Prepackaged titration packets can be utilized to carry out the first 4 days of b.i.d. dosing, which culminates in the patient achieving the lowest-approved therapeutic dosage of 6 mg b.i.d. by Day 4. The medication can be taken with or without food. The titration is as follows: Day 1 = 1 mg b.i.d.; Day 2 = 2 mg b.i.d.; Day 3 = 4 mg b.i.d.; and Day 4 = 4 mg b.i.d. If after Day 4 clinical judgment warrants an increase, titration should not exceed 2 mg twice daily (4 mg/day). Available dosing strengths are 1, 2, 4, 6, 8, 10, and 12 mg. The tablets are not a long-acting formulation (Fanapt [package insert]).

Iloperidone is metabolized by the liver-specific enzyme pathways of CYP3A4 and CYP2D6. Therefore, the dosing of iloperidone should be adjusted for patients taking other medications known to inhibit CYP3A4 or CYP2D6 systems and, therefore, inhibit metabolism (e.g., increase plasma level) of iloperidone. Common scenarios among patients treated for schizophrenia would involve patients receiving adjunctive antidepressants that are CYP2D6 inhibitors such as fluoxetine, paroxetine, and venlafaxine, for which the dose of iloperidone would be reduced by 50%. CYP3A4 inhibitors such as ketoconazole or grapefruit juice would also necessitate such a reduction in iloperidone dosing. Iloperidone can be administered with or without food.

In the first of the two large pivotal clinical trials conducted for FDA approval, a fairly rapid titration schedule was used to titrate iloperidone to a maximum dosage of 24 mg within 7 days with ziprasidone used as an active control. The second trial utilized a more flexible dosing scheme where one arm allowed dosing from 12 to 16 mg and the second arm studied dosing in the 20-to-24-mg range with risperidone used as an active control. As one might expect the more rapid titration arms achieved modest initial greater treatment response, but at the cost of a greater side-effect burden. These trials and other large multinational trials (>570 per trial) showed that iloperidone generally had better efficacy than placebo when using the PANSS or BPRS scores (Scott, 2009).

Of clinical importance is the observation that in the long-term flexible dose-maintenance study, the modal dose of iloperidone was 12 mg/day, suggesting that the lower end of the dose range may be therapeutic for many individuals stabilized on iloperidone. Also in support of lower dosing is the finding that there seems to be a clinically significant dose effect with higher doses (20 to 24 mg) associated with more weight gain than did lower doses. Overall, clinical studies have also shown that iloperidone has a very favorable metabolic profile and an excellent extrapyramidal and akathisia profile in clinical trials comparable to placebo. Iloperidone is like quetiapine in that there seems to be no dose-related EPS or akathisia signal across their therapeutic dose ranges. This makes iloperidone any appealing treatment option for any patient at risk for antipsychotic-induced parkinsonism or akathisia.

In clinical studies in adults, tolerability was excellent and the rate of discontinuation from clinical trials because of adverse effects was 5.0% for iloperidone versus 5.0% for placebo. Dizziness, dry mouth, tachycardia, and orthostatic hypotension, all of which are related to early alpha-1 antagonism along with fatigue and somnolence, were the most commonly reported adverse reactions. Orthostatic hypotension and other side effects related to noradrenergic alpha-1 antagonism are more problematic with iloperidone than most other antipsychotics. However, most of these side effects appear dose related and are transient, so they do not add to long-term burden once the initial dose-titration period is over. Although rare, priapism, is related to alpha-1 antagonism and should be addressed for its potential occurrence.

Metabolic changes (hyperlipidemia, hyperglycemia) were quite favorable, and iloperidone is considered to have insignificant effects on serum lipids or glucose. Iloperidone is not likely to cause clinically significant prolactin elevation based on study assessments. While iloperidone is associated with modest weight gain, the mean change in weight from baseline across all short-term and long-term trials up to 52 weeks was 2.1 kg, which would be medically and psychologically acceptable for most patients. The extent of weight gain related to iloperidone in the pediatric population has yet to be determined.

The issue that is concerning to clinicians initially about iloperidone is its potential for QTc prolongation, which is cited in the PI in bold lettering. The PI states that in choosing among treatments, prescribers should consider the ability of FANAPT to prolong the QT interval and the use of other drugs first. Iloperidone has some propensity like ziprasidone to prolong the QTc interval, which for some drugs has been associated with a theoretical risk of arrhythmia such as Torsade de Pointes. The safety of iloperidone has been extensively studied in a safety study where maximal doses were used and metabolic inhibitors added. The mean QTc elevation at the maximal recommended dose of 12 mg twice a day was 9.6 msec, and when iloperidone was given as a single dose of 24 mg the QTc elevation was 15.4 msec. When study patients were given 24 mg of iloperidone plus a full dose of a CYP2D6 inhibitor such as paroxetine 20 mg QD in combination with the CYP3A4 inhibitor ketoconazole 200 mg b.i.d., the QTc elevation was 19 msec, which would likely be of limited clinical relevance. Thus far, the real issue of arrhythmia risk or sudden death has not been reported since iloperidone's release into the market including overdose episodes. Like ziprasidone and paliperidone, the package insert for iloperidone suggests that clinicians consider the relatively greater QTc prolongation associated with these antipsychotics when considering iloperidone. In related fashion, iloperidone is contraindicated when the patient is already taking another medication with QTc elevation that meets "black box" labeling criteria such as thioridazine, pimozide, and droperidol.

It should be remembered that the recommended dose–titration schedule for iloperidone was developed for acutely ill, relapsing patients, where getting to therapeutic quickly was the priority to achieve FDA approval and that there is no known contraindication presently to the option of uptitrating at a slower rate to minimize the early onset risk of hypotension, dizziness, and tachycardia side effects. Indeed in outpatient practice with less acute patients, this slower titration schedule seems to be common among clinicians. One should also consider the need for reinstituting the titration schedule if an individual has an interval off FANAPT of more than 3 days.

Pending Pediatric Clinical Trials (clinicaltrials.gov)

It is doubtful that the makers of Iloperidone Novartis Pharmaceuticals will ever seek pediatric indications as the company has suspended its pediatric study "Tolerability and Pharmacokinetics of Iloperidone in Adolescent Patients." Such tolerability and pharmacokinetic studies are typically done before actual studies for specific conditions are initiated. Some pediatric clinicians will be enticed to select iloperidone for its generally favorable tolerability profile to reduce the overall long-term side-effect burden. Due to lack of pediatric studies, iloperidone should be used cautiously and not used without compelling reason in children because of the lack of clinical data and the QTc labeling precaution previously addressed.

Asenapine (Saphris)

In 2009, the FDA approved asenapine for the treatment of schizophrenia and bipolar disorder in adults. Safety and effectiveness in pediatric patients have not been established.

Asenapine belongs to the class dibenzo-oxepino pyrroles. Asenapine exhibits high affinity for serotonin $5\text{-}HT_{1A}$, $5\text{-}HT_{1B}$, $5\text{-}HT_{2A}$, $5\text{-}HT_{2B}$, $5\text{-}HT_{2C}$, $5\text{-}HT_{5}$, $5\text{-}HT_{6}$, and $5\text{-}HT_{7}$ receptors, dopamine D_2, D_3, D_4, and D_1 receptors, alpha-1- and alpha-2-adrenergic receptors, and histamine H_1 receptors. Asenapine has moderate affinity for H_2 receptors and has no appreciable affinity for muscarinic cholinergic receptors.

The recommended starting dosage for all approved indications of schizophrenia (acute and maintenance treatment) and bipolar mania (monotherapy and as an adjunct to lithium or valproate) in adults is 5 mg sublingually twice daily. The maximal recommended dose is 10 mg sublingually twice daily for all indications. The available 5- and 10-mg sublingual tablets cannot be swallowed but rather placed under the tongue and left to dissolve completely. The tablet will dissolve in saliva within seconds. Following sublingual administration, asenapine is rapidly absorbed with peak plasma concentrations occurring within 0.5 to 1.5 hours. The bioavailability of sublingual asenapine at 5 mg is 35%. There are unique absorption issues associated with sublingual dosing as increasing the dose from 5 to 10 mg twice daily (a twofold increase) results in <1.7 times increases in both the extent of exposure and maximum concentration. The absolute bioavailability of asenapine when swallowed is extremely low at <2% with an oral tablet formulation. The intake of water several (2 or 5) minutes after asenapine administration resulted in decreased asenapine exposure. Therefore, eating and drinking should be avoided for 10 minutes after administration or absorption will be markedly impaired. The original sublingual tablets had a rather offensive taste, so sublingual tablets in black cherry flavor were later released which are much more palatable.

Elimination of asenapine is primarily through direct glucuronidation by UGT1A4 and oxidative metabolism by cytochrome P450 isoenzymes (predominantly CYP1A2). To assess the potential for other drugs to affect asenapine, the potential effects of inhibitors of several of these enzyme pathways on asenapine clearance were studied. The only notable finding was that fluvoxamine (a CYP1A2 inhibitor), even at a subtherapeutic dose of 25 mg b.i.d., elevated the C_{max} by 13% and AUC by 29% for asenapine, and thus caution is advised when coadministering. *In vitro* studies indicate that asenapine weakly inhibits CYP2D6, and thus the potential for asenapine to affect other CYP2D6 substrates drugs was conducted. Coadministration of a single 20-mg dose of paroxetine (a CYP2D6 substrate and inhibitor) during treatment with 5 mg asenapine twice daily in 15 healthy male subjects resulted in an almost twofold increase in paroxetine exposure. Asenapine should be coadministered cautiously with drugs that are both substrates and inhibitors for CYP2D6. Dextromethorphan, valproic acid, and lithium predose serum concentrations collected from an adjunctive therapy study were comparable between asenapine-treated patients and placebo-treated patients, indicating a lack of effect of asenapine on valproic and lithium plasma levels. Following an initial more rapid distribution phase, the mean terminal half-life is approximately 24 hours and with multiple-dose twice-daily dosing, steady-state is attained within 3 days.

In the schizophrenia clinical studies in adults, tolerability was quite good and the rate of discontinuation because of adverse effects was approximately 9% in asenapine-treated patients compared with about 10% of placebo-treated patients. The most common adverse reactions (≥5% and at least twice the rate of placebo) reported with acute treatment in schizophrenia were akathisia, oral hypoesthesia, and somnolence. Oral hypoesthesia and/or oral paraesthesia may occur directly after administration of asenapine and usually resolves within 1 hour.

The most common adverse reactions (≥5% and at least twice the rate of placebo) reported with acute monotherapy treatment of manic or mixed episodes associated with bipolar I disorder were somnolence, dizziness, EPS other than akathisia, and weight increase. In short-term, placebo-controlled schizophrenia trials, the mean weight gain was 1.1 kg for asenapine-treated patients compared with 0.1 kg for placebo-treated patients. In a 52-week, double-blind, comparator-controlled trial of patients with schizophrenia or schizoaffective disorder, the mean weight gain from baseline was 0.9 kg.

To assess EPS in the short-term, placebo-controlled schizophrenia and bipolar mania trials, data were objectively collected on the Simpson Angus Rating Scale for EPS, the Barnes Akathisia Scale (for akathisia), and the Assessments of Involuntary Movement Scales (for dyskinesias). The mean change from baseline for the all-asenapine 5- or 10-mg twice-daily-treated group was comparable to placebo in each of the rating scale scores.

The effects on fasting serum glucose levels as well as the total cholesterol and fasting triglycerides in the short-term schizophrenia and bipolar mania trials revealed no clinically relevant mean changes. In a 52-week, double-blind, comparator-controlled trial of patients with schizophrenia and schizoaffective disorder, the mean increase from baseline of fasting glucose was 2.4 mg/dL. In a 52-week, double-blind, comparator-controlled trial of patients with schizophrenia and schizoaffective disorder, the mean decrease from baseline of total cholesterol was 6 mg/dL and the mean decrease from baseline of fasting triglycerides was 9.8 mg/dL. As is the case with other D_2 antagonists, asenapine is associated with increases in prolactin during the early phases of treatment, but in a longer-term 52-week study, there was no signal of any prolactin increase but rather a decrease, suggesting any significant elevation in prolactin levels is not sustained. Asenapine is pregnancy category C.

Although rare, asenapine may induce orthostatic hypotension and syncope in some patients, especially early in treatment, because of its alpha-1-adrenergic antagonist activity. The effects of asenapine on the QT/QTc interval were evaluated in a dedicated QT study. This trial involved asenapine doses of 5, 10, 15, and 20 mg twice daily, and placebo, and was conducted in 151 clinically stable patients with schizophrenia, with electrocardiographic assessments throughout the dosing interval at baseline and steady state. At these doses, asenapine was associated with increases in QTc interval ranging from 2 to 5 msec compared with placebo. No patients treated with asenapine experienced QTc increases ≥60 msec from baseline measurements, nor did any patient experience a QTc of ≥500 msec. Despite these small increases of 2 to 5 msec in QTc, the PI indicates the use of asenapine should be avoided in combination with other drugs known to prolong QTc including class 1A antiarrhythmics (e.g., quinidine, procainamide) or class 3 antiarrhythmics (e.g., amiodarone, sotalol), antipsychotic medications (e.g., ziprasidone, chlorpromazine, thioridazine), and antibiotics (e.g., gatifloxacin, oxifloxacin) (Saphris [package insert], 2009).

Pending Pediatric Clinical Trials (clinicaltrials.gov)

A. A Study to Evaluate the Pharmacokinetics, Safety and Tolerability of Sublingual Asenapine in a Pediatric Population with Schizophrenia or Bipolar I Disorder (P06522 AM1)—Completed Study

Results: This study determined C_{max}, T_{max}, area under the plasma concentration–time curve from 0 to 12 hours post dose (AUC0-12) of asenapine, elimination half-life ($T_{1/2}$) of asenapine, and terminal phase (elimination) half-life ($T_{1/2}$) of asenapine. No serious AEs were recorded during this study.

This study was an open-label, sequential-group, two-site, multiple-dose escalating study of sublingually administered asenapine in a pediatric population with schizophrenia or bipolar I disorder; in one study cohort (3a), participants with other conditions treatable with chronic antipsychotic medication were also enrolled. Participants received a single sublingual placebo dose on Day 1, followed by multiple sublingual doses of asenapine twice daily (b.i.d.) for 6 days (Cohorts 1 and 2), 7 days (Cohort 3b–d), or 11 days (Cohort 3a), and a final once daily administration on Day 7 (Cohorts 1 and 2), Day 8 (Cohort 3b–d), or Day 12 (Cohort 3a).

B. Extension Study of Asenapine {P06107 (NCT01244815)} for Pediatric Bipolar Disorder

Status: Not yet completed

Estimated study completion date: August 2014

Purpose: This study will investigate the safety and tolerability of a flexible dosing regimen of asenapine for the long-term treatment of manic or mixed episodes associated with bipolar disorder I in children and adolescents who completed study P06107 (NCT01244815).

Dosing strategy—one flavored asenapine sublingual tablet twice daily (b.i.d.) starting at 2.5 mg on Day 1 for 3 consecutive days. Normally on Day 4, the dose will increase to 5 mg b.i.d. beginning with the evening dose. Normally on Day 7, the dose will increase to 10 mg b.i.d. beginning with the evening dose. The dose may be uptitrated earlier than Days 4 and 7 at the investigator's discretion. Beginning on Day 8 (or after at least 1 day on 10 mg b.i.d.), asenapine dosing will be flexible (2.5, 5, or 10 mg b.i.d.) until up to Week 50.

C. Efficacy and Safety of Asenapine Treatment for Pediatric Bipolar Disorder {P06107 Has an Extension (P05898; NCT01349907)}(P06107 AM3)

Status: Not yet completed

Estimated study completion date: August 2013

Purpose: Efficacy and safety of asenapine for the treatment of bipolar I disorder (manic or mixed episodes) will be evaluated in participants between 10 and 17 years old, who are either hospitalized or nonhospitalized. In this 3-weeks, double-blind, parallel-design trial, patients eligible for participation will be randomized to receive one out of three fixed-dose levels of asenapine or placebo. Trial medication and placebo are provided as identical-looking sublingual tablets; concurrent use of psychotropics is prohibited, except use of short-acting benzodiazepines and psychostimulants approved for the treatment of ADHD. Main treatment effect is measured using the YMRS, and safety is evaluated using the recordings of AEs, routine blood panels, physical examinations (including vital signs), and electrocardiograms. Patients who complete the double-blind trial may be offered to continue (open-label) treatment with asenapine for an extended period of time. Follow-up information on safety parameters will be collected in all patients within 30 days following treatment discontinuation.

Some pediatric clinicians will be enticed to select asenapine for its generally favorable tolerability profile to reduce the overall long-term side-effect burden. Until the current pediatric studies in progress are completed, asenapine should be used cautiously and not used without compelling reason in children because of the lack of sufficient clinical and safety data.

Antidepressant Drugs

CHRISTINA WESTON

Note: In October 2004, the FDA directed manufacturers of antidepressant medications to add the following Black Box Warning to their labeling. "Warning: Suicidality in Children and Adolescents—Antidepressants increased the risk of suicidal thinking and behavior (suicidality) in short-term studies in children and adolescents with major depressive disorder (MDD) and other psychiatric disorders. Anyone considering the use of [drug name] or any other antidepressant in a child or adolescent must balance this risk with the clinical needs. Patients who have started on therapy should be observed closely for clinical worsening, suicidality, or unusual changes in behavior. Families and caregivers should be advised of the need for close observation and communication with the prescriber. [Drug name] is not approved for use in pediatric patients except for patients with [Any approved pediatric claims here]. (See Warnings and Precautions: Pediatric Use.)

Pooled analyses of short-term (4 to 16 weeks) placebo-controlled trials of nine antidepressant drugs (SSRIs and others) in children and adolescents with MDD, obsessive-compulsive disorder (OCD), or other psychiatric disorders (a total of 24 trials involving more than 4,400 patients have revealed a greater risk of adverse events representing suicidal thinking or behavior (suicidality) during the first few months of treatment in those receiving antidepressants. The average risk of such events on drug was 4%, twice the placebo risk of 2%. No suicides occurred in these trials."

Furthermore, in the labeling under "Warnings," the following is indicated: "All pediatric patients being treated with antidepressants for any indication should be observed closely for clinical worsening, suicidality, and unusual changes in behavior, especially during the initial few months of a course of drug therapy, or at times of dose changes, either increases or decreases. Ideally, such observation would include at least weekly face-to-face contact with patients or their family members or caregivers during the first 4 weeks of treatment, then biweekly visits for the next 4 weeks, then at 12 weeks, and as clinically indicated beyond 12 weeks. Additional contact by telephone may be appropriate between face-to-face visits.

Adults with MDD or comorbid depression in the setting of other psychiatric illness taking antidepressants should also be observed for clinical worsening and suicidality, especially during the first few months of treatment, or at times of dose increases or decreases."

INTRODUCTION

The selective serotonin reuptake inhibitor (SSRI) antidepressants are now the most frequently prescribed antidepressants for children and adolescents and continue to be prescribed with increasing frequency because of their significantly safer untoward-effects profile, in particular, the reduced risks of cardiotoxicity and lethality of overdose compared with the risks associated with tricyclic antidepressants (TCAs). For these reasons, Ambrosini et al. (1993) recommended prescribing SSRIs, and not tricyclics, to depressed patients with suicidal and/or impulsive tendencies. The SSRIs have also been approved for the treatment of several other psychiatric disorders and are used off-label for several additional ones. In 2005, the FDA, directed manufacturers of all antidepressants, including SSRIs, to label their package inserts with a warning of increased suicidal thoughts and behavior in children and adolescents, noting that a pooled analysis of short-term studies in subjects <18 years old showed an increase from 2% in subjects receiving a placebo to 4% in subjects receiving an antidepressant.

SUICIDAL RISK AND ANTIDEPRESSANTS

Since the FDA issued a "Black Box" warning for increased suicidal risk during treatment in young patient for all antidepressants in October 2004, there has been debate about the warnings and how they have effected the use of antidepressants in this population group. Several authors have examined SSRI prescription rates in many countries before and after the warnings were issued. The warnings were initially concerning paroxetine and a warning for this drug was issued initially in June 2003 by the UK equivalent of the FDA. This was followed by the FDA's Black Box warning more than a year later. Olfson and colleagues (2008) examined antidepressant prescription rates among three physician groups, namely, psychiatrists, primary care physicians, and other physicians during three periods, namely, prewarning, paroxetine warning, and after the Black Box warnings. Youth antidepressant use during the prewarning study period increased by 36% per year ($P < .001$), which was followed by a decrease of −0.8% and −9.6% per year during the paroxetine and Black Box warning study periods, respectively. They noted that youth paroxetine use increased during the prewarning study period (30% per year; $P < .001$) before decreasing during the paroxetine warning study period (−44.2% per year; $P < .001$). They did not find similar changes in antidepressant use in older age groups. They found that all groups of physicians increased their use of SSRIs in youth during the prewarning period. They found that use of paroxetine decreased first by psychiatrists during the prewarning period (−23.0% per year; $P = .06$) while that of primary care physicians increased (+21.2% per year; $P = 1.0$). During the paroxetine warning period, use of paroxetine decreased by −49.4% per year ($P < .001$) among psychiatrists, −38.1% per year among primary care physicians, and −32.2% per year among other physicians. This may be indicative of psychiatrists having greater knowledge of regulatory developments affecting antidepressants.

Kurian and colleagues (2007) found that during the 2 years before the UK warnings in 2003, there was no change in monthly SSRI users aged 2 to 17 years with 23 new users per 10,000 persons per month. This proportion decreased by 33% in the 21 months following the UK warnings (95% confidence interval [CI], 23% to 41%; $P < .001$). They found that the decrease was most pronounced for antidepressants, other than fluoxetine, which dropped by 54%. New users of fluoxetine, however, increased by 60%. These data suggest that warnings about the relative safety of fluoxetine in comparison with other SSRIs were headed by practitioners. Clarke and colleagues (2012) analyzed prescription rates for antidepressants in youth at a large HMO, from 2000 through 2009. They found that the rates of antidepressant prescriptions to youth ages 10 to 17 continued to decline through 2009 as had been noted by other authors. They also found that rates of prescription refills decreased, which suggests that prescribers wanted to encourage return visits to monitor for improvement and adverse effects (AEs) after the warnings were issued, which mandated close follow-up.

Kurdyak and colleagues (2007) found that in Ontario the rate of paroxetine prescriptions in children and adolescents declined by 54% immediately following the first paroxetine warnings issued in June 2003. Paroxitine prescriptions were unchanged in other age groups. Dutch researchers (Volkers et al., 2007) found that use of SSRIs prescribed by general practitioners decreased from 1.2 to 1.1 per 1,000 children and adolescents between 2001 and 2005. The use of other antidepressant types and TCAs also decreased (0.3 to 0.2 and 0.8 to 0.7, respectively). In Australia, researchers found that use of all SSRIs decreased over time in children and adolescents whereas its use increased in adults (Dean et al., 2007). This decrease in prescription rates of SSRIs have alarmed some who fear that depressed and anxious children are receiving treatment for their disorders.

The Black Box warnings have also affected research studies. The warnings were issued while the treatment of resistant depression in adolescents (TORDIA) multisite trial was recruiting subjects. Wagner et al. (2012) describe the difficulties continuing the trial after the warnings. As a result of the paroxetine warnings, no further subjects were randomized to receive paroxetine and a citalopram arm replaced it. When additional warnings and the Black Box warnings were released, additional informed consents of the new warnings were required. Recruitment to the study was adversely affected following the warnings. Gibbons and colleagues (2007) analyzed dropping SSRI prescription rates in children and adolescents and compared them with youth suicide rates. US and Dutch prescriptions rates for SSRIs were compared from 2003 to 2005, the years before and after the warnings. Suicide rates from the US through 2004 and in the Netherlands through 2005 were compared. It was found that SSRI prescriptions for youth decreased by 22% in both the US and the Netherlands after the warnings were issued. In the Netherlands, the youth suicide rate increased by 49% between 2003 and 2005. In the US, the suicide rates increased by 14% between 2003 and 2004. This was the largest year-to-year change in the suicide rate for this population ever seen since the CDC started collecting data.

Simon et al. (2006) provided an excellent and succinct review of the events leading up to the FDA's issuing a warning about increased suicidal risk in children and adolescents being treated with newer antidepressants. The authors identified 65,103 patients with 82,285 episodes of antidepressant treatment over a period of 12½ years ending June 30, 2003. The subjects were members of the Group Health Cooperative (GHC), a mixed-model prepaid health plan with about 500,000 members in the states of Washington and Idaho. An "episode" was defined as an outpatient antidepressant prescription filled (the index prescription) during the study period with no prior antidepressant prescription filed in the preceding 180 days and a ICD-9 diagnosis of unipolar major depressive disorder (MDD), dysthymia, or depressive disorder NOS made during a treatment visit within 30 days before or after the index prescription. Data were obtained from four computerized record systems, including GHC pharmacies where about 95% of members fill their prescriptions, outpatient visit registration records, hospital discharge data, and mortality records (Simon et al., 2006). A total of 11,436 patients had two or more treatment episodes and 5,107 (6.2%) of the episodes occurred in patients <17 years. Females comprised 69.5% of the sample.

The authors evaluated the risks of death by suicide and serious suicide attempts (defined as leading to hospitalization), whether these risks increased during the month after starting an antidepressant, and whether the 10 newer antidepressants (bupropion, citalopram, fluoxetine, fluvoxamine, mirtazapine, nefazodone, paroxetine, sertraline, escitalopram, and venlafaxine) initially identified by the FDA warnings were associated with higher risks of serious suicidal attempts or death by suicide compared with older antidepressants.

During the 3 months before the index prescription, a total of 73 serious suicide attempts were identified. During the 6-month follow-up period after the index prescription was filled, there were 76 (93/100,000) serious suicide attempts and 31 (40/100,000) completed suicides. The probability of death by suicide was much higher in males (OR = 6.6; 95% CI = 2.9 to 14.7) but did not vary significantly with age. The probability of serious suicide attempts was not significantly different between males and females; however, it strongly correlated with younger age ($Z = 3.18$, $P < .001$) with an absolute rate of 314/100,000 (95% CI = 160 to 468) in children and adolescents and of 78/100,000 in adults (95% CI = 58 to 98).

The highest risk of serious suicide attempts was during the month before the index prescription and was primarily because of the increased risk in the 7 days preceding the index prescription; the authors attributed this to the fact that such an attempt may result in beginning treatment with antidepressants. Compared with the month before treatment, there was a decrease in serious suicide attempts during the first month after the index prescription; however, the number of attempts during the first month was greater than in any of the following 5 months, over which a continuing gradual decline occurred. This risk of suicide death during the first month after the index prescription was not significantly higher than in the subsequent 5 months (OR = 1.2; 95% CI = 0.5 to 2.9). During the 6-month follow-up, there were a total of three suicide deaths in adolescents. The pattern of serious suicide attempts in adolescents over the 6-month period ($N = 17$) was similar to that in adults with the highest risk in the month before the index prescription, a sharp decline immediately after starting treatment and continuing to gradually decline over the next 5 months.

The authors found differences in the risks between the 10 newer antidepressants and older antidepressants (primarily tricyclics and trazodone). The risk of suicidal death over the 6-month follow-up period was 34/100,000 for the 10 newer antidepressants and 51/100,000 for the older antidepressants. The risk of serious suicidal attempts was 76/100,000 for the 10 newer antidepressants and 129/100,000 for the older antidepressants. Patients treated with the 10 newer antidepressants had the highest risk of serious suicidal behavior in the month before starting antidepressants and the risk in the first months after the index prescription was not significantly different from that in months 2 through 5 (OR = 1.6; 95% CI = 0.9 to 3.1). Patients treated with the older antidepressants had the highest risk in the first month of treatment, which was significantly higher than in months 2 through 6 (OR = 3.6; 95% CI = 1.8 to 6.9).

The authors concluded that their data did not support the contention of increased risk of suicide deaths or serious suicidal attempts during the first month of antidepressant therapy; however, the risk of serious suicidal attempts was higher during the first week of therapy. The risk of suicide deaths appeared to be relatively constant during the first 6 months of therapy. The authors found no evidence that the newer antidepressants increased the risk of suicidal deaths or serious suicidal attempts compared with the risks of older antidepressants (Simon et al., 2006).

SELECTIVE SEROTONIN REUPTAKE INHIBITORS

The SSRIs approved by the FDA for the treatment of depression only in adults are sertraline hydrochloride (Zoloft), paroxetine hydrochloride (Paxil), and citalopram hydrobromide (Celexa). Fluoxetine hydrochloride (Prozac) is approved for treating depression in individuals 8 years of age or older. Escitalopram oxalate (Lexapro) is approved for treating depression in individuals 12 years of age or older. The FDA has approved for treating obsessive-compulsive disorder (OCD) the following SSRIs: sertraline for individuals 6 years of age or older, fluoxetine for individuals 7 years of age or older, fluvoxamine maleate (Luvox) for individuals 8 years of age or older, and paroxetine only for adults. Fluoxetine, paroxetine, and sertraline are approved for treating panic disorder only in adults. Paroxetine and sertraline are approved for treating social anxiety disorder and posttraumatic stress disorder (PTSD) in adults. Fluoxetine is approved for treating bulimina nervosa disorder only in adults. Fluoxetine and sertraline are approved to treat premenstrual dysphoric disorder (PMDD) only in adults. Finally, escitalopram and paroxetine are approved to treat generalized anxiety disorder (GAD) only in adults. Table 7.1 summarizes the FDA-approved uses of these SSRIs.

With the exception of escitalopram, which is the S-enantiomer of racemic citalopram, these SSRIs are chemically unrelated to each other or to tricyclic or tetracyclic antidepressants, or to other antidepressants currently used in clinical practice (*PDR*, 2006). As the term SSRI suggests, at therapeutic levels, these drugs act primarily to inhibit serotonin reuptake; they also have relatively little effect on catecholaminergic (norepinephrine) reuptake mechanisms. At least five types and several subtypes of serotonin receptors with both distinct and overlapping functions have been identified in the central nervous system (Sussman, 1994a). These SSRIs have differing specificities in the serotonin receptors whose reuptake they inhibit, which explains their efficacy in treating disorders other than depression and the fact that they have somewhat different untoward effects. SSRI antidepressants also do not have clinically significant direct effects on the adrenergic, muscarinic, or histaminergic systems, resulting in fewer and less severe untoward effects than the TCAs. The most common untoward effects of the SSRIs parallel the symptoms caused by the administration of exogenous serotonin and include headache, nausea, vomiting, diarrhea, nervousness, sleep disturbance, and sexual dysfunction (Sussman, 1994a).

Safer and Zito (2006) conducted a meta-analysis of placebo-controlled studies, which reviewed the incidence of treatment-emergent adverse events (TEAEs) in SSRIs in children, adolescents, and adults. They found that children had a two-to-three-times higher incidence of behavioral activation and vomiting than did adolescents, with adults having the lowest rates. Behavioral activation is described as restlessness, hyperkinesis, hyperactivity, and agitation. Activation in children was seen on average in 10.7% of children on SSRIs and 3.4% of children on placebo. Adolescents had activation rates of 2.1% on SSRIs and 1.9% on placebo. They found that somnolence increased with age occurring in 3% of children on SSRIs versus 3.4% on placebo, increasing to 11.3% of adolescents on SSRIs and 5.0% on placebo. Adults had an incidence of somnolence of 16.5% on average on SSRIs and 7.6% on placebo (Safer and Zito, 2006). Gualtieri and Johnson (2006) conducted a retrospective chart review of 128 children and adolescents treated with SSRIs. They found that 28% developed behavioral side effects. Behavioral side effects are characterized as hyperactivity and disinhibition, which occurred in 17; anger and aggression, which occurred in 17 youth; and dysphoria and extreme emotional reactivity, which occurred in 13. They found self-injurious behavior occurring in 12 and suicidal ideation threats or attempts occurring in 9. They analyzed the severity of the events and found that most were managed by discontinuing the drug or lowering the dose. In all, 34 of 36 youth who developed behavioral toxicity were able to continue to be treated with antidepressants after their side effects resolved with either a lower dose of the same drug or a different agent (Gualtieri and Johnson, 2006).

Zuckerman and colleagues (2007) conducted a retrospective chart review of children below 7 years of age on SSRIs. They found 39 children who were prescribed citalopram, fluvoxamine, paroxetine, fluoxetine, or sertraline. Seven patients in the sample needed to discontinue their SSRI due to adverse events (AEs). One youth had gastrointestinal distress that resolved after discontinuation, and six youth developed

TABLE 7.1 » Summary of Selective Serotonin Reuptake Inhibitor Indications by Age for FDA-Approved Advertising

SSRI	Major Depressive Disorder (y)	Obsessive-Compulsive Disorder (y)	Panic Disorder (y)	Social Anxiety Disorder (y)	Posttraumatic Stress Disorder (y)	Bulimia Nervosa (y)	Premenstrual Dysphoric Disorder (y)	Generalized Anxiety Disorder (y)
Citalopram	≥18							
Escitalopram	≥12							≥18
Fluoxetine	≥8	≥7	≥18			≥18	≥18	
Fluvoxamine		≥8						
Paroxetine	≥18	≥18	≥18	≥18	≥18			≥18
Sertraline	≥18	≥6	≥18	≥18	≥18			

behavioral activation which required discontinuation. In their sample, 28% of youth below 7 years of age developed AEs with behavioral activation occurring in 21% (Zuckerman et al., 2007).

SSRI-induced sexual dysfunction is of particular concern in adolescents. Sharko (2004) reviewed the literature and reported a paucity of reported cases of sexual dysfunction—only 1 male of 1,346 pediatric subjects in 31 clinical studies of SSRIs reported such an AE, erectile dysfunction. During 11 years, only eight subjects, all male, were reported to MedWatch for sexual dysfunction secondary to treatment with an SSRI: four reported loss of orgasm, three reported loss in interest, and one reported loss of physical arousal. Scharko noted that in adults, on adequate doses of SSRIs, sexual dysfunction has been reported by 30% to 40% of patients and that this was probably a low estimate because of the difficulties many adults have in discussing sexual matters. He further speculated that the surprisingly low incidence reported was because it was even more difficult for adolescents to talk to their doctors/psychiatrists, but also noted that only 3 of 15 controlled clinical trials cited used ratings to assess AEs (two studies used the Systematic Assessment for Treatment-Emergent Events and one study used the Side Effects Form for Children and Adolescents) and that neither measure asks directly about sexual dysfunction and relies on self-report. In adults treated with SSRIs, it is known that relying on spontaneous self-report greatly underestimates the actual frequency of SSRI-related sexual dysfunction (Sharko, 2004). It is likely that clinicians and researchers fail to adequately address this area and do not directly ask adolescents about sex and sexual functioning as a part of their medication management. Doing this is likely to be the best way to assess sexual dysfunction of our adolescent patients (Sharko, 2004), and neglecting to do so is a disservice to them and may also increase rates of noncompliance with treatment.

A discontinuation syndrome has been identified for the SSRIs. Hosenbocus and Chahal (2011) reviewed the literature on discontinuation-emergent symptoms in children and adults taking SSRIs and noted that dizziness occurs in 60% of cases followed by nausea in almost 40% of adults. The most common symptoms seen in children are dizziness, lightheadedness, drowsiness, poor concentration, nausea, headache, and fatigue. These symptoms are seen when SSRIs are abruptly discontinued (Hosenbocus and Chahal, 2011). Rosenbaum et al. (1998) conducted a 4-week, prospective double-blind, placebo-substitution, discontinuation study of 242 adults receiving long-term maintenance (duration 4 to 24 months) with SSRIs for remitted depression (81 subjects on fluoxetine, 79 subjects of sertraline, and 82 subjects on paroxetine). Effects of the abrupt withdrawal of medication were evaluated by baseline ratings on the Symptom Questionnaire (SQ), the Discontinuation-Emergent Signs and Symptoms (DESS) Checklist, and two depression rating scales, namely, the Hamilton Depression Rating Scale (HDRS) and the Montgomery-Asberg Depression Rating Scale. Medication was abruptly interrupted for 5 to 8 days; 83% were randomly assigned to receive placebo and 17% to continue on their medication. Following this phase, all subjects on placebo resumed their usual maintenance dose of the SSRI they were previously taking. Two hundred twenty (91%) of the subjects completed the entire protocol. Following medication withdrawal during placebo, scores both on the DESS and the SQ increased significantly for patients who had been on sertraline or paroxetine ($P < .001$ for both) but not for patients who were receiving fluoxetine ($P = .578$). There were many more discontinuation-emergent symptoms reported on the DESS under inquiry than reported spontaneously; fluoxetine-treated patients reported significantly fewer such symptoms than sertraline-treated patients ($P = .001$) or paroxetine-treated patients ($P < .001$). Reported symptoms (ranked from most to least frequent) that occurred in at least 10% of the 185 subjects who underwent withdrawal from medication in decreasing frequency were the following: worsened mood, irritability, agitation, dizziness, confusion, headache, nervousness, crying, fatigue, emotional lability, trouble sleeping, dreaming, anger, nausea, amnesia, sweating, depersonalization, muscle aches, unsteady gait, panic, sore eyes, diarrhea, shaking, muscle tension, and chills. Overall, a SSRI discontinuation syndrome occurred in 14% of patients withdrawn from fluoxetine, 60% of patients withdrawn from sertraline, and 66% of patients withdrawn from paroxetine. There appeared to be a relationship between a longer half-life and the development of fewer discontinuation-emergent symptoms (e.g., patients abruptly discontinued from fluoxetine developed fewer clinically significant such effects than did patients withdrawn from sertraline or paroxetine). In addition, patients treated with either sertraline or paroxetine were rated as having a significant increase in depressive symptoms during the withdrawal period on placebo ($P < .001$). Subjects who were taking fluoxetine did not experience this reemergence of depressive symptoms. Following restabilization on medication, there were no significant rating scale differences among the three drugs (Rosenbaum et al., 1998). Discontinuation symptoms are best managed by restarting the SSRI or serotonergic noradrenergic reuptake inhibitor (SNRI) and following a more gradual tapering of the medication (Hosenbocus and Chahal, 2011). In cases where SSRIs are unable to be tapered due to reemergence of symptoms, it is possible to overlap with a longer half-life SSRI such as fluoxetine. The first SSRI is tapered off slowly and then the fluoxetine can be discontinued.

SSRIs are of great interest to child and adolescent psychiatrists for several reasons:

1. Only one double-blind, placebo-controlled study conducted with prepubertal children and no such studies with adolescents have shown TCAs to be superior to placebo in treating MDD. In that study (Preskorn et al., 1987), however, subjects receiving IMI had their dose of IMI adjusted by laboratory personnel to achieve plasma levels within the therapeutic range.
2. There have been several reports of sudden death in at least eight children and adolescents being treated with tricyclics, leading to particular concern about their cardiotoxicity in younger patients. SSRIs have a significantly safer untoward-effect profile, including decreased lethality in overdose.
3. Although significant, the untoward effects of SSRIs are more tolerable than those of tricyclic and monoamine oxidase inhibitor (MAOI) antidepressants.
4. SSRIs may be administered once daily.
5. SSRIs appear to have potential in treating a spectrum of childhood psychiatric disorders in addition to depression, including OCD with and without comorbid Tourette disorder, attention-deficit/hyperactivity disorder (ADHD), anxiety disorders, elective mutism, and eating disorders.

Fluoxetine was the first SSRI to be approved by the FDA, and there are more published reports of its use in children and adolescents than for the SSRIs that were introduced later. As additional clinical experience with the SSRIs in this age group has continued to accumulate, the SSRIs have displaced the TCAs as the agents of choice in treating children and adolescents diagnosed with depression, OCD, and other disorders where TCAs were used. Consensus guidelines on medication treatment of childhood MDD have been developed and recommend monotherapy with SSRI antidepressants as the first-line treatment (Hughes et al., 2007).

Fluoxetine Hydrochloride (Prozac, Sarafem)

Fluoxetine is an SSRI that is chemically unrelated to any current antidepressant. Fluoxetine's antidepressant effect is thought to be related to its specific and selective inhibition of serotonin reuptake by central nervous system neurons. This action appears to take place at the serotonin reuptake pump, not at a neurotransmitter receptor site, and fluoxetine appears to have no significant pharmacological effect on norepinephrine or dopamine uptake (Bergstrom et al., 1988).

Fluoxetine binds to muscarinic, histaminergic, and alpha-1 adrenergic receptors significantly less than TCAs, which may account for the relative lack of anticholinergic, sedative, and cardiovascular effects of fluoxetine compared with TCAs.

The therapeutic serum levels of fluoxetine (FLX) and its major metabolite norfluoxetine (NORFLEX) in children and adolescents has recently been evaluated. Koelch and colleagues performed therapeutic drug monitoring of 71 youth aged 8 to 19 years who were being treated with fluoxetine in doses 10 to 60 mg. They found that the serum concentrations of the active moiety (FLX + NORFLEX) ranged from 21 to 613 ng/mL. They noted that there was very high interindividual variability in the serum concentrations of FLX at each dosage level. There was no relationship between serum concentration and clinical response. The only factor that affected serum concentration was smoking. These results are similar to therapeutic drug monitoring studies of fluoxetine in adults (Koelch et al., 2012).

Several studies, including some that were placebo controlled, have found fluoxetine's therapeutic efficacy to be comparable to that of the tricyclics (IMI, amitriptyline, and doxepine) in treating adults with MDD (for reviews, see Benfield et al., 1986; Lader, 1988). Two meta-analyses of randomized controlled trials of antidepressants used to treat depression in children and adolescents concluded that fluoxetine is the only antidepressant that demonstrated efficacy in treating juvenile depression (Tsapakis et al., 2008; Usala et al., 2008).

Pharmacokinetics of Fluoxetine Hydrochloride

Peak plasma levels of fluoxetine at usual clinical doses occur after 6 to 8 hours. Food does not significantly affect the bioavailability of fluoxetine; hence, it may be administered with or without food. Fluoxetine is metabolized by the P450 2D6 system in the liver; active and inactive metabolites are excreted by the kidneys. About 95% of fluoxetine is bound to plasma proteins. The elimination half-life after chronic administration is 4 to 6 days for fluoxetine and 4 to 16 days for norfluoxetine, its active metabolite. It may take up to 4 to 5 weeks for steady-state plasma levels to be achieved, but once obtained they remain steady.

Sallee et al. (2000a) reported the death of a 9-year-old male attributed to genetic polymorphism of the CYP2D6 gene, revealed upon genetic testing of autopsy material, which resulted in impaired metabolism of fluoxetine. The case was complicated with multiple psychiatric diagnoses treated with polypharmacy, including high doses of fluoxetine, methylphenidate, and clonidine.

Contraindications for the Administration of Fluoxetine Hydrochloride

Known hypersensitivity to the drug is a contraindication.

Fluoxetine should not be administered to any patient who has received an MAOI within the preceding 2 weeks. Because of the long half-lives of fluoxetine and its metabolites, an MAOI should not be administered sooner than 5 weeks (35 days) after discontinuing fluoxetine. The manufacturer notes that it may be advisable to wait even longer before giving an MAOI if fluoxetine has been prescribed chronically or at high doses (*PDR*, 2000).

The drug should be administered with caution if impaired liver function is present; if prescribed, a lower dose or a decrease frequency of administration should be used.

Fluoxetine is secreted in breast milk, and hence nursing is not recommended while taking fluoxetine.

Interactions of Fluoxetine Hydrochloride with Other Drugs

The use of fluoxetine with other psychoactive drugs has not been systematically studied. However, because it is metabolized by the P450 2D6 enzyme system, the potential exists for interactions with other drugs metabolized by this system, including TCAs and other SSRIs.

When used with TCAs, their plasma levels may be significantly increased.

Agitation, restlessness, and gastrointestinal symptoms have occurred when used concurrently with tryptophan.

Diazepam clearance was significantly prolonged in some patients who were administered both drugs.

Elevated plasma levels and toxicity have occurred in some patients receiving carbamazepine or phenytoin when fluoxetine was added to their drug regimes.

Untoward Effects of Fluoxetine Hydrochloride

Wernicke (1985) and Cooper (1988) have reviewed the safety and untoward effects of fluoxetine. The most frequent troublesome untoward effects are nausea, weight loss, anxiety, nervousness, insomnia, and excessive sweating. They are reported more frequently, and anticholinergic effects and sedation less frequently compared with the TCAs.

Many of the untoward effects may be described as behavioral activation. Riddle et al. (1990/1991) reported the behavioral side effects of fluoxetine in 24 children and adolescents of various diagnoses (age range, 8 to 16 years). Mean dose was 25.8 ± 9.0 mg/day for the 12 subjects (including the ADHD children) who developed fluoxetine-induced behavioral side effects, such as restlessness, hyperactivity, insomnia, an internal feeling of excitation, subtle impulsive behavioral changes, and suicidal ideation (King et al., 1991; Riddle et al., 1990/1991). Bangs et al. (1994) documented significant memory impairment in a 14-year-old who was receiving 20 mg/day of fluoxetine for treatment of MDD. Hypomania, mania, and transient psychosis have also been reported to occur in children and adolescents treated with fluoxetine (Boulos et al., 1992; Hersh et al., 1991; Jafri, 1991; Jerome, 1991; Rosenberg et al., 1992; Venkataraman et al., 1992).

Simeon et al. (1990) reported that those subjects receiving fluoxetine who were depressed experienced a small but significant weight loss compared with subjects receiving placebo. As many teenagers, especially females, refuse to take TCAs because of frequently associated weight gain, this could be a clinically advantageous characteristic of fluoxetine for some patients.

The effect of fluoxetine on aggression and or hostility-related events was examined in a meta-analysis (Tauscher-Wisniewski et al., 2007). Five studies were included in the analysis in which 376 children and adolescents were treated with fluoxetine compared with 255 treated with placebo. Aggression and/or hostility-related events were identified in 2.1% of youth treated with fluoxetine versus 3.1% of placebo-treated patients; this suggests that there is not an association between fluoxetine treatment and increased risk of aggression.

Indications for Fluoxetine Hydrochloride in Child and Adolescent Psychiatry

NOTE: Review the Black Box Warning at the beginning of the chapter or in the package insert before prescribing.

Fluoxetine is approved for use in children at least 8 years of age, adolescents, and adults for the treatment of MDD; children at least 7 years of age, adolescents, and adults for the treatment of OCD; and older adolescents and adults for treatment of bulimia nervosa, panic disorder, social anxiety disorder, and PMDD. Food does not seem to affect significantly the bioavailability of fluoxetine. It is recommended that once 20 mg/day is exceeded, particularly at higher doses, the medication be taken in divided portions twice daily, in the morning and at noon.

(continued)

Indications for Fluoxetine Hydrochloride in Child and Adolescent Psychiatry *(continued)*

Fluoxetine Dosage Schedule

- *Children and adolescents ≤17 years:* Fluoxetine has been approved for the treatment of MDD in children aged 8 years and older and for the treatment of OCD in children aged 7 years and older. The safety and efficacy of fluoxetine in younger children with these disorders has not been established. At the present time, the safety and efficacy of fluoxetine for children and younger adolescents diagnosed with other disorders remains to be elucidated. However, studies including patients in this age range are appearing in the literature with increasing frequency. Riddle et al. (1992) noted that 20 mg/day may be too high a dose for some children and suggested that an initial dose of 10 mg/day of fluoxetine is the most common starting dose given to children by most clinicians. Boulos et al. (1992) found that an initial dose of 20 mg of fluoxetine too often causes unacceptable untoward effects and suggested beginning with 5 to 10 mg daily the first week; they noted that some of the subjects (ranging from 16 to 24 years of age) experienced good antidepressant response on doses as low as 5 to 10 mg daily.

Treatment of Depression

- *Children <8 years:* Not approved.
- *Children and adolescents ≥8 years through 17 years:* An initial morning dose of 10 to 20 mg/day is recommended. Because of higher plasma levels in lower weight children, both the starting and target doses should be 10 mg daily. If there is no improvement after several weeks, increasing the dose to 20 mg daily may be considered. Older and heavier children may initially be prescribed 20 mg daily; there is evidence that this may frequently be the optimal dose (Altamura et al., 1988). The full antidepressant action may take 4 weeks or longer to develop.
- *Adolescents ≥18 years and adults:* An initial morning dose of 20 mg is recommended, and this is usually the optimal dose. A dose increase may be considered after several weeks if there is inadequate clinical improvement. Such doses may be administered once or twice daily and should not exceed a maximum of 80 mg/day.

Treatment of OCD

- *Children <7 years:* Not approved.
- *Children and adolescents ≥7 years through 17 years:* In lower weight children, an initial morning dose of 10 mg/day is recommended; an increase to 20 mg may be considered after several weeks if there is inadequate clinical improvement. A dose range of 20 to 30 mg is recommended. In heavier children and adolescents, an initial dose of 10 mg is also recommended with an increase to 20 mg daily after 2 weeks. Further dose increases may be considered, if there is inadequate clinical improvement after several more weeks. A dose range of 20 to 60 mg/day is recommended.
- *Adolescents ≥18 years and adults:* An initial morning dose of 20 mg is recommended. Full therapeutic effect may take 5 weeks or longer to develop. A dose increase may be considered after several weeks if there is inadequate clinical improvement. A dose range of 20 to 60 mg/day is recommended; the maximum dose should not exceed 80 mg/day. Full therapeutic effect in the treatment of OCD may take 5 weeks or longer to develop. If adequate clinical response does not occur after several weeks, the dosage may be increased gradually to a maximum of 80 mg/day.

Treatment of Bulimia Nervosa

- *Children and adolescents ≤17 years:* Not approved. At the present time, the safety and efficacy of fluoxetine for children and younger adolescents remains to be elucidated.
- *Adolescents ≥18 years and adults:* In clinical studies of fluoxetine in fixed doses of 20 or 60 mg/day versus placebo in subjects diagnosed with bulimia nervosa, only the 60-mg dose was significantly better than placebo; hence the recommended target dose is 60 mg/day administered in the morning. It is frequently helpful to begin at a lower dose and to reach the target dose by increments of dose over a period of several days.

Treatment of Panic Disorder

- *Children and adolescents ≤17 years old:* Not recommended.
- *Adolescents ≥18 years and adults:* An initial dose of 10 mg/day with an increase to 20 mg/day after 1 week is recommended. Further increase in dose may be considered, if no significant clinical improvement has occurred after several weeks. Doses over 60 mg/day have not been systematically evaluated.

(continued)

**Indications for Fluoxetine Hydrochloride in Child
and Adolescent Psychiatry** *(continued)*

Treatment of PMDD

The recommended daily dose is 20 mg.

Fluoxetine Hydrochloride Dose Forms Available

Eli Lilly, who manufactures all four forms of the medications, states that they are bioequivalent.

- *Tablets:* 10, 20, and 60 mg (scored); Sarafem is available in 10- and 20-mg tablets.
- *Pulvules:* 10, 20, and 40 mg
- *Weekly capsules (Prozac weekly capsules):* 90 mg
- *Liquid:* 20 mg/5 mL

Reports of Interest

Fluoxetine in the Treatment of Child and Adolescent MDD

Joshi et al. (1989) reported on their treatment with fluoxetine of 14 patients (8 males, 6 females) ranging in age from 9 to 15 years (average age, 11.25 years) who were diagnosed with major depression by DSM-III-R (American Psychiatric Association [APA], 1987) criteria and who had not responded adequately to TCAs, had serious untoward effects from tricyclics, or could not be treated with tricyclics for medical reasons. Ten (71.4%) of the subjects responded favorably within 6 weeks to fluoxetine 20 mg administered in the morning. Side effects were limited to transient nausea and hyperactivity in one patient each and did not require discontinuation of the drug.

Simeon et al. (1990) reported a 7-week, double-blind, placebo-controlled fluoxetine treatment study of 40 adolescents (22 females and 18 males), aged 13 to 18 years (mean age, 16 years), who met DSM-III criteria for major depression unipolar type and had baseline Hamilton Depression Scores (Ham-D) of at least 20. In addition, the Ham-D scores of all subjects improved <20% during a preceding 1-week, single-blind placebo treatment protocol. Fluoxetine was begun at 20 mg/day, increased to 40 mg/day after 4 to 7 days, and increased to 60 mg/day during the second week. Further dosage changes were individually titrated.

At baseline, no significant differences were found between the groups. Thirty subjects completed the study divided equally between medication and control groups. About two-thirds of patients in each group showed moderate to marked clinical global improvement with significant improvement by week 3. With the exception of disturbances of sleep, all symptoms showed slightly greater improvement in subjects treated with fluoxetine than in those receiving placebo, but differences were not significant. Patients taking fluoxetine, however, experienced a small but significantly greater weight loss than those receiving placebo. Untoward effects were usually mild and transient, and none necessitated discontinuation of medication. Those most frequently reported were headache, vomiting, insomnia, and tremor. There were no significant differences in the effects of fluoxetine and placebo on heart rate or blood pressure.

Thirty-two patients were successfully followed up 8 to 46 months later (mean, 24 months) at ages 15 to 22 years (mean, 18 years). No significant differences were found between the fluoxetine and placebo groups, or between responders and non-responders to the initial clinical trial. Both groups showed further overall improvement; however, psychosocial functioning was still poor in more than one-third of the patients, and 50% of the patients' parents felt their children still required professional help. The authors noted that 10 patients were still depressed and 7 of them were still in treatment. About half of the patients who did not respond to placebo or fluoxetine during the initial 8 weeks of treatment were thought to constitute a very-high-risk group and remained very disturbed at follow-up (Simeon et al., 1990).

Boulos et al. (1992) treated, with fluoxetine, 15 adolescents and young adults diagnosed with MDD who had responded unsatisfactorily to prior treatment with antidepressants, usually including tricyclics, for a minimum of 2 months at doses associated with clinical efficacy. Seven subjects were 18 years old or younger. Eleven patients completed at least 6 weeks of treatment. Of these, 64% showed at least a 50% improvement on the HDRS, and 73% achieved scores of "much" or "very much improved" on the Clinical Global Impressions Scale (CGIS). Optimal doses ranged from 5 to 40 mg daily, and several patients received other medications concurrently. Untoward effects included headache, vomiting and other gastrointestinal complaints, insomnia, tremor, sweating, dry mouth, and hair loss.

Emslie et al. (1997) reported an 8-week, double-blind, randomized (stratified for age, ≤12 years or ≥13 years, and sex), placebo-controlled study of 96 children and adolescents (52 males, 44 females; mean age, 12.35; range, 7 to 17 years), diagnosed by DSM-III-R (APA, 1987) criteria with nonpsychotic MDD. Following a 3-week evaluation period and a 1-week, single-blind, placebo run-in during which responders were dropped, the 96 remaining subjects were randomized to 8 weeks of treatment with placebo or fluoxetine; there were 48 in each group (24 subjects aged 12 years or younger and 24 subjects aged 13 years or older in each group). Overall effectiveness was rated on the Clinical Global Impressions–Improvement (CGI-I) subscale and the Children's Depression Rating Scale–Revised (CDRS-R). In addition, the Brief Psychiatric Rating Scale–Children (BPRS-C) and the Children's Global Assessment Scale (CGAS) were used. Subjects were given 20 mg of fluoxetine or placebo daily for the entire 8 weeks unless they were dropped from the protocol because of failure to improve or untoward effects. Fourteen patients (29%) on fluoxetine discontinued the protocol, seven for lack of efficacy, four for untoward effects (three developed manic symptoms and one developed a severe rash), and three for protocol violation. Twenty-two patients (46%) on placebo dropped out, 19 for lack of efficacy, 1 for an untoward effect, and 2 for protocol violations. Fluoxetine was statistically better than placebo on the CGI-I; using the intent-to-treat (ITT) sample, 27 (56%) of the fluoxetine group versus 16 (33%) of the placebo group were rated much or very much improved ($P = .02$). Using a last-observation-carried-forward (LOCF) analysis for all 96 subjects, there was a significant drug-by-time interaction in favor of fluoxetine ($P = .01$); there was no significant drug-by-age or -sex interaction, meaning that males and females in both age groups responded equally well. After week 5, the mean CDRS-R score for the fluoxetine group became significantly lower than that for the placebo group ($P = .03$). Comparing initial and exit outcome LOCF scores on the CDRS-R for both groups, fluoxetine (initial score, 58.5 ± 10.5; exit score, 38.4 ± 14.8) was significantly better than placebo (initial score, 57.6 ± 10.4; exit score, 47.1 ± 17.0; $P = .002$). Subjects initially had relatively severe and chronic symptoms of depression and, despite their overall improvement, after 8 weeks, only 15 (31%) of the fluoxetine group and 11 (23%) of the placebo group had CDRS-R scores <28, consistent with relatively complete remission of depressive symptoms. Scores on the BPRS-C and the CGAS improved for both groups and were not significantly different. The authors concluded that fluoxetine was significantly better than placebo in acute-phase treatment of children and adolescents diagnosed with severe, persistent MDD and encouraged further studies.

The Treatment for Adolescents with Depression Study (TADS) Team (2004) conducted a randomized controlled trial in 439 patients at 13 sites (age 12 to 17 years, mean age 14.6 years; 45.6% males and 73.8% White, 12.5% Black, and 8.9% Hispanic) with a primary diagnosis of MDD by DSM-IV criteria (APA, 1994), which compared the efficacy of fluoxetine (10 to 40 mg/day) versus cognitive-behavior therapy (CBT) versus fluoxetine (10 to 40 mg/day) plus CBT versus placebo (equivalent to 10 to 40 mg/day) over a 12-week period. Medication in the fluoxetine and placebo group was administered in a double-blind fashion;

fluoxetine was administered openly in the fluoxetine plus CBT group as CBT was administered unblindly.

The 439 subjects of the study were those remaining from an initial 2,804 screened by telephone after inclusion and exclusion criteria were satisfied and those not interested in participation or withdrawing consent were eliminated. Major outcome measures were the CDRS-R and the CGI-I Score. The Reynolds Adolescent Depression Scale total score and the Suicidal Ideation Questionnaire–Junior High School Version (SIQ-Jr) total score were used as secondary outcome measures. CBT was composed of a possible 15 skills-orientated 50- to 60-minute sessions based on the premise that depression is "caused by or maintained by depressive thought patterns and a lack of active, positively reinforced behavioral patterns." The mean number of sessions completed was 11 in both groups with CBT. The mean fluoxetine dose in the fluoxetine-only group was 28.4 ± 8.6 mg/day and in the fluoxetine-plus-CBT group was 33.3 ± 10.8 mg/day; the mean placebo dose was 34.1 ± 9.5 mg/day.

Based on the improvement on the CDRS-R, combined treatment with fluoxetine and CTB was superior ($P = 001$) to treatment with placebo, but treatment with fluoxetine alone ($P = .10$) and CBT alone ($P = .40$) were not. Fluoxetine with CBT was superior to fluoxetine alone ($P = .02$) and to CBT alone ($P = .001$). Fluoxetine alone was also superior to placebo ($P = .01$).

On the CGI-I Scale, rates of positive response (a rating of 1 [very much improved] or 2 [much improved]) were fluoxetine plus CBT, 71% (95% CI, 62% to 80%); fluoxetine only, 60.6% (95% CI, 51% to 70%); CBT only, 43.2% (95% CI, 34% to 52%); and placebo 34.8% (95% CI, 26% to 44%).

After patients at high-risk for suicide were eliminated from the study because of exclusion criteria, 29% of the subjects had scores of >31, a level of suicidal thinking that requires prompt clinical attention on the SIQ-Jr at baseline; this decreased to 10.3% at 12 weeks and there was clinically significant improvement in suicidal thinking in all four groups. During the 12-week trial, 24 (5.5%) of the patients reported a suicide-related adverse event (worsening suicidal ideation or a suicide attempt) and 7 (1.6%) of patients attempted suicide but none was successful. Improvement in suicidality was greatest for the fluoxetine plus CBT group and least for the fluoxetine-only group. The authors concluded that fluoxetine is effective in the treatment of MDD and that the addition of CBT increases both clinical improvement and protection from suicidality (TADS, 2004).

The TADS study participants have been followed in a maintenance phase component from weeks 18 through 36 of the study (Stage III) and also in a naturalistic 1-year follow-up study after the end of 36 weeks of active treatment (Stage IV) (Kennard et al., 2009; March et al., 2009). In both of these studies, the remission rates were examined. Remission is defined as a return to a symptom-free state or a near symptom-free status. By 36 weeks, the estimated remission rates were as follows: combined treatment, 60%; Fluoxetine alone, 55%; CBT alone, 64%; and overall remission rate, 60% (Kennard et al., 2009). This is a significant improvement from previous reports of the TADS group remission rates of 23% after 12 weeks (Kennard et al., 2006). In the naturalistic study, TADS treatments were stopped at 36 weeks and participants received continued treatment in the community. They were assessed by the TADS researchers at 3, 6, 9, and 12 months after completion of the initial 36-week TADS study. Sixty-six percent of the original study group participated in at least one assessment and the benefits of active treatment continued during the naturalistic study period (March et al., 2009). These TADS follow-up studies suggest that the majority of adolescents with depression achieve remission and that their remission can be continued with long-term treatment (Kennard et al., 2009).

The Adolescent Depression and Psychotherapy Trial (ADAPT) study examined the effect of adding CBT to treatment with an SSRI (primarily fluoxetine). This study was funded by the UK National Health System and was conducted in community clinic settings. In contrast to the TADS study, the authors included participants with active suicidal intent, self-harm, depressive psychosis, and/or conduct disorder. Subjects were aged 11 to 17 and had moderate to severe levels of depression.

In the ADAPT study, 510 youth were screened for participation and of those 249 were eligible for the study. All participants were offered a brief initial intervention consisting of two sessions before they were referred to the study. Some participants declined to participate in the initial intervention and were enrolled in the study. Of those who participated in the intervention, 34 of 164 improved. Youth who did not respond to the brief intervention were randomized to SSRI alone (103) or SSRI plus CBT (105). The primary SSRI used in the study was fluoxetine, which was dosed at 10 mg daily for a week and then increased to 20 mg for 5 weeks. If no response was seen by 6 weeks, the dose was increased to 40 mg, and if no response was noted by 12 weeks, then the dose was increased to 60 mg. Participants who could not tolerate fluoxetine or in whom it was ineffective were given a different SSRI. Youth were followed for 28 weeks, and response was assessed at 12 and 28 weeks. Depressive symptoms decreased but no differences were detected between the two treatment arms. At the end of the 28-week study, 51% of those in the SSRI-alone group and 53% of those in the CBT-plus-SSRI group were much or very much improved (Goodyer et al., 2007).

The Treatment of SSRI-Resistant Depression in Adolescents (TORDIA) trial was funded by the National Institute of Mental Health to provide empirical evidence to guide clinical practice when initial treatment for depression is unsuccessful. Participants aged 12 to 18 were recruited, who had not responded to an initial course of SSRI treatment. They were randomized into one of four treatments: (a) switch to a second, different SSRI (fluvoxamine, citalopram, or paroxetine); (b) switch to a different SSRI plus CBT; (c) switch to venlafaxine (150 to 225 mg); or (d) switch to venlafaxine + CBT. At the completion of 12 weeks of treatment, the groups who received CBT + medication had a response rate of 54.8%. The groups with a medication switch alone had a response rate of 48.2%. There was no difference in response rates between the study drugs fluoxetine, citalopram, paroxetine, or venlafaxine (Brent et al., 2008). In a continuation study, the TORDIA study participants were continued in their treatment arm if they had responded and nonresponders received open treatment which could consist of a switch to another antidepressant, augmentation, or addition of CBT or other psychotherapy. Of the individuals enrolled in the original study, 78.1% were followed for another 24 weeks. They found that treatment type did not have any statistical differences and that all groups had similar remission rates. At 24 weeks, 38.9% had achieved remission. Of those who had remitted, it was more likely to occur in subjects who had a clinical response by week 12 (61.6% vs. 18.3%). Factors which predicted remission were lower rates of depression, hopelessness, anxiety, suicidal ideation, family conflict, and absence of comorbid dysthymia. The relapse rate among subjects who had initially responded by week 12 was 19.6% by week 24 (Emslie et al., 2010). The study ended at 24 weeks, and subjects were discharged to community care and naturalistically assessed at weeks 48 and 72. By week 72, 61.1% of the youth in the study had reached remission. Treatment group did not influence remission rate or time to remission. The study did find that the group assigned to SSRIs had a more rapid decline in self-reported depressive symptoms and suicidal ideation than the group assigned to venlafaxine (Vitiello et al., 2011).

These three large studies build on earlier research on the use of fluoxetine and SSRIs in depressed youth and have advanced knowledge to guide treatment selections in depressed youth. The TADS, ADAPT, and TORDIA studies compare the effectiveness of different treatment methods instead of comparing a treatment against placebo. Taken together, they can give physicians confidence in the continued use of medications and therapy to treat depression in adolescents.

Fluoxetine in the Treatment of Children and Adolescents with OCD or OCD and Tourette Disorder

In an open clinical study, Riddle et al. (1990) treated, with fluoxetine, 10 children (5 males, 5 females) ranging in age from 8 to 15 years (average age, 12.2 years) diagnosed with OCD only or with both OCD and Tourette disorder. Dosage ranged from 10 to 40 mg/day, with 80% of the patients receiving 20 mg/day; duration of treatment ranged from 4 to 20 weeks. Four of the patients with Tourette disorder received concomitantly additional medication for treatment of their tics. Fifty percent were considered responders to fluoxetine and were rated much improved; response rates were similar in patients with OCD only and in those with both diagnoses. The most common untoward effect was behavioral agitation/activation, characterized by increased motor activity and pressured speech. It occurred in 40% of the patients and usually started within the first few days; symptoms were most severe during the first 2 to 3 weeks but remained until medication was discontinued. No significant changes in blood pressure, pulse, weight, laboratory tests, or ECG were observed (Riddle et al., 1990/1991).

Riddle et al. (1992) reported a randomized, 20-week, double-blind, placebo-controlled, fixed-dose study with crossover after 8 weeks of fluoxetine in treating 14 subjects (6 males and 8 females; age range, 8.6 to 15.6 years; mean, 11.8 ± 2.3 years) diagnosed with OCD by DSM-III-R criteria. Subjects received 20 mg of fluoxetine or placebo. For various reasons, 13 subjects completed the first 4 weeks, 11 subjects completed the first 8 weeks, and only 6 subjects satisfactorily completed the entire 20 weeks. A comparison of between-group differences at 8 weeks was made for 13 subjects; this number of subjects was made possible by carrying the 4-week data forward to 8 weeks for the 2 subjects who dropped out during that time. The seven subjects receiving fluoxetine showed significant decreases on the Children's Yale–Brown Obsessive-Compulsive Scale (CY-BOCS) total score (mean decrease, 44%; $P = .003$), obsessions score (mean decrease, 54%; $P = .009$), and compulsions score (mean decrease, 33%; $P = .005$), and on the Clinical Global Impressions for Obsessive-Compulsive Disorder (CGI-OCD) (mean decrease, 33%, $P = .0004$). The six subjects on placebo also showed reductions in their obsessive-compulsive symptomatology on the CY-BOCS of 27% and on the CGI-OCD of 12%, but these reductions were not significant. When the two groups were compared, the improvement of subjects on fluoxetine was significantly greater than that of those on placebo on the CGI-OCD ($P = .01$) but not on the CY-BOCS ($P = .17$). The most frequently reported untoward effects were insomnia, fatigue, motoric activation, and nausea. Preexisting chronic motor tics worsened in two subjects; however, fluoxetine was continued and the tics subsided to negligible levels over the subsequent 2 years. A subject with comorbid diagnoses of MDD, separation anxiety, and oppositional disorder developed suicidal ideation, which resolved after fluoxetine was discontinued. The authors noted that 20 mg/day may be too high a dose for some children and that an initial dose of 10 mg/day of fluoxetine was the most common starting dose given to children by most child and adolescent psychiatrists.

Of the six subjects initially on fluoxetine who crossed over to placebo at 8 weeks, three dropped out at week 12 because of worsening of symptoms, with a mean increase of 53% ± 37% in CY-BOCS scores. A fourth subject was worse at week 20 on the CY-BOCS, and the remaining two showed improvement (decrease) in their CY-BOCS scores. Although three of the four subjects who crossed over from placebo to fluoxetine had shown substantial reductions in their CY-BOCS scores during the placebo period, there was further reduction in these scores at 20 weeks. Overall, these results complement findings in adults and suggest that fluoxetine is both safe and effective in treating children and adolescents with OCD for 20 weeks (Riddle et al., 1992).

Geller and colleagues (2001) examined the effectiveness of fluoxetine in children and adolescents with OCD in a double-blind placebo-controlled study

(Geller et al., 2001). One hundred three patients were enrolled in the study and were randomized to receive either fluoxetine (71) or placebo (32). Patients were initially given a 10-mg dose of fluoxetine for the first 2 weeks of treatment and then 20 mg for the next 2 weeks. After 4 weeks, their fluoxetine dose was increased to 40 mg/day if their CGI-Severity score was unchanged or worse than baseline. Three weeks later, the dose could be increased another 20 mg if the CGI-Severity score was unchanged or worse. The maximum fluoxetine dose was 60 mg/day. If subjects had difficulty tolerating a higher dose of fluoxetine, the dosage could be reduced. Improvement was primarily measured with the CY-BOCS.

The mean dose of fluoxetine in the treatment group was 24.6 mg. Sixteen (23%) had a final dose of 40 mg/day, and 15 (21%) had a final dose of 60 mg/day. Fluoxetine was associated with significantly greater improvement in CY-BOCS scores ($P = 0.26$), which indicate improvement in OCD symptoms. Patients with a 40% or greater reduction in their CY-BOCS scores were considered responders. By this criteria, 35 of 71 (49%) of the fluoxetine group and 8 of 32 (25%) of the placebo group were responders. CGI-Improvement scales in the fluoxetine treated group had 55% of patients rated as much or very much improved compared with 18.8% of the placebo group.

Fluoxetine was well tolerated. Discontinuation due to AEs occurred in 8.5% of the fluoxetine group and 6.3% of the placebo group. Discontinuation in the fluoxetine group occurred due to headache, hyperkinesia, abnormal liver function tests, manic reaction, nervousness, or somnolence. Placebo-treated patients discontinued because of hyperkinesia or nervousness. The authors conclude that fluoxetine 20 to 60 mg a day was effective and well tolerated for the treatment of OCD in the pediatric population.

Fluoxetine in the Treatment of Children and Adolescents with Anxiety Disorders

Birmaher et al. (1994) treated with fluoxetine 21 patients (age range, 11 to 17 years; mean, 14 years) diagnosed with overanxious disorder (OAD) only ($N = 6$); OAD, social phobia (SP), and separation anxiety disorder (SAD) ($N = 5$); or OAD and SP or SAD ($N = 10$), who had not responded to prior psychopharmacotherapy or psychotherapy. Subjects with a prior history of OCD, panic disorder, or current MDD were excluded. The mean fluoxetine dose after an average of 10 months (range, 1 to 31 months) on fluoxetine was 25.7 mg/day; the following distribution of doses was reported: 10 mg/day (1), 20 mg/day (15), 30 mg/day (1), 40 mg/day (2), and 60 mg/day (2).

Twenty subjects (95%) showed some improvement in anxiety, with 17 (81%) rated as moderately to markedly improved on the severity and improvement subscales of the CGIS ($P = .0001$). It is important to note that in most cases improvement did not begin until 6 to 8 weeks after initiation of fluoxetine. Although no subject fulfilled diagnostic criteria for MDD or dysthymia, 10 patients did have depressive symptoms. These symptoms also improved significantly ($P = .0001$); analysis suggested that the improvements in depressive symptoms and anxiety were independent. Only a few untoward effects, which were usually mild and transient, were reported: mild headache (one), nausea (three), insomnia (one), and stomachache (one). No significant changes in pulse, blood pressure, or ECG were found, and no subject experienced agitation, manic, or hypomanic symptoms, or suicidal ideation. These data suggest that fluoxetine may be a useful treatment for children and adolescents with anxiety disorders (Birmaher et al., 1994).

Fairbanks et al. (1997) treated with fluoxetine monotherapy on an open-label basis, 16 outpatients (8 males, 8 females; mean age, 13.0 ± 2.9 years; age range, 9 to 17 years) diagnosed by DSM-III-R (APA, 1987) criteria with mixed anxiety disorders and who were unresponsive to psychotherapy. Eleven subjects (69%) had a mean of 2.5 ± 1.5 coexisting anxiety disorders, including SAD ($N = 11$), SP ($N = 10$), GAD ($N = 7$), specific phobia ($N = 6$), and panic disorder ($N = 5$). Efficacy was assessed by ratings on the CGAS, the modified Liebowitz Social Anxiety Scale, the modified social behavior scale, the CGIS, and a side-effects checklist. Fluoxetine was initiated at a dose of 5 mg/day and subsequently increased weekly by 5 or 10 mg/day for 6 to 9 weeks until clinical improvement occurred or to a maximum of 40 mg for subjects <12 years of age or 80 mg/day for subjects ≥12 years of age.

The mean fluoxetine dose for all subjects was 35.0 ± 17.1 mg/day or 0.71 ± 0.28 mg/kg/day. The mean mg/kg/day dose was almost identical for subjects of all ages; subjects <12 years had lower optimal doses because they weighed less. Subjects with only one anxiety disorder responded to lower doses than subjects with two or more anxiety disorders. The CGIS ratings showed significant improvement in the severity of anxiety in ratings by psychiatrists, mothers, and subjects. Mean duration of time on medication until a rating of "improved," "much improved," or "completely recovered" on the CGIS was 5 weeks, with a range of 1 to 9 weeks. According to diagnoses, improvements on the CGIS were as follows: separation anxiety (N = 10): 6 much improved, 4 improved; SP (N = 10): 1 much improved, 7 improved; GAD (N = 6): 1 much improved, 4 improved; panic disorder with or without agoraphobia (N = 5): 1 much improved, 3 improved. Fluoxetine did not appear to aggravate the anxiety of any of the patients. The authors state that their outcome assessments found that SAD, SP, specific phobia, and panic disorder all responded favorably to fluoxetine but that GAD did not. The most common untoward effects were drowsiness, difficulty falling asleep or staying asleep, decreased appetite, nausea, abdominal pain, and a state of being easily excited or keyed up. None of the subjects was reported to have disinhibition, akathisia, suicidal or violent reactions, or hypomania. The authors concluded that fluoxetine is potentially effective in the short-term treatment of anxiety disorders (excluding GAD) in children and adolescents who do not have comorbid MDD, OCD, substance abuse, or medical complications and that further studies are needed.

Birmaher et al. (2003) conducted a 12-week, randomized, placebo-controlled, double-blind study to assess the efficacy and tolerability of fluoxetine in the outpatient treatment of 74 children and adolescents (age range 7 to 17 years; mean age 11.8 ± 2.8 years; 34 [45.9%] males and 40 [54.1%] females) diagnosed by DSM-IV (APA, 1994) criteria with GAD, SP, and/or SAD; most subjects were diagnosed with more than one anxiety disorder, and 24 (32%) were also diagnosed with other nonanxiety psychiatric disorders. Fluoxetine was initiated at a dose of 10 mg/day for the first week and, if tolerated, was increased to 20 mg/day for the remaining 11 weeks of the study. No other psychiatric medications were permitted for the duration of the study.

At the end of the study, on the CGI-I Scale, using an ITT analysis for all subjects, 61% (22/36) of subjects taking fluoxetine and 35% (13/37) of subjects taking placebo had scores of 1 (very marked improvement) or 2 (marked improvement) (P = .03) although the analysis for completers was even more positive for the fluoxetine group: 75% for fluoxetine versus 38.7% for the placebo group (P = .005). The authors noted that compared with SP subjects on placebo (N = 19), the subgroup with a diagnosis of SP on fluoxetine (N = 21) had significantly better outcomes on the CGI-I (12% vs. 76%, P = .001). Regarding AEs during the first 2 weeks, subjects on fluoxetine had significantly more AEs than those on placebo for abdominal pain and nausea, 46% versus 22%, P = .04; drowsiness and headaches 44% versus 14%, P = .004. For the entire duration of the study, only abdominal pain and nausea were significantly more frequent in the fluoxetine group: 44% versus 22%, P = .04. The authors also noted that during the study 11 patients (7 on fluoxetine and 4 on placebo, P = NS) experienced 20 incidents of excitement, giddiness, or disinhibition and 5 of these, all receiving fluoxetine, were dropped from the study as a result. Subjects were more severely ill at intake (scores of >30) on the Screen for Child Anxiety-Related Emotional Disorders–Child (SCARED-C) and those with positive family histories for anxiety had a poorer clinical response to fluoxetine than subjects without such histories. The authors concluded that fluoxetine is clinically effective and safe for the acute treatment of anxiety in this age group. They suggested that an increase in dose is indicated for patients with no or only partial clinical response after 4 to 6 weeks of treatment. In addition, they noted that mild to moderate agitation/disinhibition may be successfully treated by lowering the dose of fluoxetine in many cases (Birmaher et al., 2003).

In a 1-year follow-up of the 74 subjects in Birmaher et al.'s (2003) 12-week acute, controlled study of fluoxetine, an open-label, l-year extension was conducted (Clark et al., 2005). Fifty-six completed the 1-year follow-up; of these, four were not included in the analysis as they received other medications as well. Of the 52 analyzed completers, 42 were assigned to fluoxetine (of this group, 22 had been on fluoxetine during the acute 12-week trial and 20 had been on placebo) and 10 received no medication (of these 4 had been on fluoxetine during the 12-week acute study and 6 had been on placebo). Those subjects on fluoxetine were rated as significantly more improved than those on no medication on the SCARED–Parent Report ($P \leq .01$), the SCARED-C ($P < .05$); the Pediatric Anxiety Rating Scale–Parent Report (PARS-P), and the PARS–Rater Report (PARS-R) ($P = .05$). The PARS–Child Report (PARS-C) was not significantly different between the fluoxetine and the placebo groups. The group showing the greatest improvement in CGI-S was the group that was on placebo during the 12-week acute trial and on fluoxetine during the 1-year open-label extension period. The results suggest that fluoxetine continues to be of benefit for the treatment of anxiety in this group of subjects for up to 15 months (Clark et al., 2005).

Fluoxetine in the Treatment of Children and Adolescents with ADHD

Barrickman et al. (1991) reported on 19 children and adolescents (age range, 7 to 15 years) diagnosed with ADHD who were treated for 6 weeks in an open study with fluoxetine hydrochloride. Fourteen subjects had comorbid diagnoses of either conduct disorder ($N = 6$) or oppositional defiant disorder ($N = 8$). Most subjects had prior psychopharmacologic treatment that was unsatisfactory or had untoward effects on stimulants (e.g., tics) or antidepressants (e.g., sedation). Initial daily dose was 20 mg in the morning; subsequent doses were individually adjusted. Average daily dose was 27 mg (0.6 mg/kg) (range, 20 to 60 mg). Nine subjects took 20 mg/day, eight took 40 mg/day, and two took 60 mg/day. Most subjects improved within 1 week after a therapeutic dose was reached. Ratings were made on a large number of standardized instruments. Eleven subjects (58%) were rated "moderately improved" or "very much improved" after 6 weeks; eight had minimal improvement. Side effects were minimal and all remitted spontaneously or with dose reduction except mild sedation in one case. In particular, there were no reports of loss of appetite or significant changes in weight. Only one subject experienced nervousness, and none had insomnia or developed suicidal ideation.

All three children diagnosed with ADHD showed worsening of ADHD symptoms on fluoxetine in the Riddle et al. (1990/1991) study of behavioral side effects of fluoxetine discussed earlier.

Gammon and Brown (1993) reported the use of fluoxetine augmentation of methylphenidate in an 8-week open trial with 32 patients (9 to 17 years old) who were diagnosed with ADHD and one or more comorbid disorders—that is, dysthymia (78%), oppositional defiant disorder (59%), MDD (18%), anxiety disorders (18%), and conduct disorder (13%)—and who had inadequate therapeutic responses to methylphenidate alone. Addition of fluoxetine was begun with an initial dose of 2.5 or 5.0 mg/day for subjects <12 years of age and 12 years of age or older, respectively. Dose was titrated upward every 3 to 4 days in increments equal to the initial dose, to a maximum of 20 mg/day. Optimal daily dose of fluoxetine at 8 weeks ranged from 2.5 to 20 mg. The majority of subjects (19, or 59%) required 20 mg/day; 6 subjects (18%) received 10 to 15 mg/day; 4 subjects (12.5%) received 5 to 7.5 mg/day; and 3 subjects (9%) had optimal fluoxetine doses of 2.5 mg/day. No significant or lasting untoward effects were reported.

After 8 weeks of combined drug treatment, all 32 subjects showed statistically significant improvements on assessments rating attention, behavior, and affect. These improvements were also rated clinically significant in 94% (30) of the subjects. Scores on the CGAS dramatically improved ($P < .0001$). Mean scores on the Children's Depression Inventory declined from 22, which is in the clinical range for depressive symptoms, to 8, which is below that range ($P < .0001$). On the Conners Parents Rating Scale, group means improved on all six scales; on five scales improvement was significant ($P < .001$ to $P < .0001$). There was also a marked jump in student grade point average within one marking period. Parents reported substantial improvement in hyperactivity, impulsivity, anxiety, conduct, and learning problems. Augmentation with fluoxetine also produced significant further improvement in sustaining attention and concentration and helped to alleviate symptoms of anxiety, depression, irritability, and oppositionalism that had not responded adequately to methylphenidate alone. More seriously affected children showed the most significant improvements (Gammon and Brown, 1993).

Fluoxetine in the Treatment of Children Diagnosed with Bulimia Nervosa

Kotler and colleagues (2003) treated 10 subjects (age range of 12 to 18 years) who were diagnosed with bulimia nervosa in an open, 8-week study with fluoxetine 60-mg/day dose. They offered subjects a 4-week supportive psychosocial treatment phase preceding the 8-week medication trial. One subject improved significantly after therapy alone and did not receive medication. Five subjects elected to start the medication phase initially. Fluoxetine was initiated at 20 mg/day and titrated to 60 mg/day by day 7 and continued for the next 7 weeks. The subjects improved having average weekly binges decrease from 4.1 to 0. Average weekly purges decreased from 6.4 to 0.9. All patients improved their CGI-I scales with 20% rated as much improved, 50% improved, and 30% slightly improved (Kotler et al., 2003).

Fluoxetine in the Treatment of Children Diagnosed with Autism Spectrum Disorders

Given that youth with autism frequently often have repetitive behaviors similar to those seen in OCD, it is logical to believe that SSRIs could potentially help decrease compulsive symptoms in these children. One double-blind, placebo-controlled crossover study used fluoxetine in children with autism and examined its effect on global improvement. Hollander and colleagues enrolled 45 subjects with autism spectrum disorder (ASD). They defined ASD as meeting criteria for autism, Asperger syndrome, or pervasive developmental disorder not otherwise specified (PDDNOS) by Autism Diagnostic Interview. Subjects were randomized into two acute 8-week phases separated by a 4-week washout phase. Dosage began with 2.5 mg/day of liquid fluoxetine the first week and was then titrated up for the next 2 weeks up to a maximum dose of 0.8 mg/kg/day by the end of week 4. This dose was maintained for the remainder of the 8-week phases. AEs were monitored by use of the Fluoxetine Side Effects Checklist (FSEC). Clinical response was assessed by CY-BOCS and CGI-AD assessments. Thirty-nine subjects were included in data analysis ranging in age from 5 to 16 years. The dosage range of fluoxetine used was 2.4 to 20 mg. Their analysis showed that low-dose fluoxetine was superior to placebo in the treatment of repetitive behaviors by CY-BOCX compulsion scale. The effect size was in the moderate-to-large range (0.76). The improvement in CGI autism scores was only slightly superior to placebo in the fluoxetine group. The fluoxetine group did not differ significantly from placebo in treatment-emergent side effects. They did not detect any increase in suicide subscale measures, and anxiety/nervousness on fluoxetine was less than on placebo. The authors attribute the lack of side-effect differences between placebo and fluoxetine groups to their low doses and slow titration schedule. This contrasts with other studies which have found that SSRI treatment in ASD children frequently has increased side effects of behavioral activation (hyperactivity and agitation), aggression, and suicidal ideation (West et al., 2009).

Fluoxetine in the Treatment of Children Diagnosed with Selective (Elective) Mutism

Black and Uhde (1994) treated 15 subjects (age range of 6 to 11 years) who were diagnosed with elective mutism with fluoxetine in a double-blind, 12-week study. During a single-blind, 2-week placebo period preceding the study, a 16th subject who responded to placebo was dropped. Three boys and three girls (mean age, of 9.1 ± 2.3 years) were randomly assigned to fluoxetine. Three boys and six girls (mean age, of 8.1 ± 1.6 years) were assigned to placebo. Fluoxetine was given at a dose of 0.2 mg/kg/day for the first week, increased to 0.4 mg/kg for the second week, and further increased to 0.6 mg/kg for the final 10 weeks of the study. The mean maximum dose of fluoxetine was 0.60 to 0.62 mg/kg/day or 21.4 mg/day (range, 12 to 27 mg/day). The fluoxetine group improved more than the placebo group on 28 or 29 rating scales, but most of the differences were not significant. Both groups showed significant improvement from baseline over time in elective mutism, anxiety, and social anxiety as rated by parents, teachers, and clinicians. The fluoxetine group improved significantly more than the placebo group on parents', but not on teachers' or clinicians', ratings of mutism and clinical global improvement. This was consistent with earlier findings that children with elective mutism show improvements in the home setting before school and clinic settings. The authors noted that, although statistically significant, the improvements were modest and that the subjects continued to show serious impairments in their functioning. Untoward effects were minimal (Black and Uhde, 1994).

Dummit et al. (1996) reported a 9-week, open-label study of fluoxetine in the treatment of 21 children (5 males, 16 females; mean age, 8.2 ± 2.6 years; range, 5 to 14 years) who met DSM-IV (APA, 1994) criteria for selective mutism and co-morbid avoidant disorder or SP. Efficacy was assessed by ratings of the CGAS and the Liebowitz Social Anxiety Scale (LSAS). Subjects rated themselves on the social behavior scale, and parents rated their children on the same scale. Initially, fluoxetine was begun at a dose of 1.25 mg/day and gradually increased. As the authors found that none of the first 10 subjects improved on <20 mg/day and there were no problematic untoward effects at that dose, for subsequent subjects the initial dose was increased to 5 mg/day for the first week, 10 mg/day for the second week, and 20 mg/day for the third week. It was permissible to increase the dose to 40 mg/day for the sixth week and to 60 mg/day at the eighth week if clinically indicated. The mean optimal daily dose of fluoxetine was 28.1 mg/day or 1.1 mg/kg/day, and the dose ranged from 20 to 60 mg/day, with 15 subjects receiving 20 mg/day, 4 receiving 40 mg/day, and 2 requiring 60 mg/day. Overall scores on all indicators indicated significant improvement on all rating scales ($P < .001$ for clinicians' and subjects' self-ratings and $P < .005$ for parental ratings). After 9 weeks, 16 of 21 (76%) subjects were rated "improved" by their psychiatrist. Treatment outcome was inversely related to age, with 14 of 15 children <10 years improving to a clinically meaningful degree and only 2 of the 6 children ≥10 years old doing so. Four children developed excitement and behavioral disinhibition, which resulted in three of them discontinuing the medication and dose reduction in the fourth child. Most untoward effects were transient, and none was reported during the final week of treatment. The authors recommended a relatively low initial dose of

5 to 10 mg/day because of the possibility of behavioral activation and also noted that complete remission of the elective mutism often required more than 9 weeks of treatment, even in the marked treatment responders.

Sertraline Hydrochloride (Zoloft)

Sertraline hydrochloride is an SSRI that is chemically unrelated to other antidepressants currently in use. Its antidepressant effect is presumed to be related to its inhibition of neuronal serotonin uptake. Sertraline has also been approved for the treatment of OCD in patients 6 years of age and older, and for the treatment of panic disorder, social anxiety disorder, and PTSD in adults. It has only very weak effects on norepinephrine and dopamine reuptake. *In vitro*, sertraline has no significant affinity for alpha-1, alpha-2, or beta-adrenergic, cholinergic, gamma aminobutyric acid (GABA), dopaminergic, histaminergic, 5-HT_{1A}, 5-HT_{1B}, or 5-HT_2 serotonergic, or benzodiazepine receptors. Chronic administration of sertraline is thought to down-regulate norepinephrine receptors.

Pharmacokinetics of Sertraline Hydrochloride

Peak plasma levels of sertraline hydrochloride are reached between 4.5 and 8.4 hours after ingestion. Food increases the availability of sertraline slightly and peak blood levels are higher and are reached more quickly. Dosage, however, does not require adjusting and sertraline may be taken with or without food. During the first pass, sertraline undergoes extensive N-demethylation in the liver to form N-desmethylsertraline, which has a half-life of 62 to 104 hours but is significantly less pharmacologically active than sertraline. Both drug and metabolite subsequently undergo oxidative deamination followed by reduction, hydroxylation, and glucuronide conjugation. The average termination half-life of plasma sertraline is about 26 hours. Steady-state plasma levels at a given dose occur within about 7 days. Drug and metabolites are excreted in about equal amounts in the feces and urine, although all unmetabolized sertraline (about 13%) is found in the urine.

Data provided by the manufacturer suggest that patients in the pediatric age range, 6 through 17 years old, metabolize sertraline with slightly greater efficacy than do adults. Nevertheless, because of their lower body weights, lower doses than that prescribed for adults may be advisable (*PDR*, 2000).

Alderman et al. (1998) explored single 50-mg-dose and steady-state (200 mg/day) pharmacokinetics of sertraline in 61 patients (age range, 6 to 17 years of age). The authors found that all pharmacokinetic parameters for serum sertraline and desmethylsertraline levels were similar for their patients and those reported for adults when corrected for weight. They conclude that the titration regime recommended for adults was suitable and safe.

In their study of 92 children and adolescents prescribed sertraline for the treatment of OCD, March et al. (1998) reported that trough plasma levels of sertraline and its active metabolite desmethylsertraline, normalized for body weight, did not correlate significantly with age, sex, or clinical response.

Axelson et al. (2002) reported that the pharmacokinetics of sertraline varied significantly in adolescents (mean age 15.1; range 13.1 to 17.9 years) according to dose. The mean steady-state half-life at 50 mg/day was 15.3 ± 3.5 hours compared with 20.4 ± 3.4 hours at a dose of 100 to 150 mg/day. Because of this, they recommended that sertraline should be administered twice daily if adolescents were receiving <200 mg daily. The authors also measured platelet serotonin reuptake inhibition. They found that after 2 weeks' treatment with 50 mg/day of sertraline, platelet serotonin uptake was <70% in six of nine subjects and concluded that most adolescents need sertraline doses higher than 50 mg daily to achieve an adequate therapeutic response.

Alderman et al. (2006) reported the tolerability and efficacy of long-term sertraline use up to 200 mg/day in children and adolescents (Alderman et al., 2006). In this study, 16 children (6 to 12) and 27 adolescents (13 to 18) who were in a short-term study of sertraline safety and efficacy entered in a 24-week open-label phase with sertraline titrated to 200 mg/day. The mean daily dose at endpoint was 157 ± 49 mg. No significant age or gender effects or age-by-gender interactions were observed in sertraline values. Mean sertraline plasma concentrations normalized for dose and body weight did not differ significantly by age or gender. They had two patients (7%) discontinue due to AEs. Patients in the study had OCD or MDD, and both groups showed clinical improvement over 24 weeks of treatment. This study suggests that long-term treatment with sertraline in children and adolescents results in dose-normalized plasma concentration similar to that seen in adults.

Contraindications for the Administration of Sertraline Hydrochloride

Known hypersensitivity to sertraline hydrochloride is a contraindication.

Because of a possibility for serious, life-threatening reactions when administered simultaneously with an MAOI, the use of sertraline in combination with an MAOI is contraindicated. At least 14 days should elapse after stopping an MAOI before administering sertraline. Based on the half-life of sertraline, at least 14 days should elapse following its discontinuation before administering an MAOI.

Untoward Effects of Sertraline Hydrochloride

The most common side effects of sertraline in premarketing controlled studies included nausea, insomnia, diarrhea, ejaculatory delay, and somnolence. March et al. (1998) reported in a multicenter, 12-week, placebo-controlled trial of 187 children and adolescents (age range, 6 to 17 years) that 4 untoward effects occurred significantly more frequently in the subjects receiving sertraline: insomnia (37% vs. 13%; $P < .001$); nausea (17% vs. 7%, $P = .05$); agitation (13% vs. 2%, $P = .005$); and tremor (7% vs. 0%, $P = .01$). Additional untoward effects that occurred in at least 2% of the patients of the March et al. study and at least at twice the rate reported in patients on placebo were hyperkinesia, twitching, fever, malaise, purpura, weight loss, impaired concentration, manic reaction, emotional lability, abnormal thinking, and epistaxis (*PDR*, 2000). There is one case report of serotonin syndrome occurring in a 9-year-old boy following administration of a single 50-mg dose of sertraline (Phan et al., 2008).

Effects of Sertraline upon the Heart

Wilens et al. (1999) prospectively assessed cardiovascular functions (vital signs and ECG parameters) of the 187 children and adolescents diagnosed with OCD and treated with sertraline ($N = 92$) or placebo ($N = 95$) as discussed later in the report by March et al. (1998). Baseline data were contrasted with data from weeks 1, 4, and 12 of the study. There were no clinically significant differences in supine or standing heart rates or systolic or diastolic blood pressures between the two groups. There were no significant differences in PR, QRS, or QTc, and no significant new developments of sinus arrhythmias, nodal abnormalities, or intraventricular conduction abnormalities with the exception of two subjects on sertraline who developed a QTc interval of >440 msec ($P = .05$); no subject developed a QTc interval of >460 msec. The authors concluded that monotherapy with sertraline in doses of up to 200 mg/day in healthy children and adolescents was not associated with any symptomatic or asymptomatic clinically significant cardiovascular untoward effects but cautioned that the sample size precluded conclusions regarding small differences or rare events.

Indications for Sertraline Hydrochloride in Child and Adolescent Psychiatry

NOTE: Review the Black Box Warning at the beginning of the chapter or in the package insert before prescribing.

Sertraline has been approved for the treatment of depression, OCD, panic disorder, PTSD, PMDD, and social anxiety disorder in adults. It has been approved for the treatment of OCD in children 6 years of age and older, but its safety and efficacy for treating the other adult indications in the pediatric age group have not been established or approved by the FDA.

Sertraline Dosage Schedule

- *Children <6 years of age:* Not recommended.
- *Children ≥6 and adolescents through 17 years of age:*
  Treatment of OCD: In children 6 to 12 years of age, a single initial daily dose of 25 mg either in the morning or in the evening is recommended. Although the manufacturer recommends a single initial daily dose of 50 mg for adolescents aged 13 to 17 years, it is often prudent to begin with 25 mg daily, particularly in younger, less heavy adolescents, to avoid possible activation. Effective doses in clinical trials of patients 6 to 17 years of age ranged from 25 to 200 mg daily. Because of sertraline's relatively long (24-hour) elimination half-life, titration based on clinical response is recommended at intervals of at least 7 days to permit adequate assessment of clinical response at a given dosage. (See also recommendations of March et al., 1998, in the following text.)
  Treatment of MDD, panic disorder, SAD, social anxiety disorder, PTSD, and PMDD: Not recommended. The safety and efficacy of sertraline have not been established for the pediatric age group.
- *Adolescents at least 18 years of age and adults:*
  Treatment of MDD and OCD: An initial daily dose of 50 mg given either in the morning or at night is recommended. Full antidepressant response may be delayed for up to several weeks in some patients. Some patients may benefit from increases to a maximum of 200 mg/day. Because of sertraline's 24-hour elimination half-life, increments should be made at least 7 days apart to permit adequate assessment of clinical response at a given dosage.
  Treatment of panic disorder, PTSD, and social anxiety disorder: An initial daily dose of 25 mg is recommended with an increase to 50 mg daily after 7 days. Dose may be gradually increased in patients who do not have an adequate response. Effective dose range is usually between 50 and 200 mg daily. Because of sertraline's 24-hour elimination half-life, increments should be made at least 7 days apart to permit adequate assessment of clinical response to a given dosage.
  Treatment of PMDD: An initial dose of 50 mg/day is recommended to be given either throughout the menstrual cycle or during the luteal phase depending on the physician's assessment and judgment. Patients with inadequate clinical response may benefit from a 50-mg dose increase at the onset of each menstrual cycle to a maximum of 150 mg/day throughout the menstrual cycle or up to 100 mg/day if administered only during the luteal phase. If 100 mg/day is given during the luteal phase, it should be initiated with 50 mg/day and increased to 100 mg/day after 3 days of each luteal phase. Sertraline should be administered in a single morning or evening dose.

Sertraline Hydrochloride Dose Forms Available

- *Tablets (scored):* 25, 50, and 100 mg
- *Oral concentrate:* 20 mg/mL

■ *Reports of Interest*

Sertraline in the Treatment of Children and Adolescents with OCD

March et al. (1998) reported a multicenter randomized double-blind, placebo-controlled 12-week, parallel-group trial of sertraline versus placebo in 187 patients diagnosed with OCD by DSM-III-R criteria. There were 107 children aged 6 to 12 years, of whom 53 received active drug and 54 were given placebo, and 80 adolescents aged 13 to 17 years, of whom 39 received active drug and 41 were given placebo. The four main dependent-outcome measures for efficacy were the CY-BOCS, the National Institute of Mental Health Global Obsessive-Compulsive

Scale (NIMH GOCS), and the NIMH Clinical Global Impressions–Severity of Illness (CGI-S) and CGI-I rating scales. Subjects were required to have a baseline score of at least seven on the NIMH GOCS indicative of at least moderate impairment and absence of significant depression. In addition, none of the subjects responded to a week-long, single-blind placebo lead-in that was to eliminate placebo responders. Sertraline was initiated at 25 mg/day for children and 50 mg/day for adolescents and titrated upward by 50 mg weekly for 4 weeks, until a maximum of 200 mg/day or the maximum tolerated dose was achieved. Patients then continued to receive this dosage for weeks 5 through 12 of the study. Mean dose of sertraline at end point was 167 mg/day for the 92 subjects on sertraline. The number of adolescents tolerating 200 mg/day was greater than that tolerated by children: 39 (82%) versus 30 (57%).

Patients receiving sertraline improved significantly more than patients on placebo on the CY-BOCS ($P = .005$), the NIMH GOCS ($P = .02$), and the CGI-I Scale ($P = .002$), but only a trend was seen on the CGI-S Scale. Of the subjects receiving sertraline, 49/92 (53%) showed at least a 25% decrease in their CY-BOCS scores at end point versus baseline and 39/92 (42%) were rated as very much or much improved on the CGI-I rating at end point. These results were significantly better than that of the subjects receiving placebo, of whom 35/95 (37%) ($P = .03$) showed at least a 25% decrease of the CY-BOCS and 25/95 (26%) ($P = .02$) were rated as very much or much improved on the CGI-I rating at end point. Despite the significant clinical improvement, the average subject in the sertraline group was rated in the mildly ill range on the CY-BOCS at the end of the 12-week study. Untoward effects reported are described earlier; the authors note they may have increased because the protocol required the dose to be titrated upward so rapidly. There was no evidence that sertraline caused clinically significant changes in vital signs, laboratory values, or electrocardiogram (ECG).

March et al. (1998) concluded that sertraline appears to be a safe and effective short-term treatment for OCD in this age group. There was no significant difference in the untoward effects of sertraline in children compared with adolescents. The authors recommended an initial sertraline dose of 50 mg/day, titrated over a period of 6 to 8 weeks to reach maximum doses in partial or nonresponders. For an adequate clinical trial, sertraline should be taken for at least 10 to 12 weeks.

The Pediatric OCD Treatment Study (POTS) was a large multisite randomized controlled trial that examined the effect of CBT for OCD, sertraline, and combined treatment on improving OCD symptoms (March et al., 2004). In this study, 112 participants aged 7 to 17 were enrolled and randomly assigned to receive one of four treatment arms: (a) CBT alone, (b) medical management with sertraline, (c) combined treatment consisting of CBT and sertraline, or (d) a control condition pill placebo. In the medication groups, subjects were seen weekly and sertraline doses were started at 25 mg and adjusted upward up to 200 mg over 6 weeks. Subjects were followed for 12 weeks. The clinical remission rate for combined treatment was 53.6%; for CBT alone, 39.3%; for sertraline alone, 21.4%; and for placebo, 3.6%. The authors conclude that children and adolescents with OCD should begin treatment with a combination of CBT and SSRI or CBT alone rather than be treated with SSRI alone initially.

In further analysis of data from the POTS study, March and colleagues (2007a) examined the effects a comorbid tic disorder has on treatment outcome. In the POTS study, 15% of the subjects (17 of 112) had comorbid tic disorder. In patients with a comorbid tic disorder, sertraline did not differ from placebo. Combined (sertraline + CBT) treatment remained superior and CBT alone remained superior to placebo. This study suggests that tic disorders appear to adversely affect the outcome of medication management in pediatric OCD. This suggests that youth with OCD and comorbid tics should not be treated with sertraline alone and should be offered CBT alone or in combination with sertraline as their initial treatment.

Sertraline in the Treatment of Children and Adolescents with OCD or Depression

Alderman et al. (1998) treated 29 children (mean age, 10.4 ± 1.7 years; age range, 6 to 12 years) and 32 adolescents (mean age, 14.9 ± 1.4 years; age range, 13 to 17 years) who were diagnosed by DSM-III-R (APA, 1987) criteria with OCD ($N = 16$), MDD ($N = 44$), or both ($N = 1$) for 5 weeks with sertraline. All 61 subjects received an initial morning 50-mg dose of sertraline to determine single-dose pharmacokinetic parameters, followed by a 7-day washout. Following this (on day 8), subjects received either 25 mg/day of sertraline, which was force-titrated in 25-mg increments every 3 to 4 days to reach 200 mg/day on day 32, or 50 mg/day of sertraline, which was force-titrated in 50-mg increments every 7 days to reach 200 mg/day on day 29. After the titration period, both groups received 200 mg/day through day 42. Efficacy was assessed by ratings of the CY-BOCS, the NIMH GOCS, and the CGI-S and CGI-I scales.

At the end of the 5 weeks on sertraline, scores on the CY-BOCS for the 17 patients diagnosed with OCD decreased significantly from baseline (24.9 vs. 12.9; $P < .001$), scores on the NIMH GOCS declined significantly from baseline (10.2 vs. 6.7; $P < .001$), and scores on the CGI-S declined from 4.8 to 2.8 ($P < .001$). Ratings on the CGI-S for the 41 depressed patients who completed the 5-week period on sertraline declined significantly from 4.8 to 2.8 ($P < .001$). Changes in the children's and adolescents' groups were similar. The mean CGI-S for all subjects improved by 2.26, a rating signifying "much improved." Overall, 51 subjects reported at least one untoward effect but most were mild or moderate. The most commonly reported were headache (21%), nausea (21%), insomnia (21%), somnolence (15%), dyspepsia (12%), and anorexia (12%). There was no significant difference in incidence of untoward effects between children and adolescents except for dyspepsia, which was more frequent in children. Medication was discontinued in three of the depressed children because of the development of moderate hyperactivity in one, nervousness attributed to family stress in another, and severe self-mutilation in the third. The development of untoward effects did not correlate with any pharmacokinetic parameter or dose-titration schedule. The authors concluded that their results suggest that sertraline, administered as recommended for adults, is safe and effective in the treatment of subjects 6 to 17 years of age diagnosed with OCD or MDD.

Sertraline in the Treatment of Children and Adolescents with Major Depression

Tierney et al. (1995) reported a retroactive chart study of 33 inpatients and outpatients (14 males, 19 females; mean age, 13.25; range, 8.1 to 18.1 years) who were diagnosed with MDD by DSM-III-R (APA, 1987) criteria and treated with sertraline monotherapy on an open basis. Efficacy was determined by chart review ratings on the CGI-S Scale and the CGI-I Scale. Data were analyzed only for patients who completed 2 to 10 weeks of treatment in an attempt to eliminate those who had positive responses to hospitalization or spontaneous improvement. Twelve patients (including 10 inpatients) were treated for <2 weeks. The 21 patients included in the data analysis of efficacy were 9 males (mean age, 13.2; age range, 12.0 to 15.3 years) and 12 females (mean age, 14.3; age range, 9.5 to 18.1 years). Several had comorbid diagnoses but none had a history of mania or hypomania at the time of treatment. Untoward effects were tabulated for all 33 subjects. The usual initial dose of sertraline was 25 mg, with an increase to 50 mg/day within 1 week and subsequently titrated individually based on clinical response. At the end of 10 weeks, the optimal dose for 1 subject was 25 mg/day, with the other 20 patients ranging from 50 to 200 mg/day. The mean daily dose of sertraline at the end of treatment was 100 ± 53 mg or 1.6 ± 0.7 mg/kg.

The overall ratings on the CGI-S decreased significantly, from 5.83 ± 0.69 at baseline to 3.44 ± 0.17 at endpoint ($P < .01$). On the CGI-I Scale, 11 of 17 patients treated with sertraline for 2 to 10 weeks had ratings of "very much improved" or "much improved" over baseline; no subject's depression worsened. Older patients showed significantly greater improvement in depressive severity than younger patients ($P < .01$). Untoward effects were reported by 16 (48%) of the initial 33 patients. Four of the 12 who dropped out during the first 2 weeks did so because of untoward effects; 3 had behavioral activation (1 with intent to self-injure, 1 with mood lability, and 1 with symptoms [mania] consonant with bipolar I disorder) and 1 had nausea. Of the 33 subjects, 5 (15%) reported gastrointestinal symptoms (nausea, stomachache, vomiting, decreased appetite); 5 (15%), fatigue and sedation; 3 (33%), headaches; 7 (21%), behavioral activation, including 2 who developed mania (1 at 3 days and 1 after 94 days). The authors concluded that their data suggested that sertraline was clinically beneficial in some children and adolescents but noted that the potential for inducing behavioral activation and mania was of concern (Tierney et al., 1995).

McConville et al. (1996) treated with open-label sertraline 13 inpatients (3 males, 10 females; mean age, 15.1 years; range, 12 to 18 years) who were diagnosed with MDD by DSM-III-R criteria. No patient had received a psychotropic medication for at least 5 months before beginning sertraline at a mean of 6.75 days after admission. The hospitalizations of patients averaged a mean of 19 days (range, 9 to 38 days); patients were followed up after discharge and evaluated after a total of 12 weeks on medication. Of the 20 subjects who were there at the beginning of the study, 6 were dropped because of poor compliance with outpatient follow-up and 1 was dropped because he developed a manic episode after 8 days of sertraline. Efficacy was assessed by ratings on the Hamilton Rating Scale for Depression (Ham-D), the Montgomery-Asberg Depression Scale (M-ADS), the Clinical Global Impressions Scale Adapted for Depression (CGI-D), the CGAS, and the Family Global Assessment Scale (FGAS).

Sertraline was initiated at 50 mg/day and titrated weekly in increments of 50 mg based on clinical response. Two patients developed untoward effects on the initial dose and required a reduction in dosage. Mean sertraline dose at time of discharge from the hospital was 77 ± 26 mg/day or 1.5 ± 0.45 mg/kg/day. At the 12-week outpatient follow-up, the mean dose was 110 ± 50 mg/day or 2.0 ± 0.85 mg/kg/day; final optimal dose range was 25 to 200 mg/day.

Mean ratings on the three scales (Ham-D, M-ADS, and CGI-D) measuring depressive symptoms decreased significantly from premedication baseline to 12 weeks ($P < .001$ in all cases), with 11 of the 13 patients experiencing a decrease of more than 50% in their Ham-D scores. The authors noted a sharp drop in depressive symptoms during the first week on the drug, which they attributed to placebo or nondrug effects (e.g., hospitalization), so they also analyzed changes from the end of treatment week 1 to the end of treatment week 12. All were still significant (Ham-D, $P = .027$; M-ADS, $P = .022$; and CGI-D, $P = .029$). The CGAS showed a significant improvement from baseline to 12 weeks ($P = .011$) but not from week 1 to week 12, and the FGAS ratings did not improve significantly for either time interval. The most frequent untoward effects at 12 weeks were insomnia (69%), drowsiness (61%), weight change (46%), nightmares (39%), loss of appetite (31%), and headache (31%). The authors concluded that sertraline was a promising drug for the treatment of adolescent MDD (McConville et al., 1996).

Ambrosini et al. (1999) reported the combined data of six university-affiliated outpatient clinics that treated 53 adolescents (26 males and 27 females; mean age, 16 ± 2 years; range, 12.2 to 19.8 years), diagnosed with MDD with sertraline in a 10-week, open-label, acute-phase study. Thirty-seven subjects (70%) had a single episode and 16 (30%) had recurrent MDD; the mean duration of the index depressive episode was 78 ± 79 weeks, and most subjects had moderate ($N = 29$ [55%]) or severe ($N = 22$ [42%]) symptoms by DSM-III-R criteria (APA, 1987). Sixty-eight subjects participated in a 2-week, single-blind placebo washout period before beginning the protocol. Fifteen were eliminated from the study during this period, usually because they had improved clinically and no longer met study criteria for severity. Forty-one subjects completed at least 6 weeks of the study, and 34 completed the initial 10 weeks. The 26 "responders," defined as much or very much improved on the CGI-I, were eligible to continue receiving sertraline for an additional 12 weeks.

Severity of illness and efficacy were rated on the Schedule for Affective Disorders and Schizophrenia (SADS), HDRS, the CGAS, Beck Depression Inventory (BDI), and the CGI-S and CGI-I Scales. The initial dose of sertraline was 50 mg/day. Subjects were seen for evaluation of efficacy, untoward effects, and titration of medication at weeks 2, 3, 4, 6, 8, 10, and for responders, at weeks 14, 16, 18, 20, and 22. Dose could be decreased at any time for untoward effects and, beginning with week 3, could be increased by 50 mg each visit to a maximum of 200 mg. The mean sertraline dose at week 6 was 93.3 ± 20 mg/day and at week 10 was 127.2 ± 45 mg/day.

By week 2, there was significant improvement over baseline ($P = .0001$) in scores on the HDRS, the 17-item depression rating scale (part of the Mini-SADS), the BDI, and the CGI-S. Response rates improved with time throughout the study. The response rate on the 17-item scale, the most sensitive indicator of depressive symptoms, increased from 55% of subjects at 6 weeks to 76% by 10 weeks. On the HDRS, 26 (55.3%) subjects had a reduction in their scores by at least 50% by week 10. Response did not correlate with the age of the subject or baseline severity of depressive symptoms. Twenty-two of the 26 responders completed the additional 12-week period on sertraline, during which they maintained their improvement or improved further. Maximum clinician ratings of improvement occurred after the initial 10-week period. There were no clinically significant changes in vital signs, CBC, laboratory values, or ECGs. Untoward effects occurred in about 10% of the patients and were usually mild to moderate in severity. The most common were headache (36%), insomnia (26%), nausea (17%), dizziness (15%), flu-like symptoms (13%), diarrhea (13%), fatigue (11%), agitation (11%), and somnolence (11%). No patient developed manic symptoms. The only patient to discontinue sertraline did so because of akathisia.

The authors concluded that their data suggested that sertraline in doses of up to 200 mg/day was efficacious and safe in treating chronically depressed adolescent outpatients with moderate to severe MDD. They emphasized that, in the acute phase of treatment, it is important to administer sertraline for at least 10 weeks and that improvement can continue even after 10 weeks (Ambrosini et al., 1999).

Wagner et al. (2003) reported on the results of two multicenter randomized, double-blind placebo-controlled trials that were conducted at 53 sites that examined the use of sertraline for MDD. The study enrolled 367 children and adolescents aged 6 to 17 years. Subjects met the diagnostic criteria for MDD as defined by DSM-IV and as determined by K-SADS-PL at the first and third visits of a 2-week screening period. During all three visits of the screening period, patients were recruited if they had a CDRS-R score of at least 45 and a CGI-S rating of at least 4, which indicates a moderate severity of illness. Subjects enrolled in the study were randomized to receive either sertraline or placebo for a period of 10 weeks. Sertraline was dosed at 25 mg for the first 3 days and then increased to 50 mg for the end of the second week. If well tolerated, sertraline was increased by 50 mg every 2 weeks to a maximum of 200 mg/day until a satisfactory clinical response was achieved. The mean dose of patients who completed 10 weeks of double-blind treatment was 131 mg/day of sertraline and 144 mg/day of placebo equivalent.

Treatment outcomes were assessed with the CDRS-R and CGI-S measurements collected at the end of weeks 1, 2, 3, 4, 6, 8, and 10. The sertraline-treated group experienced statistically significant greater improvement than placebo patients on the CDRS-R total score. They had a mean change at week 10 of -30.24 versus -25.83, respectively, $P = .001$. Subjects with a 40% decrease in the adjusted CDRS-R total score at study end point were considered responders. Sixty-nine percent of sertraline-treated patients compared with 59% of placebo patients were considered responders ($P = .05$). Slightly greater improvement in CDRS-R scores were seen in adolescents than in children although the study was not powered to detect differences between age groups.

Sertraline was generally well tolerated by the study subjects. The majority (over 90%) of patients had AEs that were mild or moderate in intensity. The four AEs that occurred in at least 5% of the sertraline-treated subjects with an incidence of at least twice that of placebo were diarrhea, vomiting, anorexia, and agitation. Discontinuation of the study because of AEs occurred in 17 (9%) of the sertraline patients, 13 of whom were children. Five placebo-group subjects (3%) discontinued the study due to AEs. Serious adverse events (SAEs) were seen in seven sertraline-treated patients and six placebo patients. Suicide attempts were seen in two sertraline subjects and two placebo subjects. Suicidal ideation was seen in three sertraline subjects. Aggressive reaction was seen in one sertraline subject. Medical hospitalization occurred in one sertraline subject and four placebo subjects.

The authors conclude that their pooled analysis demonstrates that sertraline is an effective and well-tolerated short-term treatment for children and adolescents with MDD. They note that their study showed a drug–placebo difference similar to that found by Emslie and colleagues (2002) with fluoxetine.

Rynn and colleagues (2006) followed the subjects in this study in a long-term (24 week) open-label observational extension study (Rynn et al., 2006). Subjects in the acute study were offered enrollment in the open-label study. Two hundred twenty-one of 299 patients in the original study chose to continue. All patients were initially dosed with 50 mg of sertraline regardless of their final study-drug dose taken. Doses were flexibly titrated in the range of 50 to 200 mg/day. Subjects who had received placebo in the initial study received their first dose of sertraline in the extension study. The duration of sertraline dosing was 34 weeks for subjects initially treated with sertraline and 24 weeks for subjects initially treated with placebo. By the conclusion of the study, the mean daily dose was 109.9 mg/day. They found that patients continued to improve. The mean overall CDRS-R score at endpoint was 29.4 (SD ± 12.62), which is indicative of mild depressive symptomatology. Since the group that received sertraline in the initial study had lower mean CDRS-R scores initially, their scores dropped 6 points by endpoint, while the group who had placebo initially then received sertraline had a 9-point CDRS-R drop. By the end of the study, 86% of patients were considered CDRS-R responders and 58% had CDRS-R scores, which were indicative of remission of their depressive symptoms. They had 18 subjects discontinue their medicine related to sertraline, 9 from AEs, 1 from a laboratory abnormality (elevated liver function test), and 8 from lack of efficacy.

Sertraline Hydrochloride in the Treatment of Children Diagnosed with Anxiety

Rynn et al. (2001) examined the treatment of children with GAD with sertraline in a placebo-controlled trial. They enrolled 22 children and adolescents aged 5 to 17 who met DSM-IV criteria for GAD according to the Anxiety Disorders Interview Schedule for Children–Revised and who also had a Hamilton Anxiety Rating Scale score over 16. Subjects underwent at 2- to 3-week prestudy evaluation period in which seven subjects improved and were not able to be included in the study. Subjects were randomized to receive either sertraline or placebo. Sertraline was dosed 25 mg the first week and increased to 50 mg in the second. Subjects were followed with 9 weekly medication management visits for the 9-week treatment phase. They were not allowed to participate in CBT but were allowed to continue other psychotherapies in which they had been participating. At the end of the evaluation period, subjects receiving sertraline showed improvement in Hamilton Anxiety Scale (Ham-A) total score and CGI severity and improvement scales showed significant improvement with sertraline treatment when compared with the placebo group. Ninety percent of the patients who received sertraline were rated as improved (10 of 11) compared with only 10% of the placebo group (1 of 11). Two patients in the sertraline group were rated as markedly improved representing a likely remission rate of 18%. This study was limited by small sample size and relatively low sertraline dose (50 mg) in older adolescents but points to the usefulness of sertraline for youth with GAD.

Walkup et al. (2008) examined the use of sertraline and cognitive behavioral therapy as a treatment for children with anxiety disorders in the Child/Adolescent Anxiety Multimodal Study (CAMS). The CAMS study was designed in two phases. The first phase was a 12-week trial of short-term treatment comparing CBT, sertraline, CBT + sertraline, and a placebo drug. The second phase was a 6-month open trial of responders in the first phase. In this phase, 488 youth were randomized to receive the four treatment arms. The CBT intervention involved fourteen 60-minute sessions. The sertraline groups involved eight psychopharmacotherapy sessions and treatment with Zoloft or placebo administered on a fixed-flexible dosing schedule beginning with 25 mg/day adjusting up to 200 mg by week 8 if subjects were considered to be mildly ill or worse. Subjects receiving combination treatment received both interventions usually on the same day. Diagnosis was made using the Anxiety Disorders Interview Schedule for DSM-IV-TR, child version. Subjects who met criteria for separation, social, and/or GAD were included in the study. The mean age of study participants was 10.7 ± 2.8 years. Outcome measures were taken at screening, baseline, and at weeks 4, 8, and 12. Improvement was assessed by treatment response on the CGI-Improvement scale as well as anxiety severity measures on the Pediatric Anxiety Rating Scale (PARS).

At the end of phase 1, children rated as very much or much improved on the CGI-Improvement scales were 80.7% for the combination therapy ($P < 0.001$), 59.7% for CBT ($P < 0.001$), and 54.9% for sertraline ($P < 0.001$). All three treatment arms were superior to placebo with only 23.7% improved. Combination therapy was statistically superior to both the CBT and sertraline monotherapies. AEs included suicidal and homicidal ideation and were no more frequent in the sertraline group than in the placebo group. None of the study subjects attempted suicide. The side effects of insomnia, fatigue, restlessness, and sedation were seen more in the sertraline group than in the CBT subjects. The CAMS study has findings which have been seen in similar studies of different disorders and drugs which show that the combination of CBT and an SSRI is the most effective treatment selection for youth with internalizing (anxiety and depressive) disorders.

An analysis of remission rates seen in the CAMS trial was reported by Ginsburg et al. (2011). Remission was defined as a loss of all study-entry anxiety disorder diagnoses or by CGI-S or CGI-I measurements and varied with the loss of diagnosis having the highest remission, and the CGI-I scores have the lowest rates. They found that the combined group had the highest remission rates ranging from 46% to 68%. The sertraline group had remission rates of 34% to 46%. The CBT group had remission rates of 20% to 46%. The placebo group had remission rates of 15% to 27%. This showed that for most children in the study, some symptoms of anxiety persisted and may need additional treatment.

Sertraline Hydrochloride in the Treatment of Children Diagnosed with Selective Mutism

Carlson et al. (1999) treated five outpatients (one male, four females; age range, 5 to 11 years) diagnosed with selective mutism by DSM-IV (APA, 1994) criteria in a 16-week, double-blind, placebo-controlled trial of sertraline within a replicated multiple-baseline/across-participants research design. There were four randomly ordered treatment phases: no drug for 2 weeks, placebo for 2 to 6 weeks, 50 mg/day of sertraline for 2 weeks, and 100 mg/day of sertraline for 6 to 10 weeks (subjects who were assigned to longer placebo periods had a respectively shorter time on 100 mg/day of sertraline). Selective mutism had been present from 2 to 7 years in the subjects. Subjects had no comorbid psychiatric conditions, no prior drug treatment of their selective mutism, or ongoing psychotherapy, although all five had previously had behavioral therapy and three had had individual psycho-therapy. Efficacy was determined by ratings on goal attainment scaling to quantify the progress toward a target behavior, for example, speaking; both parents and teachers rated children on this scale. CGI-S ratings adapted for mutism, anxiety, and shyness were completed by parent, teacher, and psychiatrist. Improvement in speaking occurred within a few days of beginning sertraline in four of the five subjects as rated by parents. Two of the five subjects were speaking in school and no longer met criteria for selective mutism after <10 weeks of receiving sertraline. Parents of a third subject taking 50 mg/day of sertraline reported that their daughter was speaking in school and in other settings at follow-up 20 weeks after the study. Untoward effects were minimal and did not require dose reduction. The results suggest that sertraline may be useful in treating selective mutism in this age group.

Sertraline Hydrochloride in the Treatment of Children Diagnosed with PTSD

Given its effectiveness in adults, researchers have sought to show that sertraline is also helpful as a psychopharmacologic intervention in children and adolescents. The effectiveness of sertraline in the treatment of PTSD was examined in a double-blind placebo-controlled trial by Robb et al. (2010), which yielded negative results. In this multicenter trial, youth who met criteria for PTSD after a 2-week assessment period were enrolled in the 10-week trial and given either flexible doses of sertraline (50 to 200 mg/day) or a placebo. The University of California Los Angeles Post-Traumatic Stress Disorder Index score (UCLA PTSD-I) was used to assess presence and severity of PTSD symptoms. The Child Stress Disorder Checklist (CSDC) is a 30-item parent-rated scale that was used to assess response. CGH-S and CGI-Improvement scales and CDRS-R ratings were also used. Two hundred four patients were screened and 131 (64.2%) met criteria at the end of the 2 week screening period and were randomized to receive sertraline or placebo. The mean duration of symptoms was 2 years. The study found that there was no difference on the UCLS PTSD-I scores between the sertraline or the placebo group. Both groups had improvement in the assessment measures, but the placebo group had more improvement than the sertraline group. An interim analysis of the study data was performed, and the study was stopped for futility after 81.8% of the initially planned subject group was enrolled.

Another study by Cohen et al. (2007) found little benefit to adding sertraline to an already established effective treatment for PTSD in children: Trauma Focused Cognitive Behavioral Therapy (TF-CBT). In this study, 25 females aged 10 to 17 were randomly assigned to receive TF-CBT + placebo or TF-CBT + sertraline for 12 weeks. Both groups had significant improvement in their PTSD and clinical outcome measures. No differences were found in most measures except the CGI ratings suggested a slight improvement in the sertraline TF-CBT group. The authors conclude that sertraline could have caused some improvement in comorbid depression symptoms.

Stoddard et al. (2011) examined the effect of sertraline to prevent PTSD in burned children. In this study, 26 children aged 6 to 20 years who were admitted to a pediatric burn center were screened and randomized to receive either sertraline dosed between 25 and 150 mg or placebo in a double-blind placebo-controlled design. The subjects who received sertraline had no difference in child-reported symptoms from their peers who received placebo. The sertraline group did show a greater decrease in parent-reported symptoms over the course of the study. This suggests that sertraline may prevent the emergence of PTSD symptoms in children.

Paroxetine Hydrochloride (Paxil); Paroxetine Mesylate (Pexeva)

Paroxetine hydrochloride, an SSRI, is the hydrochloride salt of a phenylpiperazine compound. Its chemical structure is unrelated to other SSRIs and antidepressants currently in use. Studies suggest that its antidepressant action and clinical efficacy in obsessive-compulsive, panic, and social anxiety disorders are related to its being a highly potent selective inhibitor of neuronal serotonin reuptake. In addition, paroxetine has only a very weak effect on the neuronal reuptake of norepinephrine and dopamine. Paroxetine has little affinity for muscarinic alpha-1-, alpha-2-, beta-adrenergic; dopamine (D_2); 5-HT_1, 5-HT_2; and histamine (H_1) receptors.

Pharmacokinetics of Paroxetine Hydrochloride

Food slightly increases bioavailability of paroxetine; it increases maximum plasma levels and decreases the time to reach peak plasma concentration from about 6.5 to 5 hours. Paroxetine may be administered with or without food without dosage adjustment. Paroxetine is extensively metabolized in the liver, in part by the P450 2D6 enzyme system. Its principal metabolites have only one-fiftieth the potency of the parent compound in inhibiting serotonin reuptake. About two-thirds of the drug is excreted in the urine and one-third in the feces. Serum half-life ($T_{1/2}$) is approximately 21 hours. Steady-state plasma levels usually occur within 10 days.

Findling et al. (1999) studied paroxetine pharmacokinetics in 30 children and adolescents (age range, 6 to 17 years; mean age, 11.2 ± 2.9 years), 15 of each sex, who were being treated for a diagnosis of MDD. The mean half-life of paroxetine in this age group was 11.1 ± 5.2 hours, considerably shorter than that in adults; however, steady-state plasma levels were still achieved with once-daily dosing.

There has been great interest in the role of all SSRIs in contributing to suicidal thoughts and behaviors in children and adolescents. Paroxetine was the first SSRI to have suicide concerns identified. The FDA issued a statement about the possibility of paroxetine increasing risk of suicidal thinking in children below 18 years of age in June 2003. The FDA recommended that paroxetine not be used to treat depression in children and adolescents, and similar warnings were issued by the United Kingdom's Chairman of the Committee on Safety of Medicines (CSM) (Duff, 2003; FDA, 2003). A full discussion of the issue is discussed at the beginning of the chapter. An analysis of all subjects treated with paroxetine and placebo in double-blind trials was completed by Apter et al. (2006). One thousand one hundred ninety-one children and adolescents who received paroxetine or placebo in double-blind studies were blindly reviewed; incidents of AEs were reviewed and cases of suicidal or nonsuicidal behavior were examined. Incidence rates were calculated for suicide-related events and for rating scale items assessing suicidality. The authors found that suicide-related events occurred more often in paroxetine than (22 of 642, 3.4%) than placebo groups (5 of 549, 0.9%). Except for one child, all suicide-related events occurred in adolescents over 12. The authors conclude that adolescents treated with paroxetine showed an increased risk of suicide-related events.

Contraindications for the Administration of Paroxetine Hydrochloride

Known hypersensitivity to paroxetine hydrochloride is a contraindication.

Because of a possibility of serious, life-threatening reactions when administered simultaneously with an MAOI, the use of paroxetine in combination with an MAOI is contraindicated. At least 14 days should elapse after stopping an MAOI before administering paroxetine. Based on the half-life of paroxetine, at least 14 days should elapse following its discontinuation before administering an MAOI.

Paroxetine hydrochloride is secreted in breast milk, and hence nursing is not recommended while taking paroxetine.

Untoward Effects of Paroxetine Hydrochloride

In clinical trials, between 16% and 20% of patients discontinued taking paroxetine for the following reasons: asthenia, sweating, nausea, decreased appetite, somnolence, dry mouth, dizziness, insomnia, tremor, nervousness, ejaculatory and other male sexual disturbances, and female sexual disorders.

Findling et al. (1999) reported that two (6.7%) of their 30 subjects (mean age, 11.2 ± 2.9 years) diagnosed with MDD and treated with paroxetine developed hypomania requiring discontinuation of the medication. In both cases, the hypomanic symptoms remitted without complications following discontinuation.

Indications for Paroxetine Hydrochloride or Paroxetine Mesylate in Child and Adolescent Psychiatry

NOTE: Review the Black Box Warning at the beginning of the chapter or in the package insert before prescribing.

Paroxetine hydrochloride has been approved for the treatment of MDD, OCD, panic disorder, social anxiety disorder, GAD, and PTSD in adults. Its safety and efficacy for use in the pediatric age group have not been established. One manufacturer notes that three placebo-controlled studies of paroxetine in the treatment of MDD in pediatric patients did not adequately support its use in this age group (*PDR*, 2006).

Paroxetine Dosage Schedule

Paroxetine may be administered with or without food. It is recommended that it be given in a single daily dose, usually in the morning.

- *Children and adolescents ≤17 years of age:* Not recommended. Safety and efficacy have not been established in this age group.
- *Adolescents at least 18 years of age and adults:*
  Treatment of MDD: An initial single dose of 20 mg, usually administered in the morning, is recommended. Full antidepressant response may be delayed for up to several weeks. Although 20 mg/day is adequate for many patients, others may benefit from higher doses. Based on clinical response, weekly increments of 10 mg/day may be made at intervals of at least 1 week to a maximum daily dose of 50 mg.
  Treatment of OCD: The usual target dose for the treatment of OCD is 40 mg daily. The recommended initial daily dose is 20 mg, usually administered in the morning. Increments of 10 mg/day are suggested at weekly intervals to reach the recommended dose of 40 mg/day. Some patients may benefit from higher doses, and further increments, at least 1 week apart, may be made to a maximum of 60 mg/day.
  Treatment of panic disorder: The usual target dose for the treatment of panic disorder is 40 mg daily. The recommended initial daily dose is 10 mg, usually administered in the morning. Increments of 10 mg/day are suggested at weekly intervals to reach the recommended dose of 40 mg/day. Some patients may benefit from higher doses, and further increments, at least 1 week apart, may be made to a maximum of 60 mg/day.
  Treatment of social anxiety disorder: An initial single dose of 20 mg, usually administered in the morning, is recommended. Available information shows no additional benefit to patients treated with higher doses (up to 60 mg/day) for this disorder.
  Treatment of GAD: An initial single dose of 20 mg, usually administered in the morning, is recommended. Available information shows no additional benefit to patients treated with higher doses (up to 50 mg/day) for this disorder.
  Treatment of PTSD: An initial dose of 20 mg is recommended, which is the established effective dose. If there is an inadequate clinical response, weekly increases in increments of 10 mg, to a maximum of 50 mg, may be considered.

Paroxetine Hydrochloride Dose Forms Available

- *Tablets:* 10 (scored), 20 (scored), 30, and 40 mg
- *Oral suspension:* 10 mg/5 mL
- *Controlled release tablets (Paxil CR):* 12.5, 25, and 37.5 mg

Paroxetine Mesylate Dose Forms Available

- *Tablets:* 10 and 20 mg

■ *Reports of Interest*

Paroxetine in the Treatment of Children and Adolescents with MDD

Berard et al. (2006) conducted a 12-week, prospective, international (10 different countries), multicenter (33 centers), randomized, double-blind, placebo-controlled, flexible-dose, parallel-group study of the safety and efficacy of paroxetine in the treatment of outpatient adolescents, age range 12 to 19 years, diagnosed with unipolar major depression by DSM-IV criteria and confirmed by the Kiddie-Schedule for Affective Disorders and Schizophrenia for School-Age Children–Life Time (K-SADS-L), a score of >16 on the Montgomery-Åsberg Depression Rating Scale (MADRS) at screening and baseline (average score at baseline was 25.9), and a rating of <69 on the CGAS. At baseline, 33.7% of the paroxetine group and 39.3% of the placebo group were rated as markedly or severely ill. Of the 324 subjects who were screened, 286 met study criteria and were randomly assigned at a 2:1 ratio to paroxetine ($N = 187$) or to placebo ($N = 99$). This was the first major depressive episode for approximately 83% of the subjects. Analyses, based on ITT, comprised 275 subjects (age range 12 to 19 years; 92 males, 183 females) with at least one dose of study medication, and one postbaseline safety or efficacy assessment included 182 subjects in the paroxetine group and 93 in the placebo group.

All subjects received single-blind placebo for a 2-week run-in period before the 12-week study. Following this, subjects in the paroxetine group were initially prescribed 20 mg daily in the morning with food. Dosage was flexible and could be increased or decreased at a maximum of 10 mg/week but had to remain between 20 and 40 mg/day. The mean maximum paroxetine dose at the end of the 12-week study was 25.8 mg/day; 59% of subjects received 20 mg/day, the lowest permitted dose. During the study, 55 (30.2%) of the paroxetine group (including 11.8% because of AEs and 4.9% for lack of efficacy) and 24 (25.8%) of the placebo group (including 7.1% because of AEs and 6.5% for lack of efficacy) withdrew from the study.

The primary outcome measures necessary for a positive response were at least a 50% decrease from baseline in both the Montgomery-Åsberg Depression Rating Scale score and the Kiddie-Schedule for Affective Disorders and Schizophrenia for School-Age Children–Life Time depression subscale. Subjects meeting "responder" criteria on the Montgomery-Åsberg Depression Rating Scale included 60.5% of the paroxetine group and 58.2% of the placebo group, which did not differ significantly ($P = .70$) or clinically. On the K-SADS-L, the paroxetine group had a decrease of 9.3 points and the placebo group of 8.9 points, which did not differ significantly ($P = .62$) or clinically. Regarding secondary measures of efficacy, the two groups did not differ significantly on the CGI-S, the Mood and Feelings Questionnaires (MFQs), or the BDI; however, the CGI-I Scale showed a significant difference between the groups. A rating of 1 (very much improved) or 2 (much improved) was present at endpoint for 69.2% of the paroxetine group versus 57.3% of the placebo group ($P = .045$).

Berard et al. (2006) noted that older adolescents treated with paroxetine had a greater response than younger adolescents so treated. This was indicated by the fact that although the CGI-I responder rate was significant for the entire group, when it was analyzed by age subgroups, it was significant only in the older (>16 years old) adolescent group ($P = .040$).

AEs were not statistically different between the paroxetine and placebo groups, being reported in 69% of the paroxetine group and 59.1% of the placebo group. The most frequent AEs reported in the paroxetine group were nausea (24.2%), headache (18.7%), dizziness (10.4%), somnolence (9.3%), decreased appetite (7.7%), infection (7.7%), and asthenia (6.6%); however, only decreased appetite was statistically more frequent compared with the placebo group (7.7% vs. 3.2%). AEs related to suicidality occurred in 4.4% of the paroxetine group (four in adolescents ≤16 years and four in adolescents >16 years) and 2.1% of the placebo group (two adolescents ≤16 years), which was not statistically different ($P = .502$). Suicidal attempts were reported in three (1.7%) of the paroxetine group (one adolescent <16 years and two adolescents >16 years) and two (2.1%) of the placebo group with no statistical difference between the groups ($P = 1.000$).

The authors concluded that there were no significant statistical or clinical differences between paroxetine and placebo in treating this group of adolescents diagnosed with MDD on the primary outcome variables; however, the CGI-I rate was significantly greater for the paroxetine group. They also suggested that adolescents >16 years may respond more favorably to paroxetine than younger adolescents. The authors thought that paroxetine in the doses used (20 to 40 mg/day) was generally well tolerated in this age group (Berard et al., 2006).

Emslie et al. (2006) treated 206 subjects 7 to 17 years old with MDD with paroxetine or placebo for 8 weeks. In a randomized multicenter double-blind placebo-controlled trial, a 1-week screening phase was used to determine eligibility and conduct baseline depressive symptoms assessments. Patients eligible for the study were randomized to receive paroxetine (10 to 50 mg) or placebo. Paroxetine was dosed 10 mg for the first week and titrated upward in 10 mg/day increments no more than weekly until a max of 50 mg/day was reached. Patients terminating treatment at a dose of 20 mg/day or higher were required to gradually reduce study medication by 10 mg/day/week. Outcomes were measured by CDRS-R rating changes from baseline to 8 weeks as well as improvement in CGI-I scores and change from baseline of illness of the CGI-S scores. Remission in the study was defined as a CDRS-S score of ≤28 and a CGI-I score of 1 (very much improved). Three hundred five patients were screened and 206 patients were randomized in the trial. Of this group, 96 (47.3%) were children and 107 (52.7%) were adolescents; 108 (53.2%) were male and 95 (46.8%) were female.

A total of 73.4% of subjects completed the 8-week study. It was noted that a higher percentage of patients withdrew from the paroxetine group (30.7%) than the placebo group (22.5%). This pattern was not evident in the 7-to-11-year-old subgroup but was evident in the adolescent subgroup with 30.9% of patients withdrawing who received paroxetine versus 23.1% of placebo subjects. The doses used in the paroxetine group were 20.4 mg/day throughout the study (18.9 mg/day for children and 21.8 mg/day for adolescents). The study did not find any differences in depression rating scales between the paroxetine and placebo group. CDRS-R total score adjusted mean changes from baseline for patients receiving paroxetine and placebo were –22.58 (SE 1.47) and –23.38 (SE 1.60). It was noted that AEs of suicidal behavior and/or ideation while taking paroxetine was 1.92% versus placebo 0.98%. The authors conclude that paroxetine was not shown to be more efficacious than placebo for treating pediatric MDD.

Paroxetine in the Treatment of Children and Adolescents Diagnosed with Dysthymia

Nobile et al. (2000) treated seven subjects (five males, two females; mean age, 14.4 ± 2.6 years; age range, 11 to 18 years) diagnosed by DSM-III-R (APA, 1987) criteria with dysthymia, primary type, without comorbidity for MDD, for 3 months in an open-label study. Efficacy was assessed by ratings on the HDRS, the CGI-S Scale, and the CGI-I Scale. The initial dose of paroxetine was 10 mg daily. Dosage was titrated based on clinical response. A 10-mg increment was permissible after 1 week, with possible further increases to a daily maximum of 40 mg. Dose reduction was possible at any time. Clinical improvement of responders was noted within the first month of treatment and the improvement continued over the course of treatment. The mean dose of paroxetine after 3 months was 20.12 mg/day. Responders were *a priori* decided to have >50% improvement on the Ham-D and/or a CGI-I score of 1 (very much improved) or 2 (much improved).

Five (71%) of the seven completers (two subjects withdrew during the first month, one female participant was noncompliant and another female participant stopped because of nausea and stomachaches) were "responders." The five responders were maintained on medication and reassessed 6 months after beginning paroxetine; all five showed further improvement on the Ham-D (mean 6-month score was 1.2 ± 2.17), and all five were rated with "no disease" on the CGI-S and "very much improved" on the CGI-I. The most common untoward effects were nausea and stomachache (28.6%). Sedation, insomnia, behavioral activation, and inappropriate behavior were reported by one patient each. The authors noted that their data suggest that paroxetine is effective in the treatment of dysthymia in this age group and merits further study.

Paroxetine in the Treatment of Children and Adolescents Diagnosed with OCD

Rosenberg et al. (1999) conducted a 12-week, open-label trial of paroxetine in treating 20 outpatients (9 males, 11 females; ages 8 to 17 years) diagnosed with OCD by DSM-IV criteria (APA, 1994) and having a CY-BOCS rating of >16. Twelve subjects had comorbid diagnoses but only two were given additional medication (lorazepam for anxiety) during the study. Ratings on the Hamilton Anxiety Scale, the Yale Global Tic Severity Scale (YGTSS), the CGAS, and the CGIS were also used to assess efficacy. The criterion for a positive response was a reduction of OCD symptom severity by >30% on the CY-BOCS.

The initial dose of paroxetine was 10 mg/day and could be titrated upward by a maximum increase of 10 mg every 2 weeks to a daily maximum of 60 mg or until good clinical response or until untoward effects prevented further increase. At the end of the study, subjects showed significant ($P = .001$) improvement on the CY-BOCS, the CGAS, and the CGI. Patients also showed a significant decrease in anxiety ($P = .008$). Of clinical interest, one of the two subjects with tic-related OCD failed to improve and the other, diagnosed with Tourette disorder, had a worsening of OCD symptoms and a doubling of tic severity consonant with the earlier studies suggesting that tic-related OCD may be less responsive to specific serotonin reuptake inhibitors. Serious untoward effects occurred in two subjects (suicidal ideation in one and increased tics in one). Mild untoward effects included hyperactivity/behavioral inhibition that required dosage reduction in some cases (30%), headache (25%), insomnia (15%), gastrointestinal distress (15%), increased anxiety (10%), drowsiness (5%), and dry mouth (5%). There were no manic-like untoward effects or allergic reactions. Overall paroxetine was considered safe and effective in treating these particular subjects.

Gilbert et al. (2000) used volumetric magnetic resonance imaging (MRI) to measure and compare thalamic volumes in 21 psychotropic drug-naïve subjects (7 males, 14 females; mean age, 12.35 ± 2.93 years; range, 8.08 to 17.33 years) diagnosed by DSM-IV (APA, 1994) criteria with OCD whom they were treating with paroxetine with 21 matched healthy controls. After baseline assessment, including MRI, 13 of the 21 subjects were treated with paroxetine 10 mg/day that was titrated to a maximum of 60 mg/day based on clinical response; mean dose of paroxetine after 12 weeks was 51.00 ± 8.76 mg/day (range, 40 to 60 mg/day). Subjects did not receive cognitive-behavior therapy or psychotherapy other than supportive or family therapy. The other eight subjects elected not to participate in the protocol. Ten of the 13 subjects had a second MRI at time 12 weeks. (Two of the others refused a second MRI and the MRI of the third subject could not be used because of excess motion artifact.)

Based on CY-BOCS ratings, 7 of the 10 subjects were considered responders, having a 30% or greater improvement in their scores. At baseline, thalamic volumes of treatment-naïve patients with OCD were significantly greater than those of controls ($P = .01$). Thalamic volume in the 10 patients with OCD decreased significantly (19% mean reduction in volume) after 12 weeks' treatment with paroxetine (P = .01) and was no longer significantly different from that of the controls (P = .76). Reduction in thalamic volume correlated with significantly lower scores on the CY-BOCS, but the dose of paroxetine did not correlate with final thalamic volume. Repeat MRIs were also obtained in eight medication-free controls about 12 weeks after baseline; they showed less variation (a mean of ±5.6% of baseline) in volume, suggesting that the greater change in the paroxetine group was a real phenomenon. The authors' preliminary findings suggest that treatment-naïve children diagnosed with OCD have serotonergic abnormalities that result in increased thalamic volumes. During the 12-week period of treatment with paroxetine, significant reduction in thalamic volume and clinical improvement in OCD symptomatology occurred.

Geller et al. (2004) conducted a prospective, multicenter, 10-week, randomized, double-blind, placebo-controlled, flexible-dose, parallel-group trial to evaluate the efficacy and safety of paroxetine hydrochloride in treating 203 children and adolescents who were diagnosed with OCD by DSM-IV criteria. Comorbid psychiatric diagnoses were made in 35.5% (72) of the patients; the most common were ADHD (9.4%), GAD (6.9%), and enuresis (6.9%). Of the 203 patients, 56.7% (115) were children aged 7 to 11 years and 43.3% (88) were adolescents aged 12 to 17 years; 57.6% (117) were male and 42.4% (86) were female; and 88.2% were white.

The primary measure of efficacy was the change from baseline to the week 10 last-observation-carried-forward end point in total score on the CY-BOCS. Six secondary measures of efficacy were used: (a) Reduction >25% on the CY-BOCS; (b) a score of 1 (very much improved) or 2 (much improved) on the CGI-I score; (c and d) changes from baseline to endpoint scores on the Compulsions Subtest and the Obsessions Subtest of the CY-BOCS; (e) the CGI-S score; and (f) Global Assessment of Functioning (GAF) rating. Safety was assessed by monitoring AEs and vital signs at each visit, laboratory tests, physical examinations, and ECGs at baseline and endpoint.

The ITT population, consisting of the randomized patients who had at least one dose of study medication and one postbaseline assessment (N = 203) were assigned to paroxetine (N = 98) or placebo (N = 105). During week 1, patients received paroxetine 10 mg daily or placebo. Dose was then titrated in 10-mg increments based on the clinical response with a weekly maximum permitted increase of 10 mg/day. The maximum total dose permitted was 50 mg/day. The mean baseline CY-BOCS total score was 24.8 (moderate to severe OCD symptomatology); baseline CGI-S ratings were 52% moderately ill, 34% markedly ill, and 11.8% severely or among the most extremely ill.

About one-third (33.7%) of the paroxetine group and 23.8% of the placebo group did not complete the study. AEs (10.2%; N = 10) were the most common reason for this in the paroxetine group, and lack of efficacy (13.3%; N = 14) was the most common reason in the placebo group. The average length of treatment for the paroxetine group was 60 days and for the placebo group 64 days. The final (week 10 LOCF end point) mean dose of paroxetine for children was 25.4 mg/day and for adolescents was 36.5 mg/day.

The paroxetine group improved significantly more than the placebo group on the CY-BOCS total score (–8.75 vs. –5.34 points, P = .002). Patients with higher initial CY-BOCS scores had greater changes from baseline than patients with lower initial scores (P = .002) and children had greater changes from baseline than adolescents (P < .001). In addition, the three secondary measures utilizing the CY-BOCS for paroxetine were all statistically superior to those for placebo and the other three were numerically but not significantly superior.

The most frequently reported AEs in the paroxetine group were headache (24.5%), abdominal pain (17.3%), nausea (16.3%), upper respiratory infection (12.2%), somnolence (12.2%), motor hyperactivity (12.2%), and trauma (physical and accidental injuries) (10.2%); of these, only hyperactivity and trauma occurred at least twice as frequently as in the placebo group. Overall, 10.2% (eight children and two adolescents) of the paroxetine group and 2.9% of the placebo group discontinued treatment because of an AE. Serious adverse effects were reported in three children in the paroxetine group—two exhibited aggressive behavior and one was hospitalized for suicidal thoughts, which were closely related in timing to the patient's being forced out of his home by his guardian and his being sent to a youth shelter, and not related to the medication. One patient in the placebo group exhibited aggressive behavior.

During treatment discontinuation, that is the period of drug taper or follow-up during the first 2 weeks off the drug, patients who were taking paroxetine experienced nausea (2.5%) and vomiting (3.8%) compared with 1.1% and 0%, respectively, of patients who were on placebo.

The authors concluded that paroxetine had a modest overall effect in reducing symptoms on the CY-BOCS and was significantly more efficacious that placebo. Its tolerability and safety profile were similar to those observed with other SSRIs in children and adolescents being treated for OCD.

Paroxetine in the Treatment of Children and Adolescents Diagnosed with Social Anxiety Disorder

Wagner et al. (2004) conducted a 38-center, randomized, double-blind, placebo-controlled 16-week study of paroxetine in a total of 322 children (age 8 to 11) and adolescents (age 12 to 17) who met DSM-IV (APA, 1994) criteria for social anxiety disorder. The exclusion criteria for subjects included having a clinically prominent Axis I diagnosis other than social anxiety disorder, or a history of a psychotic disorder. The ITT population for statistical analysis consisted of the 319 subjects who had had at least one dose of study medication and one postbaseline follow-up assessment; of these, 28.5% (91) were children and 71.5% (228) were adolescents. The paroxetine group ($N = 163$) was 43.6% male and the placebo group ($N = 156$) was 57.1% male.

Paroxetine was begun at a dose of 10 mg and could be increased at weekly intervals to a maximum of 50 mg/day; after week 2, dose could be reduced to the prior dose in the event of an AE. At the end of the study, subjects whose daily dose was 20 mg or more were tapered off by reducing the dose by 10 mg weekly. The primary outcome measure (efficacy end point) was a rating of 1 (very much improved) or 2 (much improved) on the CGI-I Scale.

At week 16, the mean dose of paroxetine for all subjects was 32.6 mg/day; for children it was 26.5 mg/day, and for adolescents it was 35.0 mg/day. Of the subjects in the paroxetine group, 77.6% (125/161) met criteria for responders versus 38.3% (59/154) of subjects in the placebo group ($P < .001$). The benefit of paroxetine was apparent within 4 weeks. Paroxetine also showed statistically more clinical benefit than placebo ($P < .001$) on all five secondary outcome measures: The CGI-S; the GAF; the Liebowitz Social Anxiety Scale for Children and Adolescents (LSAS-CA); the Kutcher Generalized Social Anxiety Disorder Scale for Adolescents; and the Social Phobia and Anxiety Inventory (SPAI) or the SPAI for Children (SPAI-C). Remission was defined as either a >70% reduction on the LSAS-CA or a rating of 1 (very much improved) on the GCI-I; 34.6% of the paroxetine group met both criteria, whereas only 8% of the placebo group did so.

Most AEs were of mild to moderate intensity. AEs that possibly occurred as a result of treatment in >5% of subjects on paroxetine and at a rate at least twice that of placebo were as follows: insomnia, 14.1% versus 5.8% ($P = .02$); decreased appetite, 8.0% versus 3.2% ($P = .11$); and vomiting, 6.7% versus 1.9% ($P = .07$). Rates of nervousness, hyperkinesia, asthenia, and hostility also met the preceding criteria in children but not in adolescents; rates of somnolence and insomnia met these criteria in adolescents but not in children (P values were not given).

The authors concluded that paroxetine was effective in treating children and adolescents diagnosed with social anxiety disorder (Wagner et al., 2004).

Fluvoxamine Maleate (Luvox)

Fluvoxamine maleate is an SSRI that belongs to a new chemical series, the 2-aminoethyloxime ethers of aralkylketone. It is chemically unrelated to other SSRIs and clomipramine. In *in vitro* studies, the drug exhibited no significant affinity for histaminergic, alpha- or beta-adrenergic, muscarinic, or dopamine receptors.

Fluvoxamine has been approved for the treatment of OCD in patients at least 8 years of age.

Pharmacokinetics of Fluvoxamine Maleate

Food does not significantly affect the bioavailability of fluvoxamine. In volunteers, peak plasma concentrations at steady state occurred between 3 and 8 hours after ingestion of the drug and revealed nonlinear pharmacokinetics for single doses of 100, 200, and 300 mg, with higher doses resulting in disproportionately higher plasma levels (e.g., plasma levels of 88, 283, and 546 ng/mL, respectively). The mean plasma half-life at steady state for young adults taking 100 mg/day was 15.6 hours.

Labellarte et al. (2004) reported on the multiple-dose pharmacokinetics of fluvoxamine maleate in 16 children (9 males, 7 females) and 18 adolescents (9 males, 9 females) being treated for OCD. They measured serum levels >12 hours after 12 or more consecutive doses of 25, 50, 100, and 150 mg of fluvoxamine. Maximum daily dose was 200 mg/day for children and 300 mg/day for adolescents, given in two doses 12 hours apart. Compared with adolescents, children had higher mean peak plasma concentrations, higher mean area under the plasma concentration–time curve, and lower apparent oral clearance; at a dose of 50 mg twice daily, adjusted mean serum level for children was 182.45 versus 67.50 ng/mL for adolescents ($P \le .05$). Compared with male children, female children had higher mean peak plasma concentration, higher mean area under the plasma concentration–time curve and reported more AEs. Adolescents had similar pharmacokinetics to those reported for adults on 150-mg, twice-daily doses. These data suggest that children, especially female children, have a higher exposure to fluvoxamine at a given dose than adolescents and adults.

Smokers metabolize fluvoxamine maleate about 25% faster than nonsmokers.

Contraindications for Fluvoxamine Maleate Administration

Known hypersensitivity to fluvoxamine maleate is a contraindication.

Coadministration of terfenadine, astemizole, or cisapride with fluvoxamine maleate is contraindicated. This is because fluvoxamine maleate is likely to be a potent inhibitor of P450 3A4 isoenzyme, which would cause increased levels of the previously mentioned drugs and result in the lengthening of the QT interval, which has been associated with torsade de pointes–type ventricular tachycardia and fatalities.

Because of a possibility for serious, life-threatening reactions when administered simultaneously with an MAOI, the use of fluvoxamine maleate in combination with an MAOI is contraindicated. At least, 14 days should elapse after stopping an MAOI before administering fluvoxamine maleate. Based on the half-life of fluvoxamine maleate, at least 14 days should elapse following its discontinuation before administering an MAOI.

Interactions of Fluvoxamine Maleate with Other Drugs

Benzodiazepines should be coadministered with great caution. Plasma levels and half-life of alprazolam were approximately doubled when it was given together with fluvoxamine, resulting in decreased psychomotor performance and memory; if coadministered, the dose of alprazolam should be reduced by at least 50% and gradually titrated to the lowest effective dose. Coadministration of diazepam is not recommended, as fluvoxamine maleate reduces its clearance and that of its major metabolite N-desmethyldiazepam, and clinically significant increases would be expected.

Many other potential interactions, particularly with drugs that inhibit or are metabolized by cytochrome P450 isoenzymes, have been reported (package insert).

Untoward Effects of Fluvoxamine Maleate

The most frequently reported untoward effects were somnolence, insomnia, dry mouth, nervousness, tremor, nausea, dyspepsia, anorexia, vomiting, abnormal ejaculation, asthenia, and sweating. As decreased appetite and weight loss can occur with fluvoxamine, these parameters should be monitored.

Indications for Fluvoxamine Maleate in Child and Adolescent Psychiatry

NOTE: Review the Black Box Warning at the beginning of the chapter or in the package insert before prescribing.

Fluvoxamine is approved only for the treatment of obsessions and compulsions in children 8 years of age and older, adolescents, and adults diagnosed with OCD. Its safety and efficacy have not been established in children <8 years of age.

Fluvoxamine Dosage Schedule

Treatment of OCD

- *Children <8 years of age:* Not recommended. Safety and efficacy have not been established for this age range.
- *Children at least 8 and adolescents up to 17 years of age:* An initial bedtime dose of 25 mg is recommended. The dose may be titrated upward every 4 to 7 days as clinically indicated in 25-mg increments to a maximum of 200 mg to achieve maximal therapeutic response. Daily doses totaling more than 50 mg should be given in two doses; if the two doses are unequal, the larger dose should be taken at bedtime.
- *Adolescents at least 18 years of age and adults:* An initial bedtime dose of 50 mg is recommended. The dose may be titrated upward every 4 to 7 days as clinically indicated in 50-mg increments to a maximum of 300 mg to achieve maximal therapeutic response. Daily doses totaling more than 100 mg should be given in two doses; if the two doses are unequal, the larger dose should be taken at bedtime. Usual optimal doses range from 100 to 300 mg.

Fluvoxamine Maleate Dose Forms Available

- *Tablets:* 25, 50 (scored), and 100 mg (scored).

Reports of Interest

Fluvoxamine Maleate in the Treatment of Adolescents Diagnosed with MDD or OCD

Apter et al. (1994) reported treating 20 adolescent inpatients 13 to 18 years of age who were diagnosed with MDD (N = 6) or OCD (N = 14) with fluvoxamine in an 8-week, open-label protocol. Inclusion criteria for the six depressed patients included lack of response to a TCA, additional symptoms of suicidality, impulsivity or affective instability, or a comorbid major psychiatric diagnosis. Four had comorbid diagnoses of both borderline personality and conduct disorders, one had comorbid bulimia, and the sixth was diagnosed with MDD only. Eleven of the 14 patients with OCD also had comorbid diagnoses: Tourette syndrome (TS) (4), schizophrenia (4), and anorexia nervosa (3). All eight subjects diagnosed with comorbid TS or schizophrenia also received haloperidol; in addition, three of them received benzhexol, an anticholinergic drug. Fluvoxamine was increased by 50 mg weekly until either a therapeutic result was obtained or untoward effects prevented further increase. Doses ranged from 100 to 300 mg/day (mean, 200 mg/day). Sixteen patients completed the study, and four dropped out because of untoward effects; for the latter four patients, the last ratings while on medication were used in analyzing the data.

All six patients with MDD improved significantly on the BDI ($P < .0002$), but only two of the four patients with comorbid MDD and borderline personality disorder showed clinically significant decreases in impulsivity and suicidality.

As a group, the 14 patients with OCD improved significantly on the Yale-Brown Obsessive-Compulsive Scale (Y-BOCS) ($P < .0001$). However, one of the three patients with comorbid anorexia nervosa developed confusion and delirium and another developed hallucinations; both were dropped from the study at week 6. Of note, statistically significant improvement over baseline ratings on the Y-BOCS did not occur until week 6, and there was further improvement at week 8.

All subjects developed at least some mild untoward effects compared with baseline ratings on the Dosage Record Treatment-Emergent Symptom Scale (DOTES). Fluvoxamine initially caused some activating untoward effects, such as insomnia, hyperactivity, agitation, excitement, anxiety, and hypomania. These were mild and transient in most cases; however, one patient with a family history of bipolar disorder who developed hypomania was dropped during the fifth week. Nausea, tremor, and dermatitis occurred in about 75% of subjects; in one case, the drug had to be discontinued because of itchy maculopapular dermatitis. No changes in heart rate, blood pressure, ECG, or routine laboratory tests were reported. No patient showed a significant increase in ratings on the Suicide Potential or Overt Aggression Scales (Apter et al., 1994).

Fluvoxamine Maleate in the Treatment of Children and Adolescents Diagnosed with Anxiety Disorders

Walkup et al. (2001) reported findings of a multisite, double-blind, placebo-controlled trial of fluvoxamine in the treatment of 128 subjects (age range, 6 to 17 years) who were diagnosed with SP, SAD, or GAD and treated for 8 weeks with fluvoxamine or placebo. Fluvoxamine was titrated on an individual basis to a maximum of 300 mg/day. Efficacy was determined by ratings on the PARS and the CGI-I Scale. Fluvoxamine-treated subjects had significantly improved ratings on the PARS compared with subjects on placebo ($P < .001$). Their PARS scores decreased by 9.7 ± 6.9 points while the placebo group had a decrease of 3.1 ± 4.8 points. On the CGI-I, 76% of subjects on fluvoxamine were rated as responders versus only 29% on placebo ($P < .001$). These data suggest that fluvoxamine may be an effective treatment for children and adolescents diagnosed with these three anxiety disorders.

Citalopram Hydrobromide (Celexa)

The SSRI citalopram hydrobromide is a racemic bicyclic phthalane derivative that is chemically unrelated to other SSRIs or to tricyclic, tetracyclic, and other antidepressants.

Citalopram has minimal effects on the neuronal reuptake of norepinephrine and dopamine. It has no or very low affinity for 5-HT_{1A}, 5-HT_{2A}, dopamine D_1, and D_2, alpha-1, alpha-2, or beta-adrenergic, histamine H_1, gamma aminobutyric acid, muscarinic, cholinergic, and benzodiazepine receptors.

Pharmacokinetics of Citalopram Hydrobromide

Food does not affect the bioavailability of citalopram hydrobromide. Peak serum levels occur about 4 hours after ingestion. With once-daily dosing, steady-state plasma levels occur in approximately 1 week and are about 2.5 times the concentration observed after a single dose.

Metabolism occurs primarily by N-demethylation in the liver, with CYP3A4 and CYP2C19 being the primary enzymes involved. The parent compound is at least eight times more active than its metabolites, suggesting that they do not play a significant role clinically. Mean terminal half-life is about 35 hours.

Contraindications for Administration of Citalopram Hydrobromide

Known hypersensitivity to citalopram hydrobromide is a contraindication.

Because of a possibility of serious, life-threatening reactions when administered simultaneously with an MAOI, it is recommended that the drug is not used in combination with an MAOI. At least 2 weeks should elapse after stopping citalopram before administering an MAOI and, conversely, after stopping an MAOI before administering citalopram.

Untoward Effects of Citalopram Hydrobromide

Dry mouth, increased sweating, nausea, diarrhea, somnolence or insomnia, ejaculatory disturbance (in 6%, usually ejaculatory delay) have been reported in individuals taking citalopram.

In 2011, the FDA issued drug safety warnings concerning the use of citalopram. At higher doses, citalopram can cause abnormal changes to the electrical activity of the heart. These changes, known as prolongation of the QT interval, can lead to fatal changes in the heart's rhythm. The risk increases with higher dosing of citalopram and the maximum dose was lowered to 40 mg from 60 mg. They also recommend monitoring of EKG and electrolytes in cases where citalopram is an essential to treatment at higher doses. Baseline potassium and magnesium measurement and periodic monitoring are recommended as hypokalemia and/or hypomagnesemia can increase risk of QTc prolongation (Silva, 2012).

Advantages of Citalopram Hydrobromide

There was no clinically significant difference between placebo and citalopram on cardiac parameters, including electroconductivity from baseline ECG. The only significant difference was a mean decrease in cardiac rate of 1.7 beats per minute.

Indications for Citalopram Hydrobromide in Child and Adolescent Psychiatry

NOTE: Review the Black Box Warning at the beginning of the chapter or in the package insert before prescribing.

Citalopram is approved for the treatment of depression. The safety and efficacy for use in children and adolescents has not been determined. One manufacturer notes that the data from two placebo-controlled studies in which a total of 407 subjects in the pediatric age group who were diagnosed with MDD were not adequate to report a claim for citalopram's use in this age group. Citalopram is usually administered once daily, in the morning or evening, and may be taken with or without food.

Citalopram Dosage Schedule

Treatment of MDD

- *Children and adolescents ≤17 years of age:* Not recommended. Safety and efficacy have not been established for this age group.
- *Adolescents at least 18 years of age and adults:* An initial morning or evening dose of 20 mg is recommended. An increase to 40 mg daily is usual after 1 week. Doses of more than 40 mg daily are not usually recommended as increased efficacy with higher doses has not been demonstrated. A maximum dose of 60 mg/day.

Citalopram Hydrobromide Dose Forms Available

- *Tablets:* 10, 20 (scored), and 40 mg (scored)
- *Oral solution:* 10 mg/5 mL (10 mg/tsp)

Report of Interest

Citalopram Hydrobromide in the Treatment of Children and Adolescents Diagnosed with MDD

Wagner and colleagues (2004) conducted a randomized placebo-controlled trial of citalopram in the treatment of children and adolescents with major depression. Subjects were screened and given a 1-week placebo lead in period and then returned for baseline screening. Those still eligible were randomized in a double-blind fashion to receive 8 weeks of citalopram or placebo. Citalopram was initiated at 20 mg/day with the potential to increase to 40 mg after week 4 if clinically necessary. Evaluations were scheduled after 1, 2, 4, 6, and 8 weeks of treatment. The overall mean citalopram dose was 24 mg/day.

Outcome was assessed with change in baseline of CDRS at week 8 or termination from the study. Secondary measures included the CGI-I. A total of 178 patients were enrolled in the study. Citalopram treatment showed statistically significant improvement on CDRS when compared with placebo as early as week 1. Improvements continued at every observation point to the end of the study. The difference in response rate at week 8 between placebo (24%) and citalopram (36%) was statistically significant.

Side effects were mild only with nausea, rhinitis, and abdominal pain occurring in ≥10% of citalopram-treated patients. They did not have any reports of mania in this study. Two placebo-group patients were discontinued form the study because of aggravated depression, and two citalopram patients had agitation requiring discontinuation from the study. ECG results, laboratory values, and weight did not have any clinically significant change.

Shirazi and Alaghband-Rad (2005) conducted an open-label trial of citalopram in children and adolescents with depression in Iran. In their trial, 30 children aged 8 to 17 were enrolled. The mean age was 13.57 ± 2.5; 53.3% of the sample was female and 46.7% was male. Subjects diagnosed with MDD were enrolled in an open-label trial and were given citalopram 10 to 40 mg for 6 weeks. Outcomes were measured using the HDRS and CGAS. Side effects were assessed with the New York State Psychiatric Institute side-effect form. They found improvement in HDRS and CGAS in the moderate (50% to 70% improvement) to large (>70% improvement) range in 91.7% of the children in the study. They also noted that most subjects showed improvement in symptoms 102 weeks after onset of medication. They did have five subjects (16.7%), three boys and two girls, with a mean age of 12.6, develop mania, which required them to discontinue the medication. These subjects were all taking 20 mg of citalopram from the beginning of the study and developed mania by the second week. The authors caution against using celexa due to this high switch rate to mania.

Citalopram Hydrobromide in the Treatment of Children and Adolescents Diagnosed with OCD

Thomsen (1997) treated 23 subjects (11 males, 12 females; mean age 13.1 ± 2.5 years; age range 9 to 18 years) diagnosed with OCD by DSM-III-R (APA, 1987) criteria with citalopram in a 10-week, open-label study. Fifteen had comorbid diagnoses including four with MDD. Nine subjects were inpatients, 2 of whom were followed up after discharge, and 14 were outpatients. An initial dose of 10 mg of citalopram was given approximately 2 weeks after referral and gradually titrated to a target dose of 40 mg/day for 20 subjects. Because of untoward effects, the final dose for two subjects was 20 mg/day and for one subject was 10 mg/day. The mean dose of citalopram at the end of the 10 weeks was 37.0 ± 0.8 mg/day, with a dose range of 10 to 40 mg/day. Efficacy was assessed by ratings on the Y-BOCS or its version for children (CY-BOCS) <15 years old, the Children's Assessment Schedule (CAS), and the CGAS. Posttreatment (10-week) ratings on the Y-BOCS or CY-BOCS improved significantly over baseline (mean scores declined from 30.1 to 20.9; $P = .001$). Four subjects (17%) were rated as markedly improved with a >50% decrease in the rating, 14 patients (61%) were rated as moderately improved (a 20% to 43% reduction in scores), 4 patients (17%) were slightly improved (5% to 20% reduction in scores), and 1 patient showed no change. Improvement in social functioning was reflected by scores on the CGAS, which improved significantly from baseline to posttreatment ratings (mean scores increased from 59.1 to 71.0; $P = .001$). Overall, however, only six patients improved sufficiently so as to no longer meet the diagnostic criteria for OCD, and they continued to have symptoms of subclinical OCD. Mild untoward effects were reported by 13 subjects. Most, including all cases of dry mouth, headache, and tremor, were transient resolving within a few weeks. Restlessness occurred in four patients, increased anxiety in two patients, and erectile dysfunction in one patient. In no case did untoward effects necessitate discontinuation of citalopram. The findings suggested that citalopram may be effective and well tolerated in children and adolescents diagnosed with OCD at doses of up to 40 mg/day.

Alaghband-Rad and Hakimshooshtary (2009) reported on their results of a randomized controlled clinical trial of citalopram versus fluoxetine in children and adolescents with OCD. Twenty-nine subjects aged 7 to 18 with OCD were enrolled in the study and randomized to receive either citalopram 20 mg or fluoxetine 20 mg. They chose to compare citalopram to fluoxetine as the effectiveness of fluoxetine to treat pediatric OCD had been previously demonstrated in prior studies (Geller et al., 2001; Riddle et al., 1992). The study lasted 6 weeks and outcome was measured with the CY-BOCS and the CGI. At the conclusion of the study, each group demonstrated significant improvement in their CY-BOCS scores from baseline ($P < .01$), but they did not find any improvement in CGI. They also did not show any differences in safety or efficacy between citalopram and fluoxetine. They did have one subject receiving citalopram drop out after having a hypomanic episode and another subject who received fluoxetine also had a hypomanic episode.

Citalopram Hydrobromide in the Treatment of Children and Adolescents Diagnosed with Autism Spectrum Disorder

King and colleagues (2009) investigated the efficacy of citalopram in a placebo-controlled trial of children with ASD. One hundred forty-nine youth 5 to 17 years old were randomized to receive citalopram ($N = 73$) or placebo ($N = 76$). Subjects were included if they met criteria for an autism spectrum disorder which included autism, Asperger disorder, or PDDNOS. Citalopram was administered in the liquid version and was started at 2.5 mg/day and increased by 2.5 mg/week initially and then 5 mg/week increments to a maximum of 20 mg/day. Subjects were followed for 12 weeks and improvement was measured by CGI and CY-BOCS modified for pervasive developmental disorders (PDDs). The authors hypothesized that youth with high levels of repetitive behaviors would respond to citalopram in a model similar to OCD response. At the conclusion of the study, no significant difference was found in response between the citalopram and placebo groups. The citalopram group did have more side AEs. Increased energy level, impulsiveness, decreased concentration, hyperactivity, stereotypy, diarrhea, insomnia, and dry skin were seen more often in the citalopram group. They also had two subjects on citalopram have seizures. One subject had a preexisting seizure disorder and was able to remain in the study with an increased dose of anticonvulsants. The other subject developed a prolonged seizure and continued to have frequent seizures after citalopram was discontinued and was withdrawn from the study. This trial does not support the use of citalopram for the treatment of repetitive behavior in children with ASDs and also questions the safety of these drugs in this diagnostic group.

▮ Escitalopram Oxalate (Lexapro)

Escitalopram oxalate is the pure S-enantiomer, the active isomer, of racemic citalopram, an SSRI.

Pharmacokinetics of Escitalopram Oxalate

Escitalopram oxalate may be taken with or without food. Maximum plasma levels occur about 5 hours after ingestion of the drug. Escitalopram oxalate has a half-life of about 27 to 32 hours. Steady-state plasma levels occur in approximately 1 week at a given dose. Escitalopram oxalate is metabolized primarily through demethylation by the hepatic enzymes CYP3A4 and CYP2C19. About 18% is excreted in the urine.

Contraindications for the Administration of Escitalopram Oxalate

Hypersensitivity to escitalopram oxalate, any of its inactive ingredients, or citalopram is a contraindication to its administration. As escitalopram is the active isomer of racemic citalopram, the two drugs should not be administered together.

Escitalopram oxalate should not be coadministered with an MAOI or within 14 days of treatment with an MAOI being discontinued. At least 14 days should elapse after stopping escitalopram oxalate therapy before administering an MAOI.

Untoward Effects of Escitalopram Oxalate

Untoward effects included gastrointestinal disorders, especially nausea (15%), insomnia (9%), somnolence (6%), increased sweating (5%), fatigue (5%), and decreased appetite (3%). Sexual untoward effects in males include ejaculation disorder (12%, most of which was accounted for by delayed ejaculation), decreased libido (6%) and impotence (3%); in females, they include decreased libido (3%) and anorgasmia (3%). Of note, untoward effects were approximately twice as frequent in patients treated with 20 mg of escitalopram daily compared with patients treated with 10 mg daily.

No significant ECG changes were reported. There is a report of prolonged QTc interval changes in a 14-year-old girl with escitalopram overdose (Scharko and Schumacher, 2008). The youth ingested 200 mg of escitalopram and her QTc the day after ingestion was 450 msec. Two days after ingestion, it was 469 msec and normalized later that day to 420 msec.

Indications for Escitalopram Oxalate in Child and Adolescent Psychiatry

NOTE: Review the Black Box Warning at the beginning of the chapter or in the package insert before prescribing.

Escitalopram oxalate is indicated for the treatment of MDD and GAD in adults. Safety and efficacy have not been established for pediatric patients.

Escitalopram Oxalate Dosage Schedule
Children and Adolescents

Treatment of depression
  Children 8 to 11 years: Not approved
  Adolescents ≥12 years: An initial morning dose of 10 mg increased dose. If there is no improvement after 3 weeks, increasing the dose to 20 mg daily may be considered. The full antidepressant action may take 4 weeks or longer to develop.
  Adults: The recommended dose is 10 mg, once daily. An increase to 20 mg daily can be considered after a minimum of 1 week; however, a fixed-dose trial showed no increased benefit for 20 mg compared with 10 mg.

Escitalopram Oxalate Dose Forms Available

- *Coated tablets (scored):* 10 and 20 mg
- *Oral solution (peppermint flavored):* 5 mg/5 mL

Reports of Interest

Escitalopram Oxalate in the Treatment of Children and Adolescents Diagnosed with MDD

Wagner and colleagues (2006) conducted a double-blind randomized placebo-controlled trial of escitalopram in the treatment of pediatric depression. Study participants were screened and enrolled if their CDRS-R score was at least 40 at the initial screening and baseline visits. The study enrolled 268 patients, and 136 received placebo and 132 received escitalopram. The study enrolled 104 children ages 6 to 11 years and 160 adolescents ages 12 to 17 years. Outcomes were primarily assessed using the CDRS-R. Secondary outcome measures were the CGI-I, CGI-S, and the CGAS. Escitalopram dose was 10 mg for the first 4 weeks and then flexibly dosed to 10 to 20 mg/day based on clinical response and tolerability of the study medication. The mean daily dose was 11.9 ± 2.3 mg/day for escitalopram. Eighty-two percent of the subjects completed the 8-week study.

Escitalopram did not significantly improve CDRS-R scores when compared with placebo at endpoint for the total group. The data were analyzed for adolescents only (12 to 17 years) and found that escitalopram significantly improved CDRS-R scores in this group. The lack of efficacy in younger patients is attributed to the high placebo response rate (52.3%) based on CGI-I score. Wagner and colleagues hypothesize that this is due to the short-term benefit provided by the structure and support of the clinical trial. Headache and abdominal pain were the only AEs in >10% of the escitalopram group. Potential suicide-related events were observed in one escitalopram patient and two placebo patients. One placebo subject had a manic reaction and no escitalopram patients were observed to have mania. There were no completed suicides in the study. This was the first double-blind study of escitalopram that suggested some efficacy in adolescents but not children.

Emslie and colleagues (2009) complete a randomized placebo-controlled multi-site trial of escitalopram in the treatment of adolescent depression. Three hundred sixteen adolescents aged 12 to 17 were randomized to receive placebo (158) or escitalopram (158). The study started with a 2-week screening period. After an initial screening visit, patients were administered a single-blind placebo the second week. If they still met criteria after a week of placebo, they were randomized to receive either placebo or escitalopram. The escitalopram dose was initiated at 10 mg/day for the first 3 weeks and then increased to 20 mg/day at the end of week 3 or 4. Subjects were evaluated at the end of 1, 2, 3, 4, 6, and 8 weeks of the double-blind treatment. Response was assessed using the CDRS-R. Subjects needed a score of over 45 to be enrolled in the study, and decrease in CDRS-R was the main measure of improvement in depression. CGI-I, CGI-S, and CGAS were secondary outcome measures.

At the conclusion, 83% of the study subjects completed the 8 weeks of double-blind treatment. Improvement seen in the escitalopram group was significant when compared with the placebo group. The CDRS-R score for the escitalopram group was –22.1 versus –18.8 for placebo, $P = .22$. The mean dose of escitalopram was 13.2 ± 2.9 mg/day. The majority of patients in both groups had a dose increase (76.4% placebo, 68.4% escitalopram). Eighty-five percent of the eventual escitalopram responders had responded by week 4 compared with 69% of the eventual placebo responders.

AEs seen in the escitalopram group which occurred in at least 10% of the patients were headache, menstrual cramps, insomnia, and nausea. Only influenza-like symptoms occurred in at least 5% of the escitalopram group and at least twice the incidence of placebo (7.1% vs. 3.2%). Discontinuation rates caused by AEs were 2.6% for escitalopram and 0.6% for placebo. There were 12 AEs that were considered to be suggestive of self-harm; 6 occurred in each group (3.8% of placebo and 3.9% of escitalopram patients). Serious side effects were seen in 2.6% of the escitalopram group and 1.3% of the placebo patients. In the Emslie and colleagues study, escitalopram was effective and well tolerated in the treatment of depressed adolescents. This positive study, along with others, led the FDA to approve escitalopram for the treatment of depression in adolescents in March 2009.

Escitalopram Oxalate in the Treatment of Children and Adolescents Diagnosed with PDDs

Owley et al. (2005) assessed the effectiveness of escitalopram in the treatment of 28 subjects (25 [89%] males, 3 [11%] females; age range 6 to 17 years; mean age 125.1 ± 33.5 months) who were diagnosed with PDDs (autistic disorder, 20 [71%]; Asperger disorder, 5 [18%]; and PDDNOS, 3 [11%]) in a 10-week, open-label forced-titration study. Inclusion criteria included a score of >12 on the Irritability Subscale of the Aberrant Behavior Checklist–Community Version (ABC-CV). The primary outcome measures were the CGI-S Scale and the ABC-CV. A subject with a reduction of >50% on the ABC-CV irritability subscale was defined as a "responder."

Escitalopram was initiated at a dose of 2.5 mg daily with forced weekly increases to 5, 10, 15, and 20 mg as of the fifth week. If predetermined problems with sleep or significant increases in irritability or hyperactivity on the subscales of the ABC-CV occurred, the dose was reduced to that of the preceding week and maintained there for the duration of the study. Twenty-three of the subjects completed the study. Of the five withdrawals, two were for continued significant hyperactivity, one for obsessions/compulsions that required additional medications, and two subjects secondary to their developing disinhibition and aggression. At endpoint, the mean daily dose of escitalopram was 11.1 ± 6.5 mg with a range of 0 mg/day (a subject who developed disinhibition and aggression on the lowest permitted dose of 2.5 mg was dropped from the study) to 20 mg/day. Subjects' endpoint doses were unrelated to weight and corresponded only weakly to age. Five subjects had no AEs and tolerated the 20-mg/day dose. The authors noted that some patients might be able to tolerate only doses as low as 1 mg/day without developing AEs. Of the 18 subjects for whom AEs were reported, who required reduction in dose to that of the preceding week, irritability was primarily responsible in 7, hyperactivity in 6, and both irritability and hyperactivity in 5. No subjects reported suicidal ideation, and there was no evidence of increased self-injurious behavior or sleep difficulties.

The responder rate was 17/28 (61%); 7 had an optimal response at <10 mg/day and 10 had optimal responses at doses of ≥10 mg/day. On the ABC-CV Rating Scale, scores at week 10 were significantly improved on the Irritability, Lethargy, Stereotypy, and Hyperactivity subscales at $P < .001$ and on the Inappropriate Speech subscale at $P = .035$; the ABC-CV total score was also significant at $P < .001$. CGI-S mean score at baseline was 5.2 ± 1.0 and at endpoint was 4.6 ± 1.2 ($P < .001$). The authors concluded that escitalopram was useful in treating some common symptoms present in PDD and that controlled studies should be undertaken for such subjects.

OTHER ANTIDEPRESSANTS

Trazodone Hydrochloride (Desyrel)

Trazodone hydrochloride is chemically unrelated to tricyclic, tetracyclic, and other currently approved antidepressant agents. Although it is a serotonin reuptake inhibitor, it is unlike the SSRIs in that its metabolites have significant effects on other neurotransmitter systems and their receptors (Cioli et al., 1984). It is approved for the treatment of patients diagnosed with major depressive episode, both with and without prominent symptoms of anxiety. Although trazodone's antidepressant activity is not fully understood, it inhibits serotonin reuptake in the brain in animals and potentiates behavioral changes induced by 5-hydroxytryptophan. Trazodone is more commonly used "off label" as a low-dose sedative hypnotic for youth with depression and anxiety (Owens et al., 2010).

Pharmacokinetics of Trazodone Hydrochloride

It is recommended that trazodone be ingested soon after eating. When taken in this manner, up to 20% more of the drug may be absorbed than when taken on an empty stomach, and maximum serum concentration is achieved more slowly (in about 2 hours rather than 1 hour) and with a lesser peak. This appears to diminish the likelihood of developing dizziness and/or lightheadedness.

Trazodone is eliminated through the liver (about 20% biliary) and the kidneys (about 75%). Elimination is biphasic: the initial half-life is between 3 and 6 hours, which is followed by a second phase with a half-life of between 5 and 9 hours.

Contraindications for Trazodone Hydrochloride Administration

Known hypersensitivity to the drug is a contraindication.

Interactions of Trazodone Hydrochloride with Other Drugs

Increased phenytoin levels have been reported when administered concomitantly with trazodone.

Trazodone should not be administered with MAOIs because the effects of their interaction are unknown.

Untoward Effects of Trazodone Hydrochloride

The most common side effects include drowsiness, dizziness or lightheadedness, dry mouth, and nausea or vomiting.

Priapism, which has necessitated surgical intervention and resulted in some cases of permanent impairment of sexual functioning, has been reported (incidence, about 1:15,000). Male patients with a prolonged or inappropriate erection should be told to discontinue trazodone immediately and contact their physician or, if it persists, to go to an emergency room.

Indications for Trazodone Hydrochloride in Child and Adolescent Psychiatry

NOTE: Review the Black Box Warning at the beginning of the chapter or in the package insert before prescribing.

Trazodone is approved only for the treatment of MDD in individuals at least 18 years old.
The drug is not recommended for use in the pediatric age group because its safety and effectiveness have not been established for this age range.

Trazodone Dosage Schedule

United States Pharmacopeial Dispensing Information (2005) reports the following pediatric dosage guidelines when trazodone is used as an antidepressant:

- *Children <6 years:* Not determined.
- *Children 6 to 18 years of age:* Begin with 1.5 to 2 mg/kg/day in divided doses. Titrate dosage gradually at 3- to 4-day intervals to a maximum of 6 mg/kg/day.

Trazodone Hydrochloride Dose Forms Available

- *Tablets:* 50 (scored), 100 (scored), 150 (quadrisected), and 300 mg (scored to divide into three or two equal parts)

■ *Reports of Interest*

Trazodone in the Treatment of Children and Adolescents with Significant Aggressivity

Fras (1987) reported successfully treating a 15-year-old male hospitalized for recurrent violence with a daily dose of 200 mg of trazodone. Because of a misunderstanding, following discharge the dose was significantly decreased and at times omitted altogether. Repeated angry outbursts and threats of violence developed within 1 week and the patient became morose. Upon resumption of a daily dose of 200 mg, the patient returned to the previous stability and cooperativeness, and remained so for 8 months of follow-up.

Zubieta and Alessi (1992) reported an open study of 22 inpatients (18 males and 4 females; age range, 5 to 12 years; mean age, 9 ± 2 years) with severe, treatment-refractory, behavioral disturbances. They were diagnosed with disruptive behavioral and mood disorders often with comorbidity. Six of the children continued to receive neuroleptic drugs for psychotic symptoms during the trial of trazodone. An initial dose of 50 mg of trazodone at bedtime was begun on an average of 23 ± 20 days after admission. It was titrated over a period of about 1week to the maximum dose tolerated and given three times daily. The 13 children designated as responders received a mean dose of 185 ± 117 mg/day (4.8 ± 1.7 mg/kg/day) of trazodone for a mean of 27 ± 13 days. The seven nonresponders received a mean dose of 158 ± 70 mg/day (4.7 ± 2.0 mg/kg/day) for a mean of 24 ± 11 days. One patient was dropped from the study for severe orthostatic hypotension and a second for reported painful erections (not priapism). The other children tolerated any untoward effects that occurred. The most frequent was orthostatic hypotension (50%), but this effect diminished over a few days and did not require clinical intervention; 27% of children reported drowsiness; 9%, nervousness; and 9%, anger. Dizziness, increased fatigue, and nocturnal enuresis each occurred in one child (4.5%).

Target symptoms that improved most frequently were impulsivity, hyperactivity, "involvement in dangerous activities," cruelty to people, frequency of physical fights, arguing with adults, and losing one's temper. Improvement of symptoms usually occurred within a few days of the initial administration of trazodone, as contrasted with the several weeks of continuous administration typically required for its antidepressant effects to occur. In a telephone follow-up 3 to 14 months later (mean, 8.8 ± 4.2 months), 9 of the 13 responders were successfully contacted. Eight of the children continued to receive a mean trazodone dose of 241 ± 128 mg/day (range, 100 to 800 mg/day). Trazodone was the only medication being taken at follow-up, the neuroleptics that three children were taking at discharge having been withdrawn within 2 months after discharge. The ninth child had an unsatisfactory response and his medication was changed to a combination of carbamazepine and pemoline. Overall, parents rated their children's improvement at 70 ± 20 (range, 50 to 90) on a subjective overall rating of efficacy scale ranging from 0 to 100 (Zubieta and Alessi, 1992). Trazodone appears to be a potentially useful drug in treating acute and chronic behavioral disorders that have not responded to other treatments and merits further investigation.

Ghaziuddin and Alessi (1992) noted the relationship of the expression of aggression and decreased levels of serotonin in the central nervous system and the successful use of trazodone to control aggressive behavior in adults with organic mental disorders. They administered trazodone to three boys who were 7, 8, and 9 years old with primary diagnoses of severe disruptive behavioral disorders; two of the boys were hospitalized. Trazodone was initiated at doses of 25 mg once or twice daily and increased gradually. Improvement of symptoms was noted within 7 to 10 days at a mean dose of 3.5 mg/kg/day of trazodone (about 75 mg/day). In all three cases, marked deterioration of behavior occurred upon discontinuing the medication and aggressiveness decreased to former treatment levels once medication was resumed. One boy had no reported untoward effects; one experienced mild sedation during the first week, but this remitted with no change in dosage. The third experienced spontaneous erections on 100 mg/day; because of concerns about reported priapism, dosage was reduced to 75 mg daily and behavioral control deteriorated. When 1,000 mg daily of L-tryptophan (which has been subsequently withdrawn from the commercial market) was added, behavior markedly improved again. No ECG changes were noted in any of the boys. The authors note that further studies will be needed to determine the efficacy and safety of trazodone in treating aggressive children.

Trazodone for the Treatment of Insomnia in Youth with Major Depression

Shamseddeen and colleagues (2012) examined the use of trazodone as an adjunctive sleep aid in the TORDIA study described above. In the TORDIA trial, participants were randomly assigned to one of four treatments after an unsuccessful initial SSRI treatment. They were switched to a second SSRI, switched to venlafaxine, switched to a second SSRI combined with CBT, or switched to venlafaxine combined with CBT. All participants in the study received sleep hygiene education. The study allowed for the addition of a sleep agent in a nonblinded manner as it was felt that residual sleep disturbance was a common symptom in adolescents who failed to have their depression remit in acute-phase treatment (Vitiello et al., 2011). Of the 334 youth enrolled in the study, 58 (17%) received at least one adjunctive sleep medication based on the pharmacotherapist's clinical judgment. One sleep medication was used in 48 (82.2%) of the subjects, 8 (13.8%) received two medications, and 2 (3.4%) were prescribed three different medications. The most frequently prescribed sleep medication was trazodone, which was prescribed for 33 (57%), and antihistamines were prescribed to 20 (34.5%). GABA-acting nonbenzodiazepines were prescribed to 11 (19%); two agents were used—zolpidem ($N = 10$) or eszopiclone ($N = 1$).

Youth who received trazodone were six times less likely to respond than those who received no sleep medication (adjusted odds ratio [AOR] = 0.16, 95% CI = 0.05 to 0.50, $P = .001$). Subjects who received trazodone were three times more likely to experience self-harm (OR = 3.0, 95% CI = 1.1 to 7.9, $P = .03$). None of the subjects (0 of 13) cotreated with trazodone, and either paroxetine or fluoxetine had an improvement in their depression. Subjects treated with hypnotics other than trazodone had similar rates of depression response (60.0% vs. 50.4%, $P = .36$) and self-harm events (OR = 0.5, 95% CI = 0.1 to 2.6, $P = .53$) as subjects who received no sleep medication. The authors suggest that, based on their findings, the use of trazodone for the management of sleep difficulties in adolescent depression should be reevaluated. They recommend that future research on the management of sleep disturbance in adolescent depression be conducted.

Bupropion Hydrochloride (Wellbutrin, Zyban)

Bupropion hydrochloride is an antidepressant of the aminoketone class. It is not related chemically to the tricyclics, tetracyclics, or other known antidepressants.

Pharmacokinetics of Bupropion Hydrochloride

Peak plasma concentrations are usually reached in about 2 hours. The metabolism of bupropion is extensive and complex. Following peak serum levels, there is a biphasic decline; average half-life of the second (postdistributional) phase is 14 hours (range, 8 to 24 hours). Several metabolites are pharmacologically active and have long half-lives. Six hours after a single-dose, plasma bupropion levels are about 30% of peak concentration.

Based on a study of 19 subjects (11 males, 8 females; age range 11 to 17, mean age 15.2 ± 1.8 years) who were treated with bupropion sustained release (SR) for diagnoses of ADHD ($N = 16$) and depressive disorders ($N = 16$) which were comorbid in 13 subjects, Daviss et al. (2005) reported that youths metabolize bupropion SR to active metabolites faster than adults and that bupropion SR should be given to subjects in this age group in divided doses.

Contraindications for Bupropion Hydrochloride Administration

Known hypersensitivity to bupropion hydrochloride and seizure disorders are contraindications.

A current or prior diagnosis of bulimia or anorexia nervosa is also a contraindication because a higher incidence of seizures is reported when bupropion is administered to such patients.

Bupropion should not be administered concurrently with an MAOI. At least a 14-day period off MAOIs should precede initiation of treatment with bupropion hydrochloride.

Concurrent administration with any drug that reduces the seizure threshold is a relative contraindication.

Interactions of Bupropion Hydrochloride with Other Drugs

Relatively few data are available on interactions of bupropion hydrochloride with other drugs. Increased adverse experiences were reported when the drug was administered concomitantly with L-dopa. MAOIs may increase the acute toxicity of bupropion.

Although bupropion is not metabolized by the CYP2D6 enzyme, the drug and its metabolite, morpholinol, inhibit this enzyme *in vitro*. Therefore, extreme caution should be exercised when coadministering any drug metabolized by that enzyme, and initial dosage of the drug should be as low as possible.

Untoward Effects of Bupropion Hydrochloride

Of particular clinical concern is the finding that seizures have been associated with about 4 (0.4%) per 1,000 patients treated with bupropion at doses of 450 mg/day or less. This is about four times the incidence of seizures reported with other approved antidepressants, and the incidence of seizures increases with higher daily doses. Conversely, Clay et al. (1988) note that the positive effects of bupropion on memory performance may be unique among antidepressants and that other antidepressants either have no effect or a negative effect on memory performance.

During the first few days of treatment, agitation, motor restlessness, and insomnia frequently occur; starting at a lower dose and making increments gradually helps to minimize these effects.

The most common untoward effects were reported to be agitation, dry mouth, insomnia, headache, nausea, vomiting, constipation, and tremor.

Ferguson and Simeon (1984) reported no adverse (or positive) effects on cognition on a cognitive battery in 17 children with attention-deficit disorder or conduct disorders who were treated in an open trial with bupropion.

Indications for Bupropion Hydrochloride in Child and Adolescent Psychiatry

NOTE: Review the Black Box Warning at the beginning of the chapter or in the package insert before prescribing.

Bupropion hydrochloride is indicated for the treatment of MDD. Bupropion hydrochloride SR (Zyban) is indicated as an aid to smoking cessation treatment.

(continued)

**Indications for Bupropion Hydrochloride in Child
and Adolescent Psychiatry** *(continued)*

Bupropion Dosage Schedule

- *Children and adolescents ≤17 years of age:* Not recommended. Safety and efficacy have not been established for this age group.
- *Adolescents at least 18 years of age and adults:*
  Standard-release tablets: An initial dosage of 100 mg twice daily is suggested. Based on clinical response, this may be increased to 100 mg three times daily but not before day 4 of treatment. During the first few days of treatment, agitation, motor restlessness, and insomnia frequently occur; starting at a lower dose and making increments slowly helps to minimize these effects. When insomnia is problematic, administer divided doses earlier in the day and not at bedtime. If no or insufficient clinical improvement occurs within 4 weeks, dosage may gradually be increased. Because of increased risk of seizure, a dose of 150 mg should not be exceeded within a 4-hour time period. The maximum daily dosage should not exceed 450 mg.
  Sustained-release tablets: Sustained S-release tablets should be swallowed whole, and there should be at least an 8-hour interval between successive doses. See preceding text regarding pharmacodynamics of bupropion SR in older children and adolescents.
  Sustained-release tablets (in treating MDD): An initial morning dose of 150 mg is recommended. If tolerated, an additional 150 mg may be added after 4 or more days to reach the target dose of 300 mg. Sustained-release tablets should be administered at least 8 hours apart. If no or insufficient clinical improvement occurs within 4 weeks, dosage may be increased to a maximum daily dose of 400 mg (administered as 200 mg b.i.d.).
  Sustained-release tablets (Zyban, as a smoking cessation aid): An initial daily dose of 150 mg is recommended for the initial 3 days, followed by an increase to the target and maximum recommended daily dose of 150 mg twice daily.
  Extended-release tablets (in treating MDD): An initial morning dose of 150 mg is recommended. If tolerated, an increase to a single, morning target dose of 300 mg/day may be made at day 4. There should be an interval of at least 24 hours between doses (*PDR*, 2006).

Bupropion Hydrochloride Dose Forms Available

- *Tablets:* 75 and 100 mg
- *Sustained-release tablets (Wellbutrin SR):* 100, 150, and 200 mg; (Zyban) 150 mg
- *Extended-release tablets (Wellbutrin XR):* 150 and 300 mg

Reports of Interest

Bupropion Hydrochloride in the Treatment of Children Diagnosed with ADHD

Simeon et al. (1986) treated 17 male subjects (age range, 7 to 13.4 years; mean, 10.4 years) with bupropion in a 14-week, single-blind, uncontrolled study. Fourteen subjects were diagnosed with attention-deficit disorder with hyperactivity (ADDH); of these, eight were also diagnosed with conduct disorder, undersocialized aggressive type, and two with OAD. Eleven of the subjects had prior drug treatment; of these, eight had shown no improvement. Four weeks of placebo were followed by 8 weeks of bupropion and then by 2 weeks of placebo. The initial dose of bupropion was 50 mg/day; this was increased to 50 mg twice daily during the second week and to a maximum of 50 mg three times daily during the third week. None of the subjects responded to the baseline placebo. Of the subjects who were on the drug, five patients showed marked improvement, seven moderate improvement, and two mild improvement on the CGI-I ratings. Significant improvements also occurred on the Children's Psychiatric Rating Scale (CPRS), Conners Parents and Teachers Scales, and self-ratings. Although not significant, group means for all nine cognitive test variables showed improvement. Optimal dose was 150 mg/day in 15 cases and 100 and 50 mg/day in the other 2 subjects. Untoward effects were reported to be infrequent, mild, and transient.

Clay et al. (1988) reported that bupropion hydrochloride was safe and efficacious in treating prepubertal children diagnosed with ADHD. The authors' clinical impression was that children with additional prominent symptoms of conduct disorder responded particularly well to bupropion.

Thirty prepubertal children diagnosed with ADHD were enrolled in a double-blind, placebo-controlled study and individually titrated to optimal doses of bupropion (Clay et al., 1988). Optimal doses ranged from 100 to 250 mg/day (3.1 to 7.1 mg/kg/day; mean, 5.3 ± 1 mg/kg/day). Subjects receiving bupropion showed statistically significant improvement on the CGI-I and CGI-S Rating Scales, on the Self-Rating Scale, and on digit symbol and delayed recall on the Selective Reminding Test. No significant improvement was reported on the Conners Parent Questionnaire and the Conners Teacher Questionnaire. The only serious side effect noted was an allergic rash in two children.

Clay et al. (1988) also noted that some children who had previously not responded satisfactorily to stimulants had a good response to bupropion. On the other hand, some subjects who had never received stimulants and who did not respond well to bupropion responded well when methylphenidate was openly prescribed at a later time.

Casat et al. (1989) administered bupropion to 20 children and placebo to 10 children in a parallel-groups design, double-blind comparison study. All subjects were diagnosed with ADDH. Decreases in symptom severity and overall clinical improvement were noted in physician ratings, and there was a significant decrease in hyperactivity in the classroom settings on the Conners Teacher Questionnaire.

Barrickman et al. (1995) conducted a 16-week, double-blind crossover-design study comparing bupropion with methylphenidate (MPH) in the treatment of 15 outpatients (12 males, 3 females; mean age, 11.8 ± 3.3 years; range, 7 to 16 years) who were diagnosed with ADHD by DSM-III-R (APA, 1987) criteria. Following an initial 2-week washout period, subjects were randomly assigned to bupropion or MPH for a 6-week treatment period. This was followed by another 2-week washout; subjects then received the alternative medication for the next 6 weeks. Efficacy was determined by ratings on the Iowa-Conners Abbreviated Parent and Teacher Questionnaires (ICQ-P and ICQ-T), the CGI-I Scale, the CGI-S Scale, and side effects scale. Bupropion was administered at a dose of 1.5 mg/kg/day for the first week, increased to 2.0 mg/kg/day for the second week, and individually titrated clinically during the third week to achieve an optimal dose, which was then held constant for the final 3 weeks. Active doses of bupropion were usually given twice daily in the morning and at 4:00 PM. The final mean dose of bupropion was 140 ± 146 mg/day (range, 50 to 200 mg/day) or 3.3 ± 1.2 mg/kg/day (range, 1.4 to 5.7 mg/kg/day). Methylphenidate was given at a dose of 0.4 mg/kg/day for the first week and individually titrated to the optimal dose over the next 2 weeks; this dose was then maintained for the final 3-week period on the drug. The final mean dose of MPH was 31 ± 11 mg/day (range, 20 to 60 mg/day) or 0.7 ± 0.2 mg/kg/day (range, 0.4 to 1.3 mg/kg/day).

Treatment with both bupropion and MPH resulted in significantly lower scores on the ICQ–Parent ratings and the ICQ–Teacher ratings when compared with baseline ($P < .001$). There was no significant difference between the two drugs, and the order in which they were given was not significant. Ratings on some of the individual factors on the ICQ improved significantly more on methylphenidate (e.g., attention on the ICQ–parent), and all the rating scales except the R-CMAS, which had nonsignificant trends, suggesting that MPH was slightly more effective than bupropion. Untoward effects were minimal, were usually transient, and occurred primarily during the first 2 weeks of treatment. While on bupropion, nine (60%) subjects reported nine untoward effects: drowsiness (four), fatigue (three), nausea (three), anorexia (two), dizziness (two), "spaciness" (two), anxiety (one), headache (one), and tremor (one). Only five (33%) reported nine untoward effects during the period they were on MPH: anxiety (one), anger/crying (one), drowsiness (one), headache (one), insomnia (one), irritability (one), low mood (one), nausea (one), and stomachache (one). Bupropion appears to be a useful treatment option for treating ADHD but may be slightly less effective than MPH overall and have somewhat more, although usually mild, untoward effects.

Conners et al. (1996) conducted a multisite, 6-week, parallel-group random-ized, double-blind comparison of bupropion hydrochloride ($N = 72$) and placebo ($N = 37$) in 109 children diagnosed with ADDH by DSM-III criteria (APA, 1980a); none of the subjects had comorbid MDD. Subjects were 90% male, and 75% were white; their average age was about 8.5 years (range, 6 to 12 years); two-thirds were in the third grade or below.

Following an initial 1-week single-blind placebo phase, bupropion or placebo was administered at 7:00 AM and 7:00 PM daily over the 4-week flexible-dose treatment phase. Dose was initiated at 3 mg/kg/day and titrated to reach 6 mg/kg/day during days 15 to 28. Daily maximum doses of 150, 200, and 250 mg were permitted for subjects weighing 20 to 30 kg, 31 to 40 kg, and >40 kg, respectively. The sixth week was again a 1-week placebo washout for all subjects. Efficacy was assessed on several scales, including the Conners Parent and Teacher Ques-tionnaires, the Abbreviated Parent and Teacher Questionnaire (Conners 10-item "Hyperactivity Index"), CGI-S and CGI-I Scales, a short-term memory test, and a continuous performance test.

Teachers noted significant improvement in hyperactivity and conduct prob-lems after the third day on medication. Parents rated restless-impulsive behavior and conduct problems as significantly improved only at the end of the 4-week treatment period. GCI ratings by clinicians at the four settings were not signifi-cant when their data were pooled. At the end of the study, when all subjects had completed a week on placebo, teachers' ratings showed no difference between the placebo and medication groups. The authors also reported modest improvement in cognitive functions of attention and memory retrieval. Although the bupropion group improved below the subject selection cutoff of 15 points on the hyperactiv-ity index, the degree of improvement was less than that typically found with the treatment of the standard stimulants.

Overall untoward effects were infrequent. There were no clinically important differences in vital signs, ECG, or laboratory values between the two groups. EEGs at day 28 compared with baseline found that six patients on bupropion developed abnormal EEGs, including three who developed spike-and-wave discharges. No patient had evidence of clinical seizure activity during treatment. Four (6%) pa-tients receiving bupropion developed apparent allergic skin rashes with urticaria and were dropped from the study. Bupropion hydrochloride appears to be a pos-sible second-line treatment for children diagnosed with ADHD, although the mag-nitude of clinical improvement appears to be less than what is typical for standard stimulants, and there is some concern about AEs on the EEG and increased seizure potential (Conners et al., 1996).

Although confirmation of these findings is needed, bupropion may be an alter-native treatment for ADHD that does not respond to standard therapies.

Bupropion Treatment of Adolescents Diagnosed with ADHD and Comorbid Substance Abuse and Conduct Disorder

Riggs et al. (1998) treated in a 5-week, open-label study using bupropion 13 nondepressed adolescent males (mean age, 15.5 years; range, 14 to 17 years) diagnosed with ADHD by DSM-IV (APA, 1994) criteria, who were residing in a long-term, unlocked facility for treatment of their comorbid substance abuse and conduct disorders. Efficacy was determined by ratings on the Conners' Teacher Rating Scale-39 (CTRS-39), the CGI-S and the CGI-I Scales. Bupropion was started at a dose of 100 mg twice daily and increased to 100 mg given three times daily after 7 days for the final 4 weeks of the study. Final dose of all subjects was 300 mg/day (dose range, 3.9 to 5.6 mg/kg/day). Subject mean score on the CTRS-39 declined significantly by 13% ($P \leq .01$); the mean CGI-S score improved by 39% ($P < .002$); and the mean CGI-I score was rated "much" or "very much improved" for seven subjects and "minimally improved" for the remaining six. Untoward effects were reported by seven (54%) of the adolescents; most were mild and transient. One subject, however, developed hypomanic symptoms during the fifth week of the study. The symptoms resolved within 1 week after discontinuing bupropion. These initial data suggest that bupropion may be a useful treatment for such adolescents.

Bupropion in the Treatment of Comorbid ADHD and Chronic Motor Tic Disorder or TS

Spencer et al. (1993b) reported that bupropion exacerbated tics in four children with ADHD and comorbid TS. All four patients had been initially treated with stimulants, when two patients with preexisting symptoms of ADHD and TS experienced worsening of their tics and the other two developed tics and TS. Bupropion was subsequently prescribed as a possibly effective alternative treatment for children diagnosed with ADHD who did not respond satisfactorily to stimulants or could not tolerate their untoward effects. All four children experienced an exacerbation of tics over a period ranging from almost immediately to 2 months. The tics rapidly improved to pretreatment levels when bupropion was discontinued. The authors suggest that bupropion may not be a useful alternative to stimulants in treating patients with comorbid ADHD and TS.

Bupropion in the Treatment of Adolescents with Comorbid ADHD and Nicotine Dependency

In an open-label study, Upadhyaya et al. (2004) administered bupropion SR to 16 adolescents (10 males, 6 females, age range, 12 to 19 years), with nicotine dependency, 11 of whom had comorbid ADHD. Over the first week, subjects weighing 90 or more pounds were titrated to 150 mg bupropion SR b.i.d.; this dose was maintained for the next 6 weeks. Subjects weighing less than 90 lb remained on a total daily dose (TDD) of 150 mg of bupropion SR for the entire 7-week period. All subjects also received two 30-minute individual sessions on smoking cessation. Nine subjects completed at least 4 weeks on medication. Three subjects withdrew because of untoward effects; two withdrew because of pregnancy and one subject took an overdose of study medication. Five subjects (31.25%) had stopped smoking within 4 weeks of taking bupropion SR. Some subjects did not stop smoking but did reduce the number of cigarettes smoked, suggesting that bupropion SR might have a harm-reduction effect. The weights of the subjects did not change significantly; the authors noted the potential importance of this as the possibility of gaining weight was a frequent concern, especially among girls, before entering the study. Finally, ADHD symptoms did not change significantly; this is relevant as bupropion has been shown to be effective in the treatment of ADHD and there is also some evidence that nicotine may improve ADHD symptoms in adults—both smokers and nonsmokers.

Bupropion in the Treatment of Adolescents with Nicotine Dependency

Gray and colleagues (2011) examined the use of bupropion SR and contingency management (CM) in improving smoking cessation rates in adolescents. In a double-blind placebo-controlled study, 134 adolescent smokers were randomized to receive a 6-week course of one of four treatment arms. Subjects were randomized to receive bupropion SR + CM, bupropion SR + non-CM, placebo + CM, or placebo + non-CM. Subjects received treatment for 6 weeks and were assessed at 6 weeks after the conclusion of treatment (week 12). The primary outcome measure was a 7-day cotinine-verified point prevalence abstinence. The combined bupropion SR + CM group had significantly superior abstinence rates during active treatment when compared with placebo + non-CM treatment. The authors conclude that combined bupropion SR and CM appears efficacious for adolescent smoking cessation and may be superior to either intervention alone.

SELECTIVE SEROTONIN AND NOREPINEPHRINE REUPTAKE INHIBITORS

Venlafaxine Hydrochloride (Effexor)

Venlafaxine hydrochloride is chemically unrelated to other available antidepressants. Its antidepressant effects are thought to be due to its potent inhibition of the reuptake of neuronal serotonin and norepinephrine and weak inhibition of dopamine uptake (a serotonergic noradrenergic reuptake inhibitor). Venlafaxine does not have significant affinity for muscarinic, histaminergic, or alpha-1 adrenergic receptors.

Pharmacokinetics of Venlafaxine Hydrochloride

Food has no significant effect on the bioavailability of venlafaxine. The drug is extensively metabolized by the liver to O-desmethylvenlafaxine (ODV), the major metabolite, which is clinically active. Mean terminal elimination half-life is approximately 11 hours. Steady-state serum concentrations are achieved within approximately 3 days of multidose administration. The primary route of excretion of venlafaxine and its metabolites is through the kidneys.

Contraindications for Venlafaxine Hydrochloride Administration

Known hypersensitivity to the drug is a contraindication.

Because of a possibility of serious, life-threatening reactions when administered simultaneously with an MAOI, it is recommended that the drug not be used in combination with an MAOI. At least 2 weeks should elapse after stopping an MAOI before administering venlafaxine. Based on the half-life of venlafaxine, at least 7 days should elapse following its discontinuation before administering an MAOI.

Significant hepatic or renal disease may markedly decrease elimination of the drug and increase serum levels. If the clinician elects to use venlafaxine, adjustment of dosage may be necessary.

Use with caution in depressed patients with a history of hypomania or mania, as activation of either could occur.

Untoward Effects of Venlafaxine Hydrochloride

Among the most commonly reported untoward effects are anxiety, nervousness, somnolence or insomnia, nausea, anorexia, initial dose-dependent weight loss, constipation, increased sweating, dry mouth, dizziness, abnormal ejaculation/orgasm, and impotence. A sustained increase in supine diastolic blood pressure, which appeared to be dose related has been reported in some patients treated with venlafaxine. Many other untoward effects have been reported.

ECG Changes

Administration of regular venlafaxine resulted in no treatment-emergent conduction abnormalities compared with placebo, but the mean heart rate was increased by 4 beats per minute compared with baseline. On Effexor XL (brand name extended-release preparation), however, the QTc interval increased by 4.7 msec over baseline, compared with a decrease of 1.9 msec for placebo. Heart rate increased by 4 beats per minute over baseline on Effexor XL compared with an increase of 1 beat per minute over baseline for placebo.

Indications for Venlafaxine Hydrochloride in Child and Adolescent Psychiatry

NOTE: Review the Black Box Warning at the beginning of the chapter or in the package insert before prescribing.

Venlafaxine hydrochloride in its immediate-release form is indicated for the treatment of MDD only. Venlafaxine hydrochloride in its extended-release capsule form (Effexor XR) has been approved for the treatment of MDD, GAD, and social anxiety disorder. Venlafaxine's efficacy and safety in patients <18 years of age have not been established. One manufacturer notes that data from two placebo-controlled trials with extended-release venlafaxine (Effexor XR) in a total of 766 pediatric patients (ages 6 to 17 years) diagnosed with MDD and from two placebo-controlled studies in a total of 793 pediatric patients diagnosed with general anxiety disorder were not sufficient to support a claim for use in this age group (*PDR*, 2006). Data from these studies suggest that venlafaxine may adversely affect weight and height, which should be monitored if used in children. It was also noted that elevations in blood pressure and in serum cholesterol that were considered clinically relevant occurred in these subjects and that they were similar to those reported in adult patients (*PDR*, 2006).

Venlafaxine Dosage Schedule

- *Children and adolescents ≤17 years of age:* Not recommended. Safety and efficacy have not been established in this age group.
- *Adolescents at least 18 years of age and adults:*
  Treatment of MDD with immediate-release tablets: The initial recommended starting dose is 75 mg divided into two or three doses and taken with food. If clinically indicated, the dose may be titrated up to 225 mg/day for moderately depressed patients and up to a maximum of 375 mg/day in severely depressed patients. Increments of up to 75 mg may be made at intervals of at least 4 days.
  Treatment of MDD, GAD, and social anxiety disorder with extended-release capsules: Should be swallowed whole and taken with food in a single morning or evening dose at about the same time each day. Initial recommended daily dose is 75 mg, but 37.5 mg/day initially is an option. Steady-state serum levels usually occur by the fourth day. If adequate clinical response does not occur, dose may be raised by 75-mg increments at intervals of 4 days or more to a maximum of 225 mg/day.

Venlafaxine Hydrochloride Dose Forms Available

- *Tablets:* 25, 37.5, 50, 75, and 100 mg
- *Extended-release capsules:* 37.5, 75, and 150 mg

Report of Interest

Venlafaxine Hydrochloride in the Treatment of Major Depression Disorder

Emslie and colleagues (2007) reported on the use of venlafaxine in two placebo-controlled trials. In this report, the results of two similar trials comparing venlafaxine to placebo were combined. Three hundred sixty-seven subjects were enrolled: 183 were assigned to receive placebo, and 184 were assigned to receive venlafaxine ER. Venlafaxine ER was dosed at 37.5 mg for the first week. Subjects who weighed 25 to 39 kg could have the dose increased to 75 mg on day 8 and 112.5 on day 19. For subjects weighing 40 to 49 kg, the dose was automatically increased to 75 on day 8 and could be increased to 112.5 on day 15 and to 150 mg on day 29. For subjects over 50 kg, the dose was automatically increased to 75 mg on day 8 and could be increased to 150 mg on day 15 and 225 mg on day 29. The mean daily dose of venlafaxine ER was 97.1 mg/day. Among children (7 to 11 years), the mean dose was 80.4 mg/day, and among adolescents (12 to 17 years), the mean dose was 109.2 mg/day. Outcomes were measured using the CDRS-R score. The pooled data did not show any statistically significant differences between venlafaxine ER and placebo on the CDRS-R. Analysis of the pooled data showed that adolescents 12 to 17 had greater improvement on the CDRS-R with venlafaxine ER than with placebo (−24.4 vs. −19.9; $P = 0.22$). Children did not show any clinically significant improvement in CDRS-R scores. AEs commonly seen were anorexia and abdominal pain. There were more hostility and suicide-related events in the venlafaxine ER–treated subjects than in the placebo-treated subjects. There were no completed suicides. The authors conclude that venlafaxine ER may be an effective treatment in depressed adolescents, but not in depressed children.

The TORDIA study described above in the fluoxetine section used venlafaxine as one of its treatment arms in addition to the SSRIs paroxetine, citalopram, and fluoxetine in the treatment of adolescents with SSRI-resistant depression. In this study, venlafaxine had response rates similar to the other SSRIs in the study, which indicate that it is an effective treatment for depression in adolescents. In this study, 83 subjects received venlafaxine alone and 83 subjects received venlafaxine in combination with CBT. In the study, venlafaxine was dosed for weeks 1 to 3 at 37.5, 75, 112.5, and 150 mg/day for weeks 1 to 4, respectively. There was an option to increase the dose to 225 mg by week 6. If side effects developed, the venlafaxine dose was lowered to 150 mg. The mean venlafaxine dose was 205.4 mg/day. The venlafaxine group had a greater increase in diastolic blood pressure and pulse and had a more frequent occurrence of skin problems when compared with SSRI treatment. The authors conclude that since the venlafaxine had similar response rates to SSRIs and more significant side effects that a second SSRI should be selected over venlafaxine as a second-line antidepressant.

Venlafaxine Hydrochloride in the Treatment of Anxiety in Children and Adolescents

March and colleagues (2007b) reported on a double-blind placebo-controlled trial of venlafaxine ER to treat pediatric social anxiety disorder. In this study, 293 subjects ages 8 to 17 who met criteria for social anxiety disorder were randomized to receive either venlafaxine ER or placebo over 16 weeks. Venlafaxine was titrated from 37.5 mg to a maximum of 225 mg/day depending on weight and clinical response over the length of the study. The primary measures of response were the social anxiety scale, child or adolescent version (SCA-CA) and the CGI-I scores. The authors found that when compared with placebo, ITT random regression analysis indicated a statistically significant advantage for venlafaxine ER ($P = .001$) on the SAS-CA. On the CGI-I, 56% of the venlafaxine ER–treated subjects responded, which was superior to placebo at 37%. Three venlafaxine ER and no placebo patients developed treatment-emergent suicidality, and there were no completed suicides. The authors conclude that venlafaxine ER is an effective and fairly well-tolerated treatment for generalized social anxiety disorder in children and adolescents.

Venlafaxine Hydrochloride in the Treatment of ADHD in Children and Adolescents

Olvera et al. (1996) conducted a 5-week, open-label trial of venlafaxine in the treatment of 16 subjects (15 males, 1 female; mean age, 11.6 ± 2.3 years; age range, 8 to 16 years) diagnosed with ADHD without comorbid depression by DSM-IV (APA, 1994) criteria to assess efficacy, dose range, and untoward effects. Efficacy was determined by ratings on the Conners, Parent Rating Scale (CPRS) and the Conners, Continuous Performance Test (CPT). Venlafaxine was given at a daily dose of 12.5 mg for the first week. Dose was subsequently increased by 25 mg/week to reach a target dose of 75 mg/day unless prevented by untoward effects; subjects weighing <40 kg had weekly increases of 12.5 mg to a maximum of 50 mg/day. Ten subjects completed the 5-week study. Of the six noncompleters, three had behavioral activation (increased hyperactivity), one had severe nausea, and two were lost to follow-up. The mean dose of venlafaxine for the 10 completers was 60 mg/day or 1.4 mg/kg/day given in two or three divided doses.

Overall, 7 (44%) of the 16 subjects improved on the CPRS. At the end of 5 weeks, mean ratings on the CPRS impulsivity factor improved significantly ($P = .008$), and mean ratings on the CPRS hyperactivity index improved significantly ($P = .003$); there were no significant changes in mean ratings on the

CPRS conduct factor. Cognitive symptoms of ADHD as reflected in omission or commission errors or reaction time on the CPT showed no significant improvement. The most common untoward effects were drowsiness (8/16, 50%), nausea (6/16, 37.5%), irritability (5/15, 33%), and behavioral activation (worsening of hyperactivity in 5/15, 33%). The authors concluded that low doses of venlafaxine appeared to be effective in reducing behavioral but not cognitive symptoms of ADHD but that behavioral activation may be of concern (Olvera et al., 1996).

Findling and colleagues (2007c) conducted a 2-week open-label trial of venlafaxine in the treatment of ADHD in 33 males aged 5 to 17 years. The authors wanted to examine changes in symptom severity, tolerability, and pharmacodynamics of venlafaxine in youths with ADHD. The study was conducted with three dosing strata. The subjects were divided into two age groups, children ages 5 to 12 and adolescents ages 13 to 17. The first five subjects in each age group received 0.5 mg/kg of venlafaxine per day divided into two daily doses with a maximum TDD of 37.5 mg which was administered for 2 weeks. If that dose was judged to be well tolerated by the treating physician in three subjects, then the next five subjects in each age group received 1.0 mg/kg of venlafaxine per day with a TDD of 75 mg. If that dose was felt to be tolerated by at least three subjects, then the next five subjects received a dose of 2.0 mg/kg/day, TDD = 150 mg.

Effectiveness was measured by comparing parent- and teacher-completed 18-item ADHD rating scale of ADHD symptoms (ARS-IV) as well as by using CGI-S and CGI-I scores. The study enrolled 21 children and 17 adolescents. Fourteen subjects received venlafaxine at 0.5 mg/kg/day, 13 subjects received it at 1.0 mg/kg/day, and 11 subjects received it at 2.0 mg/kg/day. At the end of the study, parent ARS-IV scores were improved over baseline in total inattentive and hyperactive-impulsive subscores ($P < .001$). Teacher ARS-IV ratings for total symptoms were improved over baseline ($P = .03$). Inattentive symptoms were improved ($P = .02$) but hyperactivity-impulsivity symptoms did not reach statistical significance ($P = .06$). When response was defined by a CGI-S score of 1 or 2, only 5% of study subjects were classified as responders 2 of 17 adolescents and none of the 21 children had responded. No difference in response was found among the dosing levels. No subjects discontinued due to AEs. No suicidal behaviors were observed or reported in the study. Considering that venlafaxine requires at least 4 weeks to see an antidepressant response in adults, the length of this trial was likely inadequate to see treatment effects. The authors conclude that this open trial shows that venlafaxine may offer some benefit and appears relatively safe for the short-term treatment of ADHD.

Mirtazapine (Remeron)

Mirtazapine is a selective serotonin and norepinephrine reuptake inhibitor (SSNRI) belonging to the piperazine/azepine group. It has a tetracyclic chemical structure unrelated to other antidepressants in use. Preclinical studies showed that it acts as an antagonist at central presynaptic alpha-2-adrenergic inhibitory autoreceptors and heteroreceptors, resulting in an increase in central noradrenergic and serotonergic activity. Mirtazapine is a potent antagonist of 5-HT$_2$ and 5-HT$_3$ receptors, but has no significant affinity for 5-HT$_{1A}$ and 5-HT$_{1B}$ receptors. It is also a potent antagonist of histamine (H$_1$) receptors, which may cause its prominent sedative effects. Mirtazapine is a moderate peripheral alpha-1-adrenergic antagonist, which may cause the orthostatic hypotension that sometimes occurs. The drug also has moderate antagonistic properties at muscarinic receptors, which may explain the relatively low incidence of anticholinergic effects associated with its use.

Pharmacokinetics of Mirtazapine

Food has a clinically insignificant effect on the rate and bioavailability of mirtazapine. It is rapidly absorbed, with peak plasma concentrations occurring about

2 hours after ingestion. It is extensively metabolized in the liver by demethylation and hydroxylation followed by glucuronide conjugation. Serum half-life ranges between 20 and 40 hours and is significantly longer in females (mean, 37 hours) than in males (mean, 26 hours). Steady-state plasma levels occur within 5 days at a given dose. Elimination is about 75% via urine, with most of the remainder being excreted in the feces.

Contraindications for the Administration of Mirtazapine

Known hypersensitivity to the drug is a contraindication.

Because mirtazapine was associated with the development of severe neutropenia in about 0.1% of patients in premarketing clinical trials, whenever a patient develops sore throat, fever, stomatitis, or other signs of infection and has a low white blood cell count, mirtazapine should be discontinued and the patient closely monitored.

Because of a possibility of serious, life-threatening reactions when administered simultaneously with an MAOI, it is recommended that the drug not be used in combination with an MAOI. At least 2 weeks should elapse after stopping an MAOI before administering mirtazapine. Likewise, based on the half-life of mirtazapine, at least 2 weeks should elapse following its discontinuation before administering an MAOI.

Untoward Effects of Mirtazapine

Somnolence occurred in more than one-half of patients administered mirtazapine and resulted in discontinuation of treatment in 10.4% of 453 subjects in a controlled 6-week trial (package insert). Other untoward effects included increased appetite, weight gain, dizziness, dry mouth, and constipation. Many other untoward effects have been reported.

Indications for Mirtazapine in Child and Adolescent Psychiatry

NOTE: Review the Black Box Warning at the beginning of the chapter or in the package insert before prescribing.

Mirtazapine is approved for the treatment of depression in adults. Its safety and efficacy in pediatric patients have not been established.

Mirtazapine Dosage Schedule

- *Children and adolescents ≤17 years of age:* Not established.
- *Adolescents at least 18 years of age and adults:* An initial daily dose of 15 mg at bedtime is recommended. Effective daily doses usually range between 15 and 45 mg. Dose should be titrated upward on the basis of clinical response, but, because of the relatively long serum half-life of mirtazapine (20 to 40 hours), increments should not be made at intervals of <1 to 2 weeks in order to permit adequate assessment of therapeutic response at each dose.

Mirtazapine Dose Forms Available

- *Tablets:* 15 (scored), 30 (scored), and 45 mg

Report of Interest

Mirtazapine in the Treatment of Social Phobia

Mrakotsky and colleagues (2008) conducted an open-label pilot trial of the effectiveness of mirtazapine in children and adolescents with SP. The authors enrolled 18 children ages 8 to 17 who met DSM-IV-TR criteria for social anxiety disorder.

They initiated mirtazapine at 15 mg/day and increased to 30 mg after 1 week. The target maximum dose was 0.58 mg/kg/day or the lesser of 45 mg/kg/day. Eight patients (44.5) were on their target maximum dose of 0.8 mg/kg/day. Primary outcomes were symptom improvement based on clinician rating and self-report as well as tolerability. Fifty-six percent of youth (10/18) responded to treatment and 17% (3/18) achieved full remission. They did find that SP symptoms increased during the first 2 weeks of treatment along with symptoms of anxiety and depression. The side effects seen were increased sleepiness in the morning and irritability which were felt to be mild. By the final visit, 2 of 18 patients had moderate to severe AEs of headaches sand sleepiness. No suicidal ideation or suicide attempts were reported. Four patients discontinued due to AEs. The authors conclude that this study provides some evidence for the use of mirtazapine as a treatment for pediatric SP and encourage further studies.

Duloxetine Hydrochloride (Cymbalta)

Duloxetine hydrochloride is an SSNRI.

Pharmacokinetics of Duloxetine Hydrochloride

Duloxetine may be taken with or without food which does not affect the maximum plasma concentration, but delays it and decreases the amount absorbed by about 10%. Because the capsules contain enteric-coated pellets that prevent the drug from degrading in the stomach, there is a median delay of about 2 hours until absorption begins. Evening doses are absorbed up to 3 hours more slowly and cleared up to 33% more rapidly than morning doses. Maximum plasma levels occur about 6 hours after ingestion of the drug.

Duloxetine hydrochloride has a half-life of about 12 hours (range 8 to 17 hours). Steady-state plasma levels occur after about 3 days at a given dose. Duloxetine is extensively metabolized primarily by the hepatic P450 enzymes CYP2D6 and CYP1A2. About 70% is eliminated in the urine and 20% through the feces.

Contraindications for the Administration of Duloxetine Hydrochloride

Hypersensitivity to duloxetine hydrochloride or its components is a contraindication to its administration. Concomitant use with MAOIs is contraindicated. It should not be prescribed to patients with uncontrolled narrow-angle glaucoma. Duloxetine should not be coadministered with thioridazine.

Duloxetine should not be coadministered with an MAOI or within 14 days after treatment with an MAOI has been discontinued. At least 5 days should elapse after stopping duloxetine therapy before administering an MAOI.

Interactions of Duloxetine Hydrochloride with Other Drugs

CYP1A2 inhibitors are expected to increase duloxetine plasma levels; for example, fluvoxamine increases maximum plasma levels by 2½ times and the serum concentration by up to 6 times. Quinolone antibiotics should also be avoided for the same reason.

Potent CYP2D6 inhibitors also are expected to increase duloxetine plasma levels, for example, 20 mg of paroxetine daily reportedly increased plasma levels caused by 40 mg daily of duloxetine by 60%; fluoxetine and quinidine would also be expected to increase plasma levels of duloxetine.

Duloxetine, itself, is a moderate inhibitor of CYP2D6. Coadministration of duloxetine with other drugs that are extensively metabolized by CYP2D6, which have a narrow therapeutic index such as the TCAs nortriptyline, amitriptyline, imipramine, and desipramine; phenothiazines, and type 1C antiarrhythmics should be avoided if possible because of potentially dangerous increases in their serum levels. If coadministered, TCA serum levels should be monitored closely.

Coadministration with thioridazine is contraindicated because of the risk of ventricular arrhythmias and sudden death that has been associated with elevated thioridazine levels.

Untoward Effects of Duloxetine Hydrochloride

The most common untoward effects reported in adult placebo-controlled clinical trials were nausea (20% vs. 7%), dry mouth (15% vs. 6%), constipation (11% vs. 4%), fatigue (8% vs. 4%), decreased appetite (8% vs. 2%), somnolence (7% vs. 3%), and increased sweating (6% vs. 2%). Duloxetine was associated with a mean blood pressure increase of 2 mm Hg systolic and 0.5 mm Hg diastolic compared with levels with placebo.

Indications for Duloxetine Hydrochloride in Child and Adolescent Psychiatry

NOTE: Review the Black Box Warning at the beginning of the chapter or in the package insert before prescribing.

Duloxetine is indicated for the treatment of MDD in adults. Safety and efficacy have not been established for pediatric patients.

Duloxetine Hydrochloride Dosage Schedule

- *Children and adolescents <18 years of age:* Not recommended.
- *Adolescents ≥18 years of age and adults:* The recommended target dose is 60 mg, given in a single daily dose. Administration may be begun at 20 mg, twice daily and titrated upward. If discontinuing duloxetine, a gradual tapering down of dose is recommended to avoid possible serious untoward effects that may occur with abrupt cessation.

Duloxetine Hydrochloride Dose Forms Available

- Delayed-release capsules 20, 30, and 60 mg

Report of Interest

Duloxetine in the Treatment of Major Depression

Prakash and colleagues (2012) conducted an open-label study on the use of duloxetine in pediatric patients with major depression. Study participants with major depression were enrolled if their CDRS-R score was over 40 and their CGI-S was over 4 at three screening visits. The study was conducted as a 32-week, single-arm, flexible-dose, open-label study. There were five study periods: 2- to 4-week screening phase, 10-week dose-titration/pharmacokinetic sampling phase which included weekly study visits, 8-week acute safety and tolerability phase with visits every 2 weeks, 12-week extended safety and tolerability with visits every 4 weeks, and a 2-week taper phase. Patients were started with duloxetine at 20 mg/day if they weighed <40 kg and 30 mg/day if they weighed over 40 kg for the first 2 weeks. The dose was then flexibly escalated from 20 to 30 to 60 to 90 to 120 mg daily over the 8-week dose-titration phase. Doses were increased based on the investigator's assessment of safety and tolerability as well as an inadequate clinical response (CGI-S score ≤3). If duloxetine dose increases were not tolerated, the dose was decreased. During the 8-week safety and tolerability phase, they remained on the dose they attained during the titration period. During the 12-week extended safety trial, dose could again be titrated within the range of 20 to 120 mg based on the investigator's discretion.

Seventy-two patients were enrolled in the study and, of those, 58 (80.6%) completed the 10-week dose-titration phase, 48 (66.7%) completed the 18 weeks of acute treatment, and 42 (58.3%) completed an additional 12 weeks of extended treatment. The study enrolled 31 children 7 to 12 years and 24 adolescents 13 to 17 years. At least 85% of the subjects were compliant with the study drug at each visit. Patients CYP2D6 status was evaluated, and the majority were extensive metabolizers and four patients (5.6%) were identified as CYP2D6 poor metabolizers. The majority of patients (55.72; 76%) required dose escalation to higher doses of duloxetine (60, 90, or 120 mg/day). Typical duloxetine clearance in pediatric patients was approximately 42% to 60% higher than in adults.

Four patients (5.6%) discontinued due to TEAE. Three had nausea/vomiting, rash, or reemergence of ADHD. A fourth patient on duloxetine 120 mg/day discontinued after 5 months of treatment due to irritability. The most common TEAEs were seen in the acute treatment period. Nausea was reported in 25% of the total study population. Females experienced nausea 40%, vomiting 17.1%, and dizziness 14.3%, more frequently than males. Headaches were seen in 13.9% of the study subjects. Serious adverse events were seen in five patients (6.9%) six times, which required hospitalization during the study and occurred during the acute treatment period. Two patients had self-injurious behaviors, one felt to be nonsuicidal and one felt to be suicidal. One patient abruptly stopped duloxetine (90 mg) and had worsening of depression. One patient had worsening of oppositional defiant disorder while on 30 mg/day. Another patient experienced viral gastroenteritis on 60 mg/day. Overall, one nonfatal suicidal attempt occurred and two patients (2.8%) experienced worsening of suicidal ideation. The study included 19 patients with suicidal ideation at baseline and 17 (90%) reported improvement in suicidal ideation. Many patients (37/72, 50%) experienced clinically significant elevation in blood pressure which, in most cases (21/36, 58%), was transient.

The study did show improvement in depression measures by the end of the acute and extension treatment phases. CGI-S scores decreased from baseline to endpoint –2.11 (1.17) and –2.7 (1.07) for the acute and extension treatment phases, respectively. The mean changes in CDRS-R scores from baseline to endpoint were –35.4 (SE:1.0) (MMRM) and –35.8 (SD:10.3) (OC) for the acute treatment phase. The extension treatment phase had improvement in CDRS-R scores of –39.4 (SE:0.5) (MMRM) and –40.1 (SD:9.2) (OC). A total of 43/72 (59.7%) of subjects achieved remission at the end point of the 18-week acute treatment phase. The authors suggest that this study shows duloxetine is generally well tolerated in pediatric patients at doses from 30 to 120 mg daily. They did observe transient elevations in blood pressure in many patients, which may be clinically significant. The pharmacokinetic results suggest that adjustment of total dose based on body weight may not be necessary for pediatric patients and TDDs lower than that used in adults may not be indicated.

TRICYCLIC ANTIDEPRESSANTS

Indications for TCAs in Child and Adolescent Psychiatry

TCAs have FDA approval for the treatment of depression only in those children at least 12 years of age, although it is well established that prepubertal children can be diagnosed with MDD using research diagnostic criteria (RDC) (Spitzer et al., 1978) or *Diagnostic and Statistical Manual of Mental Disorders*, Third Edition (DSM-III; APA, 1980a) criteria (Puig-Antich, 1987).

A review of the literature on the use of TCAs in children and adolescents with major depression found them to be clinically effective in several open studies, but no double-blind placebo-controlled study has reported that tricyclics were superior to placebo (Ambrosini et al., 1993). However, the placebo-controlled double-blind study of Preskorn et al. (1987) found that desipramine (DMI) was superior to placebo when plasma levels were controlled (reviewed later). Geller et al. (1993) caution that the use of TCAs in depressed 6- to 12-year-olds may precipitate switching to mania and hasten the onset of bipolarity and perhaps increase later rapid cycling.

Imipramine (IMI) is also approved for the treatment of enuresis in those at least 6 years of age. There is, however, a considerable body of literature suggesting that IMI is effective in the treatment of ADHD, school phobia (SAD), disorders of sleep (sleep terror disorder and sleepwalking disorder), and MDD in some children treated on an open basis.

Clomipramine, another TCA, has been approved for the treatment of childhood OCD.

Currently, there are no formal criteria for the prophylactic use of TCAs in children and adolescents. The risks versus the benefits of long-term use for prevention of recurrences of mood disorders in this age group have not yet been established, and such use must be based on the physician's clinical judgment (National Institute of Mental Health/National Institutes of Health Consensus Development Panel, 1985).

Given the significant risk of death when taken in overdose and the availability of other treatment options which are better tolerated, TCAs are rarely considered as first-line treatments for childhood mental health disorders.

TCAs in the Treatment of Children and Adolescents Diagnosed with ADHD

Although the treatment of ADHD is not an approved indication, TCAs were among the second-line drugs most frequently prescribed in treating patients diagnosed with ADHD who have not responded to stimulant medication; they were used as the drug of first choice by some clinicians when comorbid diagnoses such as depression or anxiety disorder are present (Green, 1995). The use of TCAs has significantly decreased since the reports of sudden death with their use and the introduction of the SSRI antidepressants. Of the TCAs, imipramine hydrochloride (IMI) and desipramine hydrochloride (DMI) are the best studied and were the most frequently used, although nortriptyline hydrochloride, amitriptyline hydrochloride, and the antiobsessional drug, clomipramine hydrochloride, have also been found to be effective. Overall, desipramine hydrochloride appears to have a lower risk of untoward effects than IMI, amitriptyline, and clomipramine (Biederman et al., 1989a); however, cardiotoxicity is a major concern (see following text). There are few studies on long-term safety and efficacy of the TCAs in treating ADHD (Green, 1995).

The mechanism of action of TCAs in ADHD is different from that in depression. Optimal doses are usually considerably lower, and the onset of clinical response is rapid (Donnelly et al., 1986; Linnoila et al., 1979), although one study required 3 to 4 weeks for subjects treated with DMI to show significant clinical improvement compared with subjects receiving placebo (Biederman et al., 1989b). When used to treat ADHD, tricyclics improve mood and decrease hyperactivity but usually are sedating and do not appear to improve concentration (Wender, 1988). TCAs have also been reported to cause small but significant declines in motor performance, which are usually of limited clinical significance (Gualtieri et al., 1991).

The preponderance of published studies strongly suggests that TCAs are effective in the treatment of ADHD. In fact, in the early 1970s, some authors considered IMI to be the drug of choice in treating ADHD (Huessy and Wright, 1970; Waizer et al., 1974). Most double-blind studies comparing TCAs with a stimulant, a placebo, or both have found that both drugs are superior to placebo; however, the stimulant drug is usually equal or superior to the tricyclic on most of the clinically significant measures of improvement and, overall, the literature suggests that stimulants are superior (Campbell et al., 1985; Klein et al., 1980; Pliszka, 1987; Rapoport and Mikkelsen, 1978b).

Parallel to the situation with stimulants, there is evidence that patients diagnosed with ADHD may not respond to one TCA but may have a markedly positive response to another. For example, Wilens et al. (1993b) found that 31 (70%) of 44 subjects who had had unsatisfactory responses to desipramine subsequently had positive responses to nortriptyline.

One difference noted in several studies relates to the longer serum half-lives of the TCAs compared with those of methylphenidate and dextroamphetamine; the therapeutic effects last longer with the tricyclics, and behavior after school and in the evenings of subjects receiving tricyclics is typically rated better by parents and others than behavior of subjects on the stimulants. The latter is true because when the last dose of the stimulant is given at lunchtime, it loses its clinical efficacy by late afternoon (Green, 1995; Yepes et al., 1977).

Pharmacokinetics of TCAs

About 7% of the general population has a genetic variation that results in decreased activity of the drug-metabolizing enzyme cytochrome P450 2D6 (*PDR*, 1995). Such individuals metabolize TCAs more slowly than usual and may develop toxic serum levels at therapeutic doses of <5 mg/kg. Individuals taking the same oral dose of desipramine have been reported to have up to a 36-fold variation in plasma levels (*PDR*, 1995, p. 1417).

There may be large interindividual variations in steady-state plasma levels of tricyclics and their metabolites, although intraindividual levels are usually reproducible and correlate linearly with dose. Preskorn et al. (1989a) reported that steady-state IMI plus DMI levels varied 22-fold (from 25 to 553 ng/mL) among 68 hospitalized children, aged 6 to 14 years, who were prescribed a fixed daily dose of 75 mg of IMI to treat major depression ($N = 48$) or enuresis ($N = 20$); likewise, Biederman et al. (1989b) found that DMI serum levels varied up to 16.5-fold when fixed doses of DMI were administered.

Potter et al. (1982) found that about 5% of 47 subjects, including 32 enuretic males aged 7 to 13 years, were deficient DMI hydroxylators and that such subjects had two to four times the steady-state concentrations of either IMI or DMI per unit dose as the general population. Preskorn et al. (1989b) warned that persons who metabolize tricyclics slowly may develop central nervous system toxicity, which may be confused with worsening of depression, or severe cardiotoxicity when taking conventional doses of tricyclics and that deaths have occurred. Because of these variables, it is necessary to obtain plasma levels to avoid treatment failures for subtherapeutic levels or possible toxic effects from excessive levels.

Dugas et al. (1980) have recommended administering TCAs to children in two or three divided doses daily if more than 1 mg/kg/day is given to avoid or minimize untoward effects related to peak serum levels. Long-acting preparations (e.g., imipramine pamoate capsules) are designed for once-daily dosing; their use is not recommended in children and younger adolescents because of their high unit potency and the greater sensitivity of this age group to cardiotoxic effects.

Table 7.2 summarizes the development of symptoms of central nervous system toxicity. Preskorn et al. (1989b) have urged that therapeutic drug monitoring of TCAs be considered a routine standard of care for patients receiving these drugs.

TCA Discontinuation/Withdrawal Syndrome

Some children experience a flu-like withdrawal syndrome, with gastrointestinal symptoms including nausea, abdominal discomfort and pain, vomiting, headache, and fatigue. These symptoms result from cholinergic rebound and may be considered a cholinergic overdrive phenomenon. Ryan (1990) noted that because of their rapid metabolism of tricyclics, some prepubertal children and younger adolescents may show daily withdrawal effects if they receive their entire daily tricyclic medication in one dose; hence, it may be necessary to divide the medication into two or three doses.

TABLE 7.2 » Evolution of Central Nervous System Tricyclic Antidepressant Toxicity				
Affective Symptoms	**Motor Symptoms**	**Psychotic Symptoms**	**Organic Symptoms**
Mood	Tremor	Thought disorder	Disorientation
↓Concentration	Ataxia	Hallucinations	↓Memory
Lethargy	Seizures[a]	Delusions	Agitation
Social withdrawal			Confusion

[a]Seizures typically occur late but can occur earlier in the evolution.
From Preskorn SH, Jerkovich GS, Beber JH, et al. Therapeutic drug monitoring of tricyclic antidepressants: a standard of care issue. *Psychopharmacol Bull.* 1989;25:281–284.

When maintenance medication is discontinued, tapering the medication down over 10 days to 2 weeks rather than abruptly withdrawing the medication will usually avoid the development of a clinically significant withdrawal syndrome. The clinician is cautioned that in patients with poor compliance, who in essence may undergo periodic self-induced acute withdrawals, the resulting withdrawal syndrome may be confused with untoward effects of the medication, inadequate treatment, or worsening of the underlying condition.

Contraindications for TCA Administration

Known hypersensitivity to TCAs is an absolute contraindication.

TCAs are contraindicated for children and adolescents with cardiac conduction abnormalities.

TCAs should not be administered concomitantly with an MAOI. At least 14 days must pass after discontinuing an MAOI before administering a TCA.

Tricyclics may lower the seizure threshold and should be used with caution in individuals with seizure disorder.

TCAs may activate psychotic processes in schizophrenic patients.

Interactions of TCAs with Other Drugs

Hyperpyretic crises or severe convulsive seizures may occur in patients receiving MAOIs and TCAs simultaneously.

Anticholinergic effects of TCAs may be additive with those of antipsychotics and result in central nervous system anticholinergic toxicity.

The central nervous system depressive effects of TCAs may be additive with those of alcohol, benzodiazepines, barbiturates, and antipsychotics.

TCAs may diminish or reverse the efficacy of antihypertensive agents.

Cigarette smoking may decrease the efficacy of TCAs.

Many other interactions with various drugs have also been reported.

Untoward Effects of TCAs

TCAs and Cardiotoxicity

Reports of Sudden Death

At least eight sudden deaths have been reported in children taking TCAs. Although these deaths have not been proven to be cardiac related, cardiac arrhythmias, particularly tachyarrhythmias and torsade de pointes, are suspected.

Certain circumstances may increase the risk of the occurrence of torsade de pointes and/or sudden death in association with the use of drugs that prolong the QTc interval, including (a) bradycardia; (b) hypokalemia or hypomagnesemia; (c) concomitant use of other drugs that prolong the QTc interval; and (d) presence of congenital prolongation of the QT interval (*PDR*, 2005, p. 2611).

Six of the sudden deaths occurred in children taking DMI and two occurred in children taking IMI (one IMI only and one IMI and thioridazine). Four of the sudden deaths occurred after strenuous exercise (three on DMI and one on a combination of IMI and thioridazine); however, whether strenuous exertion might have been a precipitating or contributing cause was not addressed for several subjects. Six of the children who died were 9 years old or younger, one was 12 years, and one was 16 years.

A 6-year-old girl taking IMI for chronic school phobia and separation anxiety died 3 days after the dose had been raised to 300 mg (14.7 mg/kg) at bedtime (Saraf et al., 1974).

Sudden deaths were reported in three boys treated with DMI ("Sudden Death," 1990). These were two 8-year-old boys diagnosed with ADD (one received DMI for 2 years at an unknown dose and one received the same drug for 6 months at 50 mg/day) and a 9-year-old boy whose diagnosis, dose, and duration of DMI administration were not reported. All three of the boys had plasma levels in the therapeutic or subtherapeutic ranges ("Sudden Death," 1990). A fifth child, a 12-year-old girl who had been prescribed a single daily 125-mg dose of DMI for the treatment of ADD, died a few days after the dose was increased to 50 mg three times daily; she was found unconscious after playing tennis and retiring for a nap and was not successfully revived (Riddle et al., 1993). The sixth sudden death, reported by Popper and Zimnitzky (1995), was a 14.7-year-old male who was prescribed 300 mg/day of DMI. His serum level on 225 mg/day was 132 ng/mL. He was in a residential treatment facility and collapsed and died a short time after swimming in the pool. In 1997, Varley and McClellan reported yet two more (the seventh and eighth) sudden deaths: one a 9-year-old male with multiple psychiatric problems who was started on DMI for treatment of depression during an inpatient hospitalization. He died suddenly 29 days after discharge after a total of 5 weeks of treatment with DMI. At the time of his death, he was taking 50 mg twice daily (3.3 mg/kg). The other child was a 7-year-old male with disruptive behavior and multiple psychiatric diagnoses, including adjustment disorder with mixed disturbance of emotion and conduct, oppositional defiant disorder, possible PTSD, and possible MDD. Two months before his death, IMI was increased to 150 mg at bedtime, and thioridazine, 25 mg, was added for extreme agitation, to be given if needed (p.r.n.), every 2 hours. At the time of death, thioridazine was reportedly given as "25 to 75 mg at night p.r.n. for agitation"; it was not known when the last thioridazine was administered. After running several blocks home from school, the boy collapsed, went into cardiac arrest, and could not be resuscitated.

Several publications, reports, editorials, and commentaries rapidly followed the reports of these deaths. It became clear how little was known about the cardiac effects of tricyclics in prepubertal and even older subjects. Basically, the response was to be even more cautious when administering tricyclics not only to children but also to adolescents (Geller, 1991). In particular, it was recommended that a rhythm strip be obtained at baseline, during titration of medication, and at maintenance levels emphasizing measurement of the QTc to aid in identifying potentially vulnerable children (Riddle et al., 1991). Elliott and Popper (1990/1991) recommended obtaining ECGs at baseline, at a dose of about 3 mg/kg/day, and at a final dose of not >5 mg/kg/day. They also suggested using the following parameters as guidelines for cardiovascular monitoring in children and adolescents receiving TCAs.

PR interval: <210 msec
QRS interval: widening to no more than 30% over baseline
QTc interval: <450 msec

Heart rate: maximum of 130 beats per minute
Systolic blood pressure: maximum of 130 mm Hg
Diastolic blood pressure: maximum of 85 mm Hg

Although a more conservative viewpoint would be to obtain an ECG after each dose increase, Elliott and Popper (1990/1991) have pointed out that simply increasing the frequency of ECG monitoring does not necessarily reduce the risk of sudden death.

Cardiovascular toxicity of TCAs is of concern in all age groups, but especially in children and younger adolescents. Of particular concern is the slowing of cardiac conduction as reflected on the ECG by increases in PR and QRS intervals, cardiac arrhythmias, tachycardia, and heart block.

Schroeder et al. (1989) reported that the cardiovascular effects of DMI in 20children, aged 7 to 12 years, who were treated with an average dose of 4.25 mg/kg/day (maximum of 5 mg/kg/day) were a 21% increase in cardiac rate and a 2.5% increase in the QT interval. Arrhythmias and clinically meaningful blood pressure changes did not occur. The authors concluded, concerning potential cardiotoxicity, that DMI was safe in children without heart disease, although ECG monitoring was essential (Schroeder et al., 1989). Baldessarini (1990) noted that children are more sensitive to cardiotoxic effects of TCAs than adolescents and adults; he suggested that this increased vulnerability may be related to the relative efficiency with which they convert TCAs to potentially cardiotoxic 2-OH metabolites. However, Wilens et al. (1992) studied steady-state serum concentrations of DMI and 2-OH-DMI (OHDMI) in 40 child, 36 adolescent, and 27 adult psychiatric patients. Serum levels of DMI per weight-corrected (mg/kg) dose rose from 50 ng/mL in children (age range, 6 to 12 years), to 56 ng/mL in adolescents (age range, 13 to 18 years), and to 91 ng/mL in adults (age range, 19 to 67 years). Contrary to expectations, 2-OH-DMI levels also increased with age from 17 ng/mL in children to 20 ng/mL in adolescents, and to 26 ng/mL in adults. The results did not support the hypothesis that children would develop relatively higher levels of OHDMI than adolescents and adults because of more efficient hepatic oxidative metabolism of DMI. Children either were more efficient in clearing both DMI and OHDMI than adults or absorbed DMI relatively inefficiently. In fact, the data supported the clinical impression that children and adolescents usually require higher mg/kg doses of DMI than adults to reach similar serum DMI and OHDMI concentrations (Wilens et al., 1992).

In a subsequent study, Wilens et al. (1993a) analyzed the effects of serum levels of DMI and 2-OH-DMI on ECGs in 50 children, 39 adolescents, and 30 adult psychiatric patients treated with DMI. With these expanded numbers of subjects, children and adolescents continued to have lower serum levels of DMI and OHDMI for weight-corrected doses compared with adults. Children and adolescents showed no significant associations between serum drug and metabolite levels and heart rate or conduction (PR and QRS) intervals, although there was a weak relationship between sinus tachycardia and higher total DMI plus OHDMI levels. When data from all the 119 subjects were combined, there was a modest correlation among DMI, OHDMI, and DMI plus OHDMI serum levels and PR and QRS intervals; however, the authors concluded that these were not likely to be clinically significant in any age group. About 10% of the subjects had combined DMI plus OHDMI serum levels of 250 ng/mL or greater, which may increase risk of cardiovascular toxicity. They recommended monitoring serum levels and obtaining a baseline ECG and ECGs with increases in daily dose of >3 mg/kg (Wilens et al., 1993a).

Because routine ECGs may not record infrequent cardiac arrhythmias, Biederman et al. (1993) examined 24-hour ECG recordings and echocardiographic findings in 35 children and 36 adolescents receiving long-term (1.5 ± 1.2 years)

DMI therapy for psychiatric disorders. Compared with untreated healthy children, subjects' ECGs had significantly higher rates of single or paired premature atrial contractions and runs of supraventricular tachycardia and a decreased rate of sinus pauses and junctional rhythm. DMI levels correlated significantly only with paired premature atrial contractions. All echocardiographic findings but one were normal; the abnormal one was thought to be caused by a pericardial effusion of viral origin and not drug related. Overall, the data supported earlier impressions that treatment with DMI is associated with minor and benign cardiac effects (Biederman et al., 1993).

Walsh et al. (1994) reported on the effects of DMI on the autonomic control of the heart in 13 children, adolescents, and young adults (mean age, 17.5 ± 6.4 years; age range, 7 to 29 years). They noted that parasympathetic input to the heart decreases substantially with age and suggested that, because of the tricyclics' anticholinergic effects and their blockading the more active parasympathetic nervous systems of this age group, they increase supine blood pressure and pulse, notably more in children and adolescents than in middle-aged and older adults. Their study documented that DMI reduces parasympathetic input to the heart and suggested that DMI may increase the ratio of sympathetic to parasympathetic cardiac input more in younger patients because of their relatively higher pretreatment levels of autonomic activity. This may explain the findings that DMI increased the ratio of low-frequency to high-frequency variability in heart rate and overall substantial decrease in heart period variability found in their study. Because reductions in heart period variability are associated with increased vulnerability to serious arrhythmias, treatment with TCAs may increase the risk of arrhythmias in children and adolescents. The authors emphasized that their data were preliminary and that further studies were needed before clinical recommendations could be made.

In a subsequent study designed to further evaluate the cardiac effects of DMI on autonomic input to the heart, Walsh et al. (1999) obtained 24-hour ECGs from 42 subjects; 12 subjects were 7 to 18 years of age, and 30 subjects were between 19 and 66 years old. Ten of the subjects <19 years old were diagnosed with ADHD that had not responded to stimulants and one with MDD that had not responded to an SSRI. The authors assessed cardiac autonomic input using spectral analysis of the RR interval variability to determine heart rate variability. Pretreatment (off-medication) ECGs were done before administration of DMI in 41 cases. The ECG on DMI was done at optimal clinical dose, but 5 mg/kg/day could not be exceeded. Average duration on DMI was 33.1 ± 18.4 days for all ages. The mean dose of DMI was lower and the mean dose in mg/kg/day was higher in subjects <19 years old than in older subjects (148 ± 99 mg/day vs. 195 ± 57 mg/day and 3.30 ± 0.77 mg/kg/day vs. 2.80 ± 0.87 mg/kg/day, respectively).

The authors reported that DMI treatment was associated with a significant increase in heart rate and significant decreases in RR interval variability at all frequencies. DMI had no selective effect on the ratio of high-frequency bands, which are thought to reflect parasympathetic input, to low-frequency bands, which are thought to reflect sympathetic input. Hence, DMI had no impact on cardiac sympathetic/vagal (parasympathetic) balance. Although the RR interval variability was greater in the younger age group both with DMI and off medication, the magnitude of the effect of DMI on RR interval variability was similar in children, adolescents, and adults. The authors noted that the decrease in cardiac vagal modulation with DMI theoretically should increase the risk of arrhythmia because parasympathetic input to the heart generally protects against the development of arrhythmias. However, they did not resolve the issue as to whether DMI treatment would significantly increase the risk of developing a life-threatening arrhythmia.

The preceding studies appear to conclude that TCAs in the usual clinical dose range (<5 mg/kg/day) and at the usual serum drug and metabolite levels (250 to 300 ng/mL or less of DMI plus OHDMI) are usually associated with minor and clinically benign effects on cardiac function in all age ranges. They further suggest that children and adolescents are not at significantly greater risk for developing such effects compared with adults. The Ad Hoc Committee on Desipramine and Sudden Death of the American Academy of Child and Adolescent Psychiatry, established to investigate these concerns, reported at a members' forum at the 1992 Annual Convention that the risk of sudden death for children 5 to 14 years old who are treated with DMI in therapeutic doses is approximately the same as the risk of sudden death for similarly aged children in the general population, between 1.5 and 4.2/million/year ($P > .23$) (American Academy of Child and Adolescent Psychiatry [AACAP], 1992, p. 8). The matter remains controversial, however. Werry (1994), in a letter to the editor of the *Journal of the American Academy of Child and Adolescent Psychiatry*, proposed severe restrictions on the use of DMI, whereas Riddle et al. (1994) rebutted his suggestion, noting

> based on the available data, there is as yet no established cause of the deaths nor any scientific evidence that they were related to the DMI. As the number of sudden deaths is so small, the causal mechanism(s) are unknown and no specific cardiac finding has any known predictive value, clinically it should be considered mandatory to monitor both ECG changes and serum drug and metabolite levels and to keep them within recommended parameters whenever tricyclic antidepressants are prescribed.

Amitai and Frischer (2006) used the large database of the American Association of Poison Control Centers (AAPCC) Toxic Exposure Surveillance System (TESS) for the 20-year period, 1983 to 2002, to determine the relative risk of death that was associated with the ingestion of desipramine compared with other TCAs (amitriptyline [AMI], imipramine, nortriptyline, and doxepin) in younger children (<6 years old) and older children and adolescents (6 to 17 for years 1983 to 1992 and 6 to 19 for years 1993 to 2002). (The case fatality rate [CFR] was defined as the ratio of the number of deaths divided by the number of exposures, an exposure being a report to the AAPCC-TESS concerning an individual ingestion of a drug or toxin.) The authors reported that there was a total of 24 deaths in the younger group and 144 deaths in the older group during these 20 years; most ingestions in the younger group were thought to be accidental while those in the older group were usually intentional or "suicide." The authors noted that poisoning fatalities are vastly underreported to poison control centers and that the actual number of fatalities is much higher. The CFR for desipramine was significantly higher than that of the other four drugs in both groups ($P \leq .001$). Specifically, the CFR for desipramine exceeds that for amitriptyline by 7- to 8-fold, for doxepine by 4-fold; for imipramine by 6- to 12-fold; and for nortriptyline by 7- to 10-fold. The authors concluded that the reports on sudden death in children treated with desipramine coupled with its increased lethality compared with other TCAs when ingested accidently or in a suicide attempt indicate that restrictions should be place on the use of desipramine in children and adolescents (Amitai and Frischer, 2006).

Other Untoward Effects of TCAs

Untoward effects to the central nervous system may include drowsiness, EEG changes, seizures, incoordination, anxiety, insomnia and nightmares, confusion secondary to anticholinergic toxicity, delusions, and worsening of psychosis.

TCAs may cause blood dyscrasias; if patients develop fever and sore throats during treatment with tricyclics; a complete blood count should be taken.

Anticholinergic untoward effects may include dry mouth, blurred vision, and constipation.

Changes in libido, both increases and decreases, have been reported; gynecomastia and impotence have also been reported.

Preskorn et al. (1988) reported that cognitive toxicity was associated with su-pratherapeutic plasma levels of tricyclics.

TCAs, including clomipramine, may cause acute psychotic episodes if inadver-tently administered to some individuals with schizophrenia who have been incor-rectly diagnosed.

Readers are encouraged to consult the online edition for details about the use of specific TCAs (imipramine hydrochloride, nortriptyline, amitriptyline hydrochlo-ride, desipramine hydrochloride, and clomipramine hydrochloride).

MONOAMINE OXIDASE INHIBITORS

There are two forms of monoamine oxidase (MAO), which are distinguished by their substrate specificity. Type A MAO deaminates or deactivates norepinephrine, serotonin, and normetanephrine, and type B MAO deaminates dopamine and phenylethylamine (Zametkin and Rapoport, 1987).

MAOIs are primarily used in treating adults with depressive disorders that are unresponsive to antidepressant drugs of other classes. MAOIs that are presently FDA approved and marketed in the United States include phenelzine sulfate (Nardil), which has been approved for use only in individuals at least 16 years of age, and tranylcypromine sulfate (Parnate), which has been approved only for adults.

MAOIs that have been used in children and adolescents include clorgyline (a selective MAO-A inhibitor), tranylcypromine sulfate and phenelzine sulfate (mixed MAO-A and MAO-B inhibitors), and L-deprenyl or selegiline hydrochloride (Eldepryl) (a selective central MAO-B inhibitor). Because of the potentially very serious drug interactions and untoward effects of MAOIs, their use in children and adolescents is not usually recommended, and only a few reports in this age group are reviewed.

Special Considerations in Using MAOIs

It is critical to have a minimum of a 2-week washout period after stopping an MAOI and beginning a tricyclic or when changing from one MAOI to another. It is also contraindicated to add a TCA when an MAOI is already being used, although the reverse has been done; that is, an MAOI can be added to an ongoing treatment regimen to augment a tricyclic that has been only partially effective (Ryan et al., 1988b). If patients are on MAOIs and are in areas that are not rapidly accessible to medical treatment, they may be given several 25-mg chlorpromazine tablets to be taken should they accidentally ingest tyramine and become symptomatic (Ryan et al., 1988b). Pare et al. (1982) suggested that a combination of tricyclics and MAOIs might provide relative protection against tyramine-induced hyperten-sion, or "cheese effect," which may occur with dietary indiscretions while taking MAOIs; however, this is not common practice at the present time.

Contraindications for MAOI Administration

Note: Review the Black Box Warning at the beginning of the chapter or in the package insert before prescribing.

Known hypersensitivity to an MAOI, pheochromocytoma, congestive heart failure, liver disease, or abnormal liver function are contraindications.

MAOIs must not be prescribed if a TCA (however, see Ryan et al., 1988b, for a different opinion), another MAOI, or buspirone hydrochloride has been taken within the preceding 2 weeks.

Other contraindications usually found more frequently in older patients also exist. In addition, the patient must not be unreliable or be unable to keep to a strict diet (i.e., avoiding foods with high tyramine or dopamine concentrations).

Interactions of MAOIs with Other Drugs

Ingestion of tyramine can cause a hypertensive crisis. Hence, foods rich in tyramine, such as cheese, wine, beer, yeast derivatives, some beans, and others, must be avoided.

Concomitant use with TCAs should be avoided because hypertensive crises or severe seizures have been reported with such combinations (see Ryan et al., 1988b, for a different opinion).

Use with sympathomimetic drugs such as amphetamines, methylphenidate, cocaine, dopamine, caffeine, epinephrine, norepinephrine, and related compounds may cause a hypertensive crisis.

Other drug interactions occur as well.

Untoward Effects of MAOIs

MAOIs may cause significant orthostatic hypotension, dizziness, headache, sleep disturbances, sedation, fatigue, weakness, hyperreflexia, dry mouth, and gastrointestinal disturbances; other untoward effects occur as well.

Reports of Interest

MAOIs in the Treatment of Adolescent Depression

Ryan et al. (1988b) reported an open clinical trial of tranylcypromine sulfate and phenelzine sulfate, both alone and in combination with a TCA, in which 23 adolescents diagnosed with MDD who had responded inadequately to TCAs were treated with these MAOIs. Seventy-four percent (17) had a fair to good antidepressant response; however, because of dietary noncompliance, the MAOI was discontinued in 4 subjects and only 57% (13) of the subjects continued on the medication. The authors concluded that MAOIs appeared to be useful in treating some adolescents with major depression who had not responded satisfactorily to TCAs. During the study, a total of seven (30%) had purposeful or accidental dietary noncompliance, and the authors emphasized that only very reliable adolescents are suitable for treatment with MAOIs (Ryan et al., 1988b).

MAOIs in the Treatment of ADHD

Zametkin et al. (1985) conducted a double-blind crossover study of 14 boys (mean age, 9.2 ± 1.5 years) who were diagnosed with ADDH. The authors compared dextroamphetamine to either clorgyline, a selective MAO-A inhibitor (six subjects), or tranylcypromine sulfate, a mixed MAO-A and MAO-B inhibitor (eight subjects). Both MAOIs had immediate, clinically significant effects (in contrast to delayed effects when used as an antidepressant), which were clinically indistinguishable from those of dextroamphetamine.

Zametkin and Rapoport (1987) reported that M. Donnelly had administered 15 mg/day of L-deprenyl, a selective MAO-B inhibitor, to 14 hyperactive children with relatively little therapeutic effect. The authors suggested that the fact that a type A MAOI and a mixed MAOI showed therapeutic efficacy in children with ADHD, whereas a type B MAOI did not support the hypothesis that dysregulation of the noradrenergic system is important in the etiology of ADHD (Zametkin and Rapoport, 1987).

At the present time, the use of MAOIs in the treatment of ADHD is not recommended because of necessary dietary constraints.

Mood Stabilizers: Lithium Carbonate and Antiepileptics

JULIA JACKSON

LITHIUM CARBONATE (LITHOTABS, ESKALITH, LITHANE, LITHOBID) AND LITHIUM CITRATE (CIBALITH-S)

Currently, lithium carbonate is approved by the FDA for the treatment of manic episodes of bipolar disorders and for maintenance therapy of bipolar patients. Lithium carbonate is FDA approved for persons 12 years of age and older; however, pediatric approval was based solely on literature supporting its use in adults with bipolar disorder. Over the past three decades, lithium carbonate has been investigated in the treatment of many child and adolescent disorders, but especially in the treatment of children with severe aggression directed toward self or others, children with bipolar or similar disorders, and behaviorally disturbed children whose parents are known lithium responders. One major impetus for this research was that typical antipsychotic agents, which were historically used often to control severe behavioral disorders and sometimes mania, not only could cause cognitive dulling when used in sufficient dosage to control symptoms, but also carried significant risk of causing tardive dyskinesia when used on a long-term basis (Platt et al., 1984).

Pharmacokinetics of Lithium Carbonate

The lithium ion is readily absorbed from the gastrointestinal tract and is most commonly administered in the form of lithium carbonate (Li_2CO_3), a highly soluble salt. Peak plasma concentrations occur within 2 to 4 hours, and complete absorption takes place within approximately 8 hours (Baldessarini, 1990). Approximately 95% of a single dose of lithium is excreted by the kidneys, with up to two-thirds of an acute dose being excreted within 6 to 12 hours. The serum half-life is approximately 20 to 24 hours. Depletion of the sodium ion causes a clinically significant degree of lithium retention by the kidneys. Steady-state serum lithium levels typically occur within 5 to 8 days of repeated identical daily doses of lithium carbonate. Although lithium pharmacokinetics differs considerably among individuals, they are fairly stable over time for a given person (Baldessarini and Stephens, 1970).

Vitiello et al. (1988) and Malone et al. (1995) studied the pharmacokinetics of lithium carbonate in children. Both discovered a trend toward a shorter elimination half-life and a significantly higher total renal clearance of lithium. The clinical significance of this is that a steady state of lithium is reached more rapidly in children than in adults, and therapeutic levels can be achieved more quickly.

Contraindications for Lithium Carbonate Administration

Administration of lithium carbonate is relatively contraindicated in individuals with significant renal or cardiovascular disease, severe debilitation, severe dehydration, or sodium depletion because these conditions are associated with a very high risk of lithium toxicity. Patients with such disorders should be thoroughly assessed, usually in consultation with the person providing medical care, before beginning lithium therapy.

Except under urgent circumstances, adolescents who are likely to become pregnant should not be administered lithium; this is particularly true of those in early pregnancy. Lithium carbonate is associated with a significant increase in cardiac teratogenicity, especially with Ebstein's anomaly. A significantly increased incidence of other cardiac anomalies has also been reported. Kallen and Tandberg (1983) reported that 7% of the infants of women who used lithium in early pregnancy had serious heart defects other than Ebstein's anomaly. Nursing should not be undertaken during treatment with lithium as lithium is excreted in human milk.

Significant thyroid disease is a relative contraindication to lithium carbonate therapy; however, with careful monitoring of thyroid function and the use of supplemental thyroid preparations when necessary, it may be used when other drugs are not effective and the potential benefits outweigh the risks.

Interactions of Lithium Carbonate with Other Drugs

There are several reports that increased neuroleptic toxicity with an encephalopathic syndrome or neuroleptic malignant syndrome may occur when lithium and neuroleptics are used concomitantly, but this has usually been seen with high doses. The simultaneous use of lithium and neuroleptic agents, however, may be indicated in some cases of mania or schizoaffective psychoses, and many patients have received both a neuroleptic and lithium with no untoward effects.

Elevations in lithium serum concentration and increased risk of neurotoxic lithium effects may occur when carbamazepine and lithium are used simultaneously because carbamazepine decreases lithium renal clearance. Use of calcium channel blockers in conjunction with lithium treatment has resulted in neurotoxicity including ataxia, tremors, and gastrointestinal symptoms.

Many other drugs may increase or decrease serum lithium levels by influencing its absorption or excretion by the kidneys. For example, cyclooxyneganse-2 (COX-2) inhibitors, nonsteroidal anti-inflammatory drugs (NSAIDs), metronidazole, enalapril, and losartan increase plasma lithium levels. By contrast, sodium bicarbonate, alkalinizing agents, and xanthine preparations lower serum lithium concentrations. Frequent serum drug monitoring should be employed when these types of medications are used together.

Lithium Toxicity

One major difficulty associated with the administration of lithium carbonate is its low therapeutic index; lithium toxicity is closely related to serum lithium levels and may occur at doses of lithium carbonate close to those necessary to achieve therapeutic serum lithium levels. Adverse or side effects are those unwanted symptoms that occur at therapeutic serum lithium levels, whereas toxic effects occur when serum lithium levels exceed therapeutic levels. However, this is not absolute, as patients who are unusually sensitive to lithium may develop toxic signs at serum levels below 1.0 mEq/L (*Physicians' Desk Reference* [PDR], 2000).

Lithium toxicity may be heralded by diarrhea, vomiting, mild ataxia, coarse tremor, muscular weakness and fasciculations (twitches), drowsiness, sedation, slurred speech, and impaired coordination. Patients and/or their caretakers must be made familiar with the symptoms of early lithium toxicity and instructed to discontinue lithium immediately and contact their physician if such signs occur. Increasingly severe and life-threatening toxic effects, including cardiac arrhythmias and severe central nervous system difficulties such as impaired consciousness, confusion, stupor, seizures, coma, and death, may occur with further elevations in serum lithium levels.

No specific treatment for lithium toxicity is available. If signs of early lithium toxicity appear, the drug should be withheld, lithium levels determined, and the medication resumed at a lower dosage only after 24 to 48 hours. Severe lithium toxicity is life threatening and requires hospital admission, treatments to reduce the concentration of the lithium ion, and supportive measures.

Lithium's low therapeutic index and its pharmacokinetics make it necessary to administer lithium carbonate tablets or immediate-release capsules in divided doses, usually three or four times daily, to maintain therapeutic serum levels without toxicity. Even controlled-release tablets must be administered every 12 hours. It is essential that a laboratory capable of determining serum lithium levels rapidly and accurately be readily available to the clinician. For accuracy and serial comparisons, determinations of serum lithium levels should be made when lithium concentrations are relatively stable and at the same time each day. Typically, blood is drawn 12 hours after the last dose of lithium and immediately before the morning dose (trough level).

Although some patients who are unusually sensitive to lithium may exhibit toxic effects at serum levels below 1 mEq/L, for most patients mild to moderate toxic effects occur at serum levels between 1.5 and 2 mEq/L and moderate to severe reactions occur at levels of 2 mEq/L and above.

Lithium decreases sodium reuptake by the renal tubules; hence, adequate sodium intake must be maintained. This is especially important if there is significant sodium loss during illness (e.g., sweating, vomiting, or diarrhea) or because of changes in diet or elimination of electrolytes. The importance of adequate ingestion of ordinary table salt and fluids should be emphasized. Caution during hot weather or vigorous exertion has been advised, because additional salt loss and concomitant dehydration secondary to pronounced diaphoresis may cause the serum lithium levels of patients on maintenance lithium to increase and move into the toxic range. This may also be true of sweating caused by elevated body temperature secondary to infection or heat without exercise (e.g., sauna), but some evidence suggests that heavy sweating caused by exercise may result in lowered rather than elevated serum lithium levels. Jefferson et al. (1982) studied four healthy athletes who were stabilized on lithium for 1 week before running a 20-km race. At the end of the race, the subjects were dehydrated but their serum lithium levels had decreased by 20%. The authors found that the sweat-to-serum ratio for the lithium ion was approximately four times greater than that for the sodium ion. These authors concluded that strenuous exercise with extensive perspiration was more likely to decrease rather than increase serum lithium levels, and patients were more likely to require either no change or an increase, rather than a decrease, in dosage of lithium to maintain therapeutic levels. The authors do caution, however, that any conditions that significantly alter fluid and electrolyte balance, including strenuous exercise with heavy sweating, should be carefully monitored with serum lithium levels.

Untoward Effects of Lithium Carbonate

Lithium carbonate is frequently reported to have adverse effects early in the course of treatment, though most diminish or disappear during the first weeks of treatment. Studies show that side effects are more likely to occur in pediatric versus adult patients (Campbell et al., 1984a, 1991).

Early adverse effects include fine tremor (unresponsive to antiparkinsonism drugs), polydipsia, and polyuria that may occur during initial treatment and persist or be variably present throughout treatment. Nausea and malaise or general discomfort may initially occur but usually subside with ongoing treatment. Weight gain, headache, and other gastrointestinal complaints such as diarrhea may also occur. Taking lithium with meals or after meals or increasing the dosage more gradually may be helpful in controlling gastrointestinal symptoms.

Later adverse effects are often related to serum level, including levels in the therapeutic range; these include continued hand tremor that may worsen, polydipsia, polyuria, weight gain and edema, thyroid and renal abnormalities, dermatologic abnormalities (including acne), fatigue, leukocytosis, and other symptoms. As serum levels increase, toxicity increases and other, more severe untoward effects, discussed earlier under toxicity, appear.

The most common adverse effects of lithium carbonate in 61 children, aged 7 to 17 years and diagnosed with bipolar I disorder were nausea (66.7%), headache (65%), vomiting (55%), dizziness (36.7%), diarrhea (30%), upper abdominal pain/tremor (26.7%), and somnolence (18.3%) (Findling et al., 2011). This study involved an 8-week open-label trial of lithium with starting doses of either 300 mg twice daily or 300 mg thrice daily.

Abnormalities in renal functioning (diminution of renal concentrating ability) and morphologic structure (glomerular and interstitial fibrosis and nephron atrophy) have been reported in adults on long-term lithium maintenance. Occasional proteinuria was reported in a 14-year-old girl (Lena et al., 1978). Vetro et al. (1985) reported that after 1 year of lithium treatment, one child developed polyuria with daytime enuresis and impaired renal concentration. Other parameters of renal function did not change, and polyuria ceased within a few days of lithium's being discontinued. Five other children on long-term lithium therapy showed transient albuminuria that remitted spontaneously, and discontinuation of treatment was not necessary (Vetro et al., 1985). At least four cases of nephrotic syndrome related to pediatric lithium treatment have been reported (Peterson et al., 2008; Sakarcan et al., 2002). In the above cases, discontinuation of lithium resulted in resolution of symptoms. Given that reemergence of proteinuria has been reported during lithium rechallenge, this should be avoided (Peterson et al., 2008). Peterson et al. (2008) argue that because the use of lithium in the pediatric population is likely to increase, periodically monitoring for urine protein, particularly during the first year of treatment, appears reasonable.

Lithium may also interfere with thyroid function, with decreased circulating thyroid hormones and increased thyroid-stimulating hormone (TSH). Vetro et al. (1985) reported that two children developed goiter with normal function after 1.5 to 2 years of lithium therapy. Findling et al. (2011) revealed that 4 out of 61 pediatric patients experienced a treatment-emergent thyroid-related adverse event during an 8-week open-label trial of lithium—hypothyroidism ($N = 1$) and elevated TSH levels ($N = 3$). Furthermore, three patients experienced significant changes in levels of antithyroglobulin AB and thyroid peroxidase ($N = 1$) and increased thyrotropin levels ($N = 2$) (Findling et al., 2011).

Neuroleptic malignant syndrome has been reported in a few patients who were administered neuroleptic drugs and lithium simultaneously.

Dostal (1972) reported specific adverse effects of lithium in 14 developmentally delayed adolescent males that interfered with patient management despite significant therapeutic gains. Polydipsia, polyuria, and nocturnal enuresis were so severe as to alienate staff who cared for the youngsters. These symptoms remitted within 2 weeks of discontinuing lithium (Dostal, 1972).

Premedication Workup and Periodic Monitoring for Lithium Treatment

Routine Laboratory Tests

Complete Blood Cell Count with Differential

Lithium frequently causes a clinically insignificant and reversible elevation of white blood cells, with counts commonly between 10,000 and 15,000 cells/mm^3. The lithium-induced leukocytosis characteristically shows neutrophilia (increased polymorphonuclear leukocytes) and lymphocytopenia (Reisberg and Gershon, 1979). Thus, leukocytosis can usually be differentiated from one caused by infection because the increase in neutrophils is in more mature forms, whereas in infection younger forms predominate. Lithium may also increase platelet counts. Lithium-induced leukocytosis has in fact shown to be medically advantageous in some patient scenarios. For example, Mattai et al. (2009) discovered that six pediatric patients experienced a 66% increase in absolute neutrophil count (ANC) after lithium was added to their clozapine regimen, which bolstered support for the use of lithium to manage clozapine-induced neutropenia (Mattai et al., 2009).

Serum Electrolytes

Serum electrolyte levels should be determined, in particular to verify that sodium ion levels are normal, because hyponatremia decreases lithium excretion by the renal tubules.

Pregnancy Test

Lithium crosses the placenta, and data from birth registries suggest teratogenicity with increased abnormalities, including cardiac malformations, especially Ebstein anomaly. Lithium is relatively contraindicated during pregnancy, especially during the first trimester. Infants born to mothers taking lithium appear to be at increased risk for hypotonia, lethargy, cyanosis, and ECG changes (United States Pharmacopeial Dispensing Information [USPDI], 1990). All females who could be pregnant should be tested before initiation of lithium therapy and warned that, because of lithium's teratogenic potential for the fetus, they should take care not to become pregnant while taking the medication.

Renal Function Tests

Baseline assessment of renal functioning is essential because the kidney is the primary route of elimination of lithium. For healthy children and adolescents, a baseline serum creatinine, blood urea nitrogen (BUN) level, and urinalysis are usually adequate and should be monitored every 3 to 6 months during lithium therapy (Kowatch and Delbello, 2003). If kidney disease is suspected or abnormalities are found, a more thorough evaluation, including tests such as urinalysis (including specific gravity), 24-hour urine volume, and 24-hour urine for creatinine clearance and protein, should be performed and the patient should be referred to a nephrologist if necessary.

Thyroid Function Tests

Lithium causes thyroid abnormalities primarily by decreasing the release of thyroid hormones. This causes such findings as euthyroid goiter; hypothyroidism; decreased triiodothyronine (T_3), thyroxine (T_4), and protein-bound iodine (PBI) levels; and elevated ^{131}I and TSH levels between 5% and 15% of patients receiving long-term lithium therapy (Jefferson et al., 1987). Recommended baseline studies include thyroxine (T_4) and TSH levels. Hypothyroidism resulting from lithium treatment is thought to be related to preexisting Hashimoto thyroiditis, suggesting that determining antithyroid antibodies as part of the workup may also be useful (Rosse et al., 1989). Thyroid function tests should be monitored every 3 to 6 months throughout lithium treatment (Kowatch and Delbello, 2003). If there is suggestion of thyroid abnormality during symptom-based or lab screening, consultation with an endocrinologist should be considered.

Cardiovascular Function Tests

Various cardiac conduction and repolarization abnormalities (e.g., bradycardia) and reversible ECG abnormalities have been reported in a large percentage of adults receiving lithium. ECG changes commonly include benign, reversible T-wave changes (flattening, isoelectricity, and inversion of T waves), which are dose dependent, and an increase in the PQ interval (Jefferson et al., 1987). It has been hypothesized that lithium's cardiotoxic effects result from its displacing and substituting for intracellular potassium. A baseline ECG should be obtained routinely in patients >40 years of age or those who have any history or clinical suggestions of cardiovascular disease. Although not considered mandatory in young, healthy patients, a baseline ECG is justifiable and useful to have for comparison, should cardiovascular abnormalities develop at some later time. If patients have or develop cardiac abnormalities, frequent ECG monitoring should be done in consultation with a cardiologist.

Calcium Metabolism Tests

Lithium may increase renal calcium reabsorption, resulting in hypocalciuria (Jefferson et al., 1987). Lithium may also cause hyperparathyroidism with hypercalcemia and hypophosphatemia, with resulting decreased bone formation or density in children. If abnormal results occur, parathyroid hormone (parathormone) levels may be determined. Lithium may also replace calcium in bone formation, especially in immature bones (USPDI, 1990). A baseline calcium level should be determined in children and adolescents, but a baseline parathormone level is not usually recommended.

Indications for Lithium Carbonate in Child and Adolescent Psychiatry

The following boxed warning appears in the package insert.

NOTE: WARNING: Lithium toxicity is closely related to serum lithium levels, and can occur at doses close to therapeutic levels. Facilities for prompt and accurate serum lithium determinations should be available before initiating therapy.

Lithium carbonate is FDA approved for the treatment of manic episodes of bipolar illness and maintenance therapy of manic-depressive patients, with a history of mania, who are at least 12 years of age. Significant normalization of manic symptomatology may require up to 3 weeks of lithium carbonate therapy; hence concomitant use of antipsychotic medication may be initially required for more rapid control of manic symptoms. See subsequent text regarding titration of dose and recommended serum lithium levels.

Lithium Dosage Schedule

- *Children up to 11 years of age:* Not recommended (see below for studies done in this patient population).
- *Adolescents at least 12 years of age and adults:* Dosage must be individually regulated according to clinical response and serum lithium levels. As noted earlier, the pharmacokinetics of lithium carbonate makes it necessary to administer the total daily dose in smaller doses administered three or four times daily if immediate-release tablets or syrup is used, or twice daily if controlled-release capsules are used, to minimize risk of reaching toxic serum levels of lithium. (More detailed information on administering, titrating, and monitoring lithium in children and adolescents is found in the subsequent text.)

Lithium Carbonate Dose Forms Available

- *Tablets (Lithotabs):* 300 mg
- *Capsules (Eskalith):* 300 mg
- *Controlled-release tablets (Eskalith CR):* 450 mg (scored)
- *Slow-release tablets (Lithobid):* 300 mg
- *Syrup (lithium citrate):* 8 mEq/5 mL (8 mEq of lithium is equivalent to 300 mg of lithium carbonate)

Titration of Lithium Dosage (Ages 12 and Up)

Typically, doses of approximately 1,800 mg/day will achieve the serum lithium levels necessary to control symptoms during acute mania (between 1 and 1.5 mEq/L). During long-term maintenance, serum lithium levels usually range between 0.6 and 1.2 mEq/L; this usually requires a divided daily dose between 900 and 1,200 mg (GlaxoSmithKline, 2003). Berg et al. (1974), however, reported that a 14-year-old girl and her father, who were both diagnosed with bipolar manic-depressive disorder, required daily doses of lithium as high as 2,400 mg to achieve therapeutic levels.

Schou (1969) noted that early untoward effects, such as nausea, diarrhea, muscle weakness, thirst, urinary frequency, hand tremor, and a dazed feeling, may be caused by a too rapid rise in serum lithium levels. Lithium is a gastric irritant. A low initial dose of lithium taken after meals, which slows absorption, and gradual increases in dose will often avert the development of these symptoms. When they develop, they usually subside spontaneously within a few days.

Serum lithium levels should be monitored twice weekly during the acute manic phase and until both serum level and clinical condition have stabilized. In the maintenance phase of therapy during remission, serum lithium levels should be monitored every 3 to 6 months (Kowatch and Delbello, 2003). Lithium levels should be drawn 12 hours after the last dose and prior to the subsequent dose.

Patel et al. (2006) treated 27 adolescents (12 to 18 years old) with an initial lithium carbonate dose of 30 mg/kg/day (twice daily dosing; maximum starting dose of 600 mg PO twice daily), during a 6-week open-label trial of lithium for the treatment of bipolar depression. Seventy percent of subjects achieved a therapeutic level of 1.0 to 1.2 mEq/L over a mean of 18.4 days. The most commonly reported side effects were headache (74%), nausea/vomiting (67%), polyuria (33%), stomachache (30%), polydipsia (26%), and abdominal cramps (19%). Almost all of the side effects were judged to be mild to moderate in severity, and the authors concluded that lithium carbonate was relatively well tolerated in this trial (Patel et al., 2006).

Use of Lithium Carbonate in Children below 12 Years of Age

The therapeutic dosages of lithium carbonate used in treating children above 5 years of age with various disorders do not differ significantly from those used in treating older adolescents and adults, and the principles of administration are essentially the same (Campbell et al., 1984a). This higher-dose-per-body-weight ratio reflects the fact that higher renal lithium clearance occurs in children and adolescents than in adults.

Weller et al. (1986) published a guide for determining the initial total daily lithium dose for prepubertal children 6 to 12 years of age. The guide and summary of how it is used are presented in Table 8.1. Lower initial doses should be used for children diagnosed with mental retardation or organicity (central nervous system damage) (E. B. Weller, personal communication, 1990).

The purpose of this guide is to reach therapeutic serum lithium levels (0.6 to 1.2 mEq/L) as rapidly as possible using currently available tablet strengths without undue risk of reaching toxic serum levels. The authors administered lithium to 10 subjects diagnosed with manic-depressive illness and 5 subjects diagnosed with conduct disorder (CD), following these guidelines. Thirteen of the 15 subjects had serum lithium levels in the therapeutic range after only 5 days of treatment. Side effects were reported to be minimal, primarily mild nausea, abdominal pain, polydipsia and polyuria, and increase in preexisting enuresis. Most were transient, and none required discontinuation of lithium. As discussed earlier, some adverse effects of lithium appear to be related to excessively rapid increases in serum lithium level. It remains to be determined whether the use of the proposed lithium dosage guide will cause significantly more adverse effects or will increase their severity more

TABLE 8.1 » Lithium Carbonate Dosage Guide for Prepubertal School-Aged Children				
Weight (kg)	8 AM Dose (mg)	12 Noon Dose (mg)	6 PM Dose (mg)	Total Daily Dose (mg)
<25	150	150	300	600
25–40	300	300	300	900
40–50	300	300	600	1,200
50–60	600	300	600	1,500

Dose specified in schedule should be maintained at least 5 days with serum lithium levels drawn every other day 12 hours after ingestion of the last lithium dose until two consecutive levels appear in the therapeutic range (0.6 to 1.2 mEq/L). Dose may then be adjusted based on serum level, side effects, or clinical response. Do not exceed 1.4 mEq/L serum level. Lower initial dose should be used for children diagnosed with mental retardation or organicity.

From Weller EB, Weller RA, Fristed MA. Lithium dosage guide for prepubertal children: a preliminary report. *J Am Acad Child Psychiatry.* 1986;25:92–95.

than would a more gradual titration of lithium. In cases where very rapid control of symptoms is critical, however, it may be proved to be especially useful.

Findling et al. (2011) likewise studied lithium dosing in children and adolescents suffering from bipolar I disorder. In this 8-week trial, outpatients aged 7 to 17 years were started on lithium 300 mg twice daily (if <30 kg) or 300 mg twice or thrice daily (for children >30 kg). Doses were then increased by 300 mg per week unless one of the following stop criteria occurred: a therapeutic response was obtained (CGI-I Scale score ≤2 and a 50% decrease in Young Mania Rating Scale [YMRS] score from baseline), youth experienced significant adverse events, doses exceeded 40 mg/kg/day, or the serum lithium level was expected to be >1.4 mEq/L. As mentioned previously, the most commonly observed side effects during this trial were nausea (66.7%), headache (65%), vomiting (55%), dizziness (36.7%), diarrhea (30%), upper abdominal pain/tremor (26.7%), and somnolence (18.3%). The authors concluded that lithium was well tolerated and exhibited similar side-effect profiles in all dosing arms of the study, which led them to conclude that lithium dosed at 300 mg thrice daily (with an additional 300-mg increase during the first week), followed by 300-mg weekly increases until one or more stop criteria are met will be used in upcoming randomized placebo-controlled trials (Findling et al., 2011).

Reports of Interest

Lithium has been widely looked at over the years for the treatment of pediatric bipolar disorder. Older studies consisted primarily of case reports, chart reviews, and only a few small double-blind placebo-controlled trials, though studies completed over the past decade, including larger open and double-blinded controlled trials, have offered increased clarity regarding the efficacy and tolerability of lithium in the treatment of pediatric bipolar disorder.

Lithium Carbonate in the Treatment of Youth Bipolar Disorder

Geller et al. (1998) conducted a 6-week, double-blind, placebo-controlled, parallel-groups study comparing lithium and placebo in the treatment of 25 outpatients (16 males, 9 females; mean age, 16.3 ± 1.2 years) diagnosed by DSM-III-R (American Psychiatric Association [APA], 1987) criteria with a bipolar disorder or major depressive disorder with one or more predictors of future bipolar disorder and substance dependency disorder. The mean age of onset of substance abuse disorders was approximately 6 years after the mean age of onset of subjects' mood disorders. Subjects did not have to agree to stop their substance abuse to participate in the study. Thirteen subjects were assigned to the lithium group; of these, 10 completed the study. Twelve were assigned to the placebo group and 11 completed the study.

Efficacy was determined by ratings on the Children's Global Assessment Scale (CGAS) and random weekly urine drug assays. "Responders" were required to have a score of ≥65. Lithium was initiated with a 600-mg dose and was titrated to yield a serum lithium level between 0.9 and 1.3 mEq/L. The total dose was divided and given at 7:00 AM and 7:00 PM daily. The subjects on lithium improved significantly more than those on placebo based on predefined response criteria. Six (60%) of the 10 completers on lithium were "responders," compared with 1 (9.1%) of the 11 completers on placebo ($P = .024$). The mean daily lithium dose for the 10 completers was $1,733 ± 428$ mg; the responders' daily dose was significantly higher ($1,975 ± 240$ mg) than that of the nonresponders ($1,368 ± 399$ mg; $P = .02$), but there was no significant difference in their serum lithium levels (responders, $0.88 ± 0.27$ mEq/L vs. nonresponders, $0.85 ± 0.3$ mEq/L). After 3 weeks, the percentage of positive weekly random urine tests was significantly lower in the lithium group than in the placebo group ($P = .042$). When symptoms of mania and mood symptoms' persistence were studied specifically, however, lithium did not separate from placebo. The ratings of untoward effects on the acute lithium side-effects scale showed that lithium was well tolerated. Only polyuria and polydipsia occurred significantly more frequently in the lithium group than in the placebo group. The authors concluded that lithium may be effective for the treatment of adolescents with bipolar disorder and a comorbid substance use disorder, although they acknowledged that further research was needed with larger sample sizes and longer treatment durations.

Kafantaris et al. (2003) conducted a 4-week, open trial of lithium carbonate in treating acute mania in 100 adolescents (mean age, 15.23 years; age range, 12 to 18 years; 50 males, 50 females) who had been diagnosed with bipolar I disorder and met DSM-IV criteria for a current manic or mixed episode and had a score of ≥16 on the YMRS. ADHD was a codiagnosis in 31% of patients. Immediate-release lithium was rapidly titrated to therapeutic serum levels between 0.6 and 1.2 mEq/L using Cooper's technique (Cooper et al., 1973). Subjects ($N = 46$) with severe aggression and/or psychosis were treated concomitantly with antipsychotics. Mean lithium serum level at the end of week 1 was $0.90 ± 0.25$ mEq/L; at endpoint (week 4), the mean serum level was $0.93 ± 0.21$ mEq/L and the mean dose was $1,355 ± 389$ mg/day.

Subjects were rated weekly on the YMRS, Hamilton Depression Rating Scale (HDRS, 17 item), Brief Psychiatric Rating Scale (BPRS), Clinical Global Impressions–Improvement (CGI-I) Scale, and the CGAS. Responders were defined as having both a decrease of >33% from baseline YMRS score and a ≤2 rating (much or very much improved) on the CGI-I. At the end of week 4, all the ratings showed significant improvement ($P < .001$). Sixty-three patients met responder criteria by the end of week 2. Remission of manic symptoms (YMRS score <6) occurred in 26 patients by week 4 and only 4 of the 23 patients with suicidal ideation at baseline had such symptoms by week 4. The authors reported that the presence of baseline psychotic features (with antipsychotic treatment), prominent depressive symptoms, comorbid diagnoses including ADHD, early onset of mood disorders, and severity of mania at initial presentation and hospitalization did not impact significantly on response to lithium at week 4.

Adverse events present at week 4 ratings in >10% of patients included weight gain (1 to 12 lb), 55.3%; polydipsia, 33.3%; polyuria, 25.5%; headache, 23.5%; tremor, 19.6%; gastrointestinal pain, 17.6%; nausea, 15.7%; vomiting, 13.7%; anorexia, 13.7%; and diarrhea, 13.7%.

The study authors concluded that lithium appeared efficacious in the treatment of adolescent mania when used with or without concomitant antipsychotic medication (Kafantaris et al., 2003).

Findling et al. (2006a) conducted a prospective, 8-week, open-label outpatient lithium plus divalproex combination therapy trial for 38 patients ages 5 to 17 years with bipolar type I or II. The enrolled patients had a mean age of 10.5 years, were previously stabilized with lithium plus divalproex, and subsequently relapsed during treatment with either medication as monotherapy. During the randomized maintenance monotherapy trial, half of the patients received divalproex (target serum concentrations of 0.6 to 1.2 mmol/L), and the other half received lithium (target serum concentrations of 0.6 to 1.2 mmol/L). If subjects evidenced mood relapse by the unblinded physician monitor during the monotherapy phase, they were enrolled in the restabilization study and treated with both lithium and divalproex at doses previously required to achieve stabilization.

Outcome measures included the Children's Depression Rating Scale–Revised (CDRS-R), and the YMRS. The Clinical Global Impressions (CGI) Scale was used to assess bipolar symptom severity (CGI-S), and the CGAS was used to determine overall functioning at both home and school. Of the 38 patients enrolled in the restabilization phase, 35 completed all 8 weeks (92.1%), whereas 2 withdrew consent and 1 was lost to follow-up. No patients ended the study because of medication intolerance.

At the end of the 8-week restabilization study, a significant decline in YMRS, CDRS-R, CGAS, and the CGI-S scores were discovered in almost all of the enrolled patients. The authors thus concluded that most youth who initially stabilize with a combination of lithium and divalproex, and subsequently destabilize with monotherapy treatment alone, can be effectively restabilized with prior effective doses of lithium and divalproex. Limitations of the study include its open-label design, short trial duration, and subjects with comorbid diagnoses such as ADHD were allowed to receive concomitant pharmacotherapy, which may have facilitated symptom reduction during the trial, independent of the study medications (Findling et al., 2006).

Pavuluri et al. (2006) studied 38 youth, ages 4 to 17 years, with a history of preschool-onset bipolar disorder during a 12-month open-label trial. All subjects received lithium as monotherapy. Response was defined as a ≥50% decrease from baseline YMRS score. Patients who did not adequately respond to lithium monotherapy after 8 weeks, and those with symptom relapse after an initial positive response, were provided risperidone augmentation for up to 11 months. Of the 38 subjects treated with lithium monotherapy, 17 responded positively and 21 required risperidone augmentation. The response rate for youth treated with both lithium and risperidone was 85.7%. Predictors of inadequate response to lithium monotherapy included the presence of comorbid ADHD, high symptom severity at baseline, history of sexual or physical abuse, and preschool age. The authors concluded that a large percentage of youth with a history of preschool-onset bipolar disorder were either nonresponders or only partial responders to lithium when used as monotherapy. Subsequent augmentation of lithium with risperidone in these cases was judged to be effective and well tolerated during the trial (Pavuluri et al., 2006).

Only one study looked at lithium treatment for youth with bipolar depression (Patel et al., 2006). In this 6-week open-label study, 27 adolescents with an episode of depression associated with bipolar I disorder were treated with lithium 30 mg/kg (twice daily dosing), which was adjusted to achieve therapeutic serum lithium levels between 1.0 and 1.2 mEq/L. Efficacy measures included the CDRS-R and the CGI Scale for Bipolar Disorder (CGI-BP). Response rates were defined as ≥50% reduction in CDRS-R score, and remission rates were defined as a CDRS-R score ≤28 and a CGI-BP Improvement score of 1 or 2. Study results revealed a large effect size of 1.7, a lower response rate of 48%, and a remission rate of 30%. Side effects were deemed to be of mild to moderate severity, and lithium was judged to be relatively well tolerated in this study. Study authors concluded that based on this positive open-label study, lithium may be effective for the treatment of depression in adolescents with bipolar disorder. Future controlled studies are needed to replicate these findings, however (Patel et al., 2006).

Geller et al. (2012) studied 279 antimanic medication-naïve subjects, ages 6 to 15 years, with DSM-IV bipolar I disorder (manic or mixed phase) in a randomized controlled trial assessing response to lithium, risperidone, or divalproex sodium. Blinded independent evaluators conducted all assessments. Medications were increased weekly only if there was inadequate response and if the medication remained well tolerated. Maximum doses of lithium carbonate, divalproex sodium, and risperidone were 1.1 to 1.3 mEq/L, 111 to 125 μg/mL, and 4 to 6 mg, respectively, and primary outcome measures were the Clinical Global Impressions for Bipolar Illness Improvement–Mania and the Modified Side Effects Form for Children and Adolescents.

Study results revealed statistically significant higher response rates for risperidone (68.5%) versus both lithium (35.6%) and divalproex sodium (24.0%). Lithium versus divalproex sodium response rates did not differ significantly. The authors concluded that risperidone is more efficacious than lithium or divalproex sodium for the initial treatment of childhood mania (Geller et al., 2012).

More recent studies are focusing on whether lithium and other mood stabilizers have neurotrophic roles in treatment. Mitsunaga et al. (2011) sought to study morphometric characteristics of the subgenual cingulate cortex (SGC), which has been implicated in the pathophysiology of mood disorders. Twenty bipolar disorder youth with a mean age of 14.6 years, and 20 age- and gender-matched controls without bipolar disorder underwent high-resolution magnetic resonance imaging. Although no differences were discovered in SGC volumes between bipolar disorder subjects and healthy controls, further analysis revealed that bipolar disorder subjects with prior mood stabilizer exposure, compared with bipolar disorder subjects without prior mood stabilizer exposure and to healthy controls, had significantly increased SGC volumes. This finding led the authors to conclude that mood stabilizer exposure may be correlated with increases in SGC size. The authors describe many limitations to the aforementioned study, however, including a small sample size, concomitant use of atypical antipsychotic medication by study subjects, which may or may not have neurotrophic properties of its own, and the presence of comorbid ADHD in study subjects, a diagnosis which currently has an unknown effects on SGC size (Mitsunaga et al., 2011).

Lithium Carbonate in the Maintenance Treatment of Youth Diagnosed with Bipolar Disorder

Kafantaris et al. (2004), using a 2-week blinded discontinuation study design, randomized 40 prior lithium responders to either lithium or placebo. Prior to the randomized discontinuation phase, lithium responders received 4 weeks of open-label lithium treatment, which yielded average serum lithium levels of 0.99 mEq/L ± 0.21. During the discontinuation phase, 19 adolescents were maintained on lithium monotherapy and 21 received placebo after a 3-day lithium taper. Study authors reported no statistical difference in mood exacerbation rates between lithium monotherapy (52.6%) and placebo (61.9%) and concluded that lithium may be ineffective for maintenance treatment of adolescent bipolar disorder (Kafantaris et al., 2004). Study limitations including small sample sizes and a relatively short open-label treatment lead-in phase prevent firm conclusions from being drawn, and additional studies are needed.

Findling et al. (2005) compared lithium carbonate and valproic acid in the maintenance treatment of youth diagnosed with bipolar disorder and found no clinically significant differences between the two drugs for this indication. This study is summarized in the valproic acid section of the text (Findling et al., 2005).

Lithium Carbonate in the Treatment of Youth with Severe Mood Dysregulation

Severe mood dysregulation (SMD) is defined as a syndrome encompassing severe nonepisodic irritability and hyperarousal in youth (Liebenluft et al., 2003). In 2009, Dickstein et al. studied lithium for the treatment of youth ages 7 to 17 years with SMD in a randomized double-blind placebo-controlled trial (Dickstein et al., 2009). Subjects who met SMD criteria were gradually weaned off all of their outpatient psychiatric medication, in an inpatient setting, for a total of four drug half-lives. This was followed by a 2-week single-blind placebo run-in phase, after which only those who continued to meet SMD criteria ($N = 25$) were randomized to either lithium or placebo for the 6-week double-blind randomized controlled trial. The primary clinical outcome measure was a CGI-I score of <4 by the end of the trial. Results revealed not only a relatively small rate of improvement in the lithium group, but also no significance between group differences in outcome measures. This lead the authors to conclude that lithium may not be effective for youth with chronic irritability and hyperarousal. However, given the small sample size, these findings should be considered preliminary (Dickstein et al., 2009).

Lithium Carbonate in the Treatment of Disorders with Severe Aggression, Especially When Accompanied by Explosive Affect, Including Self-Injurious Behavior

In a double-blind, placebo-controlled study of 61 treatment-resistant hospitalized children (age range, 5.2 to 12.9 years) diagnosed with undersocialized aggressive CD, both haloperidol and lithium were found to be superior to placebo in ameliorating behavioral symptoms (Campbell et al., 1984b). Optimal doses of lithium carbonate ranged from 500 to 2,000 mg/day (mean, 1,166 mg/day); corresponding serum levels ranged from 0.32 to 1.51 mEq/L (mean, 0.99 mEq/L). The authors noted that lithium caused fewer and milder untoward effects than did haloperidol and that these effects did not appear to interfere significantly with the children's daily routines. There was also a suggestion that lithium was particularly effective in diminishing the explosive affect and that other improvements followed (Campbell et al., 1984b).

Campbell et al. (1995) reported a double-blind, placebo-controlled study that was designed to replicate their 1984 study. Fifty treatment-resistant inpatients (46 males, 4 females; mean age, 9.4 ± 1.8 years; age range, 5.1 to 12.0 years) diagnosed with CD, undersocialized aggressive type by DSM-III (APA, 1980a) criteria and having chronic severe explosive aggressiveness were treated with lithium carbonate only or placebo. Following a 2-week, placebo baseline period during which baseline assessments were conducted and placebo responders were eliminated, the 50 remaining subjects were randomly assigned to placebo ($N = 25$) or lithium ($N = 25$) for a 6-week period; this was followed by 2 weeks of posttreatment placebo. Efficacy was assessed by ratings on the Global Clinical Judgments (Consensus) Scale, Children's Psychiatric Rating Scale (CPRS), CGI, Clinical Global Impressions–Severity (CGI-S), and Improvement (CGI-I) Scales, Conners Teacher Questionnaire (CTQ), and the Parent–Teacher Questionnaire (PTQ). Lithium carbonate was begun at 600 mg/day and titrated individually over a 2-week period with a maximum permitted dose of 2,100 mg/day or serum lithium of 1.8 mEq/L or equivalent saliva lithium level. The mean optimal dose of lithium was 1,248 mg/day (range, 600 to 1,800 mg/day); the mean serum lithium level was 1.12 mEq/L (range, 0.53 to 1.79 mEq/L); and the mean saliva lithium level was 2.5 mEq/L (range, 1.45 to 4.44 mEq/L).

On the Global Clinical Judgments (consensus) Scale, 68% (17/25) of subjects on lithium were rated as moderately or markedly improved while only 40% (10/25) of subjects on placebo were so rated ($P = .003$). Further refining this measure, 40% (10/25) of the subjects of lithium were "markedly" improved versus only 4% (1/25) of the subjects on placebo. The CGI-I scores after 6 weeks were also significantly better for the lithium group ($P = .044$); although it was not significant whether the lithium group improved more on the CGI-S. The authors concluded that these data supported the conclusions of their earlier study and that lithium carbonate can be efficacious in treating children with CD and explosive aggressiveness who have not responded to psychosocial treatments or medication with methylphenidate or standard neuroleptics.

Vetro et al. (1985) treated 17 children, aged 3 to 12 years, with lithium, who were hospitalized for hyperaggressivity, active destruction of property, severely disturbed social adjustment, and unresponsiveness to discipline. Ten of the children had not responded to prior pharmacotherapy, including haloperidol and concomitant individual and family therapy. Lithium carbonate was titrated slowly over 2 to 3 weeks to achieve serum levels in the therapeutic range (0.6 to 1.2 mEq/L). Mean serum lithium level was 0.68 ± 0.30 mEq/L. The authors reported that 13 of the children improved enough that their abilities to adapt to their environment could be described as good, and their aggressivity had been reduced to tolerable levels. Three of the four cases that did not improve had poor compliance in taking the medication at home. The authors also noted that these children usually required continuous treatment with lithium for longer than 6 months.

DeLong and Aldershof (1987) reported that rage, aggressive outbursts, and, interestingly, encopresis responded favorably to lithium pharmacotherapy in children with behavioral disorders associated with a variety of neurologic and medical diseases, including mental retardation.

Lithium Carbonate in the Treatment of Children and Adolescents Diagnosed with CD

Malone et al. (2000) conducted a 6-week, double-blind, placebo-controlled, parallel-groups study comparing lithium carbonate and placebo in the treatment of 40 inpatients (33 males, 7 females; mean age, 12.5 years; age range, 9.5 to 17.1 years) who were diagnosed with CD by DSM-III-R (APA, 1987) criteria and hospitalized for chronic, severe aggressive behavior. Eighty-six inpatients entered the study; however, 46 were eliminated during the initial 2-week single-blind placebo baseline; 40 of this group did not meet the protocol's aggression criteria. All 40 remaining subjects entered the 4-week treatment phase and completed the protocol; 20 subjects were assigned randomly to each group.

Efficacy was determined by ratings on the Global Clinical Judgments (Consensus) Scale (GCJCS), the CGI, and the Overt Aggression Scale (OAS). Lithium was initiated with a 600-mg dose; serum lithium levels were determined 24 hours later, and an initial target dose was calculated for each subject using a nomogram. Subsequent lithium doses were increased by 300 mg daily and given in three equal doses to reach the target dose. At the end of the study, optimal mean lithium dose was 1,425 ± 321 mg/day (range, 900 to 2,100 mg/day) with a mean steady-state therapeutic lithium level of 1.07 ± 0.19 mmol/L (range, 0.78 to 1.55 mmol/L).

On the GCJCS, 16 (80%) of the lithium group versus 6 (30%) of the placebo group were rated as "marked" or "moderately" improved on the criterion for responders ($P = .004$). Significantly more of the lithium group were also rated as responders on the CGI (17 [30%] vs. 4 [20%] of the placebo group; $P = .004$). On the OAS, the lithium group continued to show improvement over the 4-week period, whereas the placebo group showed an initial decline at week 1 but then remained rather stable. The lithium group's mean decrease from baseline was significantly greater than that of the placebo group, with a significant interaction between treatment group and time ($P = .04$). Although untoward effects were frequent, they were usually mild and similar for both placebo and lithium groups. Only three adverse effects occurred significantly more on lithium: nausea in 12 of 20, vomiting in 11 of 20, and urinary frequency 11 of 20 ($P \le .05$ in all cases). The authors noted that the aggressive behavior of 40 (47.1%) of their initial 85 subjects improved significantly during the first 2 weeks secondary to hospitalization and treatment with placebo alone. For the 40 subjects who remained aggressive and entered the medication phase of the protocol, lithium was a safe and effective treatment. The authors noted that determining the long-term efficacy and safety of lithium in such subjects will require further research.

ANTIEPILEPTICS/MOOD STABILIZERS

Currently, there is robust clinical interest in the off-label use of antiepileptic drugs to treat psychiatric disorders in children and adolescents; their safety and efficacy in treating these disorders remains to be fully elucidated, however. In addition to ongoing research clarifying the question of efficacy and tolerability of antiepileptic medication in youth, research designed to delineate which specific disorders, symptoms, and patients or subgroups of patients are most likely to respond well to antiepileptic medication would be of clear value (e.g., patients with various abnormal EEG findings and patients who are mentally disabled or have other evidence of abnormal central nervous system functioning compared with affectually or behaviorally disordered patients without signs of central nervous system dysfunction).

Valproic Acid (Depakene); Divalproex Sodium (Valproic Acid and Valproate Sodium [Depakote; Depacon])

Note: The FDA has directed the manufacturers of valproic acid and its derivatives (e.g., divalproex sodium and valproate sodium) to label their products with the following Black Box warning. HEPATOTOXICITY: Hepatic failure resulting in fatalities has occurred in patients receiving valproic acid. Experience has indicated that children below the age of 2 years are at a considerable increased risk of developing fatal hepatotoxicity, especially those with congenital metabolic disorders, those with severe seizure disorders accompanied by mental retardation and those with organic brain disease. When valproic acid products are used in these patient groups, they should be used with extreme caution and as a sole agent. The benefits of therapy should be weighed against the risks. Above this age group, experience in epilepsy has indicated that the incidence of fatal hepatotoxicity decreases considerably in progressively older patient groups. These incidents usually have occurred during the first 6 months of treatment. Serious or fatal hepatotoxicity may be preceded by nonspecific symptoms such as malaise, weakness, lethargy, facial edema, anorexia, and vomiting. In patients with epilepsy, a loss of seizure control may also occur. Patients should be monitored closely for appearance of these symptoms. Liver function tests should be performed prior to therapy and at frequent intervals thereafter, especially during the first 6 months. TERATOGENICITY: Valproate can produce teratogenic effects such as neural tube defects (e.g., spina bifida). Accordingly, the use of valproate products in women of childbearing potential requires that the benefits of its use be weighed against the risk of injury to the fetus. PANCREATITIS: Cases of life-threatening pancreatitis have been reported in both children and adults receiving valproate. Some of the cases have been described as hemorrhagic with a rapid progression from initial symptoms to death. Cases have been reported shortly after initial use as well as after several years of use. Patients and guardians should be warned that abdominal pain, nausea, vomiting, and/or anorexia can be symptoms of pancreatitis that require prompt medical evaluation. If pancreatitis is diagnosed, valproate should ordinarily be discontinued. Alternative treatment for the underlying medical condition should be initiated as clinically indicated.

In addition to the Black Box warnings described above, in 2008 the FDA issued an alert advising providers to monitor patients who are taking or starting antiepileptic medication for any changes in behavior that could indicate the emergence of depression or worsening suicidal thoughts or behavior (PDR.net, 2008).

Valproic acid and divalproex sodium (a stable coordination compound of valproic acid and valproate sodium) both dissociate to the valproate ion in the gastrointestinal tract and have antiepileptic properties. These drugs are indicated for the treatment of simple and complex absence seizures and adjunctively in patients with multiple seizure types, which include absence seizures. Divalproex sodium has also been approved by the FDA for advertising as safe and effective for adults in the treatment of manic episodes associated with bipolar disorder for up to 3 weeks and the prophylaxis of migraine headaches (*PDR*, 2006).

Pharmacokinetics of Valproic Acid

Following oral administration, valproic acid and divalproex sodium dissociate to the valproate ion, which is the active agent, in the gastrointestinal tract. Administration of valproic acid with food may slow the absorption rate but does not interfere with clinical efficacy. Food does not significantly affect the total amount of valproate absorbed and may be helpful in reducing gastrointestinal irritation in some patients.

Peak plasma concentration after a single dose usually occurs between 1 and 4 hours after ingestion of valproic acid, 4 hours after ingestion of sodium valproate tablets, and 3.3 hours after taking sodium valproate "sprinkles." Valproic acid is metabolized almost entirely by the liver; the metabolites are excreted primarily in the urine. Plasma valproate half-life is between 6 and 16 hours; the more rapid metabolism rates occur most frequently in patients receiving valproic acid and other antiepileptics that induce enzymes that increase the metabolism rate of valproate.

In a retroactive chart review of 16 males (age range, 5 to 14 years; mean age, 9.3 years) hospitalized for mood stabilization, Good et al. (2001) found that a relatively conservative total loading dose of 15 mg/kg/day of divalproex sodium given in two equal doses resulted in therapeutic trough plasma valproate levels on day 5 of therapy in 13 (81.3%) cases. The initial dose was calculated for one subgroup using actual weight and for a second subgroup using adjusted ideal body weight (IBW). For the latter group, Adjusted IBW = IBW + 40% (Current Weight – IBW). All subjects were also taking atypical antipsychotics, and some were taking stimulants as well during this period. The authors noted several findings of clinical interest: Of the eight patients experiencing untoward effects (mostly sedation and nausea), six (75%) had valproate plasma levels of >90 µg/mL. Patients who were ≥15% over IBW and who were dosed according to actual body weight were significantly more likely to have supratherapeutic (>120 µg/mL) valproate plasma levels than normal-weight subjects or overweight subjects whose doses were determined by adjusted IBW. Based on this study, it would seem prudent to calculate and use adjusted IBW for significantly overweight children and adolescents if it is decided to administer a loading dose of valproate to rapidly achieve therapeutic plasma levels.

Contraindications for Valproic Acid Administration

Valproic acid can cause severe hepatotoxicity, including fatal hepatic failure. Children below 2 years of age are at increased risk. It should not be administered to anyone with hepatic disease, significant liver dysfunction, or known hypersensitivity to the drug.

Because valproic acid has been reported to cause teratogenic effects in the fetus, it should be administered with caution to women who are likely to become pregnant, and they should be warned to notify their physician immediately if they become pregnant.

Interactions with Other Drugs

Valproate may potentiate the action of central nervous system depressants such as alcohol and benzodiazepines.

Coadministration with clonazepam may induce absence seizures in patients with a history of absence-type seizures.

Coadministration with risperidone (4 mg/day) did not affect the predose or average plasma concentrations and exposure area under the curve (AUC) of valproate (a total of 1,000 mg administered in three divided doses), but there was a 20% increase in valproate peak plasma concentration after concomitant administration of risperidone.

Ambrosini and Sheikh (1998) have reported two cases in which coadministration of valproic acid and guanfacine resulted in significantly increased levels of valproic acid. It was suggested that this was secondary to drug–drug competition at the level of hepatic glucuronidation.

Other drug interactions have been reported.

Untoward Effects of Valproic Acid

The most serious side effects of valproic acid are hepatic failure and pancreatitis, which can be fatal. Hepatic failure occurs most frequently within the first 6 months of treatment. Children below 2 years of age are at increased risk. The risk of hepatotoxicity decreases considerably as patients become progressively older. Hence, liver function must be monitored carefully and frequently, especially during the first 6 months of treatment. Cases of pancreatitis while taking valproic acid have been reported after initial use as well as after several years of use. Patients should be educated to monitor for symptoms of abdominal pain, nausea, vomiting, and/or anorexia while taking valproic acid.

Hyperammonemic encephalopathy has also been reported with valproic acid treatment. An ammonia level should be checked in all patients experiencing episodes of confusion while taking valproic acid.

Valproic acid has a known ability to cause neutropenia, thrombocytopenia, and macrocytic anemia, hence patients taking valproic acid should have a complete blood count (CBC) checked periodically throughout treatment.

Nausea, vomiting, and indigestion may occur early in treatment with valproic acid and usually are transient. Mood stabilizers including valproic acid have been associated with relevant weight gain which should be monitored and addressed. Sedation may occur, and untoward psychiatric effects such as emotional upset, depression, psychosis, aggression, hyperactivity, and behavioral deterioration have been reported.

Valproate and Polycystic Ovaries

Isojarvi et al. (1993) published an article noting that there was an association between valproate use in treating epileptic women and polycystic ovaries and hyperandrogenism (elevated serum testosterone concentrations). The finding was more pronounced in women who had begun treatment with valproate before 20 years of age than in women who began valproate treatment at 20 years of age or older. Sussman and Ginsberg (1998) published a critical review of valproate and polycystic ovary syndrome (PCOS), concluding that the available evidence suggests that early and long-term treatment with valproic acid is a causal or precipitating factor in the development of PCOS in epileptic women, particularly if they are overweight; relative risk factors for nonepileptic adolescents are at present unknown. Johnston (1999) basically concurs. Piontek and Wisner (2000) have suggested clinical guidelines for the appropriate clinical management of women with reproductive capacity who are treated with valproate. Although risk of PCOS does not preclude the use of valproic acid/divalproex sodium in adolescent females, risks and benefits must be discussed, informed consent obtained, and careful monitoring maintained. Further research is needed to clarify this issue.

**Indications for Valproic Acid/Divalproex Sodium
in Child and Adolescent Psychiatry**

NOTE: Prior to prescribing review the Boxed Warning at the beginning of this chapter.

Valproic acid, valproate sodium, and divalproex sodium are approved for use alone or in combination (see exception to this in patients <2 years of age in boxed warning at beginning of chapter) with other drugs in treating patients with simple and complex absence seizures or as an adjunctive agent in patients with multiple-type seizures, which include absence seizures. Valproic acid is additionally approved for the treatment of acute mania and migraine prophylaxis in adults. It has not been evaluated for safety and efficacy in either treating pediatric mania or in the prophylactic treatment of pediatric migraine headache and is not approved by the FDA for such advertising.

(continued)

**Indications for Valproic Acid/Divalproex Sodium
in Child and Adolescent Psychiatry** *(continued)*

Dosage Schedule

- *Children <2 years of age:* Contraindicated for any indication.

Treatment of Epilepsy

- *Children ≥2 years of age, adolescents, and adults:*
  An initial daily dose of 15 mg/kg is recommended. Weekly increases of 5 to 10 mg/kg/day until seizures are controlled or untoward effects prevent further increases are recommended. The maximum recommended daily dose is 60 mg/kg. Amounts >250 mg/day should be administered in divided doses.

Treatment of Acute Mania (Divalproex Sodium Only)

- *Children and adolescents <18 years of age:* Not indicated.
- *Adolescents at least 18 years of age and adults:*
  An initial divided daily dose of 750 mg is recommended, followed by rapid titration to achieve satisfactory clinical response or reach total (trough) plasma valproate levels of 50 to 125 µg/mL, which are usually associated with clinical efficacy. The maximum recommended dosage is 60 mg/kg/day. Titration can usually be completed within 14 days.
  Plasma levels of total valproate between 50 and 100 µg/mL are usually considered to be the therapeutic range for epilepsy (and for off-label psychiatric uses); however, in the treatment of acute mania, levels up to 125 µg/mL are recommended.

Prophylactic Treatment of Migraine Headache (Divalproex Sodium Only)

Children and adolescent <16 years old: Not indicated.
  Adolescents at least 16 years of age and adults: An initial 250-mg dose of divalproex sodium administered twice daily is recommended. Some patients have benefitted from doses as high as 1,000 mg/day; however, higher doses showed no evidence of increased benefit in clinical trials.

Dosage Forms Available (Valproic Acid, Depakene)

- *Capsules:* 250 mg
- *Syrup:* 250 mg/5 mL dispensed in 16-oz bottles

Dosage Forms Available (Divalproex Sodium, Depakote)

- *Sprinkle capsules:* 125 mg
- *Delayed-release tablets (Depakote):* 125, 250, and 500 mg
- *Extended-release tablets (Depakote-ER):* 250 and 500 mg. This formulation permits once-a-day dosing

Dosage Forms Available (Valproate Sodium)

- *Injectable (Depacon):* 100 mg/mL dispensed in 5-mL single-dose vials

Reports of Interest

Valproic Acid in the Treatment of Youth Diagnosed with Bipolar Disorder

Divalproex has been shown to be effective in open studies of youth with bipolar disorder. Papatheodorou et al. (1995) reported an open-label, 7-week study in which the efficacy and safety of divalproex sodium was assessed in the treatment of 15 subjects (2 males, 13 females; mean age, 17.3 years, with 10 subjects being 15 to 18 years old and 5 being 19 or 20 years old) who were diagnosed by DSM-III-R (APA, 1987) criteria with bipolar disorder, in an acute manic phase. Efficacy was evaluated using ratings on the Modified Mania Rating Scale (MMRS), the BPRS, the Global Assessment Scale (GAS), the CGI Scale, and the Valproic Acid Side Effects Scale (VA-SES). Following a 2-day entry phase during which baseline evaluations were performed, subjects began 7 weeks of treatment with divalproex sodium. Medication was administered in three divided doses and individually titrated. Thirteen patients completed the 7-week study; one patient was discontinued for lack of clinical response and one patient withdrew because of "subjectively intolerable sedation and dizziness." All 13 completers required some additional medication for symptom control (e.g., agitation) during the study. Mean dose at the end of 7 weeks was 1,423.08 mg/day (range, 750 to 2,000 mg/day) and the mean serum valproic acid level (12 to 14 hours after the evening dose and before the morning dose) was 642.85 ± 183.08 µmol/L (range, 360 to 923 µmol/L). The 13 completers' ratings on the MMRS, BPRS, GAS, and CGI were all very significantly lower ($P < .0001$ for all four scales) than at baseline. An analysis of variance (ANOVA) found a significant reduction in the MMRS within 1 week on valproex ($P < .016$), which continued throughout the treatment period. Overall untoward effects were benign and their frequency was reported to decrease over the duration of the study, with a very low number being reported at the end of the study. Liver function tests remained normal except for one patient with transiently elevated enzyme levels that reverted to normal without change in dosage. Study authors concluded that divalproex sodium is safe and efficacious in the acute (short-term) treatment of mania in adolescents, although this study was limited by its open-label design and small sample size.

Kowatch et al. (2000) studied 42 outpatients with bipolar disorder who were randomized to receive divalproate, lithium, or carbamazepine for 6 weeks in a non-blind fashion. The mean study subject age was 11.4 years. Response was defined as having a reduction of ≥50% on YMRS scores from baseline. The divalproate response rate was calculated at 53% compared with a response rate of 38% for both lithium and carbamazepine. This small study demonstrated that divalproate may be beneficial in the treatment of youth with bipolar disorder (Kowatch et al., 2000).

Wagner et al. (2002) studied divalproex sodium in an open-label study for the treatment of forty bipolar patients aged 7 to 19 years. The duration of this open-label study varied, from 2 to 8 weeks, depending on treatment response. The mean serum valproate level at the final visit was 83.4 µg/mL. Sixty-one percent of subjects showed a ≥50% improvement in Mania Rating Scale (MRS) scores, leading the authors to conclude that divalproex sodium may be effective in the treatment of bipolar youth. The most common side effects noted were headache, nausea, vomiting, diarrhea, and somnolence. All side effects were judged to be in the mild-to-moderate-severity range, and lab data results were unremarkable. Notably, 43% of study subjects required adjunctive medication to control symptoms such as agitation, irritability, insomnia, and restlessness (Wagner et al., 2002).

Pavuluri et al. (2005) studied divalproex sodium in pediatric mixed mania during a prospective 6-month open trial involving 34 subjects with a mean age of 12.3 years. The primary outcome measures were the YMRS and the Child Depression Rating Scale–Revised (CDRS-R). Response rate, defined as both ≥50% change from baseline YMRS score and ≤40 score on the CDRS-R at the end of the study, was reported as 73.5%. Similar to findings in Wagner et al. (2002), approximately 65% of subjects completing Pavuluri's study required acute adjunctive medications (Pavuluri et al., 2005).

Redden et al. (2009) conducted a 6-month open-label study assessing the safety of divalproex sodium extended-release in 9- to 17-year-old subjects with a diagnosis of bipolar I disorder. One hundred nine subjects completed the study. The most common adverse events were weight gain (16%), nausea (9%), and increased appetite (8%). Asymptomatic elevations in mean plasma ammonia levels were observed. The mean YMRS score decreased 12.4 points from baseline to final visit, equating to a 56% response rate. The authors concluded that divalproex sodium extended-release was generally well tolerated in youth with acute mania, with a side-effect profile similar to that of adults (Redden et al., 2009).

In contrast to the apparent positive findings reported in many open-label studies of divalproex sodium for the treatment of pediatric bipolar disorder, the few controlled studies done reveal less positive findings. DelBello et al. (2006) discovered in a large double-blind randomized pilot study that quetiapine was superior to divalproex sodium for the acute treatment of adolescent mania. In this study, 50 adolescents with bipolar I disorder, manic, or mixed episode were randomized to quetiapine (400 to 600 mg daily) or divalproex sodium (serum levels of 80 to 120 µg/mL) for 28 days. The primary outcome measure was the change in YMRS score across the study period. The authors concluded that quetiapine is at least as effective as divalproex sodium in this study population and may result in a quicker reduction of manic symptoms than does divalproex sodium. The rates of adverse events were judged not to differ significantly between the two study medications (DelBello et al., 2006).

Findling et al. (2007b) conducted a double-blind, placebo-controlled trial of divalproex monotherapy for the treatment of symptomatic youth judged to be at high risk of developing bipolar disorder. Subjects were between the ages of 5 and 17 years, met DSM-IV criteria for bipolar disorder not otherwise specified (NOS) or cyclothymia, and had at least one natural parent with bipolar illness. Fifty-six subjects were randomly assigned to either divalproex sodium or placebo. The mean serum divalproex sodium concentration at the end of the study was 78.8 µg/mL. At the end of the study, there was no significant difference in outcome measures between divalproex sodium and placebo. Both groups did exhibit significant decreases in depression and mania as well as improvement in psychosocial functioning, however. The authors concluded that the relatively high response rates seen in both groups during this study were similar to response rates reported in prior open-label trials of divalproex sodium. These findings lead them to question whether positive response rates seen during open-label trials were due to divalproex sodium per se versus placebo (Findling et al., 2007).

Wagner et al. (2009) studied divalproex extended-release (ER) for the treatment of youth with bipolar disorder in a large double-blind, randomized, placebo-controlled trial. In this study, 150 patients aged 10 to 17 years were randomized to placebo or divalproex ER titrated to a serum concentration of 80 to 125 µg/mL. The primary outcome measure was change in YMRS score. The response rate for divalproex ER, defined as ≥50% reduction in YMRS scores, was 24%, which was lower than response rates reported during previous trials of divalproex in pediatric bipolar disorder. No statistically significant difference between the divalproex-ER-treated patients and the placebo-treated patients was found during this trial. The incidence of adverse events between the two study arms was similar. The authors concluded that this study does not provide support for the use of divalproex ER in the treatment of youth with bipolar I disorder, though they caution that future studies are needed to replicate or refute their findings (Wagner et al., 2009).

Pavuluri et al. (2010a) conducted a 6-week double-blind randomized trial of risperidone versus divalproex in 66 pediatric bipolar disorder patients. Subjects were randomized to either risperidone (0.5 to 2 mg daily) or divalproex (60 to 120 µg/mL). Outcome measures included the YMRS and the CDRS-R. The study authors reported that the risperidone group showed more rapid improvement than the divalproex group ($P < .05$), with response rates based on YMRS of 78.1% for risperidone and 45.5% for divalproex, which was a significant difference. The dropout rate for the risperidone group was 24%, compared with 48% in the divalproex group. Increased irritability was the most common reason for dropout in the latter group.

Geller et al. (2012) reported similar findings during an 8-week randomized controlled trial of risperidone, lithium, or divalproex sodium for the initial treatment of bipolar I disorder, manic or mixed phase, in children and adolescents. In this trial, the Treatment of Early Age Mania (TEAM) recruited 279 antimanic medication-naïve subjects with a mean age of 10.1 years. Subjects received a titrated schedule of lithium, divalproex sodium, or risperidone to mean doses of

1.09 mEq/L, 113.6 μg/mL, and 2.57 mg, respectively. Primary outcome measures were the Clinical Global Impressions for Bipolar Illness Improvement–Mania and the Modified Side Effects Form for Children and Adolescents. Higher response rates occurred with risperidone versus lithium (68% vs. 35.6%, $P < .001$) as well as with risperidone versus divalproex sodium (68% vs. 24%, $P < .001$). Response rates between lithium and divalproex sodium did not differ significantly. The authors concluded that risperidone was more effective than lithium or divalproex sodium but was associated with potentially severe metabolic side effects (Geller et al., 2012).

Valproic Acid versus Lithium in the Maintenance Treatment of Children and Adolescents Diagnosed with Bipolar Disorder

Findling et al. (2005) conducted a double-blind study to determine whether divalproex sodium (DVPX) or lithium was superior as the only drug in maintenance treatment of 139 subjects (age range 5 to 17 years; mean age 10.8 ± 3.5 years; 93 [66.9%] males, 46 [33.1%] females) who were diagnosed with Bipolar I (131, 94.2%) or Bipolar II (8, 5.8%) disorder and stabilized on a combination of lithium carbonate and valproex sodium during acute treatment. Sixty subjects who met remission criteria (CDRS score <40, YMRS score <12.5 and a CGAS score >51) for a minimum of 4 weeks were than randomized to monotherapy with either lithium ($N = 30$) or divalproex ($N = 30$) for up to 76 weeks; subjects were dropped from the study if they violated protocol or required additional clinical intervention. Subjects were tapered off the nonmaintenance/discontinued drug over a period of 8 weeks to minimize discontinuation rebound relapse. Subjects maintained on lithium were maintained at lithium serum concentrations between 0.6 and 1.2 mmol/L and those on valproate were maintained with plasma concentrations between 50 and 100 μg/mL. Primary measures of effectiveness were time to premature discontinuation due to emerging mood symptoms of relapse, *or* premature discontinuation for any reason.

Median survival time to mood relapse for subjects on lithium was 114 ± 57.4 days for lithium and 112 ± 56 days for subjects on valproex and was not statistically different ($P = .55$); overall, 38 (63.3%) subjects relapsed. There was also no significant difference between the lithium and valproex groups in the 12 (20%) who dropped out for any reason ($P = .72$). At the study's conclusion, the mean lithium serum level was 0.84 ± 0.3 mmol/L and the mean valproate plasma level was 75.3 ± 29.4 μg/mL (Findling et al., 2005). Only six subjects (10%), three in each treatment group completed the 76-week protocol, a vivid indication of the chronic and debilitating course of pediatric bipolar disorder.

Regarding adverse events, comparing lithium with valproex, emesis (30% vs. 3%), enuresis (30% vs. 6.7%), and increased thirst (16.5% vs. 0%) were significantly more frequent in the lithium group; other frequent adverse events, which were not significantly different between lithium and valproex were headache (13.3% vs. 23.3%), tremor (20.0% vs. 16.7%), stomach pain (10.0% vs. 23.3%), nausea (16.7% vs. 6.7%), diarrhea (13.3% vs. 6.7%), and decreased appetite (10% vs. 10%).

The authors concluded there was no clinically significant difference between lithium and valproex monotherapy in maintaining the youth who were stabilized on combination lithium/valproex therapy for bipolar disorder (Findling et al., 2005).

Valproic Acid in the Treatment of Aggression in Children and Adolescents

Few studies have looked at valproic acid's efficacy in treating aggression specifically. Blader et al. (2009) studied the efficacy of divalproex in the treatment of children with ADHD and aggression refractory to stimulant monotherapy. Children ages 6 to 13 years were eligible to participate if they had a diagnosis of ADHD and either oppositional defiant disorder (ODD) or CD. Children with coexisting mood, anxiety, and psychotic disorders, or pervasive developmental disorders (PDDs), Tourette syndrome, and mental retardation were excluded from the study. The Retrospective Modified OAS was used to measure severity of aggression. Parents completed this scale at baseline and weekly during the study. The Conners' Global Index–Parent Version measured severity of ADHD symptoms. During the study's lead-in phase, 74 participants received open stimulant treatment for 5 weeks. Those whose aggression persisted despite optimal control of ADHD symptoms during the lead-in phase were randomly assigned to receive double-blind, flexibly dosed divalproex or placebo along with their stimulant for 8 weeks. Given that 31 participants' aggression remitted during the lead-in phase, 10 withdrew from the study, and 3 exhibited low adherence, a total of 30 children were able to be randomized to take either divalproex or placebo. All participants received weekly behavioral therapy throughout. Target serum divalproex levels were between 80 and 110 mg/L. The mean serum valproic acid level during the study was 68.11 mg/L. By the end of the study, authors concluded that a significantly higher percentage of children receiving divalproex during the trial (57%) met aggression remission criteria compared with those assigned to placebo (15%). This study is limited by its small sample size, and additional studies are clearly needed to more accurately estimate valproic acid's efficacy in the treatment of aggression in children with ADHD and comorbid ODD or CD (Blader et al., 2009).

Barzman et al. (2006) studied the efficacy of quetiapine versus divalproex for the treatment of impulsivity and reactive aggression in adolescents with comorbid bipolar disorder and a disruptive behavior disorder (ODD or CD). Thirty-three adolescents were randomized in a double-blind fashion to 28 days of quetiapine 400 to 600 mg daily or divalproex (serum level 80 to 120 µg/mL). The primary measure of efficacy was the change in the Positive and Negative Syndrome Scale (PANSS) Excited Component (EC). The authors reported that there was no significant difference in the PANSS EC scores between the two treatment groups and thus stated that both medications appear to have similar efficacy in the treatment of impulsivity and reactive aggression in children with Bipolar Disorder comorbid with ODD or CD (Barzman et al., 2006). The absence of a placebo arm in this study is a notable limitation. Further studies are needed to replicate the above findings.

Divalproex Sodium in the Treatment of Adolescents with Explosive Mood Disorder

In an open-label, 5-week study, Donovan et al. (1997) treated 10 outpatient adolescents (8 males, 2 females; age range, 15 to 17 years) with divalproex sodium who were diagnosed by DSM-III-R (APA, 1987) criteria with disruptive behavioral disorders (7, CD; 2, ODD; and 1, ADHD). Most had comorbid drug abuse or dependency (5, marijuana abuse; 3, marijuana dependency; and 1, alcohol abuse). All 10 subjects had severe unpredictable mood swings and a low threshold/high amplitude for dyscontrol once irritable, with frequent and severe temper tantrums ("explosive mood disorder"), which preceded drug abuse by at least 1 year. Efficacy was determined based on multiple informants' (subjects, parents, and teachers) reports of temper outbursts and mood lability and the Global Assessment of Functioning (GAF; Axis V of the DSM-III-R diagnoses) Scale.

Divalproex sodium was initiated at a dose of 250 mg/day and titrated to 1,000 mg/day over a period of 2 to 4 weeks. The mean plasma valproate level after receiving 1,000 mg/day of divalproex for 1 week was 75 µg/mL (range 45 to 113 µg/mL). At the end of the fifth week, all 10 subjects showed significant improvement on all three measures; 9 subjects had no temper outbursts during the fifth week, and 6 subjects had no significant mood lability. Their mean number of temper outbursts decreased from 6.5 ± 4.5 at baseline to 0.1 ± 0.3 after 5 weeks ($P < .001$). The mean mood lability score (0 = least to 4 = greater frequency, duration, and autonomy of mood swings) decreased from 3.8 ± 0.4 at baseline to

0.5 ± 0.7 after 5 weeks ($P < .000$). The mean GAF score improved from 37.8 ± 7.0 at baseline to 65.7 ± 10.2 after 5 weeks ($P < .000$). Divalproex was well tolerated with only two patients reporting mild sedation and transient nausea. There were no serious untoward effects, and liver function tests showed no significant changes. Improvements were maintained while on medication during follow-up; however, five subjects independently discontinued medication for at least 5 days and rapidly relapsed; improvement recurred within a few days of resuming medication. A sixth patient took medication sporadically during follow-up and maintained gains for approximately 6 weeks, when partial relapse occurred. These data suggest that divalproex sodium may be safe and efficacious in such adolescents though further studies should be undertaken (Donovan et al., 1997).

Donovan et al. (2000) conducted a 12-week, randomly assigned, double-blind, placebo-controlled, crossover study of divalproex sodium in the treatment of 20 outpatients (16 males, 4 females; mean age, 13.8 ± 2.4 years; age range, 10 to 18 years), all of whom were diagnosed with CD or ODD by DSM-IV (APA, 1994) criteria and chronic explosive temper (more than four episodes monthly of rage, property destruction, or fighting with minimal provocation) and mood lability (multiple daily unpredictable shifts in mood from normal to irritable and withdrawn to boisterous behavior). Four subjects were diagnosed with comorbid ADHD and six with marijuana abuse. Efficacy was assessed by ratings on the Modified OAS and on six items from the anger-hostility subscale of the Symptom Checklist-90 (SCL-90); it was decided *a priori* that "responders" had to have a $\geq 70\%$ reduction from baseline scores on both rating scales. The first 6 weeks of the study consisted of a parallel-groups design, with 10 subjects randomly assigned to valproate or placebo. Divalproex was gradually titrated to 10 mg/lb/day over the first 2 weeks; if the plasma level of valproate was <90 µg/mL at that time, a single increase of 250 mg/day was added. (To preserve the blind, a similar number of increases were made in the placebo group.) Doses ranged from 750 to 1,500 mg/day, and the mean plasma valproate level was 82.2 ± 19.1 µg/mL. At the end of this 6-week phase, 8 (80%) of the 10 patients receiving divalproex were rated as responders versus no responders in the 10 subjects on placebo ($P < .001$). Seventeen subjects completed phase I (during the first 2 weeks, one subject on divalproex dropped out as he was incarcerated for parole violation and two subjects on placebo dropped out for lack of clinical improvement). Fifteen subjects (eight responders to divalproex and seven nonresponders to placebo) entered the crossover phase of the study (weeks 7 to 12), and all completed it. Six (86%) of the seven placebo nonresponders during phase I responded to divalproex during phase II. Six of the eight responders to divalproex during phase I began relapsing between 1 and 2 weeks into phase II, and at the end of week 12, their average Modified OAS score had worsened to only 33% over baseline and their average anger-hostility scores on the subscale of the SCL-90 declined to 27% over baseline. Of the 15 subjects completing the entire study, 12 met "responder" criteria only during the medication phase, suggesting that divalproex is significantly better than placebo ($P = .003$) in this population.

Valproic Acid in the Treatment of Children and Adolescents Diagnosed with Mental Retardation and Mood Disorders

Kastner et al. (1990) reported treating three patients with valproic acid, a 16-year-old male with moderate mental retardation and two girls with profound mental retardation (ages 8 and 13 years). All three patients had symptoms of a comorbid mood disorder, including self-injurious behaviors such as face gouging and head banging, irritability, aggressiveness, hyperactivity, sleep disturbance, and paroxysms of crying. All had unsatisfactory responses to trials of several other medications. All three patients showed excellent response to valproic acid and at follow-up had maintained their gains for 7 to 10 months. Maintenance doses were 2,700 mg/day (plasma level, 109 µg/mL) for the 16-year-old, 3,000 mg/day (plasma level, 75 µg/mL) for the 13-year-old, and 1,500 mg/day (plasma level, 111 µg/mL) for the 8-year-old. The authors noted that the plasma levels were high or just above the typical therapeutic upper range and that no hepatic abnormalities developed in their patients.

In a 2-year prospective study, Kastner et al. (1993) administered valproic acid to 21 patients diagnosed with mental retardation who also had behavioral symptoms of irritability, sleep disturbance, aggressive or self-injurious behavior, and behavioral cycling that were interpreted as symptomatic of an affective disorder. Eighteen patients completed the study. (Two were lost to follow-up, and one developed acute hyperammonemia and was dropped from the study.) Twelve of the patients completing the study were 18 years old or younger; the degree of mental retardation ranged from moderate to profound. Valproic acid was titrated upward until symptoms remitted or untoward effects prevented further increase, to plasma levels between 50 and 125 µg/mL. Patients' ratings on the CGI-S Scale after 2 years on medication were significantly improved ($P < .001$) from ratings at baseline. Patients with a diagnosis of epilepsy or a suspicion of seizures correlated with a positive response ($P < .005$). Of note, 9 of the 10 patients who were receiving neuroleptic drugs at the beginning of the study were no longer being prescribed these drugs at the study's completion.

Divalproex Sodium in the Treatment of Children and Adolescents Diagnosed with PDDs

Hellings et al. (2005) conducted a double-blind, placebo-controlled study to evaluate the efficacy of valproate (VPA) in treating aggressive symptoms in 30 subjects (20 male and 10 female; age range 6 to 20 years) who were diagnosed with a PDD by DSM-IV criteria (27 were diagnosed with autistic disorder, 1 with PDDNOS, and 2 with Asperger disorder). Comorbid diagnoses, with the exception of Tourette disorder were permitted. No other psychotropic medications or antiseizure medications were permitted. Subjects exhibited significant aggression toward themselves or others, or to property, a minimum of three times weekly. Twenty-six subjects had IQs in the mentally retarded range. Subjects were randomly assigned to liquid placebo ($N = 14$) or liquid VPA ($N = 16$) for a period of 8 weeks, following a 1-week lead-in on placebo. In the VPA group, the liquid placebo was gradually replaced by liquid VPA beginning with a 250 mg/5 mL dose. VPA liquid (250 mg/5 mL) was added every 3 days to reach a target dose of 20 mg/kg/day. A psychiatrist not involved in ratings adjusted the VPA to achieve trough plasma levels of 70 to 100 µg/mL after measurement at the end of 2 and 4 weeks. Mean VPA trough plasma levels were 75.5 µg/mL at week 4 and 77.8 µ/mL at week 8.

There were no statistically significant differences between the two groups on the primary outcome measure, the Aberrant Behavior Checklist–Community Scale (ABC-C; $P = .65$), or the secondary outcome measures, the Clinical Global Impressions–Improvement subscale (CGI-I; $P = .16$), and the OAS ($P = .96$). The CGI–Severity subscale (CGI-S) also showed no statistical difference between the groups ($P = .96$).

Adverse effects were usually mild. One subject on VPA developed a rash and dropped out of the study. Increased appetite was the only adverse effect that was significantly greater in the VPA group ($P = .03$). Gastrointestinal complaints, sedation, headache, chills, and fever did not differ. Two subjects on VPA had elevations of ammonia above the normal range of 21 to 50 µmol/L, and the parent of one of these subjects reported cognitive slowing and slurred speech at times (ammonia was 98 µmol/L at the end of the study).

The authors noted that there was high intrasubject variability with large differences in the frequency and severity of aggression in different weeks, and high intersubject variability with large standard deviations for each of the outcome measures, which weakened study power. Following completion of the study,

10 subjects on VPA elected to continue on the drug and 6 on placebo elected to an open trial of VPA. Ten of these 16 subjects continued to demonstrate a positive and sustained response. The authors concluded that although this study did not demonstrate efficacy of VPA, there might be a subgroup of aggressive children and adolescents with PDD who respond favorably to VPA and that a larger, multisite study is indicated.

Hollander et al. (2006) studied divalproex sodium for the treatment of repetitive behaviors in autism in an 8-week double-blind placebo-controlled trial involving 13 patients with autism spectrum disorder (ASD). The average age of subjects was 9.5 years (12 subjects were child/adolescent patients and 1 subject was 40 years old). Nine subjects were randomized into the treatment group and four into the placebo group. The primary outcome measure was the Children's Yale-Brown Obsessive Compulsive Scale (C-YBOCS), Compulsion subscale. The mean serum divalproex level at the end of the study was 58.23 ± 21.63 μg/mL. Authors reported a significant improvement in repetitive behavior scores for subjects taking divalproex (average improvement of 0.889 points), and a worsening of behavior scores with patients taking placebo (average worsening of 2.5 points). A large effect size of $d = 1.53$ was reported for divalproex sodium. Ultimately, none of the patients in the placebo group maintained or improved their C-YBOCS scores, while 77% of the divalproex group did. There were no statistically significant differences in adverse effects between the two study groups. The authors concluded that this study provides preliminary support for the successful use of divalproex sodium in the treatment of repetitive behaviors in patients with ASD (Hollander et al., 2005). The small sample size and short study duration are important limitations to consider with this study, however.

Hollander et al. (2010) also conducted a 12-week randomized double-blind, placebo-controlled trial studying the efficacy of divalproex sodium for the treatment of irritability in 27 youth with ASDs. Primary outcome measures included the Clinical Global Impression–Improvement Scale (CGI-I) focusing on irritability and the irritability subscale of the Aberrant Behavior Checklist (ABC). Sixteen subjects were randomized to active treatment and 11 subjects to placebo. The study authors reported that 62.5% of the subjects randomized to active treatment showed a reduction in irritability according to CGI-I scores versus only 9.09% in the placebo arm. Analysis of ABC–irritability subscale scores revealed that subjects receiving divalproex sodium benefitted from a drop of >0.53 points/week compared with subjects who were randomized to placebo. It was noted that treatment responders had higher mean valproate levels (89.77 μg/mL) than nonresponders (64.33 μg/mL). Response noted per the CGI–Irritability Scale was found to be dose dependent in this study. For example, subjects with valproate levels between 87 and 110 μg/mL showed a 100% response rate, whereas subjects with levels <87 μg/mL had a reduced response rate of 60%. Subjects with valproate levels >110 μg/mL experienced the lowest response rate (33%). Divalproex sodium was well tolerated overall, with side effects ranging from mild to moderate, and no serious adverse events were reported. The study authors concluded that this study suggests valproate may be beneficial for the treatment of irritability associated with ASD, though larger studies are needed to support or refute findings (Hollander et al., 2010).

Carbamazepine (Tegretol; Carbatrol; Equetro)

Note: The FDA has directed that Black Box warnings be added to the labeling of carbamazepine products indicating that the risk of developing APLASTIC ANEMIA AND AGRANULOCYTOSIS is five to eight times greater than in the general population, although the incidence is very low. Most cases of leukopenia do not progress to the more serious aplastic anemia or agranulocytosis. However, complete pretreatment hematologic testing should be obtained as a baseline. If low or decreased white blood cell or platelet count occurs during treatment, close monitoring should be implemented and discontinuing carbamazepine should be seriously considered if there is any evidence of bone marrow depression. Carbamazepine also carries the risk for SERIOUS DERMATOLOGICAL REACTIONS including toxic epidermal necrolysis (TEN) and Stevens-Johnson syndrome (SJS). These reactions are estimated to occur in 1 to 6 per 10,000 new users in countries with predominantly Caucasian populations. The risk for TEN and SJS is estimated to be approximately 10 times higher in some Asian countries. Studies in patients with Chinese ancestry revealed a strong association between the HLA-B*1502 allele and the risk of developing serious dermatological reactions while taking carbamazepine. It is recommended that patients with at-risk ancestry be screened for the presence of HLA-B*1502 prior to initiating carbamazepine treatment. Patients who are positive for this allele should not be treated with carbamazepine unless the benefit carefully outweighs the risk.

In addition to the Black Box warnings described above, in 2008 the FDA issued an alert advising providers to monitor patients who are taking or starting antiepileptic medication for any changes in behavior that could indicate the emergence of depression or worsening suicidal thoughts or behavior (PDR.net, 2008).

Carbamazepine is an anticonvulsant indicated for the treatment of psychomotor and grand mal seizures. It is also a specific analgesic for trigeminal neuralgia.

Pharmacokinetics of Carbamazepine

Peak serum levels occur 4 to 5 hours after ingestion of standard carbamazepine tablets. Initial serum half-life values range from 25 to 65 hours; however, carbamazepine is an autoinducer of its own metabolism. Autoinduction stabilizes over 3 to 5 weeks at a fixed dose, with half-life decreasing to 12 to 17 hours. In children, there is a poor correlation between dose and serum level of carbamazepine.

Contraindications for Carbamazepine Administration

Known hypersensitivity to carbamazepine or tricyclic antidepressants, a history of previous bone marrow depression, and the ingestion of a monoamine oxidase inhibitor (MAOI) within the previous 14 days are contraindications. Coadministration with nefazodone or lurasidone is also contraindicated.

Interactions of Carbamazepine with Other Drugs

Carbamazepine is both a CYP3A4 substrate and an inducer. As such, it will reduce plasma levels of other CYP3A4 substrates (clozapine, benzodiazepines, hormonal contraceptives, warfarin, etc.). Other CYP3A4 inhibitors will raise carbamazepine levels (cimetidine, azoles, macrolides, etc.). When coadministered with risperidone (6 mg/day) over a 3-week period, plasma concentrations of risperidone and 9-hydroxyrisperidone were decreased by approximately 50%. Plasma levels of carbamazepine did not appear to be effected. Carbamazepine also reduces serum levels of haloperidol and aripiprazole.

When coadministered with olanzapine, carbamazepine in doses of 200 mg twice daily caused approximately 50% increase in the clearance of olanzapine. This was thought to be secondary to carbamazepine's being a potent inducer of CYP1A2 activity. Higher daily doses of carbamazepine may cause an even greater increase in olanzapine clearance.

Carbamazepine serum levels are markedly reduced by the simultaneous use of phenobarbital, phenytoin, or primidone.

Increased lithium serum concentrations and increased risk of neurotoxic lithium effects may occur when carbamazepine and lithium are used simultaneously because carbamazepine decreases lithium renal clearance.

Carbamazepine may cause thyroid dysfunction when used with other anticonvulsants and may result in increased isoniazid-induced hepatotoxicity when used with isoniazid (PDR.net, 2012).

The FDA has advised that carbamazepine may lose up to one-third of its potency if stored under humid conditions such as in a bathroom. Supplies should be kept tightly closed and in a dry location.

Untoward Effects of Carbamazepine

Evans et al. (1987) attributed the increased interest in the use of carbamazepine in child and adolescent psychiatry in part to both the increased awareness of the serious untoward long-term complications of standard neuroleptic drugs and the finding that the untoward effects of carbamazepine are less formidable than initially thought. In particular, the serious blood dyscrasias, agranulocytosis, and aplastic anemia are very rare. The risk of developing these disorders when treated with carbamazepine is five to eight times that of the general population. Agranulocytosis occurs in approximately six per million and aplastic anemia in approximately two per million of the untreated general population (*PDR*, 2000).

The most frequently reported untoward effects are dizziness, drowsiness, unsteadiness, nausea, and vomiting. These are more likely to occur if treatment is not begun with the low doses recommended. As noted earlier, aplastic anemia and agranulocytosis, although rare, have been reported. Hence, a complete baseline hematologic evaluation must be done and complete blood cell count with differential and platelets must be repeated and monitored closely throughout the treatment. Liver dysfunction, cardiovascular complications, and hyponatremia have been reported.

Carbamazepine is classified as pregnancy category D and should not be prescribed to those who are pregnant or nursing. Carbamazepine use in pregnancy has been associated with neural tube defects, craniofacial abnormalities, growth retardation, and cardiac defects.

Pleak et al. (1988) reported that adverse behavioral and neurologic reactions developed in 6 of their 20 male subjects, aged 10 to 16, who were diagnosed with various disorders, but primarily with ADHD and CD, and who were participating in an ongoing protocol evaluating the efficacy of carbamazepine in treating severe aggressive outbursts in child and adolescent inpatients. The untoward effects included a severe manic episode in a 16-year-old, hypomania in a 10-year-old, and increased irritability, impulsivity, and aggressiveness and/or worsening of behavior in two subjects aged 14 and 15. Two 11-year-old boys developed EEG abnormalities, with sharp waves and spikes. One of these boys improved behaviorally but had his first two absence seizures in several years. The authors caution that patients must be monitored carefully for the development of adverse neuropsychiatric effects.

Carbamazepine and the Induction of Mania

Three additional cases of carbamazepine-induced mania have been reported in children (Myers and Carrera, 1989; Reiss and O'Donnell, 1984). Myers and Carrera speculated that when adverse behavioral effects such as irritability, insomnia, agitation, talkativeness, and prepubescent hypersexuality occur with carbamazepine administration, they may be symptoms of an unrecognized hypomania or mania.

Indications for Carbamazepine

Carbamazepine is approved for use in patients at least 6 years of age for the treatment of various seizure types. Patients diagnosed with partial seizures with complex symptomatology (psychomotor or temporal lobe) tend to benefit the most from carbamazepine, but patients with generalized tonic-clonic (grand mal) seizures or a mixed seizure pattern may also improve. Absence (petit mal) seizures are not controlled by

(continued)

Indications for Carbamazepine *(continued)*

carbamazepine. Patients with trigeminal and glossopharyngeal neuralgias have shown reduction in pain when treated with carbamazepine. There are no FDA-approved psychiatric indications for carbamazepine.

Carbamazepine Dosage Schedule

The following are doses recommended for treatment of epilepsy. It is recommended that carbamazepine be taken with meals.

- *Children under 6 years of age:* 10 to 20 mg/kg/day b.i.d. or t.i.d. Increase the dose weekly to achieve optimal clinical response, t.i.d. or q.i.d. The maximum daily dose is 35 mg/kg/24 hour.
- *Children 6 through 12 years of age:* Begin with a dose of 100 mg twice daily (or 50 mg four times daily if suspension is used). The dose may be increased weekly by increments of 100 mg (b.i.d. regimen for carbamazepine XR, and a t.i.d. or q.i.d. regimen for other formulations) to obtain optimal response. The daily dose should not usually exceed 1,000 mg. Usual maintenance daily dose is 400 to 800 mg.
- *Patients >12 years old:* Begin with a dose of 200 mg twice daily (or 100 mg four times daily if suspension is used). The dose may be increased weekly by increments of 200 mg as clinically indicated to obtain optimal response. Carbamazepine XR tablets may be dosed b.i.d., whereas all other preparations should be dosed t.i.d. or q.i.d. The daily dose should not usually exceed 1,000 mg for children ages 12 to 15, or 1,200 mg daily for children older than 15 years. Usual maintenance daily dose is 800 to 1,200 mg. Usual therapeutic carbamazepine plasma levels are 4 to 12 μg/mL.

Carbamazepine Dose Forms Available

- *Tablets:* 200 mg
- *Chewable tablets:* 100 mg
- *Suspension:* 100 mg/5 mL
- *Extended-release tablets (Tegretol-XR):* 100, 200, and 400 mg
- *Extended-release capsules (Carbatrol; Equetro):* 100, 200, and 300 mg

---

▌ *Reports of Interest*

Carbamazepine Use for Nonspecific Pediatric Behavioral Symptoms

Remschmidt (1976) reviewed data from 28 clinical trials (seven double-blind and 21 open studies) with a total of >800 nonepileptic child and adolescent subjects who were treated with carbamazepine. Positive clinical results were found for target symptoms of hyperactivity or hypoactivity, impaired concentration, aggressive behavioral disturbances, and dysphoric mood disorders. In addition to these behavioral effects, Remschmidt suggested that these patients experienced positive mood changes, increased initiative, and decreased anxiety.

Groh (1976) reported on 62 nonepileptic children treated with carbamazepine for various abnormal behavioral patterns. Of the 27 who showed improvement, most had a "dysphoric or dysthymic syndrome," the most important features of which were emotional lability and moodiness, which were thought to cause most of the other behavioral abnormalities.

Kuhn-Gebhart (1976) reported symptom improvement in a large number of nonepileptic children who were treated with carbamazepine for a wide variety of behavioral disorders. The author reported that 30 of the last 50 patients treated showed good or very good responses, 10 had discernible improvement, 9 had no change in behavior, and 1 deteriorated. The author noted that the more abnormal the EEGs of these nonepileptic patients are in general, the better the response; that many of the good responders came from stable homes; and that poorer results were more frequent in subjects from unfavorable homes.

Puente (1976) reported an open study in which carbamazepine was administered to 72 children with various behavioral disorders who did not have evidence of neurologic disease. Fifty-six children completed the study. The usual optimal dose was 300 mg/day (range, 100 to 600 mg/day). Carbamazepine was given for an average of 12 weeks (range, 9 to 23 weeks). Twenty symptoms were rated on a severity scale at the beginning and end of the treatment. Individual symptoms were present in as many as 55 and in as few as 2 of the 56 children. Over the course of treatment, a decrease in symptom expression of 70% or more occurred in 17 of 20 symptoms in at least 60% of the subjects. Interestingly, all 6 children (100%) with night terrors responded positively, as did 16 (94%) of the 17 children with other sleep disturbances. Anxiety, present in 47 children, improved in 34 (72%). Enuresis improved in 8 of 9 children (89%), and aggressiveness, present in 46 children, improved in 32 (70%). The most frequent untoward effects were transient drowsiness (20%), nausea and vomiting (4%), and urticaria (4%).

Carbamazepine in the Treatment of Juvenile-Onset Bipolar I Disorder

Woolston (1999) reported three cases diagnosed with bipolar I disorder whom he treated successfully with carbamazepine. One case, a 16-year-old female, had experienced several cycles of mania followed by depression that was managed with various neuroleptics and lithium for approximately 4 years. The patient was noncompliant with lithium at least three times, resulting in manic episodes within a month that were followed by severe depression. Following the last of these episodes, she was started on carbamazepine, 150 mg/day, which was increased to 300 mg/day 3 weeks later and continued at that dosage. Her serum carbamazepine level was 7 µg/mL. The patient became euthymic within 3 weeks and remained so on 300 mg/day of carbamazepine over the next 4 years, with the exception of three brief hypomanic episodes that responded to the addition of a short course of haloperidol 1 mg/day. No untoward effects were reported and blood counts and liver function remained within normal limits.

A 14-year-old male with mania who was treated with lithium for approximately 2 years discontinued his lithium because it made him tired and dysphoric. He subsequently developed another manic episode. Carbamazepine was initiated at a dose of 100 mg/day and was increased to 200 mg/day 5 days later. His mania improved significantly within 15 days and he did not experience the unpleasant symptoms he associated with lithium. His carbamazepine serum level was 8 µg/mL. He remained euthymic on carbamazepine 200 mg/day for the next 3 years with serum levels ranging from 6 to 9 µg/mL. No untoward effects were reported and blood counts and liver chemistries remained normal throughout his treatment.

The third case was a 12.5-year-old girl, also diagnosed with spastic cerebral palsy and mild mental retardation. She was treated briefly with risperidone for persistent euphoric mood, decreased need for sleep, and intermittent hallucinations. After 3 weeks, she had increased manic symptoms with flight of ideas, pressured speech, motor restlessness, and nearly continuous visual hallucinations with poor reality testing. Risperidone was discontinued and carbamazepine 100 mg/day was begun. After 1 week, she showed improvement in sleep and reality testing and no untoward effects. Carbamazepine was then increased to 200 mg/day. Six days later, hallucinations had totally remitted, she was euthymic, had no evidence of a thought disorder, and her normal sleep pattern returned. Her serum carbamazepine level was 8 µg/mL. The patient was continued on maintenance carbamazepine, 200 mg/day. Over the next 2 years, she developed two brief periods of hypomania, both of which responded rapidly to an additional 50 mg of carbamazepine. She remained euthymic on her final maintenance daily dose of 300 mg of carbamazepine.

Craven and Margaret (2000) reported a case of a 16-year-old boy with cerebral palsy and comorbid bipolar disorder who had a favorable response to carbamazepine treatment. At the age of 9 years, this patient began to experience mood instability. His mood varied between depression and inappropriate elation, and he spoke of seeing monsters. During depressive episodes, he would refuse to eat and would become uncommunicative. Extensive medical work-ups were negative. He was initially diagnosed with a depressive disorder. A trial of imipramine proved ineffective and so was discontinued. A trial of Prozac was then started, which resulted in restlessness, insomnia, and an objectively elated mood. His diagnosis was later changed to bipolar disorder and carbamazepine 200 mg twice daily was started. Within 1 month of starting carbamazepine, his mood returned to baseline, and at the time of the case report, he was reported to have remained stable for a period of 18 months (Craven and Margaret, 2000).

Davanzo (2003) conducted a retrospective review of clinical changes during the hospitalization of 44 preadolescent bipolar youth, who were treated with either lithium, carbamazepine, or divalproex sodium. Four trained clinicians, who were blinded to the treatment group, reviewed daily progress notes and discharge summaries and rated them according to the Clinical Global Impression–Improvement (CGI-I) scale. Length of hospitalization, severity of illness at admission, and comorbidity did not differ between treatment groups. Each group approached serum therapeutic levels for their respective medication at day 7 of hospitalization. The author reported that the mean CGI-I scores were systematically higher, or worse, for carbamazepine compared with lithium and divalproex. This difference was statistically significant by week 2 of the hospitalization. The author concluded that carbamazepine may be less effective than lithium or divalproex sodium for the treatment of preadolescent patients with bipolar disorder though acknowledged numerous limitations of this retrospective study (Davanzo, 2003).

In an open trial, Kowatch et al. (2000) studied 42 outpatients with bipolar disorder who were randomized to receive divalproate, lithium, or carbamazepine for 6 weeks in a nonblind fashion. Response rates were calculated at 53% for divalproate and 38% for both lithium and carbamazepine. All had large effect sizes (1.63 for divalproex sodium, 1.06 for lithium, and 1.00 for carbamazepine) (Kowatch et al., 2000). This study is summarized in the valproic acid section of this book.

Joshi et al. (2010) conducted an 8-week prospective open-label trial of extended-release carbamazepine (CBZ-ER) for the treatment of 27 youth with bipolar disorder (9.1 ± 1.9 years of age). CBZ-ER doses averaged 788 ± 252 mg/day. Three subjects continued their long-standing stimulant medication for comorbid ADHD. The YMRS, CGI-I, Child Depression Rating Scale (CDRS), and BPRS were used to assess response to treatment. Response was identified as having a >30% reduction in YMRS scores or by being rated "improved" or "very much improved" on the CGI-I for mania. At the end of the study, 52% of subjects had a 30% reduction in YMRS scores and 44% had a 50% reduction in YMRS scores. Thirty-three percent of subjects were judged to be "improved" or "very much improved" on CGI-I scores. Based on the defined response criteria (either a 30% reduction on YMRS or CGI-Mania Improvement score of ≤2), the rate of antimanic response was 63%. Investigators concluded that CBZ-ER treatment resulted in statistically significant, but modest, improvements in YMRS scores, and resulted in significant improvement in symptoms of depression, ADHD, and psychotic symptoms. CBZ-ER was deemed well tolerated during the trial. Two subjects had to discontinue the medication due to rash, though in both cases the rash was nonprogressive and resolved within 1 week of discontinuing CBZ-ER. The most common adverse events reported were headache (23%), gastrointestinal complaints (18%), cold symptoms (15%), dizziness (8%), aches and pains (8%), and insomnia (4%). No lab abnormalities were detected. Study authors concluded that based on this open study, CBZ-ER may be effective for the treatment of pediatric bipolar disorder, though acknowledged modest response rates compared with atypical antipsychotic medication (Joshi et al., 2010).

Carbamazepine in the Treatment of Children Diagnosed with CD

Kafantaris et al. (1992) reported an open pilot study in which 10 children (9 male, 1 female; age range, 5.25 to 10.92 years; mean, 8.27 years), diagnosed with CD and hospitalized for symptoms of explosive aggressiveness, were treated with carbamazepine. Five of the subjects previously failed to respond to lithium. One week after enrollment, carbamazepine was administered in three divided doses, beginning with 200 mg/day and titrated over 3 to 5 weeks to a maximum of 800 mg/day, or a serum level of 12 µg/mL. Optimal dose range was 600 to 800 mg/day (mean, 630 mg/day) with serum levels from 4.8 to 10.4 µg/mL (mean, 6.2 µg/mL). Target symptoms of aggressiveness and explosiveness declined significantly on all measures compared with baseline ratings. On the Global Clinical Consensus Ratings, four subjects were rated as markedly improved, four as moderately improved, one as slightly improved, and one as not improved. Three of the lithium nonresponders showed marked improvement, and one showed moderate improvement; the fifth did not respond to either drug. Untoward effects during regulation and at optimal dose included fatigue (2 of 10 cases), blurred vision (2 of 10), and dizziness (1 of 10). Untoward effects above optimal dose included diplopia (2 of 10), mild ataxia (2 of 10), mild dysarthria (1 of 10), headache (2 of 10), and lethargy (1 of 10). One child experienced worsening of preexisting behavioral symptoms and loosening of associations, which were thought to be manifestations of behavioral toxicity. Overall, the untoward effects were transient and were decreased or eliminated by carbamazepine dose reduction. White blood cell counts remained within normal limits, although four children had reductions from baseline determinations.

Cueva et al. (1996) reported a 9-week, double-blind, placebo-controlled study comparing carbamazepine and placebo in 22 children (20 males, 2 females; mean age, 8.97 years; age range, 5.33 to 11.7 years) who were diagnosed with CD, solitary aggressive type by DSM-III-R (APA, 1987) criteria and who required hospitalization for treatment-resistant aggressiveness and explosiveness. Thirty-eight children who met protocol criteria entered the initial 2-week placebo washout period. At the end of this period, 14 were eliminated because they no longer met study or aggression criteria. Of the 24 subjects who entered the treatment phase of the study, 13 were assigned to carbamazepine and 11 to placebo; 22 subjects completed the study. Efficacy was measured using the Children's Psychiatric Rating Scale, the NIMH CGI-S and, CGI–Improvement (CGI-I) scales, the OAS, and the Global Clinical Judgments (Consensus) Scale, with a blind rating by all clinical staff occurring just before the code is broken. Medication was dispensed in two capsules given three times daily throughout the study. Carbamazepine was initiated at a dose of 200 mg/day and increased over a 2-week period in predetermined steps of 200 mg/dose to a maximum of 1,000 mg/day or until therapeutic effects were observed or untoward effects prevented further increase. For the 11 subjects for whom values were available, the mean optimal dose of carbamazepine was 683 mg/day (range, 400 to 800 mg/day), and the mean serum carbamazepine level was 6.81 µg/mL (range, 4.98 to 9.1 µg/mL).

The results showed no significant differences in the clinical improvement of aggression between carbamazepine and placebo on any of the rating scales. Both groups improved on the aggression factor of the Children's Psychiatric Rating Scale over time and both improved similarly on the Global Clinical Judgments (Consensus) Scale as rated by clinical staff. Carbamazepine treatment resulted in significantly more untoward effects than placebo. Twelve of the 13 subjects on carbamazepine reported a total of 57 untoward effects, whereas only 6 of 11 subjects on placebo reported six untoward effects. Two subjects on carbamazepine developed marked leukopenia (2,000 to 3,000 WBC/mm^3), and four developed moderate leukopenia (3,000 to 3,500 WBC/mm^3); one subject on placebo also developed moderate leukopenia. Leukopenia was transient in all seven cases. Other untoward effects experienced by the treatment group subjects included dizziness ($N = 7$, 54%), rash ($N = 6$, 46%), headache (46%), diplopia ($N = 5$, 38%), drowsiness ($N = 4$, 31%), nausea (31%), ataxia ($N = 3$, 23%), and vomiting (23%) (Cueva et al., 1996).

Carbamazepine in the Treatment of Children and Adolescents with Symptoms of ADHD

Silva et al. (1996) searched the world literature for reports in which carbamazepine was used to treat children and adolescents with behavioral problems and hyperactivity. Twenty-nine such reports were located; 10 of them provided information suitable for a meta-analysis. Seven studies, with a total of 189 patients, were open; 70% of subjects experienced at least a marked improvement in target symptoms (significance ranged from $P < .001$ to $P = .05$). There was a significant correlation between longer treatment and positive outcome. In the three double-blind studies, 53 subjects were assigned to carbamazepine and 52 to placebo. Thirty-eight (72%) subjects on carbamazepine and 14 (27%) subjects on placebo were rated as moderately to markedly improved. Meta-analysis of these three studies found carbamazepine significantly ($P = .018$) more efficacious than placebo in diminishing target symptoms. The most common untoward effects in the studies reviewed were sedation and rash. The authors concluded that carbamazepine merited further study as a possible second-line treatment for children and adolescents with ADHD that is not responsive to stimulant medication or when stimulant medication cannot be tolerated.

Note: The FDA has directed that Black Box Warnings be added to the labeling of carbamazepine products indicating CARDIOVASCULAR RISK WITH RAPID IV INFUSION.

Phenytoin, Diphenylhydantoin (Dilantin)

Note: In 2008, the FDA issued an alert advising providers to monitor patients who are taking or starting antiepileptic medication for any changes in behavior that could indicate the emergence of depression or worsening suicidal thoughts or behavior (PDR.net, 2008).

Contraindications for Phenytoin Administration

Known hypersensitivity to the phenytoin or a related drug is a contraindication.
Phenytoin is classified as pregnancy category D and is not for use in nursing.

Interactions of Phenytoin with Other Drugs

Acute alcohol intake may increase serum phenytoin levels, whereas chronic alcohol use may decrease levels.

Tricyclic antidepressants may precipitate seizures in susceptible patients, necessitating increased phenytoin doses.

Specific drugs have been reported to increase, decrease, or either increase or decrease phenytoin levels. Obtaining serum phenytoin levels may help clarify the situation when necessary. Some drugs that increase phenytoin levels are alcohol (when acutely ingested), benzodiazepines, phenothiazines, salicylates, and methylphenidate. Some drugs that decrease phenytoin levels are carbamazepine, alcohol (with chronic abuse), and molindone.

Interactions of phenytoin and phenobarbital, valproic acid, and sodium valproate are unpredictable, and serum levels of the drugs involved may either increase or decrease.

Reports of Interest (Phenytoin)

Three double-blind, placebo-controlled studies that treated children and adolescents with phenytoin (diphenylhydantoin) for psychiatric disorders reported that it was not significantly better than placebo.

Lefkowitz (1969) reviewed some of the earlier literature in which phenytoin was administered, primarily on an open basis, to nonepileptic children with psychiatric disorders with discrepant results. Lefkowitz compared the efficacy of placebo and phenytoin in treating disruptive behavior in male juvenile delinquents (mean age, 14 years, 11 months; range, 13 to 16 years, 3 months) in a residential treatment center. Each group contained 25 subjects. Phenytoin or placebo was administered in doses of 100 mg twice daily for 76 days. Both groups showed marked reductions in disruptive behavior. Phenytoin, however, was not significantly better than placebo on any of the 11 behavioral measures. In fact, placebo was significantly more efficacious than phenytoin in diminishing distress, unhappiness, negativism, and aggressiveness. The author suggested that mild toxic effects of phenytoin, such as insomnia, irritability, quarrelsomeness, ataxia, and gastric distress, may have accounted for the superiority of placebo.

Looker and Conners (1970) administered phenytoin to 17 children and adolescents (mean age, 9.1 years; range, 5.5 to 14.5 years) who had severe temper tantrums and suspected minimal brain dysfunction. Eleven subjects had normal EEGs, three had mildly abnormal EEGs, and three had abnormal EEGs, but no subject had clinical seizures. Subjects were placed on a 9-week, double-blind, placebo-controlled, crossover protocol, and phenytoin was titrated to achieve blood levels of at least 10 µg/mL. Twelve of the 13 subjects had adequate levels to suppress epileptic discharge. Scores on the Continuous Performance Test, the Porteus Maze Test, parent questionnaires for all subjects, and school questionnaires for 11 subjects showed no statistically significant differences between phenytoin and placebo. The authors noted, however, that some individual subjects appeared to respond positively and rather dramatically to phenytoin.

Conners et al. (1971) treated 43 particularly aggressive or disturbed delinquent males (mean age, 12 years; range, 9 to 14 years) living in a residential training school with phenytoin (200 mg/day), methylphenidate (20 mg/day), or placebo administered for 2 weeks in a double-blind protocol. Although the authors noted some limitations in their study, they found no significant difference between drugs and placebo on ratings by cottage parents, teachers, clinicians, and scores on the Rosenzweig Picture Frustration Test and Porteus Maze Test.

Overall, although there are individual patients without seizure disorder who appear to benefit from phenytoin, as yet there is no convincing evidence for the effectiveness of phenytoin prescribed for psychiatric symptoms.

Gabapentin (Neurontin)

Note: In 2008, the FDA issued an alert advising providers to monitor patients who are taking or starting antiepileptic medication for any changes in behavior that could indicate the emergence of depression or worsening suicidal thoughts or behavior (PDR.net, 2008).

Pharmacokinetics of Gabapentin

Gabapentin is not significantly metabolized in humans. It is eliminated unchanged by renal secretion, which is directly proportional to creatinine clearance. Half-life is 5 to 7 hours, and food has no effect on its absorption or excretion. Bioavailability of gabapentin decreases with dose, with a greater percentage of lower doses being available; at doses of approximately 600 mg/day and higher, it stabilizes at approximately 60% of the dose being available.

Contraindications for the Administration of Gabapentin

Gabapentin is contraindicated for patients with known hypersensitivity to the drug.

Interactions of Gabapentin with Other Drugs

Antacids, calcium carbonate, iron, magnesium, and ginkgo may decrease gabapentin's efficacy. Naproxen sodium may increase gabapentin levels. Gabapentin may decrease levels of hydrocodone in a dose-dependent manner.

Untoward Effects of Gabapentin

The most common untoward effects reported somnolence, dizziness, ataxia, fatigue, and nystagmus. Many other effects have been reported.

Gabapentin Mechanism and Indications

Gabapentin is an anticonvulsant whose mechanism of action is unknown. Gabapentin is indicated as adjunctive therapy in the treatment of partial seizures with and without secondary generalization in persons >12 years old, as adjunctive therapy in the treatment of partial seizures in pediatrics 3 to 12 years old, and for management of postherpetic neuralgia (PHN) in adults. Gabapentin is not approved for any psychiatric indication at this time. The manufacturer notes that it is not necessary to monitor serum levels to optimize therapy (PDR.net, 2012).

Dosage Schedule

- Because of its short serum half-life, gabapentin should be given three times daily, with the time interval between any two doses no longer than 12 hours.
- *Dose reduction/substitution/withdrawal:* Gradually over a minimum of 1 week.
- *Children <3 years of age:* Not recommended. Safety and efficacy have not been evaluated in this age group.
- *Children 3 years through 12 years of age:* A starting dose of 10 to 15 mg/kg/day in three divided doses is recommended. Increase to an effective dose over 3 days. The recommended effective dose for 3- and 4-year-old patients is 40 mg/kg/day divided t.i.d., whereas for patients ages 5 years and older, the typical effective dose is between 25 and 35 mg/kg/day, divided t.i.d. The maximum daily dose for children ages 3 to 12 years is 50 mg/kg/day.
- *Adolescents >12 years of age and adults:* An initial daily dose of 900 mg (300 mg t.i.d.) is recommended. The usual effective dose is between 900 and 1,800 mg/day. Based on clinical response, the dose may be titrated upward to 2,400 mg/day. Higher doses have been tolerated by some patients with epilepsy. The recommended maximum dose is 3,600 mg/day.

Gabapentin Dose Forms Available

- *Capsules:* 100, 300, and 400 mg
- *Tablets (scored):* 600 and 800 mg
- *Oral solution:* 250 mg/5 mL dispensed in 470 mL bottles.

Reports of Interest (Gabapentin)

Controlled trials of gabapentin use in adults with mania have failed to demonstrate efficacy, and data supporting its use for pediatric mania are considerably limited. Soutullo et al. (1998) reported on a 13-year-old boy with bipolar I disorder, manic episode, and comorbid ADHD, who was treated with gabapentin 1,500 mg/day as an add-on medication to carbamazepine. Within 1 month of adding gabapentin, he experienced a marked improvement and subsequently remained stable for 7 months. This patient had previously failed a trial of divalproex and was unable to tolerate lithium. Monotherapy with carbamazepine was not adequate to control his symptoms (Soutullo et al., 1998).

Lamotrigine (Lamictal)

Note: The FDA has directed that a Black Box warning be added to the labeling of lamotrigine indicating that SERIOUS RASHES including Stevens-Johnson syndrome, toxic epidermal necrolysis, and/or rash-related death. Serious rashes may require hospitalization or discontinuing of the medication. The incidence of these rashes is approximately 8/1,000 (0.8%) in pediatric patients ages 2 to 16 years old (vs. 0.3% incidence in adults), who receive lamotrigine as adjunctive therapy for epilepsy. The incidence of serious rash may be increased by coadministration of valproate, exceeding the recommended dose, or exceeding the recommended dose escalation for lamotrigine. Lamotrigine should be discontinued at the first sign of rash, unless the rash is clearly not drug related. Discontinuing lamotrigine may not prevent a rash from becoming life threatening or permanently disabling or disfiguring. [This is a summary; see the package insert or current *PDR* for the complete warning.]

In 2008, the FDA also issued an alert advising providers to monitor patients who are taking or starting antiepileptic medication for any changes in behavior that could indicate the emergence of depression or worsening suicidal thoughts or behavior (PDR.net, 2008).

Pharmacokinetics of Lamotrigine

Lamotrigine is absorbed quickly, has an absolute bioavailability of 98%, and is not affected by food intake. Time to peak plasma concentrations is between 1.4 and 4.8 hours. The elimination half-life for adults when prescribed alone is 32.8 hours for single-dose lamotrigine and 25.4 hours for multiple-dose lamotrigine. Lamotrigine's elimination half-life varies when certain other medication are taken concurrently and are summarized in the package insert. Population pharmacokinetic analyses reveal that lamotrigine's clearance is predominantly influenced by total body weight and concurrent antiepileptic therapy. The oral clearance of lamotrigine is higher in youth than in adults, based on body weight. Patients weighing <30 kg may need a 50% increase in maintenance lamotrigine doses to maintain therapeutic levels. Lamictal clearance does not appear to be altered by age.

Contraindications for the Administration of Lamotrigine

Lamotrigine is contraindicated when patients have a hypersensitivity to lamotrigine or its ingredients.

Interactions of Lamotrigine with Other Drugs

The clearance of lamotrigine is affected by coadministration of several medications. Valproate, for example, increases lamotrigine levels by approximately two-fold. Oral estrogen containing contraceptives, oxcarbazepine, and carbamazepine, by contrast, reduce lamotrigine levels. Oral progestin-only contraceptives may not protect as well against pregnancy when used concurrently with lamotrigine, which patients should be made aware of. Many other drug interactions are summarized in the package insert and should be considered prior to prescribing lamotrigine. In some instances, dose adjustments will need to be made.

Untoward Effects of Lamotrigine

See the summary of the Black Box warning above for information regarding the risk of serious rash with lamotrigine. Common side effects of lamotrigine include nausea/vomiting, somnolence, headache, dizziness, and tremor. There have been reports of blood dyscrasias, and suicidal ideation and behavior should be monitored for, as is the case of all antiepileptic medication.

Lamotrigine is classified as pregnancy category C. It is present in breast milk, so caution must be taken if prescribing lamotrigine to a nursing patient.

Indications for Lamotrigine

Lamotrigine is an antiepileptic drug of the phenyltriazine class and is chemically unrelated to antiepileptic drugs currently in use. Its mechanism of action is unknown. Lamotrigine is approved for use in the adjunctive treatment of partial seizures, primary generalized tonic-clonic seizures, and generalized seizures of Lennox-Gastaut syndrome, in patients ≥2 years old. Lamotrigine is also approved for use in adults with partial seizures who are being treated with a single hepatic enzyme-inducing antiepileptic drug (EIAED; e.g., carbamazepine, phenytoin, phenobarbital, primidone, or valproate) to convert them to monotherapy with lamotrigine. Lamotrigine is further indicated for the maintenance treatment of bipolar I disorder to decrease the frequency of mood episodes (depression, mania, hypomania, mixed episodes) in patients at

(continued)

Indications for Lamotrigine *(continued)*

least 18 years old who are being treated for an acute mood episode with standard therapy. Lamotrigine has not been proved effective in treating acute mood episodes. There are no definitive indications or conclusive empiric support for lamotrigine in child and adolescent psychiatry.

Dosage Schedule

- *Children <2 years old:* Not recommended.
- *Children ≥2 years old, adolescents, and adults:* The initial, titration, and target doses for lamotrigine vary considerably according to age and which other medications the patient is taking. The package insert or current *PDR* should be consulted for the appropriate medication protocol.

Dosage Forms Available (Lamotrigine)

- *Tablets (scored):* 25, 100, 150, and 200 mg
- *Chewable dispersible tablets:* 2, 5, and 25 mg
- *Orally disintegrating tablets:* 25, 50, 100, and 200 mg

Reports of Interest

Lamotrigine for Youth with Bipolar Disorder

Carandang et al. (2003) reported a retrospective study of nine adolescents with mood disorders refractory to previous pharmacotherapy who responded positively to lamotrigine. Six of the youth had bipolar depression, two had unipolar depression, and one was diagnosed with mood disorder NOS. Three patients received lamotrigine as monotherapy, whereas the others received lamotrigine in conjunction with concurrent pharmacotherapy (antidepressants, antipsychotics, a second mood stabilizer, anxiolytics, or sedative-hypnotics). The mean age of subjects was 16.4 years, and the mean lamotrigine dose was 141.7 mg (ranging from 25 to 250 mg/day). Eight of nine subjects demonstrated improvement as measured by the Clinical Global Impressions–Bipolar Version overall illness rating. Seven were deemed "much improved," and one was judged to be "very much improved." One subject had to discontinue lamotrigine after developing an erythematous rash, which resolved a few days after stopping lamotrigine. While the findings were positive, the study authors emphasized the need for additional trials to support or refute findings (Carandang et al., 2003).

Soutullo et al. (2006) published a small open retrospective review of five adolescent patients diagnosed with bipolar disorder, who were treated with adjunctive lamotrigine in their outpatient clinic. Three of the patients were diagnosed with bipolar disorder NOS, one with bipolar I disorder, and one with bipolar II disorder. All five were depressed at baseline, and failed to demonstrate an adequate treatment response to their current medication regimen. The average lamotrigine dose was 100 ± 87.5 mg/day and the mean treatment duration was 28 ± 28 weeks. Treatment response was rated using the Clinical Global Impression–Improvement (CGI-I) scale. The study authors reported a marked or moderate improvement in four patients (80%) and minimal improvement in one patient (20%). No skin rashes were reported, though one patient complained of dizziness. Lamotrigine was determined to be well tolerated in this small sample; however, given numerous inherent methodological limitations, definitive conclusions regarding lamotrigine's efficacy were unable to be determined. Regardless, the findings were regarded as provisional positive results for adjunctive use of lamotrigine in adolescents with bipolar depression (Soutullo et al., 2006).

In an 8-week open-label trial, Chang et al. (2006) prospectively studied the efficacy of lamotrigine as adjunctive or monotherapy for 20 adolescents with bipolar depression. The subjects were between 12 and 17 years (mean 15.8 years) and were diagnosed with bipolar I disorder, bipolar II disorder, or bipolar NOS. Subjects who were taking antidepressant medication were tapered and discontinued off the medication over 2 to 4 weeks, after which time they were reassessed for entry criteria. Lamotrigine was started at 12.5 to 25 mg daily and was gradually titrated to a mean dose of 131.6 mg/day. Primary response criteria was a 1 or 2 on the Clinical Global Impression–Improvement (CGI-I) by the end of the study. At least a 50% reduction in CDRS-R ratings served as a secondary response criteria. Seven subjects were on other psychotropic medication during the trial (mood stabilizers, antipsychotics, stimulants, strattera) though could enter the trial only if no changes were made to these medications within 1 month of enrolling. A total of 18 subjects completed the study. Eighty-four percent of subjects responded by primary response criteria and 63% by secondary response criteria. Scores on the YMRS and OAS–Modified also significantly decreased. By the end of the study, 58% of subjects were judged to be in remission (score of 28 or less on the CDRS-R and a CGI-S score of 1 or 2). Lamotrigine was weight-neutral during the trial, and no rash or other adverse events were noted. The authors concluded that lamotrigine may decrease depression, mania, and aggression in adolescents with bipolar depression though acknowledged that larger placebo-controlled studies are needed to confirm this (Chang et al., 2006).

Pavuluri et al. (2009) studied lamotrigine's efficacy and tolerability for the maintenance treatment of pediatric bipolar disorder in a 14-week open-label trial with 46 subjects who presented with mania or hypomania (ages 8 to 18 years, mean age 13.3 years). Prior to the start of the study, all subjects underwent a 1- to 4-week washout period of their previous medications. This was followed by acute stabilization with a second-generation antipsychotic (SGA) and concurrent gradual titration of lamotrigine over an 8-week period. It was planned to have all subjects achieve an endpoint Lamictal dose of 150 mg if ≤30 kg body weight, or 200 mg if >30 kg body weight by week 6 of the 8-week titration phase. The SGA was tapered off over 2 to 4 weeks between weeks 4 and 8, such that all subjects were on lamotrigine monotherapy by the end of the 8-week dosing period of the trial. Subjects were then maintained on Lamictal monotherapy for an additional 6 weeks. By the end of the 14-week trial, the depression response rate on the CDRS-R was 82%, the YMRS response rate was 71%, and the remission rate was 56%. Authors noted that depressive symptoms continued to improve over the 14-week period and that aggression and irritability (measured via the OAS) declined over the initial 8-week period and maintained during the additional 6 weeks with lamotrigine monotherapy. Lamotrigine was determined to be well tolerated in this trial, with the most common side effects being sedation (23.8%), stomachache (19.6%), increased urination (10.9%), and increased appetite (10.9%). There was no significant weight gain, no cases of serious skin rashes, and no increase in suicidal ideation. The dropout rate due to adverse events was 6.4%, all due to benign skin rashes that ultimately resolved without incident. Two rashes were treated with prednisone to assist in their resolution. Investigators concluded that lamotrigine was overall well tolerated and appeared effective as a monotherapy agent in maintaining control of manic, hypomanic, and depressive symptoms, for 6 weeks following acute stabilization with an SGA (Pavuluri et al., 2009).

Biederman et al. (2010) studied the use of lamotrigine as monotherapy for youth with bipolar disorder in a 12-week, open-label, prospective trial. Thirty-nine bipolar youth were enrolled, and 56% completed the trial. Several participants stopped the trial due to skin rash, though in all cases the rash resolved once lamotrigine was discontinued. During this trial, lamotrigine was titrated to 160.7 ± 128.3 mg in the 22 children younger than 12 years of age, and to 219.1 ± 172.2 mg/day for the 17 children ages 12 to 17 years. The study authors reported statistically significant improvements in YMRS scores associated with lamotrigine treatment and concluded that lamotrigine was well tolerated and may be efficacious for youth with bipolar disorder. An improvement in symptoms of depression, ADHD, and psychosis were also reported in this small trial (Biederman et al., 2010).

During the same year, Pavuluri et al. (2010) studied the impact of lamotrigine treatment on the neurocognitive profile of youth with bipolar disorder. Twenty-four healthy controls and 34 matched and unmedicated youth with manic, mixed, or hypomanic episodes were administered a neurocognitive battery at baseline. The youth with bipolar disorder were then treated for 14 weeks with lamotrigine, after which time both groups were readministered a neurocognitive battery. Although overall cognitive performance in the pediatric bipolar disorder group remained impaired relative to healthy controls, the study authors noted that global neurocognitive function improved with lamotrigine treatment over time. Working and verbal memory were most prominently improved in patients treated with lamotrigine, such that these cognitive domains were no longer significantly impaired relative to healthy controls. Improvements in executive functioning were noted in the lamotrigine-treated group, but continued to lag behind the performance of healthy controls. Attention did not improve in the lamotrigine-treated group, and comorbid ADHD was an exclusionary criteria for this study. Authors reported that no significant results (P > .05) were found to be related to improvements seen in the YMRS and CDRS-R scores, supporting that the cognitive improvements seen in this study were not solely due to symptomatic improvement. Ultimately, the investigators concluded that lamotrigine may reduce some of the cognitive deficits associated with PBD (Pavuluri et al., 2010).

Lamotrigine for Youth with PDDs

Belsito (2001) reported a negative double-blind placebo-controlled trial of lamotrigine for treatment of autistic disorder. Twenty-eight youth ages 3 to 11 years with a diagnosis of autistic disorder received either placebo or lamotrigine. Lamotrigine was gradually titrated upward over 8 weeks to a mean maintenance dose of 5.0 mg/kg/day and was dosed twice daily for an additional 4 weeks. Outcome measures included the Autism Behavior Checklist, the Aberrant Behavior Checklist, and the Vineland Adaptive Behavior scales. The study demonstrated no significant difference between lamotrigine and placebo on the outcome measures used (Belsito, 2001). A more recent case report suggested a positive treatment response to lamotrigine in an adolescent patient with autistic disorder and comorbid bipolar disorder, however (Howell et al., 2011). Additional studies are needed before firm conclusions can be drawn.

Oxcarbazepine (Trileptal)

Note: In 2008, the FDA also issued an alert advising providers to monitor patients who are taking or starting antiepileptic medication for any changes in behavior that could indicate the emergence of depression or worsening suicidal thoughts or behavior (PDR. net, 2008).

Pharmacokinetics of Oxcarbazepine

Oxcarbazepine is an antiepileptic drug and a 10 keto-analogue of carbamazepine; pharmacologic activity is exerted primarily through its 10-monohydroxy metabolite (MHD). Its mechanism of action is unknown; however, *in vitro* studies have indicated that oxcarbazepine and MHD produce blockade of voltage-sensitive sodium channels resulting in stabilization of hyperexcited neural membranes. Oxcarbazepine taken orally is completely absorbed and extensively metabolized to MHD. The half-life of oxcarbazepine is approximately 2 hours, and the half-life of MHD is approximately 9 hours. Food does not appear to affect the bioavailability of either oxcarbazepine or MHD. The median peak plasma level is 4.5 hours (range, 3 to 13 hours) for film-coated tablets and 6 hours for the oral suspension preparation; both preparations have similar bioavailability. Steady-state plasma concentrations are achieved in 2 to 3 days when a given dose is administered twice daily. Clearance of oxcarbazepine and its metabolites is primarily (above 95%) through the kidneys. Clearance in children below 8 years of age is 30% to 40% greater than in older children and adults, and in a controlled clinical trial, such patients had the highest maintenance doses.

Contraindications for the Administration of Oxcarbazepine

Hypersensitivity to oxcarbazepine or its components is a contraindication to the administration of oxcarbazepine. Approximately 25% to 30% of patients who had hypersensitivity reactions to carbamazepine are likely to do so with oxcarbazepine; hence, they should be asked about any such prior exposure.

Interactions of Oxcarbazepine with Other Drugs

Oxcarbazepine can inhibit CYP2C19 and induce CYP3A4 and CYP3A5, which can potentially significantly affect plasma concentrations of other drugs. Drugs that induce cytochrome P450, including some other antiepileptic drugs, can result in decreases in plasma levels of oxcarbazepine and MHD. Plasma levels of phenytoin increased by up to 40% when oxcarbazepine was given in doses >1,200 mg/day; however, phenobarbital levels increased by only 15%. Carbamazepine, phenytoin, and phenobarbital, which are all strong inducers of cytochrome P450 enzymes, decreased the plasma level of MHD by 29% to 40%.

Coadministration of oxcarbazepine with an oral hormonal contraceptive decreased plasma concentrations of ethinylestradiol and levonorgestrel, which may decrease the effectiveness of the contraceptive.

Untoward Effects of Oxcarbazepine

The most common untoward effects reported in pediatric patients being treated for a partial seizure disorder include fatigue, vomiting, nausea, headache, somnolence, dizziness, ataxia, nystagmus, diplopia, vision abnormalities, and emotional liability. One manufacturer noted that approximately 9.2% (14) of 152 pediatric patients who were treated with oxcarbazepine, but had not been treated previously with antiepileptic drugs, discontinued the drug because of untoward effects. Although relatively infrequent (<1%), "rash" was responsible for 5.3% (8) and "maculopapular rash" for 1.3% (2) of those discontinuing. In a second group of 456 pediatric patients who were being treated with oxcarbazepine as monotherapy or adjunctive therapy, and who were previously treated with antiepileptic drugs, 11% (50) discontinued the drug because of untoward effects. Patients discontinued for the following reasons: somnolence 2.4% (11), vomiting 2.0% (9), ataxia 1.8% (8), diplopia 1.3% (6), dizziness 1.3% (6), fatigue 1.1% (5), and nystagmus 1.1% (5).

Oxcarbazepine has a reduced risk for leukopenia, rashes, drug interactions, and enzyme autoinduction compared with carbamazepine (see references cited by Teitelbaum, 2001).

Hyponatremia

Clinically significant hyponatremia (sodium <125 mmol/L) may occur during treatment with oxcarbazepine. This usually occurs within 3 months of initiation of therapy but may also occur after over a year of treatment. In 14 studies with a total of 1,524 patients, 38 (2.5%) developed a sodium of <125 mmol/L sometime during treatment compared with no patients on placebo or active control (other antiepileptic drugs). Symptoms that may reflect hyponatremia such as nausea, malaise, headache, lethargy, confusion, obtundation, or increase in seizure frequency or severity should prompt checking of sodium plasma levels. Periodic monitoring of sodium levels during treatment should be considered. Precaution should be taken when prescribing oxcarbazepine along with other medications known to reduce sodium levels.

Indications for Oxcarbazepine

Oxcarbazepine is indicated as monotherapy or adjunctive therapy in the treatment of partial seizures in adults, as monotherapy in youth ages ≥4 years with epilepsy, and as adjunctive therapy in children ≥2 years with partial seizures. There are no definitive child and adolescent psychiatric indications for oxcarbazepine.

Oxcarbazepine Dosage Schedule Initiation of Monotherapy

- Total daily dose should always be administered in two divided doses (b.i.d.)
- *Children 4 years of age through adolescents 16 years of age (not taking other antiepileptic drugs):* An initial daily dose of 4 to 5 mg/kg b.i.d. is recommended. The dose should be increased by 5 mg/kg every third day to reach recommended weight-specific maintenance doses (see the package insert for complete dosing guidelines).
- *Adults, and adolescents 17 years of age and older (not taking other antiepileptic drugs):* An initial dose of 300 mg twice daily (600 mg/day) is recommended. Dose may be increased by 300 mg/day every third day to a dose of 1,200 mg/day. Many patients are unable to tolerate doses of 2,400 mg/day.

Oxcarbazepine Dosage Schedule as Adjunctive Treatment or to Convert to Monotherapy

- See the package insert or the current *PDR* for guidelines.

Dosage Forms Available (Oxcarbazepine)

- *Film-coated tablets:* 150, 300, and 600 mg
- *Oral suspension:* 300 mg/5 mL (store in original container; shake well before using). The oral suspension preparation and film-coated tablets are interchangeable at equal doses.

Reports of Interest

Oxcarbazepine for the Treatment of Pediatric Bipolar Disorder and Aggression

Teitelbaum (2001) described a case of a 6-year-old female diagnosed with bipolar I disorder who responded favorably to oxcarbazepine treatment. This patient was hospitalized four times in the preceding year with extreme aggression and destruction of property. She failed prior trials of lithium, lamotrigine (some benefit but discontinued because of rash), valproate, gabapentin, clonidine, guanfacine, risperidone, olanzapine, quetiapine, fluoxetine, and methylphenidate (worsened symptoms). She improved significantly when oxcarbazepine was added to her medication regimen of 3 months, which consisted of lithium carbonate 150 mg three times daily (0.7 mEq/L serum level) and guanfacine 0.5 mg three times daily. Oxcarbazepine was started at an initial dose at 150 mg twice daily, and she achieved full mood stabilization after 6 weeks of treatment. Three months later, her lithium dose was decreased to 150 mg twice daily, and she maintained good symptom control for an additional 7 months. The author noted that the girl experienced transient mild symptom exacerbations during a school vacation, and again during a viral illness, but was ultimately able to maintain on lithium 150 mg twice daily, guanfacine 0.5 mg twice daily, and oxcarbazepine 150 mg twice daily, with overall good effect (Teitelbaum, 2001).

Staller et al. (2005) conducted a retrospective chart review of 14 outpatients (ages 6 to 17 years; 6 males and 8 females) who were prescribed oxcarbazepine to address moderate to severe problems with anger, irritability, and aggression. Many subjects had additional symptoms including depression, mania, anxiety, disruptiveness, oppositionality, and psychosis. Subjects were rated as moderately ill (6), markedly ill (7), and severely ill (1) on the CGI-S Scale. Subjects' Axis I diagnoses, including multiple diagnoses in 11, included bipolar disorder (5); other mood disorders (3); ADHD (4); disruptive behavior disorder (3); and PDD spectrum disorders (2). Ten (71.4%) of the subjects failed to respond adequately to prior drug trials. During treatment, 70% of subjects received oxcarbazepine in combination with other medication, including atypical antipsychotics (7), SSRIs (4), stimulants (2), alpha agonists (2), antihistamines (2), beta blocker (1), and valproate (1). The average daily dose of oxcarbazepine was 878 mg (ranged from 600 to 1,800 mg/day). Duration of oxcarbazepine treatment averaged 9.8 months (ranged from 0.5 to 30 months). Clinical improvement was rated on the CGI-I Scale. Moderate clinical global improvement was reported in 50% of patients treated with oxcarbazepine. Mild AEs including dizziness, muscle aches, and tremors resulted in discontinuation of only two (14%) of the subjects studied, and oxcarbazepine was generally considered well tolerated.

Wagner et al. (2006) completed a double-blind, randomized, placebo-controlled trial of oxcarbazepine as monotherapy in the treatment of pediatric bipolar disorder and concluded that oxcarbazepine is not significantly superior to placebo. In this trial, 116 pediatric outpatients, aged 7 to 18 years of age, with bipolar I disorder, manic or mixed, were randomized to receive flexibly dosed oxcarbazepine ($N = 59$) or placebo ($N = 57$) for 7 weeks. The mean dose of oxcarbazepine used in the trial was 1,515 mg/day and the median duration of treatment was 48 days. Subjects ages 7 to 12 years averaged 1,200 mg/day, while those ages 13 to 18 years averaged 2,040 mg/day. The dose titration was fairly rapid during this trial, with subjects receiving 300 mg increment increases every 2 days, until a maximum weight-based dose of 900 to 2,400 mg/day was reached by week 2 of the study. The primary outcome measure included the change in YMRS scores from start to endpoint. Adverse effects that occurred at least twice as often in the oxcarbazepine group as in the placebo group were dizziness, nausea, somnolence, diplopia, fatigue, and rash. Each were reported in at least 5% of patients in the oxcarbazepine group. Six patients in the oxcarbazepine group, versus zero in the placebo group, experienced serious psychiatric adverse events, all of which required hospitalization. These adverse events included exacerbation of bipolar disorder ($N = 3$), aggressive outburst ($N = 1$), suicide attempt ($N = 1$), and inappropriate sexual behavior ($N = 1$). Investigators determined that only three of these adverse events (exacerbation of bipolar disorder, aggressive behavior, and suicide attempt) were related to the study medication itself. The study authors ultimately concluded that oxcarbazepine did not separate from placebo during this trial and noted a higher incidence of psychiatric adverse events for both the oxcarbazepine group and placebo group than seen in epilepsy populations (Wagner et al., 2006). Additional controlled studies are needed to support or refute these findings.

Oxcarbazepine for the Treatment of Youth with Autistic Disorder

Kapetanovic (2007) reported three cases of patients with autistic disorder who responded favorably to treatment with oxcarbazepine. In the first case, a 13-year-old Hispanic male with poor sleep and frequent aggression, who failed prior trials of risperidone and olanzapine, responded positively to oxcarbazepine 300 mg in the morning and 600 mg at night (titrated up over 7 days). His mother reported improved compliance, school reports, sleep, aggression, and attention after 2 weeks of treatment with oxcarbazepine, and he remained stable for 4 months. In the second case, a 19-year-old Caucasian female with dysfunctional compulsive routines, head banging, and violence, whose compulsive symptoms improved with fluoxetine 20 mg daily over 2 months, but whose aggressive and self-injurious symptoms persisted despite a trial of risperidone, was started on oxcarbazepine and titrated to 600 mg b.i.d. Two months later, her tantrums and head banging were notably reduced and her level of cooperation improved. She remained stable on fluoxetine and oxcarbazepine for 6 months. In the third case, a 4½-year-old Hispanic child with problematic head banging, property destruction, aggression, hyperactivity, and irregular sleep, who failed prior trials of methylphenidate and amphetamine salts (increased agitation), risperidone, and guanfacine, was started on oxcarbazepine, which was titrated to 150 mg every morning and 300 mg every night over a 2½-month period. The addition of oxcarbazepine resulted in improved sleep, reduced aggression, and improved cooperation, which maintained for 3½ months. None of the three patients developed hyponatremia or other adverse effects, and the author expressed hope that these preliminary positive findings would encourage future research into the efficacy of oxcarbazepine for the treatment of autistic disorder (Kapetanovic, 2007).

Topiramate (Topamax)

Note: In 2008, the FDA issued an alert advising providers to monitor patients who are taking or starting antiepileptic medication for any changes in behavior that could indicate the emergence of depression or worsening suicidal thoughts or behavior (PDR.net, 2008).

Topiramate, an antiepileptic drug, is a sulfamate-substituted monosaccharide. The mechanisms responsible for its antiepileptic and migraine prophylaxis effects have not been elucidated; however, preclinical studies suggest that at clinically effective concentrations, topiramate blocks voltage-dependent sodium channels, augments the activity of the neurotransmitter gamma-aminobutyrate at some subtypes of the GABA-A receptor, antagonizes the AMPA/kainate subtype of the glutamate receptor, and inhibits the carbonic anhydrase enzyme, particularly isoenzymes II and IV (package insert).

Pharmacokinetics of Topiramate

The bioavailability of topiramate is not affected by food. Peak plasma concentrations occur in approximately 2 hours. Mean plasma elimination half-life is 21 hours after single or multiple doses and steady state occurs in approximately 4 days at a given dose. Topiramate is not extensively metabolized, and approximately 70% is eliminated unchanged through the kidneys. Pediatric patients, aged 4 to 17 years, have approximately a 50% higher clearance than adults. Consequently, such patients have a shorter elimination half-life than adults and their plasma concentration of topiramate may be lower than that of adults receiving the same dose.

Contraindications for the Administration of Topiramate

Topiramate is contraindicated in patients with a history of sensitivity to topiramate or any of the components included in the pill. Clearance may be significantly reduced in patients with renal or hepatic impairment.

Interactions of Topiramate with Other Drugs

Hyperammonemia with or without encephalopathy has been associated with the combined use of topiramate and valproic acid in patients who have not developed these symptoms when treated with either drug alone. Patients who develop symptoms such as acute alterations in the level of consciousness or cognitive functioning in combination with lethargy or vomiting, which may be associated with hyperammonemic encephalopathy, should have their serum ammonia levels determined. Oligohydrosis and hyperthermia have been reported, primarily in pediatric patients, and may be more likely to occur when topiramate is used in conjunction with other medications that predispose to heat-related disorders, such as carbonic anhydrase inhibitors or drugs with anticholinergic activity. Decreased sweating and elevated body temperatures need to be monitored for. Topiramate may decrease the efficacy of oral contraceptives. Topiramate can decrease the AUC and maximum serum concentration of lithium by up to 20% and can also reduce levels of warfarin and benzodiazepines. Many other drug interactions are possible (see package insert).

Untoward Effects of Topiramate

Topiramate is associated with hyperchloremic, non–anion gap metabolic acidosis, which if chronic and untreated may cause osteomalacia/rickets and may reduce growth rate and maximal stature in pediatric patients. Treatment-emergent adverse events in children in the age group 10 through 16 years who were being treated with monotherapy (400 mg/day) for epilepsy that occurred with an incidence of at least 5% and which were more frequent than those at lower doses (50 mg/day) included fever (9%), paresthesias (16%), diarrhea (11%), weight loss (21%), anorexia (14%), mood problems (11%), difficulty with concentration/attention (9%), and alopecia (5%). Topiramate may cause cleft lip or palate in infants when used during pregnancy and is a category D medication for pregnancy. Nephrolithiasis has been reported with the use of topiramate.

Indications for Topiramate

Topiramate is approved for use as monotherapy or adjunct therapy in patients ≥2 years of age with partial onset or primary generalized tonic-clonic seizures; as an adjunctive therapy in patients ≥2 years of age with partial onset seizures, primary generalized tonic-clonic seizures, or seizures associated with Lennox-Gastaut syndrome; and for the prophylaxis of migraine headache in adults.

Topiramate Dosage Schedule for Monotherapy (Epilepsy)

- *Children 2 to <10 years of age:* Maintenance dose is based on weight (see product insert for details). An initial dose of 25 mg/day in the evening is recommended. After 1 week, increase to 25 mg twice daily as tolerated. May increase by 25 to 50 mg/day each week as tolerated. Titrate to the minimum weight-based maintenance dose over a total of 5 to 7 weeks.
- *Children ≥10 years of age, adolescents, and adults:* An initial dose of 25 mg, twice daily is recommended. Dose should be increased as tolerated by 50 mg weekly to reach a recommended target dose of 200 mg, twice daily (total dose, 400 mg/day).

Topiramate Dosage Schedule for Prophylaxis (Migraine Headache)

- *Children and adolescents <18 years of age:* Not recommended.
- *Adolescents ≥18 years of age and adults:* An initial evening dose of 25 mg is recommended. Dose should be increased as tolerated by 25 mg weekly (week 2, 25 mg b.i.d., week 3, 25 mg in the morning and 50 mg in the evening to a recommended target dose of 50 mg b.i.d. during week 4; total dose, 100 mg/day).

Topiramate Adjunct Dosage Schedule for Treating Partial Onset Seizures, Primary Generalized Tonic-Clonic Seizures or Lennox-Gastaut Syndrome

- See package insert.

Dosage Forms Available (Topiramate)

- *Tablets:* 25, 50, 100, and 200 mg.
- *Sprinkle capsules:* 15- and 25-mg sprinkle capsules may be swallowed whole or opened and put on a small amount of soft food, which should be swallowed without chewing immediately and not stored for future use.

Reports of Interest

Topiramate for the Treatment of Pediatric Bipolar Disorder

Two small retrospective chart reviews provided preliminary evidence that adjunctive topiramate may be beneficial for the treatment of pediatric bipolar disorder (Barzman et al., 2005; DelBello et al., 2002). Delbello et al. (2002) looked at outpatient medical charts of 26 youth diagnosed with bipolar disorder, type I or II, who were treated with adjunctive topiramate. The CGI and Clinical Global Assessment Scale (CGAS) were used to rate response to treatment. The mean duration of topiramate treatment was 4.1 ± 6.1 months, and the average daily dose was 104 ± 77 mg/day. The authors concluded that the response rate (defined as a CGI-I score of ≤ 2 at endpoint) was 73% for mania and 62% for overall illness. CGAS scores were significantly improved, and no adverse events were reported. Barzman et al. (2005) completed a records review of 25 hospitalized children and adolescents with bipolar I disorder who were treated with adjunctive topiramate at a mean dose of 126 mg/day. The CGI-S score was used as the primary outcome measure. The authors concluded that 64% of patients responded positively to adjunctive topiramate, based on significantly improved CGI-S scores. No adverse events were recorded (Barzman et al., 2005).

DelBello et al. (2005) reported a 4-week, multicenter, randomized, double-blind, placebo-controlled, parallel-group trial of topiramate monotherapy in treating mania in 56 children and adolescent means age 13.8 ± 2.56 years (range 6 to 17 years), who were diagnosed with bipolar disorder type I; 33 subjects (58.9%) had codiagnoses of ADHD. This study was originally designed to enroll approximately 230 subjects, but was curtailed early after learning of negative studies of topiramate for the treatment of acute mania in adults. The primary outcome measure was the YMRS scores at baseline and 4, 7, 14, 21, and 28 days of treatment. Secondary outcome measures included baseline and weekly scores on the Clinical Global Impressions–Improvement Scale, the Brief Psychiatric Rating Scale for Children (BPRS-C), the CGAS, and the CDRS.

The baseline YMRS score for the topiramate group ($N = 29$) was 31.7 ± 5.53, and it was decreased by -9.7 ± 9.65 at endpoint. The baseline YMRS score for the placebo group ($N = 27$) was 29.9 ± 6.01, and it was decreased by -4.7 ± 9.79 at endpoint, less than one-half the improvement seen in the topiramate group. However, there was no significant group difference at any visit for the change in YMRS score, the total BPRS-C score, total CDRS score, or CGAS score. Treatment-emergent adverse events occurring in >10% of subjects and greater for topiramate than for placebo included decreased appetite (27.6% vs. 0%), nausea (24.1% vs. 0%), diarrhea (13.8% vs. 7.4%), paresthesia (13.8% vs. 3.7%), somnolence (13.8% vs. 3.7%), insomnia (10.3% vs. 3.7%), and rash (10.3% vs. 3.7%). Mean change in body weight from baseline to endpoint was significantly different, with the topiramate group losing a mean of -1.76 ± 2.03 kg and the placebo group gaining a mean of 0.95 ± 1.45 kg ($P < .001$). No subject experienced a serious adverse event. This study was ultimately deemed inconclusive due to inadequate sample sizes stemming from the early discontinuation of the study.

Wozniak et al. (2009) studied 40 outpatients, ages 6 to 17 years, who were diagnosed with bipolar disorder, in 2 partially concurrent 8-week open-label trials of either olanzapine monotherapy ($N = 17$) or olanzapine augmented with topiramate ($N = 23$). Olanzapine was initiated at 2.5 mg/day and increased by 2.5 to 5 mg weekly as indicated, to a maximum dose of 20 mg daily. Topiramate was started at 25 mg/day and increased by 25 mg/day each week as tolerated, to the maximum dose of 100 mg daily. Primary outcome measures included the YMRS and the CGI-I mania scales. Investigators discovered that both groups showed a clinically and statistically significant reduction in YMRS scores. Weight gain in the olanzapine plus topiramate group, however, was statistically significantly lower (2.6 ± 3.6 kg) than in the olanzapine monotherapy group. Investigators concluded that while topiramate as augmentation of olanzapine did not lead to improved mania over olanzapine alone, it did lead to reduced weight gain in this trial (Wozniak et al., 2009).

Topiramate for the Treatment of Prader-Willi Syndrome

Smathers et al. (2003) completed an open-label study in which topiramate was used to treat youth with a diagnosis of Prader-Willi syndrome (PWS). Eight patients between the ages of 10 and 19 years were titrated, as indicated and tolerated, to a dose of topiramate 100 to 600 mg/day. Mood and behavior were assessed by parental questionnaires and phone surveys. Three patients experienced somnolence, which resolved with continued treatment or dose reduction. Seven patients completed the trial (one discontinued after 3 months due to perceived lack of benefit), all of whom were reported to have a positive change in mood, evidenced by increased interactions with others and improved self-esteem. All seven were reported to have decreased aggressiveness, violence, and acting out. Two patients stopped self-injurious skin picking after 2 months of treatment, and most had reduced obsessive behaviors such as hair brushing or hair washing. One patient had worsened skin picking and hair pulling, which necessitated the use of another medication. Parents reported reduced food foraging and hoarding, and all patients who completed the study either maintained or lost weight. Study authors opined that although this small and unblinded study provides preliminary positive support for efficacy of topiramate in treating problematic features of PWS, larger and controlled trials are needed to further support or refute this finding (Smathers et al., 2003).

Topiramate for the Treatment of Autistic Disorder

Mazzone et al. (2006) described five boys with autistic disorder (ages 9 to 13 years), who were referred for severe behavioral problems (mean IQ 54 ± 27.2). Two previously failed a trial of at least one typical antipsychotic medication. Topiramate was started at 0.5 mg/kg/day for 2 weeks, after which time it was increased by 0.5 mg/kg/day at 2-week intervals to a maximum of 2.5 mg/kg/day. The average topiramate dose was 2.1 mg/kg/day, and the mean duration of treatment was 22 ± 8.33 weeks. Treatment response was assessed by CGI-I and CBCL scores. Two patients were judged to be responders, defined as receiving a 1 or 2 on the CGI-I, and three patients showed no improvement. The authors concluded that clinical response to topiramate in severely impaired autistic disorder appears variable and that additional studies are needed (Mazzone et al., 2006).

Topiramate for the Treatment of Tourette Syndrome

Jankovic et al. (2010) completed a randomized, double-blind, placebo-controlled, parallel-group study of topiramate for the treatment of Tourette syndrome. Twenty-nine patients (mean age 16.5 years; range 7 to 65 years) with moderate to severe symptoms, based on a Yale Global Tic Severity Scale (YGTSS) of ≥ 19, were randomized to receive either topiramate (mean dose 118 mg/day) or placebo. The primary endpoint was the Total Tic Score, which improved 14.29 points by day 70 in the topiramate-treated group, compared with an improvement of only 5 points by day 70 in the placebo group. Secondary measures, including the CGI and premonitory urge CGI, also showed improvements in the treatment group. Adverse events between groups did not differ. The study authors concluded that this study provides evidence that topiramate may be efficacious in the treatment of moderate to severe Tourette syndrome (Jankovic et al., 2010).

Antianxiety Drugs

JULIA JACKSON

BENZODIAZEPINES

Benzodiazepines, introduced into clinical practice in the early 1960s, were the most frequently prescribed drugs in the United States between 1968 and 1980. In 1978 alone, 68 million prescriptions for benzodiazepines were written for approximately 10 million individuals; more than half of these were for diazepam (Ayd, 1980). Greenblatt et al. (1983) noted that by 1980, however, the trend toward increasing use of benzodiazepines reversed, perhaps due to negative publicity regarding the potential for abuse and dependency with these medications. In 1989, in response to these concerns, New York State mandated that all benzodiazepine prescriptions be written on triplicate forms, as was required for other controlled drugs. Many experts at the time, however, felt the dangers of benzodiazepines were "greatly exaggerated" (Simeon and Ferguson, 1985). In a summary statement, the American Psychiatric Association (APA) Task Force opined that "benzodiazepines, when prescribed appropriately, are therapeutic drugs with relatively mild toxic profiles and low tendency for abuse" (Salzman, 1990, p. 62). An exception to this occurs among substance abusers, however. Benzodiazepine abuse is very frequent among alcoholics, cocaine, narcotic, and methadone abusers, who use benzodiazepines to "augment the euphoria (narcotics and methadone users), decrease anxiety and withdrawal symptoms (alcoholics), or to ease the 'crash' from cocaine-induced euphoria" (Salzman, 1990, p. 62).

Little was known at the time about the efficacy of benzodiazepine medications for child and adolescent psychiatric disorders. In a 1974 monograph, after reviewing the use of benzodiazepines in youth, Greenblatt and Shader stated, "At present it is doubtful that the benzodiazepines have a role in the pharmacotherapy of psychoses or in the treatment of emotional disorders in children" (p. 88). Werry concluded that if pharmacotherapy is necessary for certain childhood sleep disturbances, including insomnia, night waking, night terrors, and somnambulism, benzodiazepines are "probably" indicated, and for some kinds of anxiety they are "possibly" indicated (Rapoport et al., 1978b).

In 1983, Coffey et al. reported that benzodiazepines appeared to be prescribed to both older adolescents and adults for relief of anxiety and tension, muscle relaxation, sleep disorders, and seizures. In children, however, they were used primarily for treatment of sleep and seizure disorders and were used much less commonly for their anxiolytic and muscle-relaxant qualities.

The literature concerning benzodiazepine use in children was reviewed by both Campbell et al. (1985) and Simeon and Ferguson (1985). Most published reports appeared in the 1960s, involved open studies composed of diagnostically heterogeneous subjects and resulted in discrepant findings. The most common drugs studied were diazepam and chlordiazepoxide.

At present, the childhood psychiatric conditions that have the most convincing rationale for the use of a benzodiazepine as the drug of choice are sleep terror disorder (pavor nocturnus) and sleepwalking disorder (somnambulism). These conditions are not usually treated with pharmacotherapy, however, unless they are unusually frequent or severe. Both sleep terror disorder and sleepwalking disorder typically occur "during the first third of the major sleep period (the interval of non-rapid eye movement [NREM] sleep that typically contains EEG delta activity, sleep stages 3 and 4)" (APA, 1987, pp. 310–311). Because benzodiazepines decrease stage 4 sleep, they are thought to be of value in these conditions. Reite et al. (1990) suggested that either 2 mg of diazepam or 0.125 mg of triazolam at bedtime may decrease the frequency of night terrors or somnambulism in children with severe cases. Conversely, benzodiazepines were hypothesized to be contraindicated in treating sleep disturbance associated with psychosocial dwarfism (psychosocially determined short stature) due to concern that they may further compromise nocturnal secretion of growth hormone, which occurs maximally during sleep stages 3 and 4, slow-wave sleep (Green, 1986).

It is well known that if a benzodiazepine is used as a hypnotic, consideration of the serum half-life of the drug is important. Flurazepam (Dalmane), temazepam (Restoril), and triazolam (Halcion) can all be used for treating sleep disorders. Flurazepam is a long-acting benzodiazepine with a half-life (for it and its metabolites) of 47 to 100 hours. The manufacturer notes that this pharmacokinetic profile may explain the clinical observation that flurazepam is increasingly effective on the second or third night of use and that after discontinuing the drug, both sleep latency and total wake time may still be decreased. Because of flurazepam's long half-life, it appears to be most useful in persons with both insomnia and significant daytime anxiety. Temazepam and triazolam, by contrast, are short-acting benzodiazepines, with a relatively rapid onset of action and half-lives of only 9.5 to 12.4 hours (temazepam) and 1.5 to 5.5 hours (triazolam). Triazolam's notably short half-life renders it a drug of choice for sleep-onset insomnia and for times when daytime sedation is of concern.

Triazolam's manufacturer warns that all benzodiazepines used to induce sleep can cause an anterior-grade amnesia, in which the person may not recall events occurring for several hours after taking the drug. Triazolam is more likely than the other benzodiazepines to cause such amnesia, particularly if a person is awakened before the drug is metabolized or excreted sufficiently to eliminate the effect. This phenomenon is referred to as "traveler's amnesia," as many travelers, especially on long flights, take medication to induce sleep and are subsequently awakened before the effects of the drug wear off. Triazolam should not be used in such situations. Because of triazolam's short half-life, patients should also be warned of the increased likelihood of experiencing a withdrawal effect, which may entail increased wakefulness during the last third of the night, and/or increased daytime anxiety or nervousness.

Wysowski and Barash (1991) compared postmarketing adverse behavioral reactions of triazolam and temazepam reported through the FDA's spontaneous reporting system. Triazolam was associated with significantly more frequent reports of confusion than did temazepam (133 vs. 2), of amnesia (109 vs. 3), of bizarre behavior (59 vs. 2), of agitation (58 vs. 4), and of hallucinations (40 vs. 1). The incidence of adverse events was quite low, however, because during the period of comparison, 13.5 million prescriptions were written for triazolam and 19.1 million prescriptions were written for temazepam. The authors noted that adverse reactions to triazolam tended to occur at higher doses (0.25 mg and higher) and in the elderly.

Klein et al. (1980) suggested that a low dose of a benzodiazepine (e.g., diazepam 5 mg) might be useful in treating residual anticipatory anxiety in school-phobic youngsters whose separation anxiety had been alleviated by treatment with imipramine. Simeon and Ferguson (1985) reported that some overly inhibited children may show lasting behavioral improvement following brief (not exceeding 4 to 6 weeks) treatment with a benzodiazepine. They attributed the improvement to an interaction between disinhibition facilitated by the medication and social learning. Consistent with this finding, they noted that children and adolescents with impulsivity and aggression, who were under significant environmental stress, should not be treated with benzodiazepines because the disinhibition could result in a worsening of behavior (Simeon and Ferguson, 1985).

Most of the literature suggests that benzodiazepines worsen symptoms in psychotic children and provide little benefit for hyperactive youth. In studies comparing dextroamphetamine, placebo, and chlordiazepoxide or diazepam in treating hyperactive children, chlordiazepoxide and diazepam were both less effective than dextroamphetamine, and placebo was rated better than diazepam (Zrull et al., 1963, 1964).

Contraindications and Cautions for Benzodiazepine Administration

Known hypersensitivity to benzodiazepines and acute narrow-angle glaucoma are usually considered absolute contraindications.

Persons predisposed to substance abuse or alcoholism should not be prescribed benzodiazepines unless the benefits clearly outweigh the increased risk for physical and psychological dependence in this patient population. Benzodiazepines should not be abruptly discontinued after extended therapy, as this may result in withdrawal symptoms.

Adolescents who are likely to become pregnant or who are known to be pregnant should not be prescribed benzodiazepines, as there is a risk of congenital malformations particularly during the first trimester of pregnancy. Maternal abuse of benzodiazepines may cause a withdrawal syndrome in the newborn (Rall, 1990). Simeon and Ferguson (1985) concluded that benzodiazepines are relatively contraindicated in children and adolescents with significant impulsivity, aggressiveness, and environmental stress, as negative disinhibiting drug effects may occur.

Interactions of Benzodiazepines with Other Drugs

Additive effects, when combined with other sedative or hypnotic drugs, including alcohol (ethanol), are clinically important drug interactions to consider when prescribing benzodiazepine medication. Phenothiazines, narcotics, barbiturates, monoamine oxidase inhibitors (MAOIs), tricyclic antidepressants, and cimetidine (Tagamet) may potentiate benzodiazepines. The rate of absorption of benzodiazepines, and the resulting central nervous system depression, are both increased by ethanol (Rall, 1990). CYP3A inhibitors, such as oral antifungals, may increase benzodiazepine levels. Benzodiazepines are relatively safe drugs, and even large overdoses are infrequently fatal unless taken in combination with other drugs (Rall, 1990).

Flumazenil (Romazicon) is a benzodiazepine receptor antagonist that reverses the sedative effects of benzodiazepines. Flumazenil does not reverse hypoventilation or respiratory suppression caused by benzodiazepines, however. In pediatric patients, flumazenil is indicated for the reversal of benzodiazepine-induced conscious sedation (ages 1 to 17 years). It is also indicated for the management of benzodiazepine overdose in adults. In cases of benzodiazepine overdose in adults, flumazenil is administered intravenously in doses of 0.2 mg (2 mL) over a 30-second period. A second dose of 0.3 mg may be administered over 30 seconds, and additional doses of 0.5 mg over 30 seconds, at 1-minute intervals to a maximum of 3 mg, may be given until the desired level of consciousness is obtained. Only rarely do patients benefit from higher doses. Due to its relatively short half-life, resedation may occur. In such cases, additional flumazenil may be given at 20-minute intervals (max of 1 mg/dose and 3 mg/hour).

Untoward Effects of Benzodiazepines

Given that benzodiazepines are central nervous system depressants, the most common untoward effects are oversedation, fatigue, drowsiness, and ataxia. Confusion progressing to coma may occur at high doses. When targeting daytime symptoms such as anxiety, benzodiazepines should be administered in divided doses to minimize sedation.

"Paradoxical reactions," or episodes of marked dyscontrol and disinhibition, have been reported in children and adolescents. Symptoms have included acute excitation, increased anxiety, increased aggression and hostility, rage reactions, loss of all control, hallucinations, insomnia, and nightmares.

Psychiatric and behavioral disturbances, including suicidality, have also been attributed to clonazepam use. For example, Kandemir et al. (2008) reported that a 9-year-old boy with no personal or family psychiatric history, experienced excessive anger, irritability, and suicidal thinking and behavior after being prescribed clonazepam 1.5 mg/day by his neurologist to treat blepharospasm. On the fourth day of treatment with clonazepam, he developed suicidal thoughts and admitted to cutting his arms and chest with a razor in response to these thoughts. His parents reported he had no history of like behavior prior to treatment with clonazepam and stated he was taking no other medication. They described him as a "calm, well adjusted, and happy" child at baseline. A complete medical work-up, including head imaging, was negative. After clonazepam was decreased and stopped over a 3-day period, his psychiatric symptoms resolved entirely. At follow-up 6 months later, he had no recurrence of symptoms (Kandemir et al., 2008).

Use of Benzodiazepines in Child and Adolescent Psychiatry

In general psychiatry, benzodiazepines are indicated for the management of anxiety disorders, or for short-term relief of anxiety and/or sleep disorders. They are also used to treat acute symptoms of alcohol withdrawal. The effectiveness of benzodiazepines for chronic treatment (lasting >4 months) has not been assessed in systematic clinical studies.

At present, randomized controlled trials do not suggest efficacy of benzodiazepine medication for the treatment of childhood anxiety disorders. In clinical practice, benzodiazepines are used at times in youth, however, to acutely reduce severe anxiety until more effective medications, such as selective serotonin reuptake inhibitors (SSRIs), achieve therapeutic effect. If used, manufacturers' clinical recommendations for children should not be exceeded. Table 9.1 gives usual daily dosages for some representative benzodiazepines, an estimate of the serum half-life of the parent compound and/or its significant active metabolites, the youngest age for which the FDA has approved their use for any purpose, and when applicable, suggested dosages for their use in child and adolescent psychiatric disorders.

The need for benzodiazepines should be reassessed frequently, and long-term, chronic use should be avoided.

TABLE 9.1 » Some Representative Benzodiazepines		
Benzodiazepine (Trade Name) (Estimated Serum Half-Life)	**Minimum Age Approved for Any Use**	**Usual Daily Dosage**
Alprazolam (Xanax) (12–15 h)	18 y	See product insert
Chlordiazepoxide (Librium) (24–48 h)	6 y	5 mg 2–4 times/d, maximum 30 mg/d
Clonazepam (Klonopin) (18–50 h)	Not specified	See product insert
Clorazepate (Tranxene) (approximately 48 h)	9 y	For children 9–12 y old, maximum initial dose of 7.5 mg twice daily. Maximum weekly increase, 7.5 mg. Maximum total dose, 60 mg
Diazepam (Valium) (30–60 h)	6 mo	See product insert
Estazolam (ProSom) (10–24 h)	18 y	1–2 mg at bedtime
Flurazepam (Dalmane) (47–100 h)	15 y	15–30 mg at bedtime
Lorazepam (Ativan) (12–18 h)	12 y	See product insert
Oxazepam (Serax) (5.7–0.9 h)	12 y	10–15 mg t.i.d.–q.i.d., max 30 mg t.i.d.–q.i.d.
Quazepam (Doral) (73 h)	18 y	7.5–15 mg at bedtime
Temazepam (Restoril) (9.5–12.4 h)	18 y	15–30 mg at bedtime
Triazolam (Halcion) (1.5–5.5 h)	18 y	0.125–0.25 mg at bedtime

As previously mentioned, there is a relative paucity of studies examining the use of benzodiazepines in youth. The few studies done are reviewed below, although many entail older, uncontrolled studies or case reports.

Chlordiazepoxide (Librium)

Reports of Interest

Chlordiazepoxide in the Treatment of Behaviorally Disordered Children and Adolescents of Various Diagnoses

Krakowski (1963) treated 51 emotionally disturbed children and adolescents 4 to 16 years of age with chlordiazepoxide. Criteria for inclusion were the presence of anxiety (especially with coexisting hyperactivity), irritability, hostility, impulsivity, and insomnia. Nine children had concurrent individual therapy, and seven received other medications, mainly antiepileptics. Chlordiazepoxide was administered initially in divided doses totaling 15 mg and individually titrated. Maintenance dosage for periods of up to 10 months ranged from 15 to 40 mg/day (mean, 26 mg/day). Twelve patients (23.5%) showed complete remission of psychiatric symptoms, and 22 (43.1%) improved moderately. Children with adjustment disorders were particularly likely to improve; specifically, 11 of 18 with conduct disorders, 2 of 3 with habit disturbances, and all 4 with neurotic traits showed marked or moderate remission of symptoms. Of 12 developmentally delayed patients, 3 improved moderately and 3 improved markedly. Untoward effects were relatively infrequent and included drowsiness, fatigue, muscular weakness, ataxia, anxiety, and depression. These effects were alleviated to a satisfactory degree by dosage reduction in all but one case.

Kraft et al. (1965) prescribed chlordiazepoxide to 130 patients (99 males, 31 females) who ranged in age from 2 to 17 years (112 were between 7 and 14 years of age). The most common diagnoses were primary behavior disorder (50), school phobia (18), adjustment reaction of adolescence (17), and chronic brain damage (14). Most subjects had marked hyperactivity and neurotic traits. Doses ranged from 20 to 130 mg/day and were administered in divided doses; 94 subjects (72%) received 40 mg or more daily. Moderate or marked improvement occurred in 53 subjects (40.8%). Forty subjects (30.8%) had either no or insignificant improvement, and 37 (28.5%) worsened. The diagnostic group showing the greatest improvement was school phobia (77%). Only 38% of the primary behavior disorder subjects and 41.2% of the adolescent adjustment disorder subjects improved to a moderate or marked degree. Of those with organic brain damage, 50% worsened, 28.6% showed minimal or no benefit, and none had an excellent response. Across diagnoses, symptoms of hyperactivity, fear, night terrors, enuresis, reading and speech problems, truancy, and disturbed or bizarre behavior were moderately or markedly improved in 40.8% of the 130 subjects. The authors concluded that chlordiazepoxide was effective in decreasing anxiety and "emotional overload" (Kraft et al., 1965). The authors also reported that 22 of the 130 had untoward effects of sufficient severity to interfere with treatment results and that 14 other subjects had milder untoward effects that were transient or responded to a lowering of the dose.

Breitner (1962) administered chlordiazepoxide, 20 to 50 mg/day, to more than 50 juvenile delinquents between 8.5 and 24 years of age. He reported that the drug produced cooperativeness, released tension, created a feeling of well-being, and made the subjects more accessible to psychotherapy.

D'Amato (1962) treated nine children 8 to 11 years of age, who were diagnosed with school phobia, with 10 to 30 mg/day of chlordiazepoxide for 5 to 30 days. The children were also seen in psychotherapy. Only one child did not attend school regularly after the second week of treatment. The author compared these 9 children with 11 others, aged 5 years to 12 years, also diagnosed with school phobia, who were treated over the six preceding years with psychotherapy only. Only 2 of these 11 children returned to school within 2 weeks, and 9 remained out of school for 1 month or longer. The author thought that this strongly suggested that chlordiazepoxide was an effective adjunct to psychotherapy in mobilizing children with school phobia to return to school.

Petti et al. (1982) treated nine boys (7 to 11 years of age) with chlordiazepoxide who failed to respond to 3 weeks of hospitalization and treatment with placebo. The subjects' diagnoses were conduct disorder (five, three of whom had borderline features), personality disorder (three, one of whom had borderline features), and schizophrenia (one). Verbal IQs on the Wechsler Intelligence Scale for Children (WISC) ranged from 71 to 110. Target symptoms were anxiety, depression, impulsivity, and explosiveness. The initial dose of chlordiazepoxide was 15 mg, administered in divided doses. The optimal dose was determined by individual titration and ranged from 15 to 120 mg/day (0.58 to 5.28 mg/kg/day). Children's ratings on optimal dose were compared with baseline ratings. Marked improvement was noted in two boys, improvement in four, and no change or worsening in three. The major improvements were increased verbal production, increased rapidity of thought associations, and a shift from blunted affect or depressed mood, to a more animated appearance and feeling subjectively better. The authors noted that chlordiazepoxide had the most positive effect on children who were withdrawn, inhibited, anergic, depressed, or anxious. The child with schizophrenia had a worsening of psychotic symptoms, and two children with severe impulsive aggressiveness experienced a worsening of behavior. The authors suggest that chlordiazepoxide's use may be contraindicated in such children (Petti et al., 1982).

Diazepam (Valium)

Reports of Interest

Diazepam in the Treatment of Children and Adolescents with Various Psychiatric Diagnoses

Lucas and Pasley (1969), in one of the few double-blind, placebo-controlled studies of benzodiazepines in this age group, administered diazepam to 12 subjects, 7 to 17 years of age (mean, 12.3 years) who were diagnosed as psychoneurotic ($N = 10$) or schizophrenic ($N = 2$). All subjects were inpatients or in a daycare program. Target symptoms included moderate to high anxiety levels, highly oppositional behavior, poor peer relationships, and aggression. The initial dose of diazepam was 2.5 mg twice daily. The drug was increased until a satisfactory therapeutic response or untoward effects occurred. The maximum dose achieved was 20 mg/day. The study lasted 16 weeks, during which subjects were assigned randomly to four different sequences of drug and placebo. Subjects were rated on 10 items: hyperactivity, anxiety and tension, oppositional behavior, aggressiveness, impulsivity, relationship to peers, relationship to adults, need for limit setting, response to limit setting, and participation in program. There was no significant difference between diazepam and placebo on any item for the nine patients who completed the study (the two patients with schizophrenia and one other patient dropped out). However, when scores on all 10 items were combined, diazepam scored significantly better than placebo ($P < .05$), although clinically the difference was not very apparent. Eleven of the 12 children, who participated in the study long enough, were rated on a global rating scale. Five subjects showed no change, two were somewhat more anxious, and four were definitely worse, with increased anxiety and deterioration in their behavior on diazepam compared with placebo. From this study, and their clinical experience with diazepam, the authors concluded that diazepam was not clinically effective in reducing anxiety or acting-out behavior in children and young adolescents. Older adolescents appeared to react similar to adults, and diazepam was thought to be useful in treating their anxiety.

Diazepam in the Treatment of Sleep Disorder

In an open study, three children with somnambulism and night terrors (pavor nocturnus) and four children with insomnia were treated with 2 to 5 mg of diazepam near bedtime, and all seven responded favorably (Glick et al., 1971).

Alprazolam (Xanax)

Reports of Interest

Alprazolam in the Treatment of Night Terrors (Pavor Nocturnus)

Cameron and Thyer (1985) successfully treated night terrors in a 10-year-old girl with alprazolam. She was initially prescribed 0.5 mg of alprazolam at bedtime for 1 week. The dose was increased to 0.75 mg nightly for the next 4 weeks, after which alprazolam was tapered off. Night terrors ceased on the first night and at follow-up 9 months later had not occurred.

Alprazolam in the Treatment of Anxiety Disorders

Pfefferbaum et al. (1987) used alprazolam to treat anticipatory and acute situational anxiety and panic in 13 patients, ages 7 to 14 years, who were being treated with stressful procedures for concomitant cancer. Alprazolam treatment was initiated 3 days before and continued through the day of the stressful procedures. This study was conducted under an Investigational New Drug permit, and the maximum dose allowed was 0.02 mg/kg/dose or 0.06 mg/kg/day, with the exception of one child who the FDA granted approval to receive a total of 0.05 mg/kg/dose, or 0.15 mg/kg/day. In this study, alprazolam was initiated at 0.005 mg/kg or lower and was titrated upward based on efficacy and tolerability. Typical total daily doses ranged from 0.375 to 3 mg (0.003 to 0.075 mg/kg/day). Subjects were rated on four scales measuring anxiety, distress, and panic. The subjects' improvement was statistically significant ($P < .05$) on three scales and reached borderline significance on the fourth scale. Mild drowsiness was the most frequently reported adverse effect. Overall, untoward effects were minimal in this small study.

Klein and Last (1989) reported Klein's unpublished data from a clinical trial of alprazolam in children and adolescents, whose separation anxiety disorder did not respond to psychotherapy. Alprazolam was clinically effective when administered to 18 subjects (ages 6 to 17 years) for 6 weeks in daily doses of 0.5 to 6 mg/day (mean dose 1.9 mg/day). Parents and the psychiatrist judged that >80% of the subjects improved significantly, whereas only 65% of the subjects rated themselves as improved.

Simeon and Ferguson (1987) administered alprazolam openly to 12 children and adolescents (8.8 to 16.5 years of age; mean, 11.5 years) diagnosed with overanxious and/or avoidant disorder. After 1-week of treatment with placebo, to which none of the subjects responded, alprazolam was titrated individually over a subsequent 2-week period to maximum daily doses of 0.50 to 1.5 mg. The total period of active treatment was 4 weeks. Seven of the 12 youth showed at least a moderate improvement on several rating scales, and no child worsened. Clinician ratings showed significant improvement of anxiety, depression, and psychomotor excitation; parents reported significant improvement of anxiety and hyperactivity on questionnaires, and teachers reported significant improvement on an anxious–passive factor. Parents frequently reported improvement in the subjects' sleep problems. Simeon and Ferguson (1987) observed that subjects with good premorbid personalities and prominent symptoms of inhibitions, shyness, and nervousness responded best to alprazolam and showed continued improvement after the medication was discontinued. By contrast, patients with poor premorbid personalities and poor family backgrounds were more commonly observed to develop undesirable symptoms of disinhibition, such as increased aggressiveness and impulsivity, especially at higher doses, and were more apt to relapse following drug withdrawal. The few untoward effects noted in this small study were mild and transient. Ferguson and Simeon (1984) reported no adverse effects of alprazolam on cognition or learning when used at therapeutically effective doses.

Simeon et al. (1992) reported a double-blind placebo-controlled study of alprazolam in 30 children and adolescents (23 males and 7 females; ages 8.4 to 16.9 years; mean age 12.6 years) who had primary diagnoses of overanxious disorder ($N = 21$) or avoidant disorder ($N = 9$). Clinical impairment ranged from moderate to severe. Placebo was administered for 1 week and was followed by random assignment to a 4-week period of either placebo or alprazolam. Medication was tapered with placebo substitution during the fifth week. During the sixth week, all subjects received only placebo. Patients who weighed <40 kg received an initial dose of 0.25 mg of alprazolam, whereas heavier patients received an initial dose of 0.5 mg. The maximum daily dosage permitted was 0.04 mg/kg. Alprazolam was increased at 2-day intervals until an optimal dose was achieved. At completion of the active drug phase, the average daily dose of alprazolam was 1.57 mg (range 0.5 to 3.5 mg). Untoward effects were few and minor (e.g., dry mouth and feeling tired) and did not appear to interfere with academic performance.

Simeon et al. (1992) noted a strong treatment effect in both placebo and alprazolam groups during this trial. Overall, alprazolam was judged to be superior to placebo based on clinical global ratings, but the differences were not statistically significant. There were strong individual responders in both groups. At study completion, there was a slight relapse of original symptoms among subjects receiving alprazolam, whereas subjects who took placebo showed no change in symptoms and/or continued to improve. The authors commented that doses employed in this study were relatively low and were administered for only 4 weeks. They suggested that higher doses and longer trials be investigated in the future and recommended that alprazolam be tapered more gradually over a period of several weeks in the future (Simeon et al., 1992).

Bernstein et al. (1990) similarly discovered that alprazolam did not separate from placebo (or imipramine) in a small placebo-controlled double-blind study of youth with anxiety disorders. In their study, 24 youth (ages 7 to 18 years old) with diagnoses of school refusal and separation anxiety disorder were randomized to receive either placebo, imipramine (50 to 175 mg/day), or alprazolam (0.75 to 4.0 mg/day). The authors concluded that there was no significant difference between the three treatment groups by the end of the study (Bernstein et al., 1990).

Clonazepam (Klonopin)

Clonazepam is approved for the treatment of seizure disorders in pediatrics.

Reports of Interest

Clonazepam in the Treatment of Panic Disorder

In an open clinical trial, Kutcher and MacKenzie (1988) treated four adolescents (three females and one male; average age 17.2 years; range 16 to 19 years) diagnosed with panic disorder by DSM-III criteria, with a fixed dose of clonazepam (0.5 mg twice daily). Average ratings on the Hamilton Anxiety Rating Scale fell from 32 at baseline, to 7.5 at week 1 and 5.7 at week 2. The number of panic attacks fell from an average of 3 to 0.5 per week after 1 week to 0.25 per week after 2 weeks. One adolescent complained of initial drowsiness that resolved within 4 days, and no other untoward effects were reported. At follow-up examinations 3 to 6 months later, all four patients continued to take clonazepam and appeared to maintain improved functioning in school and interpersonal relations.

Clonazepam in the Treatment of Childhood Anxiety Disorders

Graae et al. (1994) treated 15 subjects (8 males, 7 females; age range 7 to 13 years; mean 9.8 ± 2.1 years) diagnosed with various anxiety and comorbid disorders, with clonazepam in an 8-week, double-blind, placebo-controlled, crossover study. Diagnoses included separation anxiety disorder ($N = 14$), overanxious disorder ($N = 6$), social phobia ($N = 5$), oppositional disorder ($N = 3$), avoidant disorder ($N = 2$), conduct disorder ($N = 1$), and attention-deficit/hyperactivity disorder (ADHD) ($N = 1$). Clonazepam was initiated with a 0.25-mg dose at breakfast and increased by 0.25 mg every third day to a total dose of 1.0 mg/day. Subsequent increments of 0.25 mg were made every other day until a dose of 2 mg/day was reached or until untoward effects or compliance issues prevented it. After receiving clonazepam at a maximum of 2 mg/day for 4 days, subjects' clonazepam was gradually tapered off by the end of the 4-week period.

Three boys dropped out while on active medication, two because of serious disinhibition including marked irritability, tantrums, aggressivity, and self-injurious behavior and the other because of noncompliance. Nine children were rated as clinically improved (five had good/marked improvement and four had some/moderate improvement), and three children showed no improvement of anxiety or overall functioning while on clonazepam. Although there was no statistically significant difference between clonazepam and placebo for the 12 subjects, the authors thought individual patients made significant clinical improvements while on clonazepam. The most common untoward effects were drowsiness, irritability, lability, and oppositional behavior. Overall, 10 (83%) children had untoward effects on clonazepam compared with 7 (53%) on placebo. The difference was not statistically significant, however. Disinhibition was not seen in the placebo-treated group, and the two boys taking clonazepam who dropped out because of this effect were not included in the data analysis. Study authors suggested that a slower upward dose titration might reduce the untoward effects seen with clonazepam, including disinhibition (Graae et al., 1994).

Clonazepam in the Treatment of Obsessive-Compulsive Disorder

Ross and Piggott (1993) treated a 14-year-old male with clonazepam who was hospitalized with severely disabling obsessive-compulsive disorder. The patient did not respond adequately to prior trials of clomipramine, thioridazine, alprazolam, fluoxetine, or diazepam, either alone or in various combinations. Clonazepam was administered at an initial dose of 0.5 mg twice daily and increased to 1.0 mg twice daily after 1 week. Behavioral improvement was noted by week 2 on the medication, and he was able to be discharged home after taking clonazepam for 11 weeks.

Leonard et al. (1994) reported the use of clonazepam as an augmenting agent in a 20-year-old who had severely disabling obsessive-compulsive disorder with onset at age 7. He was treatment-resistant to prior trials of clomipramine, desipramine, fluoxetine, fluvoxamine, and buspirone augmentation, either alone or in various combinations. He experienced marked clinical improvement with at least 75% reduction in symptom severity on a combination of 60 mg/day of fluoxetine and 4 mg/day of clonazepam, which was maintained for approximately 1 year. The authors suggested that clonazepam might be efficacious and safe when used to augment specific serotonin reuptake inhibitors in treating obsessive-compulsive disorder in children and adolescents.

AZASPIRODECANEDIONES

Buspirone Hydrochloride (Buspar)

Buspirone hydrochloride is a drug with anxiolytic properties that is chemically distinct from benzodiazepines, barbiturates, or other sedative or anxiolytic medication. It has a high affinity for 5-HT$_{1A}$ serotonin receptors, an affinity associated with clinical anxiolytic properties and anticonflict activity in animals (Sussman, 1994b). Buspirone has moderate affinity for brain D$_2$-dopamine receptors. It does not have significant affinity for benzodiazepine receptors, nor does it affect gamma-aminobutyric acid (GABA) binding. Furthermore, buspirone has no cross-tolerance with benzodiazepines, will not suppress panic attacks, and lacks anticonvulsant activity (Sussman, 1994b); hence, it does not block the withdrawal syndrome that may occur when benzodiazepines and other common sedative hypnotic drugs are abruptly discontinued. At therapeutic doses, buspirone is less sedating than benzodiazepines. It does not result in physical or psychological dependence or notable withdrawal when discontinued, and due to its low abuse potential it is not classified as a controlled (Schedule II) substance.

Buspirone is approved by the FDA for the management of anxiety disorders, including short-term relief of the anxiety symptoms. However, unlike benzodiazepines, which have an immediate anxiolytic effect, buspirone may take as long as 1 to 2 weeks for its antianxiety effect to develop fully (Sussman, 1994b). Symptom improvement may continue for at least 4 weeks with psychic symptoms of anxiety improving sooner than somatic symptoms of anxiety (Feighner and Cohen, 1989).

Pharmacokinetics of Buspirone Hydrochloride

Buspirone is rapidly absorbed, with peak plasma levels occurring between 40 and 90 minutes after an acute oral dose of buspirone. Average elimination half-life after single doses of 10 to 40 mg of buspirone is usually between 2 and 3 hours. In a 21-day open-label, multisite, dose-escalation study comparing buspirone pharmacokinetics in children ($N = 13$, ages 6 to 12 years), adolescents ($N = 12$, ages 13 to 17 years), and adults ($N = 14$, ages 18 to 45 years), Salazar et al. (2001)

demonstrated that mean plasma concentrations of buspirone are equal to or higher in youth compared with adults. Furthermore, 1-pyrimidinylpiperazine (1-PP), buspirone's primary metabolite, was significantly higher in children compared with both adolescents and adults in all four dosing arms (5, 7.5, 15, and 30 mg b.i.d.) (Salazar et al., 2001).

Contraindications for Buspirone Hydrochloride Administration

A known hypersensitivity to buspirone hydrocholoride is a contraindication for its use.

Interactions of Buspirone Hydrochloride with Other Drugs

Buspirone should not be used concomitantly with MAOIs, as this may result in hypertension. Buspirone is a CYP450 3A4 substrate, and hence CYP450 3A4 inducers (phenytoin, carbamezapine, modafinil, etc.) may decrease buspirone concentrations. Similarly, CYP450 3A4 inhibitors (ketoconazole, ritonavir, etc.) may increase buspirone concentrations. Due to additive effects, buspirone may increase the risk of serotonin syndrome when used concomitantly with other serotonergic medications (SSRIs, tramadol, triptans, etc.).

Untoward Effects of Buspirone Hydrochloride

The untoward effects most frequently reported by adults taking buspirone include dizziness (12%), drowsiness (10%), nausea (8%), headache (6%), insomnia (3%), and lightheadedness (3%). Of note, however, drowsiness and insomnia were reported to occur with approximately equal frequency in subjects taking placebo; hence, these effects may not have been related to buspirone per se (PDR, 2000). In a 3-week dose-escalation study, Salazar et al. (2001) discovered that the most commonly reported adverse events in youth (ages 6 to 17 years) were lightheadedness (67% of subjects), headache (50% of subjects), and dyspepsia (21% of subjects), whereas in adults (ages 18 to 45 years) the most commonly reported adverse events were somnolence (21.4% of subjects), and lightheadedness, nausea, vomiting, and diarrhea (all 14.3% of subjects). In this particular study, buspirone was dosed as follows for all study participants: buspirone 5 mg b.i.d. (days 1 to 3), 7.5 mg b.i.d. (days 4 to 7), 15 mg b.i.d. (days 8 to 14), and 30 mg b.i.d. (days 15 to 21) (Salazar et al., 2001).

Indications for Buspirone Hydrochloride in Child and Adolescent Psychiatry

Buspirone is approved only for treatment of anxiety disorders and the short-term relief of anxiety in individuals at least 18 years of age. There are no definitive child and adolescent psychiatric indications for this medication, and its use in youth is necessarily "off-label."

Buspirone Dosage Schedule

- *Children and adolescents up to 17 years of age:* Not approved. Coffey (1990), however, suggested the following doses if a clinician elects to use buspirone in this age group:

    Prepubescent children: An initial total daily dose of 2.5 to 5 mg with increases of 2.5 mg every 3 to 4 days to a maximum of 20 mg/day.

    Younger adolescents: An initial total daily dose of 5 to 10 mg with increases of 5 to 10 mg every 3 to 4 days to a maximum of 60 mg/day. In a small dose-escalation study, Salazar et al. (2001) discovered that buspirone was generally safe and well tolerated in doses up to 30 mg b.i.d. in adolescents (*N* = 12, ages 13 to 17 years) and adults (*N* = 14, ages 18 to 45 years), though it was less well tolerated in children (ages 6 to 12 years) when used at doses higher than 7.5 mg b.i.d. Specifically, 2 of the 13 children withdrew from the study due to mild or moderate adverse effects

(continued)

when taking buspirone at the higher doses (15 and 30 mg b.i.d.). Study authors hence concluded that buspirone appeared well tolerated in youth ages 6 to 12 years at doses up to 7.5 mg b.i.d. (Salazar et al., 2001).

- *Adolescents at least 18 years of age and adults:* Initiate treatment with 7.5 mg twice daily. Titrate to optimal therapeutic response by increases of 5 mg every 2 to 3 days to a maximum daily dose of 60 mg. Usual optimal doses in clinical trials were 20 to 30 mg/day in divided doses.

Buspirone Hydrochloride Dose Forms Available

- *Tablets (scored):* 5, 7.5, and 10 mg
- *Dividose (scored for bisection or trisection):* 15 and 30 mg

Reports of Interest

Buspirone Hydrochloride in the Treatment of Anxiety Disorders in Children and Adolescents

Kranzler (1988) reported a single case study in which a 13-year-old adolescent diagnosed with overanxious disorder (now defined as DSM-IV-TR GAD), school refusal, and intermittent enuresis was administered buspirone. A previous trial of desipramine yielded some improvement, but was discontinued at the patient's request due to untoward effects. Buspirone was initially administered at 2.5 mg three times daily. At doses of 5 mg three times daily, she experienced morning drowsiness, so buspirone was decreased to 5 mg twice daily. Scores on the Hamilton Anxiety Rating Scale dropped from 26 to 15, and improvements were noted in phobic anxiety, insomnia, depressed mood, cardiovascular symptoms, and anxious behavior, though enuresis did not improve.

Simeon et al. (1994) treated 15 children (10 males, 5 females; age range, 6 to 14 years; mean age, 10 years) diagnosed with separation anxiety disorder (5), overanxious disorder (2), comorbid separation anxiety and overanxious disorders (4), separation, overanxious, and avoidant disorders (1), separation, overanxious, and obsessive-compulsive disorders (1), and overanxious disorder and ADHD (2). Subjects were rated moderately to severely impaired on the Clinical Global Impressions Scale (CGI). A single-blind placebo was administered for the initial 2 weeks, which was followed by 4 weeks of treatment with buspirone, administered initially at 5 mg daily and increased weekly by 5 mg increments as needed to a maximum of 20 mg/day (mean dose 18.6 mg/day). No subjects improved significantly on placebo. After 4 weeks on buspirone, subjects' ratings on the CGI showed marked improvement (3), moderate improvement (10), and minimal improvement (2). Repeated measures of multivariate analysis of variance (MANOVA) showed a statistically significant treatment effect after 2 weeks on medication ($P < .016$), which increased in significance to $P < .001$ after both 3 and 4 weeks on medication. Significant improvements were also seen on several rating scales as reported by parents, teachers, and subjects themselves. Untoward effects, which were mild and appeared to follow dose increases, included nausea or stomach pain ($N = 5$), headache ($N = 4$), occasional sleepwalking, sleep talking, or nightmares, and daytime tiredness ($N = 8$).

Zwier and Rao (1994) reported treating a hospitalized 16-year-old male with social phobia and schizotypal personality disorder using buspirone, initially at 5 mg/day, followed by 5 mg dose increases every 3 days, to a total daily dose of 20 mg. At 12 days of buspirone treatment, scores on the Hamilton Anxiety Rating Scale dropped from 5 to 0, at which time the patient was discharged. Over the subsequent year, buspirone was tapered to 5 mg/day, the patient's mild psychotic symptoms resolved, and he was reported to have maintained his treatment gains.

Realmuto et al. (1989) treated four autistic children, 9 to 10 years of age, with buspirone 5 mg administered three times daily for 4 weeks, followed by a week-long washout period and 4 weeks of 10 mg twice daily of either fenfluramine or methylphenidate. Two of the four children showed decreased hyperactivity while on buspirone. None of the children experienced adverse untoward effects from buspirone.

In a 3-week, double-blind, placebo-controlled crossover study, McCormick (1997) studied the safety and efficacy of buspirone for the treatment of hyperactivity in a patient with autistic disorder. The child received placebo for 3 weeks, followed by buspirone treatment for 3 weeks. The Conners abbreviated parent and teacher questionnaires, as well as the number of daily performance tasks completed by the child at school, were used as primary outcome measures. Buspirone was ultimately determined to be safe and efficacious for reducing hyperactivity and increasing school-based performance tasks. The author concluded that buspirone may be a beneficial medication for autistic patients, though cautioned that further study is needed (McCormick, 1997).

Buitelaar et al. (1998) evaluated the efficacy and safety of buspirone in a 6- to 8-week, open-label study treating chronic manifest pervasive anxiety, irritability, and/or affect dysregulation in 22 inpatients (20 males, 2 females; age range, 6 to 16 years), 20 of whom were diagnosed with pervasive developmental disorder not otherwise specified (PDDNOS) and two of whom were diagnosed with autistic disorder by DSM-III-R criteria (APA, 1987). Target symptoms were anxiety in 14 patients, irritability in 1, and both anxiety and irritability in 7. Efficacy was determined by ratings on the Clinical Global Impressions (CGI) Scale, using subscales CGI–Anxiety and CGI–Irritability, and the CGI–Severity (CGI-S) and the CGI–Improvement (CGI-I) Scales. Buspirone was initiated at a dose of 5 mg three times daily and individually titrated based on clinical response, to a maximum dose of 45 mg/day, which could be achieved within 3 weeks. Eighteen subjects received buspirone only, and four subjects continued to receive one additional drug. Twenty-one subjects completed 6 to 8 weeks on buspirone, whereas one subject dropped out earlier due to a lack of clinical response. Therapeutic improvement was apparent after 2 to 3 weeks of treatment in many subjects (mean daily dose was 29.3 mg/day). Overall on the CGI-I, 16 (76%) of 21 patients were responders (9 "marked" improvement, 7 "moderate" improvement) with clinically significant reductions of overwhelming anxiety, irritability, and temper tantrums. Six subjects did not experience therapeutic benefit. Of the 21 patients with targeted anxiety, 16 were responders (9 "marked" and 7 "moderate"), and of the 8 patients with "irritability" 5 were responders (2 "marked" and 3 "moderate"). Mild untoward effects were reported in 5 subjects and included initial sedation ($N = 2$), mild agitation ($N = 2$), and initial nausea ($N = 1$). All 16 responders continued to receive buspirone, were followed for 2 to 12 months, and maintained all therapeutic gains. One child, however, developed abnormal involuntary movement of the mouth, cheeks, and tongue after receiving 20 mg/day of buspirone for 10 months. The authors considered this a buspirone-associated orofacial-lingual dyskinesia and discontinued medication. The abnormal movements completely remitted within 2 weeks. This study suggests buspirone may be therapeutically useful in treating anxiety and irritability in some children and adolescents with pervasive developmental disorders.

Buspirone Hydrochloride in the Treatment of Aggression

Quiason et al. (1991) treated a hospitalized 8-year-old boy with conduct and ADHDs with buspirone hydrochloride. Buspirone was initially administered at 5 mg three times per day and titrated gradually to 15 mg three times a day.

By day 10, there was a notable decrease in aggressive and assaultive behavior, and the need for timeouts or seclusion ceased altogether.

Pfeffer et al. (1997) treated 25 anxious and moderately aggressive prepubertal inpatients (19 males, 6 females; ages 5 to 11 years, mean age, 8.0 ± 1.8 years) with buspirone. Subjects' DSM-III-R (APA, 1987) diagnoses included mood disorder ($N = 9$), disruptive behavior disorder ($N = 21$), anxiety disorders ($N = 8$), and specific developmental disorders ($N = 9$). This 11-week study began with a 2-week baseline evaluation phase that was followed by 3 weeks of active buspirone treatment. Buspirone was dosed initially at 5 mg/day and was increased by 5 to 10 mg every 3 days to a maximum of 50 mg/day. Subjects were then maintained at their optimal dose of buspirone for an additional 6 weeks. Efficacy was determined by analysis of ratings on the Child Depression Inventory (CDI); the Revised Children's Manifest Anxiety Scale (RCMAS); the Measure of Aggression, Violence, and Rage in Children (MAVRIC); the Suicidal and Assaultive Behavior Scales (SABS); the Overt Aggression Scale (OAS); the Children's Global Assessment Scale (CGAS); and the Udvalg for Kliniske Undersogelser (UKU) Side Effects Rating Scale (Lingjaerde et al., 1987).

During the second week of titration, four children developed behavioral toxicity (agitation and increased aggressivity) and were terminated from the study. Of the 21 subjects who entered the maintenance phase, 2 were terminated because they developed severe euphoric symptoms, increased impulsivity, and maladaptive behavior. Thus, only 19 (76%) subjects completed the 11-week study. The mean dose for completers was 28 mg/day, administered in two divided doses. For the 19 completers, there was a significant decrease ($P = .001$) in CDI scores from baseline (19 ± 8.2) to endpoint (9.2 ± 7.5). This level of improvement was achieved during the sixth week on buspirone. Seven of the 10 completers with clinically significant depression at baseline (CDI score > 18) had a CDI score of <12 (i.e., below the cutoff for nonclinically significant depression). There was a significant reduction in the number of restraints and/or seclusions used ($P = .01$), and the duration of time children spent restrained and/or secluded decreased significantly ($P = .02$). Although there was a significant decrease ($P = .02$) in the MAVRIC at endpoint, subjects continued to exhibit clinically significant levels of aggression. Similarly, CGAS scores, reflecting clinical global functioning, improved from 40.68 ± 10.49 at baseline to 54.47 ± 14.18 at endpoint ($P = .01$), and significant clinical impairments persisted. Three children improved sufficiently to continue on buspirone following completion of the study. Overall, although significant, the therapeutic efficacy on aggression and anxiety was limited, and clinically significant aggression, anxiety, and global impairment remained. Furthermore, six patients terminated prematurely from the study due to significant untoward effects. The study authors concluded that overall, the results of this study were not very promising (Pfeffer et al., 1997).

Buspirone Hydrochloride in the Treatment of ADHD

McCormick et al. (1994) conducted a 4-week, double-blind, placebo-controlled, crossover study in which buspirone hydrochloride was administered to 10 males ranging in age from 11 years, 3 months to 16 years, 10 months (mean age, 13 years, 7 months) who were diagnosed with ADHD by DSM-III-R criteria (APA, 1987). The only comorbid diagnoses were learning disorders, which occurred in four (40%) of the subjects. Each subject was randomly assigned to *receive* buspirone or placebo for 2 weeks, after which the conditions were reversed for an additional 2 weeks. On school days only, subjects received either buspirone 5 mg (at 8:00 and 11:00 AM), or placebo. During weekly telephone interviews with subjects' families, the 10-item Conners' Abbreviated Teacher Rating Scale was completed. Analysis showed no significant carryover effect between the two conditions.

The mean Conners' baseline score of 20.2 decreased to 19.3 during the second week of placebo therapy and decreased to 14.8 during the second week of buspirone therapy. Nine of the 10 subjects improved on buspirone compared with placebo, which was a significant treatment effect ($P < .025$). The only reported untoward effect for buspirone was 3 days of nausea experienced by one subject.

In a 6-week open-label trial, Malhotra and Santosh (1998) treated 12 outpatients (10 males, 2 females; mean age, 8.2 years; age range, 6 to 12 years) diagnosed with ADHD with buspirone. The Conners' Parent Abbreviated 10-item index (CPAI) and the Children's Global Assessment Scale (CGAS) at baseline, and 1, 2, 4, 6, and 8 weeks (i.e., after 2 weeks off medication) were used to assess efficacy. Subjects were administered an initial buspirone dose of 0.5 mg/kg/day (dose range, 15 to 30 mg/day) divided into two doses, which was continued for 6 weeks. No other medication was administered during the study. The mean CPAI improvement at day 7 was significant ($P < .001$). Clinical improvement continued over the 6-week period, and at the end of the study, at day 42, all four domains of the CPAI (inattention, hyperactivity, impulsivity, and behavior) improved significantly ($P < .0001$ for each domain). Based on reduced symptom severity of >50% and significant clinical improvement, all 12 patients were deemed responders. The CGAS scores improved significantly from baseline by day 7 ($P < .0001$) and by day 42 ($P < .0001$). All 12 subjects experienced symptom relapse within 2 weeks of discontinuing buspirone (the mean CPAI score returned nearly to baseline), and all families elected to restart their children on buspirone. Only two subjects reported untoward effects, with both experiencing mild transient dizziness during the first week of treatment. The authors concluded that buspirone was safe and effective in reducing the symptoms of ADHD in this group of subjects.

In a double-blind and randomized trial, Davari-Ashtiani et al. (2010) studied buspirone versus methylphenidate for the treatment of ADHD. Thirty-four youth were randomized to receive buspirone (0.5 mg/kg/day) or methylphenidate (0.3 to 1 mg/kg/day) for 6 weeks. The principal outcome measures were the parent and teacher ADHD Rating Scale scores. At week 6, both groups' parent and teacher ADHD Rating Scale scores significantly declined from baseline ($P < .001$), which correlated with significant improvements in ADHD symptoms. No significant differences between total scores occurred between groups, though methylphenidate was found to be superior to buspirone for inattentive symptoms. The author noted that buspirone had a more favorable side-effect profile than methylphenidate and opined that while these preliminary findings are positive, larger trials are needed before definitive conclusions can be drawn (Davari-Ashtiani et al., 2010).

Buspirone Hydrochloride for the Treatment of Bruxism

Sabuncuoglu et al. (2009) reported a case of an adolescent with fluoxetine-induced bruxism that was successfully treated with buspirone. The authors hypothesized that buspirone, as a 5-HT$_{1A}$ agonist, reduces serotonergic activity and increase dopaminergic activity, which may help with the theorized SSRI-led dopamine depletion that manifests as nocturnal bruxism (Sabuncuoglu et al., 2009).

Orsagh-Yentis et al. (2011) reported a case of a 7-year-old boy with PDD-NOS and moderate mental retardation, who presented with significant bruxism, predominantly diurnal, but also nocturnal. His severe bruxism led to his teeth being ground flush with his gum-line. Due to concern that his bruxism may represent internal distress, he was started on buspirone 2.5 mg daily for 1 week, which was then increased to 2.5 mg twice daily. After 2 weeks on this dose, he showed no improvement in symptoms, so buspirone was increased to 5 mg twice daily. Due to only brief improvement over the subsequent 2 months, an additional dose increase to 5 mg three times daily was made. On this dose, his parents reported that his bruxism ceased during both days and nights. At follow-up 9 months after starting buspirone, he remained overall improved, though his afternoon bruxism recurred, which prompted a final buspirone dose increase to 7.5 mg three times daily. Within weeks, his bruxism again remitted. While buspirone was considered overall effective for bruxism in this patient, it was associated with daytime sedation and sleep disturbance, which did not respond to melatonin and only partially responded to trazodone (Orsagh-Yentis et al., 2011). Future studies are warranted.

Other Drugs

RICK BOWERS

ANTIHISTAMINES

Diphenhydramine (Benadryl) and hydroxyzine (Atarax, Vistaril) are the antihistamines most frequently used in treating children and adolescents with emotional disorders. Chronologically, they were also among the earliest drugs used in child and adolescent psychopharmacotherapy, and they remain among the safest medications ever employed.

Contraindications for Antihistamine Administration

Known hypersensitivity to antihistamines is a contraindication for their prescription.

Infants born prematurely and infants are especially sensitive to the stimulating effects of antihistamines, and overdose may cause hallucinations, convulsions, or death. Because antihistamines may be secreted in breast milk, nursing mothers should also avoid taking antihistamines.

Narrow-angle glaucoma, stenosing peptic ulcer, pyloroduodenal obstruction, and symptomatic prostatic hypertrophy or bladder-neck obstruction are relative contraindications. The anticholinergic effects of antihistamines and the additional atropine-like effect of diphenhydramine hydrochloride may cause drying and thickening of bronchial secretions; hence, they should be used with caution in patients with clinical symptoms of asthma or poorly controlled asthma.

Interactions of Antihistamines with Other Drugs

Diphenhydramine and hydroxyzine have potentiating effects when used in conjunction with other central nervous system depressants, such as alcohol, narcotics, nonnarcotic analgesics, barbiturates, hypnotics, antipsychotics, and anxiolytics.

Monoamine oxidase inhibitors prolong and intensify the drying effect (an anticholinergic action) of antihistamines.

Diphenhydramine Hydrochloride (Benadryl)

Diphenhydramine hydrochloride has been used for more than 50 years to treat psychiatrically disturbed children (Effron and Freedman, 1953). Although such use is still not approved for advertising by the U.S. Food and Drug Administration (FDA), it is reviewed here because some child psychiatrists continue to find it clinically effective.

Fish (1960) reported that diphenhydramine is most effective in behavioral disorders associated with anxiety and hyperactivity but that it could also be useful in moderately (not severely) disturbed children with organic or schizophrenic (including autistic) disorders. A later study of 15 children, however, found no significant difference in behavioral improvement between diphenhydramine in doses of 200 to 800 mg/day and placebo (Korein et al., 1971).

Diphenhydramine is also effective as an anxiolytic, reducing anxiety before producing drowsiness or lethargy, in children up to approximately 10 years of age. However, it shows a marked decrease in efficacy when administered to older children; their response is similar to adults with untoward effects of malaise or drowsiness. Therefore, for older children diphenhydramine is useful primarily as a bedtime sedative for insomnia and/or nighttime anxiety (Fish, 1960).

Diphenhydramine has also been used to treat children with insomnia and/or children who wake up after falling asleep and have marked difficulty falling asleep again. Russo et al. (1976) compared diphenhydramine and placebo administered to 50 children, aged 2 to 12 years, who had difficulty falling asleep or problems with night awakenings. Diphenhydramine 1 mg/kg was significantly better than placebo in decreasing sleep-onset latency and decreasing the number of awakenings over a 7-day trial period. Total sleeping time, however, was not significantly increased. Side effects were minimal.

Contraindications for the Administration of Diphenhydramine Hydrochloride

The administration of diphenhydramine is contraindicated in premature infants and infants.

Untoward Effects of Diphenhydramine Hydrochloride

The most frequent untoward effects are anticholinergic effects and sedation. Children do seem more tolerant of the sedative effects of diphenhydramine, but the clinician should still be alert to any cognitive dulling that may interfere with learning. Young children may sometimes be excited rather than sedated by diphenhydramine. It is cautioned that overdose may cause hallucinations, convulsions, or death, particularly in infants and young children.

Diphenhydramine Hydrochloride Dosage Schedule for Treatment of Children and Adolescents

- *Premature infants and infants below 20 lb:* The use of diphenhydramine is contraindicated.
- *Infants >20 lb (9.1 kg) and older children:* Administer initially a 12.5- or 25-mg dose and titrate upward with 12.5- or 25-mg increases for optimal response. A maximum dose of 300 mg/day or 5 mg/kg/day, whichever is less, is recommended. Maximum activity occurs in about 1 hour, and the effects last about 4 to 6 hours; therefore, the drug is usually administered three to four times daily. Young children appear to tolerate a higher dose per unit of weight than do adolescents and adults. Fish (1960) found a dose range from 2 to 10 mg/kg/day, with an average daily dose of 4 mg/kg, to be most effective in treating behaviorally disturbed youngsters.

Diphenhydramine Hydrochloride Dose Forms Available

- *Capsules:* 25 and 50 mg
- *Elixir:* 12.5 mg/5 mL
- *Injectable preparations:* 10 and 50 mg/mL

Hydroxyzine Hydrochloride (Atarax), Hydroxyzine Pamoate (Vistaril)

Hydroxyzine is an antihistamine that is absorbed rapidly from the gastrointestinal tract. Its clinical effects usually become evident within 15 to 30 minutes of oral administration. It has been used widely as a preanesthetic medication in children and adolescents because it produces significant sedation with minimal circulatory and respiratory depression. It also produces bronchodilation; decreases salivation; has antiemetic, antiarrhythmic, and analgesic effects; and produces a calming, tranquilizing effect (Smith and Wollman, 1985).

Use in Child and Adolescent Psychiatry

One manufacturer stated that "hydroxyzine has been shown clinically to be a rapid-acting, true ataraxic with a wide margin of safety. It induces a calming effect in anxious, tense, psychoneurotic adults, and also in anxious, hyperkinetic children without impairing mental alertness" (*PDR*, 1990, p. 1858); this statement has been deleted from the more recent *PDR*s (*PDR*, 1995, 2000, 2006). Hydroxyzine is approved for the symptomatic relief of anxiety and tension associated with psychoneurosis and as an adjunct in organic disease states in which anxiety is manifested. Its efficacy for periods longer than 4 months has not been demonstrated by systematic clinical studies.

Although not specifically indicated in the manufacturer's labeling, the sedation caused by hydroxyzine (as with diphenhydramine) has been utilized in the short-term treatment of insomnia and frequent night awakening in children.

Untoward Effects of Hydroxyzine

The most common untoward effects of hydroxyzine are sedation and dry mouth.

Hydroxyzine Hydrochloride Dosage Schedule for Treating Children and Adolescents

- *Children below 6 years old:* Medication should be titrated individually and administered four times daily to a maximum of 50 mg/day.
- *Children 6 years of age and older and adolescents:* Medication should be titrated individually and administered three to four times daily to a maximum of 100 mg/day.

Hydroxyzine Dose Forms Available

- *Tablets (hydroxyzine hydrochloride):* 10, 25, 50, and 100 mg
- *Capsules (hydroxyzine pamoate):* 25, 50, and 100 mg
- *Syrup (hydroxyzine hydrochloride):* 10 mg/5 mL
- *Oral suspension (hydroxyzine pamoate):* 25 mg/5 mL
- *Intramuscular injection (hydroxyzine hydrochloride):* 25 and 50 mg/mL

OPIATE ANTAGONISTS

Opiate antagonists have been investigated in the treatment of mentally retarded persons with self-injurious behavior (for review, see Sokol and Campbell, 1988) and in the treatment of autistic disorder. Deutsch (1986) has given a theoretical rationale for the use of opiate antagonists in the treatment of autistic disorder.

Naltrexone Hydrochloride (Trexan, Revia)

Naltrexone hydrochloride is a pure opioid antagonist. It is a synthetic congener of oxymorphone without any opioid agonist properties and completely blocks or markedly attenuates the subjective effects of intravenous opioids and precipitates withdrawal symptoms in subjects with physical tolerance to opioids.

Pharmacokinetics of Naltrexone Hydrochloride

Naltrexone is almost completely absorbed from the gastrointestinal tract and undergoes substantial first-pass metabolism by the liver to 6-beta-naltrexol. Peak plasma levels of naltrexone and 6-beta-naltrexol occur within 1 hour of an oral dose. Both compounds are biologically active and are excreted primarily by the kidneys. Serum half-life of naltrexone is approximately 4 hours and that of 6-beta-naltrexol is approximately 13 hours.

Contraindications for Naltrexone Hydrochloride Administration

The main contraindications are hypersensitivity, any liver abnormalities, and the concomitant use of any opiate-containing substances, legal or illegal.

Interactions of Naltrexone Hydrochloride with Other Drugs

Serious adverse effects (e.g., a severe, precipitous withdrawal syndrome) may occur if naltrexone is administered to individuals taking opioids.

Indications for Naltrexone Hydrochloride in Child and Adolescent Psychiatry

Naltrexone hydrochloride is approved for the treatment of alcoholism and for the blockade of the effects of exogenously administered opiates. It is not approved for any other psychiatric disorders.

Naltrexone Dosage Schedule

- *Children and adolescents up to 17 years of age:* Not recommended. Safety and efficacy have not been determined for this age group.
- *Adolescents at least 18 years of age and adults:* Usual recommended dose in the treatment of alcoholism or opioid dependency is 50 mg/day. (Read package insert carefully before using.)

Naltrexone Hydrochloride Dose Forms Available

- *Tablets:* 25 and 50 mg

Reports of Interest

Naltrexone in the Treatment of Autistic Disorder

Campbell et al. (1989) administered naltrexone on an open basis to 10 hospitalized children aged 3.42 to 6.5 years (mean age, 5.04 years). The study lasted 6 weeks. Following a 2-week baseline, single doses of 0.5, 1, and 2 mg/kg/day were administered at 1-week intervals. Ratings were made 1, 3, 5, 7, and 24 hours after each dose and 1 week after the last dose. Subjects showed diminished withdrawal at all three dose levels. Verbal production increased at 0.5 mg/kg/day, and stereotypies decreased following the 2 mg/kg/day dose. Symptoms such as aggressiveness and "self-aggressiveness" showed little improvement. The major untoward effect was mild sedation, which occurred in 70% of the subjects. Laboratory measurements, including liver function tests and electrocardiograms (ECGs), showed no significant change from baseline. Overall, raters considered 80% of the children to be positive responders for some symptoms (Campbell et al., 1989).

Campbell et al. (1990) subsequently conducted a double-blind, placebo-controlled study of naltrexone in 18 children, aged 3 to 8 years, diagnosed with autistic disorder. The study consisted of a 2-week placebo baseline phase, random assignment to placebo or naltrexone for 3 weeks, and a posttreatment 1-week placebo phase. The initial naltrexone dose was 0.5 mg/kg/day; this was increased to 1 mg/kg/day, if no adverse effects occurred. Nine children received naltrexone; the optimal dose was 1 mg/kg/day. Six subjects receiving naltrexone were rated moderate (five) or marked (one) in improvement on Clinical Global Consensus Ratings, whereas only one child on placebo achieved a moderate rating and none was markedly improved. The difference was significant ($P = .026$). In contrast, no reduction in symptoms occurred on the Children's Psychiatric Rating Scale or Clinical Global Impressions. Naltrexone did not appear to affect discrimination learning in an automated laboratory. The authors also reported that overall symptom reduction seemed better in older autistic children than in younger ones.

Although there are case studies and open studies with some encouraging data, the 1993 report of Campbell et al.—an 8-week double-blind study in which 41 hospitalized children (2.9 to 7.8 years of age; mean, 4.9 years) diagnosed with autistic disorder were treated with naltrexone or placebo—did not support the efficacy of naltrexone in this population. All their subjects received placebo during the first 2 weeks while baseline data were obtained. Following this phase, subjects were randomly assigned to naltrexone or placebo for the next 3 weeks. During the final week, all subjects again received placebo. Twenty-three patients were assigned to the naltrexone group and 18 to the placebo group. The initial dose was 0.5 mg/kg/day of either placebo or active drug given in the morning; dose was increased to 1.0 mg/kg/day after 1 week and maintained at that level because untoward effects were minimal and did not require a reduction in dose. Naltrexone did not improve the core symptoms of autism. The only significant finding was a modest decrease in hyperactivity on three different measures. It did not improve discrimination learning significantly more than placebo. Naltrexone was no better than placebo in reducing self-injurious behavior, but six of eight subjects who had a severity rating of mild or above on the Aggression Rating Scale who received naltrexone experienced rebound (increase) in symptoms during the final placebo period; only one child in the placebo group exhibited worsening of self-injurious behavior during that time. The authors concluded that it remains to be determined whether naltrexone is efficacious in treating moderate-to-severe self-injurious behavior and that its use cannot be recommended as a first-line treatment for patients diagnosed with either autistic disorder or self-injurious behavior (Campbell et al., 1993).

In a 7-week, double-blind, placebo-controlled, crossover study, Feldman et al. (1999) evaluated the efficacy of naltrexone in improving communication skills, a core deficit, in 24 children (mean age, 5.1 years; range, 3 to 8.3 years) diagnosed with autistic disorder by DSM-III-R criteria (American Psychiatric Association [APA], 1987) who had previously shown modest behavioral improvement on naltrexone in previous studies by the authors (Kolman et al., 1995, 1997). Communication skills of the subjects at baseline ranged from preverbal to nearly normal for age. During the active drug phase, 1 mg/day of naltrexone was administered.

There was no significant improvement in communication skills with naltrexone treatment, including number of utterances, total number of words, number of different words, or reduction in echolalia in these subjects who had shown some behavioral improvement on naltrexone. Also, the authors reported that use of parental language with the patient did not change according to whether the child was receiving naltrexone. The authors suggested that medications that improve core deficits and target symptoms of autistic disorder should be preferred over those that improve only associated symptoms.

Naltrexone in the Treatment of Trichotillomania

De Sousa (2008) conducted an open pilot study to evaluate the safety and efficacy of naltrexone in the management of 14 patients with childhood onset trichotillomania (TTM). The mean age of the children was 9 years, and the mean age of onset of symptoms in the group was around 7 years. The children in the study were initially started on naltrexone at 25 mg/day for 1 week and if tolerated well were increased to a maximum of 100 mg on the basis of symptom evaluation and response over a period of 2 weeks. Once enrolled into the study, the children were evaluated clinically using the CGI–Severity (CGI-S) for improvement every 2 weeks. Liver function was evaluated monthly for the first 2 months and every 2 months thereafter. A mean dose of 66.07 ± 22.23 mg/day naltrexone was well tolerated; 11 out of 14 (78.57%) subjects showed a positive response ($P < .0001$), and 3 of those responders reported no hair pulling at all. No abnormality in liver function was noted in the study. No adverse effects were reported by the children in the study.

BETA-ADRENERGIC BLOCKERS

Propranolol Hydrochloride (Inderal)

Although initially used primarily in controlling hypertension, angina pectoris, various cardiac arrhythmias, migraine prophylaxis, and other medical disorders, there has been considerable interest in the use of propranolol in general psychiatry.

Propranolol is a nonselective beta-adrenergic receptor-blocking agent with no other autonomic nervous system activity. Propranolol and other beta-adrenergic blocking agents reduce peripheral autonomic tone, thereby lessening somatic symptoms of anxiety such as palpitations, tremulousness, perspiration, and blushing. There is some evidence that the beta-adrenergic blocking agents significantly reduce these peripheral, autonomic, physical manifestations of anxiety, but may not affect the psychological (emotional) symptoms of anxiety (Noyes, 1988). Noyes (1988) concludes from his review of the literature that beta-blockers are relatively weak anxiolytics compared with benzodiazepines and should be used for generalized anxiety disorder, primarily in patients for whom the use of benzodiazepines is contraindicated.

In adults, propranolol has been investigated in treating anxiety disorders, including generalized anxiety, performance anxiety (stage fright), social phobia, posttraumatic stress disorder (PTSD), panic disorder and agoraphobia, and episodic dyscontrol and rage outbursts (Hayes and Schulz, 1987; Noyes, 1988). It has also been used in treating schizophrenia. Propranolol is effective in the treatment of some antipsychotic-induced akathisias (Adler et al., 1986).

Pharmacokinetics of Propranolol Hydrochloride

Propranolol is almost completely absorbed from the gastrointestinal tract. Peak serum values occur within 60 to 90 minutes; serum half-life is approximately 4 hours.

The manufacturer recommends using weight to determine propranolol doses for children, as this usually results in plasma levels comparable to those in the therapeutic range for adults.

The manufacturer notes that higher-than-expected serum levels of propranolol have occurred in patients diagnosed with Down syndrome (trisomy 21), suggesting that its bioavailability may be increased in such patients.

Contraindications for Propranolol Administration

Known hypersensitivity to propranolol is a contraindication.

Patients with bronchospastic diseases (bronchial asthma), cardiovascular conditions, diabetes, hyperthyroidism, or other medical disorders should have their medical status carefully reviewed (consultation with the physician providing care for the medical condition is recommended) before prescribing propranolol. Gualtieri et al. (1983) have cautioned that propranolol is contraindicated in children and adolescents with a history of cardiac or respiratory disease, those who have hypoglycemia, or those who are being medicated with a monoamine oxidase inhibitor. Because significant depression has been reported as an untoward effect, propranolol is not recommended for children and adolescents who are already depressed.

Interactions of Propranolol with Other Drugs

Propranolol may interact with many drugs. Three interactions among those most likely to be seen in child and adolescent psychiatric practice are (a) if used concomitantly with chlorpromazine, plasma levels of both drugs are increased over what they would be if used separately; (b) alcohol slows the rate of absorption of propranolol; and (c) phenytoin, phenobarbital, and rifampin accelerate propranolol clearance.

Untoward Effects of Propranolol

There are few reports of untoward effects in children or adolescents who received propranolol for psychiatric indications. Of greatest concern have been cardiovascular effects, which are detailed in the subsequent text. Propranolol has also been reported to cause significant depression of mood, manifested by insomnia, lethargy, weakness, and fatigue. Vivid dreams, nightmares, and gastrointestinal symptoms have also been reported.

Indications for Propranolol Hydrochloride in Child and Adolescent Psychiatry

There are no approved uses of propranolol in psychiatrically disturbed children and adolescents.

Propranolol Dosage Schedule

- *Children and adolescents up to 17 years of age:* Manufacturer's recommendations for treating hypertension in this age group are an initial twice-daily dose of 0.5 mg/kg followed by individual titration based on clinical response. Usual dose range is 2 to 4 mg/kg/day in two divided doses. Doses of >16 mg/kg/day should not be used.
- *Adolescents at least 18 years of age and adults:* Manufacturer's recommendations for treating hypertension are an initial dose of 80 mg daily in two divided doses followed by individual titration based on clinical response. The usual dose range is 120 to 240 mg/day. Some patients may require higher doses and some will need three-times-daily dosing.

Propranolol Discontinuation/Treatment Withdrawal

Because of the possibility of rebound in blood pressure, the dose of propranolol should be gradually tapered over 7 to 14 days when discontinued.

Propranolol Hydrochloride Dosage Forms Available

- *Tablets:* 10, 20, 40, 60, and 80 mg
- *Long-acting capsules (Inderal LA):* 60, 80, 120, and 160 mg

---

Reports of Interest

Propranolol in the Treatment of Children and Adolescents with Brain
Dysfunction, Uncontrolled Rage Outbursts, and/or Aggressiveness

Williams et al. (1982) administered propranolol to 30 subjects (11 children, 15 adolescents, and 4 adults) with organic brain dysfunction and uncontrolled rage outbursts who had not responded to other treatments. The subjects had various psychiatric diagnoses, including 15 with diagnoses of both conduct disorder, unsocialized, aggressive type, and attention-deficit disorder with hyperactivity; 7 with comorbid diagnoses of conduct disorder, unsocialized, aggressive type, and attention-deficit disorder without hyperactivity; 3 with conduct disorder only; 3 with intermittent explosive disorders; and 2 with pervasive developmental disorders. Thirteen had IQs in the retarded range, and eight had borderline IQs. The authors reported that 80% of their subjects demonstrated moderate to marked improvement on follow-up examination between 2 and 30 months (mean, 8 months) later. Optimal dosages of propranolol ranged from 50 to 960 mg/day (mean, 160 mg/day). All untoward effects were transient and reversible with dosage reduction. Most of the patients were additionally treated with other medication: 13 subjects received anticonvulsants; 6, antipsychotics; and 3, stimulants. Twenty-one had ongoing psychotherapy (Williams et al., 1982).

Kuperman and Stewart (1987) treated openly with propranolol 16 subjects whose mean age was 13.4 years (8 patients were 4 to 14 years old, 4 were between 14 and 17, and 4 were 18 to 24 years old). Seven subjects were diagnosed with conduct disorder, undersocialized aggressive type, five had infantile autism with varying degrees of mental retardation, two had moderate mental retardation only, one had borderline intellectual functioning, and one had attention-deficit disorder. All subjects exhibited significant physically aggressive behavior that had not responded adequately to behavior therapy and/or psychotropic medication. Propranolol was administered initially at 20 mg twice daily and increased by 40 mg every fourth day until symptom improvement occurred or standing systolic blood pressure fell below 90 mm Hg, diastolic blood pressure fell below 60 mm Hg, or resting pulse fell below 60 beats per minute. The average dose of propranolol was 164 ± 55 mg/day. Ten patients (62.5%) were rated moderately or much improved, based on concurrence of ratings by parents, teachers, and clinicians. Responders and nonresponders did not differ significantly regarding age, sex, IQ, vital signs, or dosage. The authors noted that, although not significant, six of their eight patients who were mentally retarded responded favorably, which is consistent with earlier findings in adults that suggest that aggressive patients with suspected central nervous system damage respond best. Nonresponders as a group tended to develop bradycardia, which may have prevented them from reaching potentially therapeutic doses of propranolol. The authors additionally noted that before considering propranolol a therapeutic failure, a patient should receive the maximum therapeutic dose tolerated for at least 1 month. When propranolol is discontinued, it should be tapered gradually over a 2-week period to avoid rebound tachycardia (Kuperman and Stewart, 1987).

Two 12-year-old boys treated with propranolol for episodic dyscontrol and aggressive behavior showed marked improvement (Grizenko and Vida, 1988). Dosage was initiated at 10 mg three times daily and was gradually increased to 50 mg three times daily.

Propranolol in the Treatment of Children Diagnosed with PTSD

Famularo et al. (1988) reported that 11 children (mean age, 8.5 years old) diagnosed with PTSD, acute type, had significantly lower scores on an inventory of PTSD symptoms during the period when they were receiving propranolol, compared with scores before and after the drug. Dosage was initiated at 0.8 mg/kg/day and administered in three divided doses; it was increased gradually over 2 weeks to approximately 2.5 mg/kg/day. Untoward effects prevented raising dosage to this level in only three cases. Propranolol was maintained at this level for 2 weeks and then tapered and discontinued over the fifth week. The authors emphasized that their subjects had presented in agitated, hyperaroused states and that propranolol might be useful during this particular stage of the disorder (Famularo et al., 1988).

At present, although there are some encouraging initial data, the use of propranolol and the beta-blockers in children and adolescents must be further investigated. In particular, the use of propranolol in anxiety disorders remains to be elucidated.

Pindolol (Visken)

Pindolol is a synthetic, nonselective beta-adrenergic receptor-blocking agent that has sympathomimetic activity at therapeutic doses but does not possess quinidine-like membrane-stabilizing activity (package insert).

It is approved for use in treating hypertension, but its safety and effectiveness have not been established in children.

Report of Interest

Buitelaar et al. (1994a) conducted a double-blind, placebo-controlled comparison of pindolol and methylphenidate in 52 subjects (age range, 6 to 13 years) diagnosed with attention-deficit/hyperactivity disorder (ADHD). Treatment periods were of 4 weeks' duration. For the first 3 days, a morning dose of 10 mg of methylphenidate or 20 mg of pindolol or placebo was given. This was increased to 10 mg twice daily of methylphenidate or 20 mg twice daily of pindolol or placebo for the remainder of the period. Subjects were rated on various Conners' Scales by parents and teachers. After 4 weeks, teachers rated students receiving methylphenidate as significantly better on impulsivity/hyperactivity, inattentiveness, and conduct than subjects receiving either pindolol or placebo. Parental ratings did not show a significant difference between pindolol and methylphenidate on improvements in impulsivity/hyperactivity or conduct, although both were better than placebo. The authors thought that the main effect of pindolol was to improve behavioral symptoms and conduct and that the drug was only modestly effective in treating ADHD.

Untoward effects of pindolol were of particular concern and limit the potential usefulness of this drug in children. Paresthesias were reported in 10% of children during treatment with pindolol and none while receiving placebo or methylphenidate ($P < .05$). Although hallucinations and nightmares were not significantly more frequent in children on pindolol, they were of significantly greater intensity ($P < .01$) and caused so much distress that the children's daily functioning was affected adversely. These adverse effects totally remitted within 1 day after discontinuation of pindolol. The authors note that some children may be particularly sensitive to these distressing untoward effects, further limiting the usefulness of pindolol in ADHD and requiring the clinician to be very cautious whenever prescribing pindolol to children (Buitelaar et al., 1994a, 1994b).

BARBITURATES AND HYPNOTICS

At the present time, the barbiturates and hypnotics have little, if any, place in treating psychiatric disorders in children and adolescents. Today barbiturates, especially phenobarbital, are used in children and adolescents primarily for their antiepileptic properties. Behaviorally disordered children frequently may worsen when given barbiturates. As long ago as 1939, Cutts and Jasper (1939) administered phenobarbital to 12 behavior-problem children with abnormal EEGs. Behavior worsened in nine (75%), with increased irritability, impulsivity, destructiveness, and temper tantrums. The authors concluded that phenobarbital was contraindicated in the treatment of such children. For sleep disorders, diphenhydramine and benzodiazepines, which are much safer to use, are now the drugs of choice.

Clinically, barbiturates have a disinhibiting and disorganizing effect on many psychiatrically disturbed children, including psychotic children. Cognitive dulling, an untoward effect of barbiturates, is also of major concern in children and adolescents. In adults, phenobarbital was found to decrease speed of access to information in short-term memory, and short-term memory itself was highly sensitive to phenobarbital levels (MacLeod et al., 1978). The authors noted that this effect could impair the ability of children and adolescents to maintain attention in the classroom and interfere with their learning new information.

Clinically, it is also important for the child and adolescent psychiatrist to remember that phenobarbital may contribute to disturbed behavior in some patients with seizure disorder in whom it is being used to control seizures. This is also the case in some younger children when phenobarbital is being used prophylactically (e.g., after febrile seizures). Some such children may show behavioral and cognitive improvement when they are switched to other antiepileptic medications or when they are gradually tapered off medication after a sufficiently long seizure-free period.

SLEEP AGENTS

Many clinicians typically think of adults when discussing sleep disorders, but clinicians in the field of child psychiatry can attest that early, middle, and late sleep complaints from parents about their children is a common and often very concerning complaint that is presented in sessions. Indeed, pediatric sleep study programs are now common in pediatric hospitals. Due to limited data regarding the use of FDA-approved adult sleep hypnotics in children, most pediatric clinicians initially utilize "natural" agents such as 3 to 9 mg of melatonin 1 to 2 hours before bedtime or over-the-counter agents such as diphenylhydramine. While these agents may be clinically useful for some, for many others the sleep complaints continue to be problematic and other agents are trialed. Clinical experience has led to the use of select antidepressants by clinicians in an attempt to address these sleep issues. Antidepressants are known to work through the modulation of monoamine neurotransmitters including dopamine, norepinephrine, and serotonin as well as other neurotransmitters such as muscarinic ACh, alpha-1-adrenergic, and histamine which are all known to effect sleep regulation, wakefulness, and sleep architecture. NE and SER are involved in suppressing REM sleep, whereas ACH has a role in the initiation of REM sleep.

Trazodone

Although not FDA approved as a sleep hypnotic for pediatrics or adults, low-dose trazodone used as a hypnotic may be the most common off-label use of any psychotropic. Trazodone is an example of what psychopharmacologists refer to as a dose-dependent "multifunctional drug"—a drug that has more than one therapeutic mechanism. Trazodone at low dosages of 25 to 150 mg has hypnotic actions due to total blockade of 5-HT_{2A} receptors as well as alpha-1-adrenergic receptors and H_1 receptors to a significant but lesser degree. Low-dose trazodone seems to not only promote sleep onset but also aid sleep maintenance. Trazodone was compared with the sedating tricyclic antidepressant trimipramine in a small double-blind crossover study in six healthy young men. Only trazodone significantly increased deep sleep without otherwise altering the normal architecture of sleep (Ware and Pittard, 1990).

At high dosages of 300 to 450 mg, trazodone is a strong serotonin transporter (SERT) inhibitor in addition to the aforementioned serotonin receptor blocker activity resulting in unique antidepressant actions.

The immediate release (IR) formulation at low dosages is the preferred trazodone agent for hypnotic usage. A new controlled-release formulation of trazodone (XR) designed to avoid sedation and improve tolerability when used as an antidepressant would theoretically be less useful as a hypnotic. There are surprisingly few controlled studies on the efficacy of trazodone for improving sleep onset and sleep architecture, and potential bothersome side effects include sedation, dizziness, and psychomotor impairment. A well known but rare side effect associated with trazodone is priapism which should be discussed with patients for early identification. There is some evidence of tolerance associated with chronic usage. Although at times one hears of street abuse of trazodone, typically trazodone does not cause dependence and its relatively short half-life make it attractive as a sleep hypnotic.

Prazocin

As stated above, alpha-1-adrenergic antagonist agents are known to effects sleep regulation, wakefulness, and sleep architecture. Clinical experience has led to the use of these agents in alleviating nightmares, a feature of REM disruption, and other sleep disruptions associated with trauma and PTSD. More recent clinical research into the use of the antihypertensive agent prazosin to alleviate nightmares and sleep disruptions such as insomnia in US military personnel deployed in Afghanistan and Iraq has been ongoing and supports the prior clinical usage of such agents for sleep complaints in trauma patients. In a small study of 34 veterans, prazocin corrected dream characteristics typical of trauma-related nightmares to those more typical of normal dreams (Raskind, et al., 2007). In animal models, prazosin protects REM sleep from disruption by adrenergic agonists, which has clinical relevance in PTSD models and in regard to medications used in psychiatry.

Typically clinicians may start with 0.5 mg for smaller children or 1.0 mg for larger children 1 hour before bedtime. Positive efficacy is usually evident in the first night or two. In most cases, an increase in dosage will be needed but the majority of patients respond to 5 mg or less. Rare cases may require dosing up to 10 mg in the evening. Prazocin has a fairly short half-life of 2 to 3 hours, but daytime flashbacks may be significantly reduced even when bedtime only dosing is implemented. Occasionally, these persistent flashbacks may require an additional morning dose. Prazocin is an antihypertensive, and thus a baseline BP and HR is recommended as well as follow-up assessments at each visit. If dosing is gradual, SEs such as hypotension and lightheadedness should be minimal. Baseline EKG monitoring may be indicated as polypharmacy is not uncommon in such a patient population.

Doxazocin

Because trauma and PTSD patients often have symptoms during the day as well the night, investigators and clinicians have begun to utilize other longer acting formulations of alpha-1 antagonists to address these issues as well as minimize the need for slower titration and side effects of drowsiness or dizziness that may occur when initiating agents such as prazocin with its short half-life. A controlled-release formulation of the selective alpha-1 antagonist antihypertensive medication doxazosin (Cardura XL) has a half-life of 16 to 30 hours. In a small open-label study utilizing subjective sleep measures, 12 adult PTSD patients initiated at 4 mg for 4 weeks increased to 8 mg thereafter showed statistically significant benefit in PTSD Scale symptoms of recurrent distressing dreams and difficulty falling or staying asleep (de Jong et al., 2008). Placebo-controlled trials will need to be conducted to confirm the efficacy of this agent in PTSD.

OBESITY IS A HUGE PROBLEM IN PSYCHIATRY

Obesity in our current culture is occurring at an alarming rate with some estimates that more than 50% of the American population is overweight or obese. In fact, obesity in the pediatric population is at such a staggering level that this generation will reportedly be the first generation to not outlive the lifespan of their parents. A poor diet coupled with a sedentary lifestyle often associated with excessive TV watching and video game watching is far too common for many teenagers, especially males. Given this scenario, it is understandable that the utilization of atypical antipsychotics for the treatment of mental health conditions in the present pediatric population is fraught with potential health-related perils. Most second-generation antipsychotic medications as well as first-generation antipsychotics can cause weight gain. Weight gain can lead to decreased adherence to treatment and consequently increase the risk of psychotic relapse in addition to the associated increased risks of diabetes and cardiovascular disease. Antipsychotics exhibit

TABLE 10.1 » Risk of Weight Gain and Metabolic Issues/Diabetes with Atypical Antipsychotic Medications		
Medication (Trade Name)	**Risk of Significant Weight Gain**	**Risk for Metabolic Issues/Diabetes**
Clozapine (Clozaril)	+++	+
Olanzapine (Zyprexa)	+++	+
Quetiapine (Seroquel)	++	+
Risperidone (Risperdal)	++	+
Paloperidone (Invega)	++	+
Aripiprazole (Abilify)	+	−
Ziprasidone (Geodon)	+/−	−
Asenapine (Saphris)	+	[a]
Iloperidone (Fanapt)	+	[a]
Lurasidone (Latuda)	+/−	[a]

[a]Limited data available and therefore predictive confidence for Asenapine, Iloperidone, and Lurasidone as newly released.
Adapted from Schumann A, Ewigman B. Can metformin undo weight gain induced by antipsychotics? *J Fam Pract.* 2008;57(8):526–530.

variability in the amount of weight gain and diabetic/metabolic risk they may impose on a given patient (Table 10.1). Olanzapine and clozapine definitely increase the risk for diabetes. The association of diabetes with risperidone and quetiapine is probable while the experience with aripiprazole and ziprasidone thus far does not indicate an increased risk of diabetes (Newcomer, 2007). Although it is clear that there is no "magic potion" or pill that produces long-term weight loss, it is much more accepted now that there are medical interventions in addition to lifestyle changes involving diet and exercise that may have potential in maintaining a healthy weight and the most promising options will be discussed.

Weight-Control Agents

Topiramate

Topiramate was approved by the FDA in 1996 as an add-on treatment for treatment-resistant partial seizures in adults and pediatric seizures in children above the age of 2 years, and more recently for migraine headache prophylaxis in adults. In fact, it is presently the most prescribed medication for migraines in adults because of its efficacy and overall very tolerable side-effect profile. Topiramate does have potential noteworthy side effects, however. The anorectic and cognitive-blunting side effects of topiramate in particular have been well known for years to neurologists prescribing this medication in the pediatric population for seizure control. It was a logical corollary, therefore, for clinicians to trial topiramate in overweight patients, but this intervention in isolation has found limited success (Faulkner et al., 2007). In July 2012, the FDA approved three different formulations of a combination drug of topiramate combined with an extended-release formulation of the stimulant appetite-suppressant phentermine (called Qsymia) as an addition to a reduced-calorie diet and exercise for chronic weight management in adults. The patients must qualify to meet criteria for obesity with either a body mass index (BMI) of at least 30 kg/m^2 or a BMI of 27 plus a comorbid condition such as type 2 diabetes. At 56 weeks, 39% of patients taking the upper strength (phentermine 15 mg/topiramate 92 mg) of (Qsymia) + lifestyle modification achieved the composite goal of a >5% weight loss from baseline, an HbA$_{1c}$ level lower than 6.5%, and a systolic BP lower than 130 mm Hg versus 12% of patients on lifestyle modification + placebo. When looking at a goal of >10% weight loss, 31% of patients on the upper strength dose achieved this goal versus only 4% of controls – medication + lifestyle modification was approximately eightfold more effective than lifestyle modification alone.

While the combination drug of topiramate and an extended-release formulation of phentermine is only currently approved for adults, there is an extensive history of topiramate usage in pediatrics with much relevant data available about its side-effect profile in the pediatric population. The use of topiramate for weight loss in pediatrics is an off-label use, but given the problem of childhood obesity and the propensity of most atypical and antiepileptic mood stabilizers to cause weight gain, topiramate is popular in child psychiatry as an add-on medication for weight loss in dosages typically in a range of 100 to 400 mg/day. Topiramate has mild CNS side effects overall, such as fatigue, somnolence, dizziness, ataxia, irritability, altered taste sensation, renal stones, glaucoma, and mental slowing that appear to be titration and dose related. This mental-slowing side effect actually only occurs infrequently but is well known to clinicians and is often referred to as "topadope" or "topadumb," as when present can be quite impairing to the patient. Sometimes, this bothersome side effect can be alleviated by dose lowering or by its own resolution over a period of weeks to months if manageable. Many of these side effects are minimized by slow weekly titration. Monotherapy of topiramate should be titrated rather slowly starting at 25 to 50 mg/day for the first week and increasing 50 mg/week utilizing b.i.d. dosing up to 100 to 200 mg/day depending on effect and tolerability. For larger children/adolescents who are not experiencing benefit and without side effects, subsequent 50-mg increases per week up to an efficacious dosage of 400 mg/day are reasonable. BID dosing may be utilized, and most patients respond to dosages of 400 mg/day or less for weight loss (dosages as high as 1,600 mg have been used in adults for seizures). There are other potential concerning psychiatric side effects such as depression and psychosis, which may occur early or after years of treatment. If the overweight patient has ADHD and is treated with a stimulant, one can expect an augmenting anorectic effect to topiramate when used in combination. The medication did poorly in trials as a mood stabilizer, but is still used occasionally as a mood stabilizer in refractory affective disorders. It has also been proposed for use in bulimia nervosa and in chronic pain syndromes, but studies are very limited.

Metformin

Another medication that may be utilized in the battle to combat weight gain with psychotropics and the subsequent development of metabolic syndromes is metformin. Metformin is approved by the FDA to promote weight loss in youth with diabetes and has been effective in reducing weight in youth taking SGAs.

While the Faulkner et al. (2007) review was disappointing, a more recent study from China by Wu et al. (2008), which was a well-designed, randomized controlled trial conducted in 128 adults aged 18 to 45 with a first psychotic episode of schizophrenia, is more encouraging. To enter the study, patients had to have gained more than 10% of their pretreatment body weight during the first year of treatment with an antipsychotic medication (clozapine, olanzapine, risperidone, or sulpiride [not approved for use in the United States]). Unfortunately, patients with diabetes, cardiovascular disease, liver or renal dysfunction, substance abuse, or psychiatric diagnoses other than schizophrenia were excluded. This patient group was then randomized to 1 of 4 groups for the 12 weeks of the study:

- Metformin alone, 250 mg three times daily
- Placebo alone
- Lifestyle intervention plus metformin
- Lifestyle intervention plus placebo

Interested readers can read the full details, but the results evidenced that participants in all three intervention groups showed significant decreases in the mean fasting glucose, insulin levels, and insulin resistance index (IRI). Compared with baseline, weight decreased by 4.9% in the metformin-only group and by 2.2% in the lifestyle-only group. The best result was observed in the lifestyle changes plus metformin cohort, where weight decreased by 7.3%. In the placebo group, weight increased by 4.8%.

In an actual pediatric study, Klein et al. (2006) conducted a randomized placebo-controlled trial of metformin titrated weekly up to 850 mg/day dosed with meals in 39 children ages 10 to 17 whose weight had increased more than 10% on atypical antipsychotic therapy. The children treated with placebo gained a mean of 4 kg and increased their mean BMI by 1.12 kg/m^2 during 16 weeks of treatment, whereas those in the metformin group did not gain weight and decreased their mean BMI by 0.43 kg/m^2.

Shin et al. (2009) conducted a 12-week, open-label trial to evaluate metformin's effectiveness and safety for weight management as monotherapy. Eleven subjects, ages 10 to 18 years, participated in the study. Patients were instructed not to change their baseline diet or activity level during the study. Each subject was initiated with metformin at 500 mg/day for 1 week and then titrated in increments of 500 mg/week as tolerated up to a target dose of 2,000 mg/day. Primary outcome measures included weight, BMI, and waist circumference with secondary outcome measures assessing serum glucose, insulin, and fasting lipid profile. The authors were disappointed that the mean reduction in weight, waist, BMI, serum glucose, and serum insulin was not statistically significant. However, 5 out of 11 patients lost weight (mean, –2.82 kg +/–7.25), and overall the sample did not continue to gain weight. Notably, metformin did not improve insulin sensitivity and showed a trend toward increasing both LDL and cholesterol. Triglyceride levels did improve. Metformin was fairly well tolerated with the following side effects reported in order of decreasing frequency: decreased appetite, irritability, constipation, decreased attention, drowsiness, anxiety, abnormal taste, and musculoskeletal pain. This study requested subjects not to change their diets or energy levels which may have accounted for subpar results. This med-only intervention with metformin supports the need for a comprehensive approach to significant weight loss.

However, before adding topiramate or metformin to help with weight loss, clinicians may consider switching from a medication with a higher risk for weight gain, such as olanzapine, risperidone, or quetiapine to one with a lower risk, such as aripiprazole or ziprasidone, as Weiden (2007) demonstrated this strategy can result in significant weight loss.

Metformin hydrochloride is indicated as an adjunct to diet and exercise to improve glycemic control in adults and children with type 2 diabetes mellitus. Promising evidence indicates that metformin alone and in combination with lifestyle changes is superior to lifestyle changes alone or placebo. The dosages used in these predominantly adult studies for weight loss vary across the adult FDA recommended dosage range of 500 to 2,550 mg in two or three divided doses. In children aged 10 to 16 years, the maximal dosage is 2,000 mg in divided dosages. There are no clear established dosing recommendations thus far for the purpose of weight loss in adults or pediatrics.

After reviewing the literature, Schumann and Ewigman (2008) recommend initiating metformin 250 mg three times a day, along with lifestyle modifications, to promote weight loss and decrease insulin resistance in patients who gain more than 10% of their pretreatment body weight on antipsychotic medications.

The Klein et al. (2006) pediatric study initiated metformin 500 mg with the evening meal for 1 week, and then increased to 500 mg b.i.d. with meals for a week before titrating to a target dosage of metformin 850 mg b.i.d. dosed with meals at week 3. It would appear a safe strategy to initiate low dosing in a b.i.d. or t.i.d. fashion and titrate to effect in weekly increments of no more than 500 mg/week.

Contraindications

Metformin should not be prescribed to patients with serum creatinine concentrations of more than 1.5 mg/dL or those with unstable heart failure, due to the risk of lactic acidosis.

The short story about metformin is that as monotherapy it may help to minimize the trajectory of weight gain, but the weight loss is usually less than with topiramate. Some clinicians who specialize in the treatment of diabetes at times utilize metformin with topiramate, especially in prediabetic conditions. For both medications, unless lifestyle changes are enacted, weight loss efforts will be disappointing.

Uncommonly or Rarely Prescribed Drugs

FIRST-GENERATION/TYPICAL ANTIPSYCHOTICS

Thioridazine

Thioridazine has been shown to prolong the QTc interval in a dose-related manner, and drugs with this potential, including thioridazine, have been associated with torsade de pointes–type arrhythmias and sudden death. Because of its potential for significant, possibly life-threatening proarrhythmic effects, thioridazine should be reserved for use in the treatment of schizophrenic patients who fail to show an acceptable response to adequate courses of treatment with other antipsychotic drugs, either because of insufficient effectiveness or because of the inability to achieve an effective dose due to intolerable adverse effects from those drugs.

Currently, thioridazine no longer has U.S. Food and Drug Administration (FDA) approval for treating severe behavioral problems marked by combativeness and/or explosive hyperexcitable behavior, or for the short-term treatment of hyperactive children who show excessive motor activity with accompanying conduct disorders consisting of some or all of the following symptoms: impulsivity, difficulty sustaining attention, aggressivity, mood lability, and poor frustration tolerance. Use of thioridazine in child and adolescent psychiatry would not only be "off-label" but would also be ignoring the new recommendations and warnings and cannot be recommended. Further information about the history of the use of this agent is contained in previous editions of this book.

Thiothixene (Navane)

Indications for Thiothixene (Navane)

Thiothixene (Navane) is a typical antipsychotic drug of the thioxanthene class used in the treatment of psychosis in adults.

Thiothixene Dosage Schedule

- *Children younger than 12 years of age:* Not recommended.
- *Adolescents aged at least 12 years of age and adults:* For milder conditions, an initial dose of 2 mg three times daily with titration to 5 mg three times daily if needed is usually effective. For more severe

(continued)

Thiothixene Dosage Schedule (*continued*)

conditions, use an initial dose of 5 mg twice daily. The usual optimal dose is 20 to 30 mg/day; occasionally, up to 60 mg/day are required. Daily doses of >60 mg rarely increase the beneficial response (*PDR*, 2000).

Thiothixene Dose Forms Available

- *Capsules:* 1, 2, 5, 10, and 20 mg
- *Concentrate:* 5 mg/mL
- *Intramuscular injectable preparation:* 2 and 5 mg/mL

Report of Interest

Thiothixene in the Treatment of Adolescents Diagnosed with Schizophrenia

Realmuto and colleagues (1984) assigned 21 adolescent inpatients (mean age, 15.1 years; range, 11.75 to 18.33 years) diagnosed with chronic schizophrenia, to either thiothixene or thioridazine. Optimal dose was individually titrated over a period of approximately 2 weeks. For the 13 patients who received thiothixene, the mean optimal dose was 16.2 mg/day (range, 4.8 to 42.6 mg/day) or 0.30 mg/kg/day for 4 to 6 weeks. Hallucinations, anxiety, tension, and excitement decreased the most during the first week. Cognitive disorganization improved more slowly. There were no significant differences between the two drugs in rapidity of symptom improvement or extent of improvement at the end of the study. Approximately 50% of patients improved, regardless of the medication. There was a suggestion, however, that untoward effects, particularly drowsiness, were less severe with thiothixene than with thioridazine and that because of this, high-potency antipsychotics may be preferable to the more sedating low-potency antipsychotics in treating adolescents with schizophrenia (Realmuto et al., 1984).

Loxapine Succinate (Loxitane)

Indications for Loxapine Succinate in Child and Adolescent Psychiatry

Loxapine is a dibenzoxazepine compound with antipsychotic properties used in treating psychotic disorders. The manufacturer does not recommend its use in persons younger than 16 years of age.

Loxapine Dosage Schedule

- *Children and adolescents younger than 16 years of age:* Not recommended.
- *Adolescents at least 16 years of age and adults:* An initial dose of 10 mg twice daily is recommended and is titrated according to clinical response. The usual therapeutic and maintenance dose ranges from 60 to 100 mg daily. A maximum of 250 mg/day is recommended.

Loxapine Succinate Dose Forms Available

- *Capsules:* 5, 10, 25, and 50 mg
- *Oral concentrate:* 25 mg/mL
- *Injectable preparation (intramuscular):* 50 mg/mL

Report of Interest

Loxapine Succinate in the Treatment of Adolescents Diagnosed with Schizophrenia

Pool and colleagues (1976) conducted a 4-week, double-blind study comparing the efficacies of loxapine, haloperidol, and placebo in 75 adolescents, 13 to 18 years of age, diagnosed with acute schizophrenia or chronic schizophrenia with an acute exacerbation. Loxapine was begun at a dose of 10 mg daily and titrated to a maximum of 200 mg daily (average daily dose, 87.5 mg). Extrapyramidal reactions, most commonly parkinsonian muscular rigidity, were the most frequent untoward effects of loxapine and occurred in 19 of 26 subjects. The second most frequent untoward effect, sedation, occurred in 21 of the 26 subjects. Both loxapine and haloperidol were significantly superior to placebo in diminishing schizophrenic symptoms. The authors concluded that loxapine was relatively safe and efficacious in the treatment of adolescent schizophrenia.

Pimozide

Pharmacokinetics of Pimozide

Peak serum levels usually occur 6 to 8 hours after ingestion of pimozide. Pimozide is metabolized primarily in the liver; the drug and its metabolites are excreted primarily through the kidneys. There are wide interindividual variations in half-life and in peak serum levels for equivalent doses. Mean serum half-life in patients with schizophrenia is approximately 55 hours. There are few correlations between plasma levels and clinical findings. The cytochrome P4503A4 enzyme system (CYP 3A) is important in the metabolism of pimozide, and it should not be taken simultaneously with drugs that may inhibit CYP 3A. Likewise, patients taking pimozide should avoid drinking grapefruit juice, which may inhibit the metabolism of pimozide by CYP 3A. As CYP 1A2 may also be involved in the metabolism of pimozide, clinicians should be alert to the potential for drug interactions with CYP 1A2 inhibitors.

Untoward Effects of Pimozide

Pimozide prolongs the QT interval of the electrocardiogram (ECG). An ECG should be done at baseline and monthly during the period of dose titration. Increase of the QT interval beyond an absolute limit of 0.47 second in children or 0.52 second in adults or >25% above the patient's original baseline should be considered a mandate for no further increase in dose and possibly for lowering it. Because hypokalemia is associated with ventricular arrhythmias, potassium levels should be monitored during therapy.

Contraindications for Pimozide Administration

In addition to considerations for antipsychotics in general, pimozide is contraindicated in the treatment of simple tics or tics other than those associated with Tourette disorder. Pimozide should not be given together with other drugs (e.g., stimulants) that may cause tics. An ECG should be performed before initiating treatment with pimozide, which should not be given to patients with congenital long QT intervals or a history of cardiac arrhythmias or to those who are taking drugs that prolong the QT interval. Pimozide is contraindicated in patients receiving drugs that inhibit cytochrome P450 3A (CYP 3A) enzyme system, which may impede pimozide metabolism, including macrolide antibiotics, azole antifungal agents, protease inhibitors, nefazodone, and zileuton. Two sudden deaths have occurred when pimozide and the antibiotic clarithromycin, a P450 inhibitor, were administered simultaneously (*PDR*, 2000).

TRICYCLIC ANTIDEPRESSANTS

Imipramine Hydrochloride (Tofranil), Imipramine Pamoate (Tofranil-PM)

Because imipramine hydrochloride has been the most widely used clinically and has been more thoroughly studied in children and adolescents than the other tricyclics, it will serve as the prototype.

Untoward Effects of Imipramine

Imipramine (IMI) has many untoward effects, some of which are potentially life threatening. Cardiovascular effects, including arrhythmias, tachycardia, blood pressure changes, impaired conduction and heart block, and a decreased seizure threshold, are particularly worrisome.

IMI in the Treatment of Enuresis

Although the pharmacological treatment of enuresis has been shown to be effective (Poussaint and Ditman, 1965; Rapoport et al., 1980b), it should not be employed until possible organic etiologies have been ruled out by appropriate physical examination and tests. It should be emphasized that behavioral therapies (e.g., conditioning with an alarm and pad apparatus) are the treatments of choice for functional enuresis. There is a tendency for some children to become tolerant of IMI's antienuretic effects, and many children relapse after medication withdrawal. Desmopressin acetate (DDAVP, a synthetic analog of the natural hormone, arginine vasopressin) nasal spray or tablets may be effective in some cases of enuresis that do not respond satisfactorily to other treatments.

IMI's antienuretic effect occurs rapidly and appears to be unrelated to its antidepressant effects; it may directly inhibit bladder musculature and increase outlet resistance (American Medical Association, 1986). It also appears that the IMI plus DMI plasma level required for the effective treatment of enuresis is lower than that required for treating MDD. DeGatta et al. (1984) treated 90 enuretic patients, aged 5 to 14 years, with IMI and reported that the minimum efficient serum concentration of IMI plus DMI in most cases was 80 ng/mL. However, about 20% of the subjects did not respond satisfactorily to IMI even with adequate serum levels.

Fritz et al. (1994) reviewed prior studies of plasma levels of IMI and DMI, its metabolite, in enuretic children treated with IMI and reported on levels in 18 additional patients. The therapeutic efficacy of IMI was moderately but significantly related to increasing levels of mg/kg dosage. Intersubject plasma combined IMI and DMI levels varied at least sevenfold at every dosage. The combined IMI and DMI levels at 2.5 mg/kg averaged 136.0 ng/mL (range, 35 to 170 ng/mL) for complete responders, 116 ng/mL (range, 37 to 236 ng/mL) for partial responders, and 96.0 ng/mL (range, 60 to 157 ng/mL) for nonresponders. The authors noted that despite the lack of a clear therapeutic window, serum-level monitoring is useful in identifying subjects with low serum levels and suboptimal responses. In such cases, the dose of IMI may be raised before concluding that the medication is ineffective. Knowledge of the serum level is essential, however, to avoid the danger of further dose increases resulting in toxic serum levels in nonresponsive subjects who have relatively high serum levels.

A trial of IMI may occasionally be indicated when safer and more efficacious methods have failed and the symptom is psychologically a handicap or distressing to the patient, or perhaps when rapid control is essential to permit a child to go to summer camp or to travel.

The most frequent untoward effects reported in the treatment of enuretic children with IMI are nervousness, sleep disorders, tiredness, and mild gastrointestinal disturbances (PDR, 1995). DeGatta et al. (1984) reported that 40% of their 90 enuretic subjects had at least one side effect; 42% had loss of appetite, 16% had light sleep, 11% had abdominal pains, 8% had dry mouth, and 8% had headaches.

In clinical practice, initial ECGs often have not been done for the treatment of enuresis because the final total daily dosage of IMI usually remains below 2.5 mg/kg and the risk of cardiotoxicity is low. In the light of the several sudden deaths reported in children receiving tricyclic antidepressants, even in usual doses, the author recommends a baseline ECG to screen for cardiac abnormalities that may increase the risk of conduction disorders secondary to tricyclic administration. It is suggested that bedwetters who void soon after falling asleep benefit if IMI is given earlier and in divided doses (e.g., 25 mg in midafternoon and 25 mg before bed) (PDR, 1995). A maximum dose of 2.5 mg/kg should not be exceeded because of the possibility of developing ECG abnormalities. Doses of more than 75 mg/day do not increase efficacy and do increase untoward effects (PDR, 1995).

Indications for Imipramine Hydrochloride

NOTE: Review the Black Box Warning at beginning of chapter or in package insert before prescribing.

IMI is approved for use in treating symptoms of depression in adolescents and adults. Its use in children is restricted to the treatment of enuresis in children who are at least 6 years old. Manufacturers state that a maximum dose of 2.5 mg/kg should not be exceeded in children (*PDR*, 1995).

IMI Dosage Schedule

* *Children ≤11 years of age:*
  Treatment of depression: Not recommended (however, see the relevant reviews later of the use of IMI in this age group).
  Treatment of enuresis: Not recommended for children <6 years.
  For children 6 years through 11 years of age, begin with 25 mg 1 hour before bedtime. If not effective within 1 week, increase to a maximum dose of 50 mg.
  Treatment of attention-deficit/hyperactivity disorder: No official recommendations for age or dose exist. Based on the literature and experimental protocols, the following is suggested for children >6 years of age: monitoring prerequisites for IMI should be followed. Begin with a low dose, either 25 mg/day or 0.5 mg/kg/day, and slowly titrate upward with increases of 25 mg once or twice weekly.
* *Adolescents ≥12 years of age and adults:*
  Treatment of depression: An initial dosage of 30 to 40 mg with gradual titration upward is suggested. It is generally not necessary to exceed 100 mg/day (manufacturer's package insert) (however, see the discussion in the following text on treating adolescents and the importance of determining serum levels.)
  Treatment of enuresis: Begin with 25 mg 1 hour before bedtime. If not effective within 1 week, increase to 50 mg with a maximum recommended dose of 75 mg.
  Treatment of attention-deficit/hyperactivity disorder: No official recommendations for age or dose exist. Based on the literature and experimental protocols, the following is suggested: Begin with a low dose, either 25 mg/day or 0.5 mg/kg/day, and slowly titrate upward with increases of 25 mg once or twice weekly. Monitoring prerequisites for IMI should be followed.

Imipramine Hydrochloride Dose Forms Available

* *Tablets (imipramine hydrochloride):* 10, 25, and 50 mg
* *Capsules (imipramine pamoate):* 75, 100, 125, and 150 mg. These capsules are designed for once-daily dosing. Because of their high unit potency and the greater sensitivity of children to the cardiotoxic effects of IMI, their use is not recommended in children and younger adolescents.

Reports of Interest

IMI in the Treatment of Childhood (Prepubertal) Major Depressive Disorder

IMI and nortriptyline were the only tricyclics approved by the FDA for investigational use in the treatment of MDD in children 12 years of age and younger. FDA guidelines for ECG changes during treatment with either drug were as follows:

1. The PR interval should not exceed 0.21 second.
2. Resting heart rate should be <130 beats per minute.
3. The QRS interval should not exceed 0.02 second more than the baseline interval.

The blood pressure of children receiving IMI, which can both elevate the blood pressure and produce orthostatic hypotension, should not be permitted to exceed 145/95 mm Hg (Geller and Carr, 1988). IMI levels above 5 mg/kg are not usually permitted in investigational protocols (Hayes et al., 1975).

Baseline studies that should be completed before initiating treatment with a tricyclic antidepressant include sitting and supine blood pressure, complete blood count with differential, electrolytes, thyroid function tests, blood urea nitrogen (BUN), serum creatinine, urinalysis with osmolality, liver function tests, and an ECG.

Several investigators have noted that in clinical practice an absolute upper-dose maximum for tricyclic antidepressants is not very useful because of the marked intersubject variability in pharmacokinetics (e.g., metabolism and elimination) and the fact that, although children as a group tend to metabolize and/or eliminate tricyclic antidepressants more rapidly than do older adolescents and adults, some children, perhaps genetically slow hydroxylators, may reach very high serum levels on doses well below the recommended maximum (Biederman et al., 1989b). Hence, careful clinical monitoring, including serum levels, is essential.

Puig-Antich et al. (1987) investigated the use of IMI in prepubescent children diagnosed with MDD. In a double-blind placebo-controlled study of 38 subjects, there was no significant difference between response to IMI (56%; 9 of 16 subjects) and response to placebo (68%; 15 of 22 subjects).

These authors also studied total maintenance plasma levels (IMI plus DMI) in 30 prepubescent children and found a positive correlation between plasma level and clinical response. Responders had significantly higher ($P < .007$) mean maintenance total plasma levels (284 ± 225 ng/mL) than nonresponders (145 ± 80 ng/mL). The authors reported that a maintenance total plasma level of 150 ng/mL was the most important differentiating point between responders and nonresponders. Eighty-five percent (17) of 20 subjects whose values were above 150 ng/mL had positive responses, but only 30% (3) of 10 children with lower values responded positively. The authors also found nothing, including dosage, that predicted plasma levels (Puig-Antich et al., 1987). This is consonant with the finding that combined IMI and DMI steady-state plasma levels varied sixfold (from 56 to 324 ng/mL) in 11 boys receiving 75 mg/day of IMI (Weller et al., 1982).

Other important findings of Puig-Antich et al. (1987) were (a) the more severe the pretreatment depressive symptoms on the Kiddie-Schedule for Affective Disorders and Schizophrenia (K-SADS) nine-item depressive score, the less likely was a favorable response to IMI ($P < .008$); (b) prepubescent children with the Research Diagnostic Criteria (RDC) psychotic subtype of MDD were much less likely to have a favorable response to IMI than nonpsychotic depressed children ($P < .05$); and (c) some children would require dosages of more than 5 mg/kg/day to reach plasma levels in the range associated with positive response.

These authors also reported that the following untoward effects were found in more than 30% of the children treated with IMI: excitement, irritability, nightmares, insomnia, headache, muscle pain, increased appetite, abdominal cramps, constipation, vomiting, hiccups, dry mouth, bad taste in the mouth, sweating, flushed face, drowsiness, dizziness, tiredness, and restlessness. Similar untoward effects were present in the placebo group, although at lower frequencies. The untoward effects were severe enough in 17 of the 30 children to prevent upward titration to 5 mg/kg/day; cardiac side effects were responsible in 10 of these cases. Nine children had increases in the PR interval to the maximum, and one child's resting heart rate reached 130 beats per minute. No child on placebo showed ECG changes from baseline, whereas nearly every child receiving IMI had at least minor changes (Puig-Antich et al., 1987).

Preskorn et al. (1987) reported a double-blind, randomly assigned, placebo-controlled study of 22 hospitalized, prepubertal depressed children aged 6 to 12 years; IMI was found to be statistically better than placebo ($P < .05$) by 3 weeks, when IMI plus DMI plasma levels were used by laboratory workers to adjust dosage of IMI to reach a therapeutic range of 125 to 250 ng/mL. Doses of IMI could range between 25 and 150 mg/day. The authors also noted that dexamethasone suppression test (DST) nonsuppressors showed greater improvement than DST suppressors. Total plasma levels below 125 ng/mL yielded a response rate only somewhat better than placebo, and levels above 250 ng/mL were associated with a lower response rate and an increased incidence of toxic untoward effects. The latter included prolongation of intracardiac conduction, increased blood pressure and heart rate, and mental confusion. The authors noted that, in a prior study in which clinicians were unaware of plasma levels and further increased dosages resulting in some children developing total IMI plus DMI plasma levels >450 ng/mL, the antidepressant response was poor and several children developed toxic confusion that was incorrectly interpreted as a worsening of the depressive condition. This underscored the importance of monitoring plasma drug levels because a reduction in dosage, not an increase, would be indicated.

Based on their own data and those of Puig-Antich et al., Preskorn et al. (1989a) concluded that plasma IMI plus DMI levels ranging from 125 to 250 ng/mL were both efficacious and safe in treating MDD in children. These authors suggested using an initial oral dose of 75 mg IMI daily and then determining the combined plasma concentration of IMI plus DMI 7 to 10 days later, when steady-state levels would be expected. Based on their experience, 78% of children initially had plasma levels outside of the therapeutic range; 66% were below 125 ng/mL and 12% were above 250 ng/mL. Because intraindividual plasma levels were reproducible and linearly correlated with dose, the authors used the following formula to adjust the dosage:

$$\text{New dose} = (\text{Initial dose/Initial level}) \times \text{Desired level}$$

The desired level was 185 ng/mL, the midpoint of the optimal range. Using this strategy, 84% of their patients achieved levels within the therapeutic range. The remaining 16% had subtherapeutic levels, possibly requiring additional adjustments (Preskorn et al., 1989a).

IMI in the Treatment of Comorbid Prepubertal Major Depressive Disorder and Conduct Disorder

Puig-Antich (1982) reported that 16 of 43 prepubertal males accepted for treatment of MDD had a codiagnosis of conduct disorder. These subjects did not differ on significant demographic and clinical variables from subjects diagnosed with MDD only. Approximately one-third of each group had auditory hallucinations consistent with RDC criteria for psychotic subtype major depression. A history of major depression was found to precede the onset of conduct disorder in 14 (87%) of the 16 cases. Thirteen of the 16 patients who completed the study had a full antidepressant response between 5 and 18 weeks after beginning medication. Although this was a double-blind study, only one patient had a full response during the 5-week double-blind period; the others received either IMI openly or were switched to DMI and titrated upward. Dosage of 5 mg/kg/day was the desired dosage, but doses above and below this were administered; exact dosage was not reported for these patients. Of particular interest, however, was the fact that 11 of the 13 boys who definitely recovered from the major depression also experienced total remission of their conduct disorders. In a majority of cases, conduct disorders reappeared following recurrence of another major depressive episode. In six of these patients, who were treated with the same drug and dosage associated with remission, conduct disorders persisted in two (33%) following remission of the depressive symptoms. Puig-Antich (1982) emphasized the potential importance of treating these comorbid disorders and avoiding the recurrence of the depression during childhood and adolescence in significantly improving the prognosis of this subgroup of conduct disorders, which appear to develop following the onset of major depression.

IMI in the Treatment of Adolescent MDD

Thirty-four adolescents with MDD treated with IMI in an open study with monitoring of plasma IMI levels showed some differences from prepubescent children (Ryan et al., 1986). IMI was titrated to a dose of 5 mg/kg/day; the adolescents had an overall positive response rate of 44% (15) of 34, but there was no relationship between positive response and higher plasma IMI levels. Another difference between the adolescents and prepubertal children with MDD was that, as a group, nonpsychotic subjects did not respond more favorably than the psychotic subtype. The authors hypothesized that adolescents with MDD were less responsive to IMI because of an antagonistic effect of sex hormones, levels of which increase during adolescence (Ryan et al., 1986).

Strober et al. (1990) treated 35 adolescents (mean age, 15.4 years; age range, 3 to 18 years) openly with IMI; they had been hospitalized and diagnosed by RDC criteria with MDD with at least probable certainty. Ten of the adolescents also met criteria for delusional subtype. After failing to improve after 1 week's hospitalization, subjects were treated for 6 weeks with IMI. Six (17.7%) of the 34 subjects who completed the study were unable to achieve the target dose of 5 mg/kg/day because of untoward effects. Average daily dose was 222 ± 49 mg/day, and steady-state IMI plus DMI levels varied 11-fold (mean, 237 ± 168 ng/mL; range, 79 to 888 ng/mL). Eight (33%) of the 24 nondelusional subjects and 1 (10%) of the 10 delusional subjects were considered responders, suggesting greater refractoriness in patients with psychotic features. None of the responders had a plasma IMI plus DMI level below 180 ng/mL, but the difference between responders and nonresponders was not significant. Overall, only 10 (29.4%) patients were rated very much improved or much improved on the Clinical Global Impressions–Improvement (CGI-I) Scale.

Lithium Augmentation in Adolescents Diagnosed with Major Depressive Disorder Who Were Treatment Resistant to IMI

Ryan et al. (1988a) reported in a retrospective chart review their treatment of 14 adolescents, aged 14 to 19 years (mean, 16.9 years), who were diagnosed by RDC with nonbipolar MDD; these patients had not responded to treatment with various tricyclic antidepressants (for a period of at least 6 weeks in 12 cases and for 4 weeks in 2 cases) by lithium augmentation while continuing treatment with amitriptyline, DMI, or nortriptyline. Lithium carbonate was titrated to achieve therapeutic serum levels. Six patients (43%) were responders and improved to the extent that they had, at most, mild symptoms of depression and were no longer being functionally impaired by their depression. Most responders improved gradually over the first month after the addition of lithium treatment. Their serum lithium level was 0.65 ± 0.06 mEq/L and was not significantly different from that of the nonresponders. The authors suggested that the addition of lithium carbonate could be a useful adjunct to the treatment of some adolescents with major depression who do not respond satisfactorily to treatment with tricyclic antidepressants (Ryan et al., 1988a).

Strober et al. (1992) treated 24 adolescents diagnosed with MDD who had not responded to 6 weeks of treatment with IMI by augmentation with lithium. The dosage of IMI at the end of the sixth week was held constant, and lithium was added on an open basis for a 3-week period beginning with doses of 300 mg three times a day that were then titrated upward based on clinical response to a final mean serum lithium level of 0.89 mEq/L. As a comparison group, the authors used 10 patients diagnosed with MDD in an earlier study who did not respond to IMI during the first 6 weeks and who continued receiving IMI only for the subsequent 3 weeks. Both groups improved significantly during the final 3 weeks of treatment as measured on the Hamilton Rating Scale for Depression (Ham-D). Although the group receiving lithium showed greater improvement, the difference between the two groups was not significant. Two patients (8.3%) in the lithium-augmented group were rated as "marked responders," as evidenced by a decrease of at least 50% in the Ham-D and a final score of <10, between 2 and 7 days after addition of lithium. Eight additional patients (33.3%) showed partial improvement over a period of 14 to 21 days following lithium administration. The authors noted that lithium's efficacy as an adjunct in adolescents with tricyclic-resistant major depression appears to be much less compared with that in adults, in whom up to 70% respond favorably. They also suggested that a small subgroup of adolescents may show an initial robust positive effect and that other adolescents may show gradual but less improvement over time. A trial of longer than 3 weeks may be necessary to determine if additional adolescents might benefit and whether further clinical gains would occur in adolescents who showed some improvement. The authors noted that Thase et al. (1989) reported on a subgroup of adults who showed improvement only after 4 to 6 weeks of lithium augmentation.

IMI in the Treatment of Attention-Deficit/Hyperactivity Disorder

A considerable body of literature attests to the clinical efficacy of IMI in the treatment of ADHD, although most studies find stimulants superior (for review, see Campbell et al., 1985; Rapoport et al., 1974, 1978c). Although IMI does not have FDA approval for use in the treatment of ADHD, some clinicians consider IMI or DMI the next drug of choice if a patient does not respond to stimulants. Wender (1988), however, notes that when used to treat ADHD, tricyclics improve mood and decrease hyperactivity but usually are sedating and do not appear to improve concentration.

The mechanism of action of IMI in ADHD is different from that in depression; it is rapidly effective, and lower doses are often required. Mean dosages reported in the literature have ranged from 20 to 173.7 mg/day. The development of tolerance by some children to the therapeutic effects of IMI within about 6 weeks presents difficulties.

Rapoport et al. (1974) compared IMI and methylphenidate in a double-blind placebo-controlled study of 76 hyperactive boys. Mean daily dose of IMI was 80 ± 21 mg (maximum, 150 mg), and mean daily dose of methylphenidate was 20 mg (maximum, 30 mg). Although both drugs were significantly better than placebo, most measures favored the stimulant drug. Some tolerance to the therapeutic effects of IMI appeared to develop after about 10 weeks of treatment.

In a double-blind, placebo-controlled, crossover-design study of 30 hyperactive children, Werry et al. (1980) found IMI to be statistically more effective than methylphenidate in its overall therapeutic effect. Untoward effects of IMI, however, were greater and more troublesome than those of methylphenidate. Methylphenidate was given in doses of 0.40 mg/kg; IMI was given in doses of 1 and 2 mg/kg/day. The authors found few significant differences between the two IMI doses but thought that the lower dose resulted in a slightly better clinical response and milder side effects (Werry et al., 1980).

A 1-year follow-up study of 76 hyperactive boys treated with IMI or methylphenidate found that significantly more subjects on IMI discontinued the medication because of lack of benefit or untoward effects, but that subjects in both treatment groups who continued on either drug improved equally (Quinn and Rapoport, 1975). The large dropout rate is a considerable clinical disadvantage in using IMI. It appears that tolerance to IMI may develop, resulting in deterioration after an initial improvement (Gross, 1973; Klein et al., 1980; Quinn and Rapoport, 1975; Waizer et al., 1974).

IMI in the Treatment of Separation Anxiety Disorder (School Phobia/School Refusal)

Gittelman-Klein and Klein (1971) reported a double-blind, placebo-controlled study using IMI to treat 35 children diagnosed with school phobia (separation anxiety). Of the 45 children between 6 and 14 years of age who entered the study, 35 (19 females and 16 males; mean age, 10.8 years) completed the 6-week protocol. Dosage was administered in the morning and evening for a total of 75 mg/day for the first 2 weeks and then adjusted weekly. At the completion of the study, doses ranged from 100 to 200 mg/day (mean, 152 mg/day). Also, all subjects were treated simultaneously with a multidisciplinary treatment program.

Dry mouth was much more frequent in the active drug group, occurring in 50% of the subjects ($P < .003$). One child developed orthostatic hypotension requiring reduction of dosage, but all other side effects reportedly disappeared without dosage adjustment. The authors noted that doses of IMI <75 mg/day were indistinguishable from placebo in this study.

Using "return to school regularly within 6 weeks" as the criterion, there was no statistical difference between IMI and placebo at the 3-week mark, but by 6 weeks, IMI was significantly ($P < .05$) better than placebo (Gittelman-Klein and Klein, 1971).

Klein et al. (1980) emphasize that IMI is effective in reducing separation anxiety but that anticipatory anxiety may continue to be problematic. IMI doses of between 75 and 200 mg/day were effective for school-phobic children between 6 and 14 years of age; however, children with severe separation anxiety without school phobia sometimes responded to doses as low as 25 to 50 mg/day. School-phobic children who responded to IMI were found to show at least some improvement when doses reached 125 mg/day; once improvement began, further dose increases usually produced additional benefit. Response was usually maximal within 6 to 8 weeks. It was suggested that maintenance be continued for a minimum of 8 weeks following remission of symptoms and then tapered and discontinued (Klein et al., 1980).

Klein et al. (1992) compared the efficacy of IMI and placebo in a double-blind, randomized study of 21 children (14 males and 7 females; age range, 6 to 15 years; mean, 9.5 ± 0.8 years) diagnosed with separation anxiety disorder by DSM-III criteria. Nine subjects (43%) were diagnosed with comorbid DSM-III anxiety disorders, overanxious disorder being the most frequent. The 21 subjects comprised the nonresponders of a larger group ($N = 45$) who were treated for the month preceding entry into the study with vigorous behavioral therapy. Behavioral treatment continued throughout the 6-week treatment period, during which 11 patients received IMI and 10 patients received placebo.

IMI was begun at 25 mg/day for 3 days, increased to 50 mg for the next 4 days, and then titrated to a maximum dose of 5 mg/kg/day. Baseline ECGs were obtained, with subsequent ECGs recorded after every dose increase above 50 mg/day. Daily doses of IMI ranged from 75 to 275 mg/day (mean, 153 mg/day or 4.67 mg/kg) at the completion of the study. Children treated with IMI had significantly more untoward effects than those who received placebo. Irritability or angry outbursts occurred in five (45%), dry mouth in five (45%), and drowsiness in two (18%) of the children receiving IMI. ECG changes occurred, but no dosage reductions were required because they did not exceed the recommended maximum values or changes from baseline (Klein et al., 1992).

There were no significant differences between the IMI and placebo groups on any measure; both groups showed about 50% overall improvement. These results are strikingly different from those in the earlier study (Gittelman-Klein and Klein, 1971). The authors note that although IMI may still be useful in treating separation anxiety disorder, its efficacy appears to be considerably less than previously thought (Klein et al., 1992).

Bernstein et al. (2000) conducted a double-blind, placebo-controlled study of 63 adolescents (mean age, 13.9 ± 3.6 years; 38 females, 25 males) with school refusal and comorbid anxiety and MDDs, who were treated randomly for 8 weeks with either IMI or placebo; in addition, all subjects received concurrent, manual-based, monitored cognitive-behavioral therapy (CBT). Adolescents with conduct disorder were excluded from the study. The study period was preceded by a 1-week single-blind placebo washout; no subjects were eliminated because of improvement during this period. Efficacy was assessed by clinicians using the Anxiety Rating for Children–Revised (ARC-R) and Children's Depression Rating Scale–Revised (CDRS-R). IMI was administered twice daily and gradually increased every 3 to 5 days to reach a target dose of 3 mg/kg/day by the end of the second week. A nonblind psychiatrist monitored serum blood levels at week 3 and recommended increases or decreases in dose if levels were outside the therapeutic range of 150 to 300 µg/L; to maintain the blind, a similar number of patients receiving placebo were instructed to increase or decrease the dosage. The mean IMI dose after 3 weeks was 184.6 ± 33.3 mg/day and the mean IMI plus DMI blood level was 246.6 ± 227.6 µg/L. Eight subjects had levels <150 µg/L, and seven subjects had levels >300 µg/L. At completion of the study, mean IMI dose was 182.3 ± 50.3 mg and the mean IMI plus DMI blood level was 151.2 ± 90.2 µg/L; nine subjects had levels <150 µg/L, including three with no detectable drug or metabolite; the mean IMI plus DMI level was 58.0 ± 51.4 µg/L. Subjects receiving IMI with concomitant CBT improved significantly more than subjects on placebo and CBT in weekly hours of school attendance (70.1 ± 30.6 vs. 27.6 ± 36.1 hours; $P = .017$) and in decreased depression as rated on the CDRS-R (34.6 ± 8.9 vs. 45.7 ± 16.5; $P = .037$). There were no significant differences between the groups on the ARC-R and two self-report measures. The authors noted that although recent studies had shown CBT to be efficacious in school refusal without medication, the present study suggests that a multimodal approach (i.e., CBT plus pharmacotherapy) results in a superior response. The authors also noted that many subjects remained with significant symptoms at the end of the 8-week study despite their improvement. Only a little more than half of the subjects receiving IMI plus CBT were attending school 75% of the time. Follow-up to see if further improvement occurred, gains were maintained, or school attendance worsened was being pursued but the results are not yet available (Bernstein et al., 2000).

Three children with panic disorder who also had severe separation anxiety and agoraphobia responded well to a combination of IMI and alprazolam, a benzodiazepine (Ballenger et al., 1989).

IMI in the Treatment of Somnambulism and Night Terrors

Four children with night terrors, two children with somnambulism, and one child with both disorders were treated with IMI (10 to 50 mg at bedtime). The sleep disorders remitted completely in all children (Pesikoff and Davis, 1971).

▌ Nortriptyline Hydrochloride (Pamelor)

Untoward effects of nortriptyline and other tricyclic antidepressants are discussed earlier in the introduction to the tricyclic antidepressants. Untoward effects of nortriptyline are also discussed later in the summaries of its use in children and adolescents.

Indications for Nortriptyline Hydrochloride

NOTE: Review the Black Box Warning at beginning of chapter or in package insert before prescribing.

Nortriptyline is approved by the FDA for the treatment of symptoms of depression in adolescents and adults. The drug is not recommended for use in the pediatric age group because its safety and effectiveness have not been established in children.

Nortriptyline Dosage Schedule

- *Children and adolescents ≤17 years of age:* Not recommended. Safety and efficacy have not been determined for this age group.
- *Adolescents at least 18 years of age and adults:* Manufacturer recommends giving a total of 30 to 50 mg/day. One should start at a low dose and titrate upward based on clinical response. (However, see recommendations of Geller et al. in the subsequent text, on the usefulness of serum levels.)

Nortriptyline Hydrochloride Dose Forms Available

- *Capsules:* 10, 25, 50, and 75 mg

Nortriptyline Dosage Schedule for Children and Adolescents

Pharmacokinetic studies of tricyclic antidepressants in adults have shown that their elimination half-lives are sufficiently long to permit the frequent practice of giving a single bedtime dose once titration is completed (Rudorfer and Potter, 1987). Geller et al. (1987b), however, noted that 41 children, aged 5 to 12 years, had a significantly shorter mean nortriptyline plasma half-life (20.8 ± 7.2 hours; range, 11.2 to 42.5 hours) than did 32 adolescents aged 13 to 16 years (31.1 ± 19.8 hours; range, 14.2 to 76.6 hours). Geller et al. (1985) also found that correlations between the mg/kg dose of nortriptyline and steady-state plasma levels were not significant in 33 children and adolescents aged 5 to 16 years. The clinical significance of these data, including the interindividual variation of half-life by as much as six- or sevenfold, prompted Geller et al. (1987b) to advise that nortriptyline should be administered twice daily for all patients up to 16 years of age and that plasma-level monitoring is essential to ensure achieving therapeutic plasma nortriptyline levels.

Geller et al. (1985) have used a single test dose of nortriptyline to predict steady-state plasma levels and to determine the initial dose of nortriptyline and presented tables suggesting daily doses to reach therapeutic nortriptyline plasma levels (Table A.1).

To use this method, the clinician must have access to a laboratory that can reliably assay nortriptyline levels of <20 ng/mL. To use this table clinically, Geller et al. (1985) and Geller and Carr (1988) suggested the following:

1. At 9:00 AM, administer a single dose of 25 mg to patients aged 5 to 9 years or 50 mg to patients aged 10 to 16 years.
2. Twenty-four hours later (9:00 AM the next day), draw blood to determine the plasma nortriptyline level.

TABLE A.1 » Suggested Nortriptyline Hydrochloride Dose Schedules for Children and Adolescents

24-h Plasma Level (ng/mL)	Suggested Total Daily Dose (mg)
Predicted doses from 24-h plasma levels after a single dose of 25 mg administered to 5- to 9-y-olds.[a]	
6–10	50–75
11–14	35–40
15–20	25–30
21–25	20
Predicted doses from 24-h nortriptyline plasma levels after a single dose of 50 mg administered to 10- to 16-y-olds[a]	
10–14	75–100
15–19	50–75
20–24	40–50
25–29	35
30–34	30
35–40	25
>40	20

[a]Total daily dose should be divided and given twice daily because of relatively short half-life.

Adapted from Geller B, Cooper TB, Chestnut EC, et al. Child and adolescent nortriptyline single dose kinetics predict steady state plasma levels and suggested dose: preliminary data. *J Clin Psychopharmacol.* 1985;5:154–158.

3. Use the table to determine the suggested medication dose for the patient's nortriptyline level and age.
4. Seven days later, determine plasma nortriptyline level 9 to 11 hours after a dose. If the level is not in the therapeutic range (60 to 100 ng/mL), adjust the dosage using the following equation (Geller and Carr, 1988):

$$\text{Day 7 plasma levels/current dose} = 80 \text{ ng/mL/adjusted dose}$$

Geller et al. (1987b) have recommended that nortriptyline withdrawn gradually over approximately 10 days to 2 weeks to avoid withdrawal symptoms. Only 6 of 30 children and adolescents 6 to 16 years old developed withdrawal symptoms when this was done. In all cases symptoms were mild, and in five subjects they were limited to the gastrointestinal system and consisted of stomachache, nausea, and/or emesis.

Reports of Interest

Nortriptyline in the Treatment of Major Depressive Disorder in Children and Adolescents

Geller et al. have studied pharmacokinetic parameters of nortriptyline and its use in treating children and adolescents diagnosed with MDD (Geller et al., 1985, 1986, 1987a, 1987b, 1989, 1990, 1992). There are no double-blind, placebo-controlled studies establishing nortriptyline's superiority over placebo in treating MDD in children or adolescents.

In an open study, Geller et al. (1986) found that therapeutic efficacy correlated with nortriptyline plasma levels. Twenty-two children, aged 6 to 12 years, diagnosed with MDD were treated on an outpatient basis with fixed doses of either 10 mg twice daily or 25 mg twice daily for 8 weeks. Initial dose was based on individual subjects' rate of metabolism of nortriptyline, as determined by baseline single-dose kinetics, with the slower metabolizers receiving the lower fixed dose. Fourteen subjects (63.6%) responded favorably to nortriptyline. Responders were not significantly different from nonresponders in terms of age, sex, weight, social class, duration of illness, or baseline or 2-week Children's Depression Rating Scale scores. Responders, however, had significantly higher mean mg/kg daily doses (1.02 ± 0.21 mg/kg; range, 0.64 to 1.57 mg/kg) than nonresponders (0.82 ± 0.51 mg/kg; range, 0.40 to 2.01 mg/kg). The mean nortriptyline steady-state plasma level was also higher in responders (60.31 ± 20.90 ng/mL; range, 18.8 to 111.5 ng/mL) than in nonresponders (30.86 ± 17.64 ng/mL; range, 12 to 54.3 ng/mL). Twelve of the 13 subjects who received at least 0.89 mg/kg/day responded. All subjects with steady-state nortriptyline plasma levels of at least 60 ng/mL responded, as did four of seven children with levels ranging from 40 to 59 ng/mL. At the end of the 8-week protocol, seven of the eight nonresponders recovered when the dose was increased to achieve steady-state nortriptyline plasma levels of 60 to 100 ng/mL. Overall, 21 of the 22 subjects had good clinical response with minimal and transient side effects, and all ECGs remained within recommended parameters for prepubertal children. The authors thought that because children's plasma nortriptyline levels are stable over time, ECGs need to be performed only at baseline and once at steady-state plasma levels if they remain within recommended parameters (Geller et al., 1986).

Geller et al. (1989, 1992) enrolled 72 prepubescent children, aged 6 to 12 years, who were diagnosed with MDD, nondelusional type, by RDC (Spitzer et al., 1978) and DSM-III (American Psychiatric Association [APA], 1980a) criteria in a double-blind, placebo-controlled study of the efficacy of nortriptyline. The study design was a 2-week, single-blind, placebo washout phase followed by an 8-week random-assignment, double-blind, placebo-controlled phase. All subjects were outpatients, and most had coexisting separation anxiety. The children were chronically depressed: 96% had been ill for at least 2 years, and 50% had MDD for 5 or more years before entering the study. Of the 72 subjects entering the study, 12 (16.7%) responded during the placebo phase, 10 were discontinued for various reasons during the active treatment phase, and 50 (24 on placebo and 26 on nortriptyline) completed the study.

Using Table A.1, the initial dose necessary to achieve a steady-state nortriptyline level of 80 ± 20 ng/mL was determined from 24-hour plasma levels. Any necessary adjustments to obtain mean steady-state plasma levels of nortriptyline and of total, trans-10-hydroxynortriptyline, and cis-10-hydroxynortriptyline (10-OH-NT) were made during the first 4 weeks of the double-blind phase.

Both the nortriptyline and the placebo groups had a low rate of positive response (30.8% on nortriptyline and 16.7% on placebo), and there was no significant difference between them. There was no significant correlation between mean nortriptyline plasma level and response or between mean nortriptyline plus mean total, cis-10-OH-NT, or trans-10-OH-NT plasma levels and response. Because of the poor response rate and the unlikelihood of finding a statistical difference between the placebo and active groups if the protocol were completed, Geller et al. (1989, 1992) stopped their study at this point.

Geller et al. (1990) enrolled 52 postpubertal adolescents, aged 12 to 17 years and diagnosed with MDD by RDC (Spitzer et al., 1978) and DSM-III (APA, 1980a) criteria in a random-assignment, double-blind, placebo-controlled study of nortriptyline. Adolescents with delusional symptoms were not enrolled. Subjects had scores on the Children's Depression Rating Scale (CDRS) and the Kiddie Global Assessment Scale (KGAS) placing them in the severe range of pathology. Of the 31 subjects completing the study, 27 (87.1%) had a duration of symptoms of at least 2 years (10 [32.3%] between 2 and 5 years and 17 [54.8%] more than 5 years). The study comprised a 2-week, single-blind, placebo washout phase and an 8-week, double-blind, placebo-controlled phase. Using Table A.1, the initial dose necessary to achieve a steady-state nortriptyline level of 80 ± 20 ng/mL was determined from 24-hour plasma levels. Mean nortriptyline plasma level was 91.1 ± 18.3 ng/mL.

Of the 52 subjects enrolled, 17 (32.7%) responded to placebo by the end of week 2, and 4 additional subjects dropped out for other reasons. Of the 31 completing the study, 12 were assigned to nortriptyline and 19 to placebo. The results of the study showed such a low rate of response to nortriptyline that the study was terminated early. Only 1 (8.3%) of 12 subjects receiving nortriptyline responded, whereas 4 (21.1%) of the 19 subjects on placebo responded. (The one responder to nortriptyline went on to have a bipolar course.) Subjects with higher nortriptyline levels achieved significantly worse scores on the CDRS ($P = .002$). There were, however, no significant differences between the two groups on final CDRS or KGAS scores.

It is most interesting that 17, or about one-third, of enrolled patients with chronic and severe depression responded to placebo within 2 weeks. However, 13 of the 17 placebo responders relapsed, 9 of them within 1 to 4 weeks (Geller et al., 1990).

Nortriptyline in the Treatment of Children and Adolescents Diagnosed with ADHD

Saul (1985) treated 60 patients diagnosed with attention-deficit disorder (ADD) (age range, 9 to 20 years) with nortriptyline. The first group of 30 subjects was diagnosed with ADD and scored more than 9 points on the Kovacs Children's Depression Inventory (KCDI). The second group of 30 subjects had ADD but scored 9 or less on the KCDI. They were initially prescribed stimulant medication but responded poorly and were switched to nortriptyline. Nortriptyline for both groups was begun at 10 mg nightly for 2 weeks. Because no patients experienced difficulty at this dose level, the dose was then increased to 25 mg twice daily. Fifty-four (90%) of the 60 subjects had positive responses. Satisfactory clinical response usually occurred at 50 mg daily; 75 mg/day was the maximum dose given. Within 5 to 6 weeks, typically there was a marked change in attitude followed by an increase in attention span and a decrease in impulsivity. The most clinically significant untoward effects at the initial dose were dizziness and sleepiness; their inconvenience was minimized by administering the drug around bedtime.

Wilens et al. (1993b) conducted a retrospective chart review of 58 patients (mean, 12.1 ± 2.9 years; age range, 7 to 18 years) who were diagnosed with ADHD and received nortriptyline. All but 9 subjects had comorbid diagnoses, including 34 with mood disorder, 18 with oppositional defiant disorder (ODD), and 5 with conduct disorder. These were treatment-resistant patients who had not responded satisfactorily to an average of four prior medication trials. About half of the subjects were also receiving one or two other medications concomitantly. Nortriptyline was administered for a mean of 11.9 ± 14.0 months (range, 0.4 to 57.9 months) in mean daily doses of 73.6 ± 33.1 mg (range, 20 to 200 mg/day) or a mean weight-corrected daily dose of 1.94 ± 0.99 mg/kg (range, 0.4 to 4.5 mg/kg). Overall, 28 patients (48%) were rated as marked responders and 16 (28%) as moderate responders. Subjects with and without comorbidity responded equally well; all five subjects with comorbid conduct disorder responded favorably.

There were no significant differences between responders and nonresponders in mean daily dose (74.8 ± 31.9 vs. 70.0 ± 38.0 mg), in weight-corrected mean daily dose (1.9 ± 0.9 vs. 2.1 ± 1.2 mg/kg), or serum nortriptyline levels (96.3 ± 51.6 vs. 83.4 ± 43.1 ng/mL). Significantly more ($P < .03$) of the "markedly improved" subjects had serum nortriptyline levels between 50 and 150 ng/mL. Untoward effects were usually mild and necessitated stopping nortriptyline in only one child who became agitated. No clinically significant conduction abnormalities were noted on ECG follow-up assessment.

Prince et al. (2000) conducted a two-phase, 9-week, controlled study of 35 subjects (28 males, 7 females; mean age, 9.8 ± 2.6 years) diagnosed with ADHD by DSM-IV (APA, 1994) criteria. Nineteen (59%) had lifetime comorbid ODD and four (13%) had lifetime comorbid conduct disorder. During the first 6-week, open-label phase, subjects were administered nortriptyline in divided doses (before school and after dinner) that were individually titrated up to a maximum of 2 mg/kg/day over the first 2 weeks (unless clinical efficacy was achieved at a lower dose or untoward effects prevented further increase) and then maintained for the subsequent 4 weeks. Responders were determined *a priori* by ratings on the Clinical Global Impressions ADHD Improvement Scale of 1 ("very much improved") or 2 ("much improved") or by a reduction of >30% on the DuPaul ADHD DSM-IV symptom checklist. ODD symptoms were rated on a DSM-IV checklist of ODD symptoms.

Mean nortriptyline dose at the end of week 4 was 79 ± 36 mg/day or 1.9 mg/kg/day, with a mean serum nortriptyline concentration of 81 ± 66 ng/mL (range, 10 to 316 ng/mL). At the end of 6 weeks, the mean nortriptyline dose was 77 ± 35 mg/day or 1.8 mg/kg/day. Thirty-two subjects completed the first phase; two subjects had dropped out because of untoward effects and one because of nonresponse. By the end of week 6, there was an overall mean reduction in the ADHD symptom checklist of 53% ($P < .001$); 29 subjects (84%) had reductions of >30% of their baseline ratings. Opposition defiant symptoms also significantly decreased by 48% ($P < .001$) during the 6-week open phase, with 25 subjects (71%) having a >30% reduction compared with baseline ratings. There was no significant correlation between dose or serum level of nortriptyline and improvement in ADHD or opposition symptoms.

Twenty-five of the 29 responders elected to participate in the 3-week double-blind discontinuation phase; of the 23 subjects who completed this phase, 12 had been randomized to nortriptyline and 11 to placebo. The subjects who continued to receive nortriptyline had significantly lower scores on the DSM-IV ADHD checklist compared with subjects receiving placebo ($P < .04$). Overall, subjects randomized to nortriptyline maintained their clinical improvements in ADHD and ODD symptoms, whereas those randomized to placebo had a significant reexacerbation of these symptoms and their week-9 ratings were not significantly different from baseline. During the study, heart rate increased by 18% ($P < .05$) but there were no clinically significant changes in blood pressure, in PR, QRS, QTc, or any new ECG abnormality. The data suggest that nortriptyline is efficacious in treating both ADHD and oppositional symptoms in ADHD and ADHD with comorbidity (Prince et al., 2000).

Nortriptyline in Comorbid Attention-Deficit/Hyperactivity Disorder and Chronic Motor Tic Disorder or Tourette Syndrome

In a retrospective study of 12 children and adolescents (age range, 5 to 16 years; mean, 10.9 ± 1.0 years) diagnosed with ADHD and comorbid chronic motor tic disorder ($N = 2$) or Tourette syndrome ($N = 10$), Spencer et al. (1993c) reported that 8 (67%) subjects were rated as being markedly or very much improved ($P = .01$) in their movement disorders, and 11 (92%) were rated much or very much improved ($P = .0001$) in their ADHD symptoms. The average dose of nortriptyline was 105 ± 11.7 mg/day or 2.8 ± 0.3 mg/kg/day. Mean serum nortriptyline level was 122.7 ± 12.1 ng/mg for the 10 patients for whom such values had been determined. There were few untoward effects. The only cardiac symptom was a mild tachycardia in one patient; no clinically significant changes occurred in EEGs.

Amitriptyline Hydrochloride (Elavil, Endep)

Amitriptyline hydrochloride is a tertiary amine tricyclic antidepressant. Although the tricyclic antidepressants block reuptake of both norepinephrine and serotonin, evidence suggests that the tertiary amine tricyclics block the reuptake of serotonin more than the reuptake of norepinephrine, whereas the secondary amine tricyclics may block norepinephrine uptake more than serotonin uptake.

Pharmacokinetics of Amitriptyline Hydrochloride

Untoward effects of amitriptyline are discussed earlier in "Untoward Effects of Tricyclic Antidepressants" as well as in the summaries of its use in children and adolescents later.

Indications for Amitriptyline Hydrochloride

NOTE: Review the Black Box Warning at the beginning of the chapter or in the package insert before prescribing.

Amitriptyline is approved to treat symptoms of depression. It is noted that endogenous depression is more likely to be alleviated than other depressive states.

Amitriptyline Dosage Schedule

- *Children ≤11 years of age:* Not recommended because of limited experience with treating this age group.
- *Adolescents at least 12 years of age and adults:* An initial dose of 25 mg/day titrated upward in 25-mg increments is suggested. Ten milligrams three times daily and 20 mg at bedtime may be adequate for adolescents who do not tolerate higher doses. Adequate therapeutic response may take up to 30 days to develop. Usual maintenance is 50 to 100 mg/day.

Amitriptyline Hydrochloride Dose Forms Available

- *Tablets:* 10, 25, 50, 75, 100, and 150 mg
- *Injectable:* 10 mg/mL

Reports of Interest

Amitriptyline Hydrochloride in the Treatment of Children and Adolescents Diagnosed with Attention-Deficit/Hyperactivity Disorder

Yepes et al. (1977) administered amitriptyline, methylphenidate, or placebo to 50 children diagnosed with hyperkinetic reaction of childhood for randomly determined 2-week periods during which each drug was titrated. The initial dose of amitriptyline was 25 mg three times daily; dose was titrated to achieve optimal clinical response. Dose range was 50 to 150 mg/day; the mean was 92.1 mg/day. Amitriptyline was, with few exceptions, comparable to methylphenidate in effectiveness in reducing hyperactivity and aggression in both the home and school environments. The authors noted, however, that amitriptyline was more sedating than IMI and that, frequently, doses of amitriptyline sufficiently high to control symptoms could not be tolerated. Sedation remained a problem throughout the 2-week period on amitriptyline. In an earlier study (Krakowski, 1965), however, 50 children with various diagnoses with hyperkinesis received maintenance doses of 20 to 75 mg/day (i.e., about one-half that used in the preceding study) for up to 9 months with positive results, and only one instance of severe sedation occurred. (The other subjects developed tolerance or the sedative effect disappeared with reduction of dosage.)

Amitriptyline Hydrochloride in Children Diagnosed with Major Depressive Disorder

Kashani et al. (1984) performed a double-blind, crossover study comparing amitriptyline and placebo in nine prepubertal children diagnosed with MDD. Dosage ranged from 45 to 110 mg/day. Six (66.7%) of the subjects improved on amitriptyline, a finding that was not significant ($P < .09$).

Amitriptyline Hydrochloride in Adolescents Diagnosed with Major Depressive Disorder

Kramer and Feiguine (1981) compared the efficacy of amitriptyline and placebo in treating 20 adolescents diagnosed with depression. Age range was 13 to 17 years. Amitriptyline was initially given in 25-mg doses four times daily and increased within 3 days to a maximum of 200 mg/day in divided doses. The length of the study was 6 weeks. Both placebo and active medication groups improved over the 6-week period, and there was no significant difference between the two groups. Although this pilot study suggests that amitriptyline is no more effective than placebo in treating adolescent depression, more studies and larger numbers are necessary before coming to this conclusion definitively.

Amitriptyline Hydrochloride in Adolescents with "Treatment-Resistant" Major Depression

Birmaher et al. (1998) conducted a 10-week, randomized, double-blind, placebo-controlled, flexible-dose study of amitriptyline (AMI) in 27 hospitalized adolescents (19 females, 8 males; mean age, 16.2 ± 1.4 years) diagnosed by DSM-III-R (APA, 1987) criteria with nonpsychotic MDD. All subjects were taking antidepressants, and seven were also taking lithium at the time of hospitalization. They underwent a 4-week period of withdrawal and still met MDD criteria before beginning the study protocol. Amitriptyline was begun at 50 mg/day in divided doses and titrated, based on clinical response, upward by 50 mg/week to a maximum of 5 mg/kg/day, a total of 300 mg/day, or AMI plus nortriptyline (NTP) serum levels of 300 ng/mL. The average dose of amitriptyline at the end of the study was 173.1 ± 56.3 mg/day or 2.8 ± 1.0 mg/kg/day and the average total AMI plus NTP blood levels were 226.2 ± 80.8 ng/mL. Both the placebo and the AMI groups had clinically significant reductions in scores on the Hamilton Depression Rating Scale, the Beck Depression Inventory, and the National Institute of Mental Health Clinical Global Impressions–Improvement and Clinical Global Impressions–Severity of Illness (CGI-S) Scales, but there was no significant difference between the two groups. Overall, about 70% to 80% of these chronically depressed patients who were admitted to a state hospital as treatment failures showed similar significant symptomatic improvement on both placebo and AMI. Approximately 30% of the subjects continued to meet criteria for MDD, and 60% had subsyndromal symptoms of MDD. The dose of AMI or blood level of AMI plus NTP was not related to clinical outcome or untoward effects. The only untoward effect reported significantly more frequently with AMI was dry mouth. Patients in the AMI group had significantly higher resting and orthostatic heart rates at the end of the study.

Desipramine Hydrochloride (Norpramin, Pertofrane)

Desipramine is a secondary amine tricyclic antidepressant. Although the tricyclic antidepressants block reuptake of both norepinephrine and serotonin, evidence suggests that the secondary amine tricyclics block the reuptake of norepinephrine more than the reuptake of serotonin, whereas tertiary amine tricyclics may block serotonin uptake more than norepinephrine uptake.

Pharmacokinetics and Adverse Effects of Desipramine Hydrochloride

Pharmacokinetics and adverse effects of DMI, including sudden death, are discussed earlier under "Pharmacokinetics of Tricyclic Antidepressants" and "Untoward Effects of Tricyclic Antidepressants" and later under the "Reports of Interest" for DMI that follow.

Indications for Desipramine Hydrochloride

NOTE: Review the Black Box Warning at the beginning of the chapter or in the package insert before prescribing.

Desipramine is indicated in the treatment of symptoms in various depressive syndromes, especially endogenous depression.

Desipramine Dosage Schedule

- *Children and adolescents <18 years of age:* Not recommended. Its efficacy and safety have not been established in the pediatric age group.
- *Adolescents at least 18 years of age and adults:* Usual dose is between 25 and 100 mg/day. One should start at a lower dose and titrate according to clinical response. A dose of 150 mg/day should not be exceeded. Adequate treatment response may take 2 to 3 weeks to develop. Therapeutic total plasma levels of IMI plus DMI are usually considered to range between 100 and 300 ng/mL.

Desipramine Hydrochloride Dose Forms Available

- *Tablets:* 10, 25, 50, 75, 100, and 150 mg

Reports of Interest

Desipramine Hydrochloride in the Treatment of Adolescent Major Depressive Disorder

From 113 adolescents referred for depression, Boulos et al. (1991) identified a group of 52 who were diagnosed with nonpsychotic MDD by DSM-III criteria and who did not have an eating disorder, had not been treated with psychiatric medication, and had ratings of at least 17 on the Hamilton Rating Scale for Depression (Ham-D) and of at least 16 on the Beck Depression Inventory. These subjects were enrolled in single-blind placebo washout for 1 week. The 43 subjects whose rating scores continued to fulfill the preceding criteria then entered a 6-week double-blind protocol in which they received either placebo or DMI in identical capsules. Desipramine was initiated at a dose of 100 mg at bedtime.

Additional doses of 50 mg were added the next two mornings to achieve a daily dose of 200 mg (100 mg twice daily), which was maintained for the duration of the study. Thirty patients completed the study; 12 received DMI and 18 received placebo. Seven patients dropped out for "personal reasons" and six because of untoward effects. A positive treatment response was reported if there was a reduction of at least 50% in the pretreatment score on the Ham-D. There was no significant difference ($P < .59$) between the placebo group (6 [33%] of 18) and the DMI group (6 [50%] of 12). No significant differences between the groups in subjective untoward effects were reported. However, major adverse effects that necessitated discontinuing medication in six patients occurred only in the DMI group ($P < .05$) and included an allergic-type pruritic maculopapular rash (three patients), vomiting and laryngospasm (one), and orthostatic hypotension (two). ECG abnormalities, including tachycardia, sinus arrhythmia, and nonspecific T-wave changes, occurred only in the DMI group, but were clinically nonsymptomatic and did not require withdrawal from the study. Serum metabolite levels were not reported.

Kutcher et al. (1994) enrolled 70 adolescents who were diagnosed with MDD in a fixed-dose, placebo-controlled DMI protocol. During the initial single-blind, 1-week placebo period, 10 subjects were judged to be placebo responders and were dropped. The remaining 60 subjects (42 females, 18 males; age range, 15 to 20 years; mean age, 17.8 years) were assigned randomly to 6 weeks of placebo ($N = 30$) or DMI ($N = 30$). Desipramine was begun with a 100-mg 8:00 PM dose, and 50 mg was added at 8:00 AM the second day and increased to 100 mg on the third day. Desipramine was continued at 100 mg twice daily throughout the remaining 6 weeks.

Eighteen subjects dropped out. Significantly, more of these were on active medication (13 [72%] of 18), and 10 of them did not complete the study because of untoward effects. Nine (90%) of the 10 were receiving DMI; five subjects had allergic-type reactions (four had maculopapular rashes and one had mild laryngospasm), two patients had clinically significant orthostatic hypotension, and two had significant gastrointestinal complaints. The patient receiving placebo dropped out because of severe agitation. At the completion of the protocol, 2 of the 26 items on the Side Effects Scale were rated significantly higher among subjects in the DMI group: trouble sleeping ($P = .03$) and delay in urinating ($P = .007$). Although heart rate significantly increased in the DMI group, there were no significant differences in systolic blood pressure while seated or standing, diastolic blood pressure while seated, or PR and QRS intervals on the ECG between the DMI and placebo groups.

Forty-two subjects completed the protocol; the ratings of 15 subjects (36%) decreased by at least 50% from baseline on the Hamilton Depression Rating Scale at the end of week 6. There was no significant difference ($P = .53$) between improved subjects receiving IMI ($N = 8$ [47%] of 17) and placebo ($N = 7$ [28%] of 25).

Mean combined DMI level (205.06 ng/mL) plus 2-OH-DMI level (70.01 ng/mL) was 275.07 ng/mL. There was no significant correlation between DMI, 2-OH-DMI, or combined serum levels and the outcome of treatment. In fact, the 17 subjects receiving DMI who did not improve had higher mean values of DMI, 2-OH-DMI, and combined serum levels than the 8 subjects who improved. The authors concluded that their data were consonant with other studies of tricyclic medication in depressed adolescents, which did not show the significant treatment benefit seen in adults but did show a relatively high rate of significant and unpleasant untoward effects (Kutcher et al., 1994).

Desipramine Hydrochloride in the Treatment of Enuresis

Rapoport et al. (1980b) found that 75 mg of DMI at bedtime had a short-term antienuretic effect that was not statistically different from that of IMI.

Desipramine Hydrochloride in the Treatment of Attention-Deficit/Hyperactivity Disorder

Garfinkel et al. (1983) studied 12 males (mean age, 7.3 years; range, 5.9 to 11.6 years) who were diagnosed with ADD and required day hospital or inpatient treatment for the severity of their symptoms of impulsiveness, inattention, and aggression. The subjects received placebo, methylphenidate, DMI, and clomipramine in a double-blind, crossover experiment. The mean dose of DMI was 85 mg/day and did not exceed 100 mg/day or 3.5 mg/kg/day for any subject. Methylphenidate was significantly better than the other three conditions in improving overall classroom functioning as rated on the Conners Scale by teachers ($P < .005$) and program child care workers ($P < .001$).

In an open study, Gastfriend et al. (1984) treated 12 adolescents (age range, 12 to 17 years) who were diagnosed with ADD with DMI for 6 to 52 weeks. Eleven of them had previously responded poorly to stimulants or had intolerable untoward effects. Although these were outpatients, their symptoms were so severe that residential schooling or hospitalization had been considered for many of them. Desipramine was initiated with a dose of 10 or 25 mg/day and increased weekly to a maximum of 5 mg/kg or until an optimal clinical result was obtained or untoward effects prevented further increase. The mean daily dose after 4 weeks was 1.57 mg/kg (range, 0.58 to 2.63 mg/kg); 11 of the 12 patients improved, and 5 were rated "much" or "very much" improved on the Clinical Global Impressions (CGI) Scale. Ten patients were followed for 21 to 52 weeks; their optimal daily doses ranged from 0.93 to 5.95 mg/kg. Nine of the 10 patients sustained their improvement for more than 6 months, and 8 of these were rated "much" or "very much" improved. Plasma levels for a given dose varied as much as 10-fold. Untoward effects were most troublesome during the first month; six patients (50%) experienced drowsiness; three (25%), postural dizziness; three (25%), weight loss and/or decreased appetite; two (16%), headache; one (8%), insomnia; and one (8%), racing thoughts. The untoward effects lessened in all cases following reduction in dosage.

Subsequently, in another open study, Biederman et al. (1986) treated 18 children diagnosed with ADD with DMI for 4 to 52 weeks. Initial dose was 10 or 25 mg of DMI, and the dose was titrated weekly. Dose at 4 weeks ranged from 0.7 to 4 mg/kg/day (mean, 2.0 ± 0.9 mg/kg/day); on later follow-up, doses were significantly higher, ranging from 1.3 to 6.3 mg/kg/day. Improvement at follow-up time (mean time at follow-up, 22.9 ± 15.9 weeks) was also significantly greater than at 4 weeks. Although there was sufficient time for tolerance to medication to have developed, it was not observed.

Biederman et al. (1989a, 1989b) reviewed earlier work in this area and studied the efficacy of DMI in treating 42 children and 20 adolescents diagnosed with ADD with hyperactivity ($N = 60$) or without hyperactivity ($N = 2$). Sixty-nine percent of their subjects had responded poorly to earlier treatment with stimulants. The subjects were randomly assigned to a 6-week, double-blind, parallel-groups, placebo-controlled protocol. Desipramine was titrated upward to an average daily dose of 4.6 ± 0.2 mg/kg, a relatively high dose. This high dose was selected because of inconsistent findings in studies using lower doses of DMI in subjects with ADD (Biederman et al., 1989a). Patients treated with DMI had statistically significant improvement in symptoms rated on the Conners Abbreviated Parent and Teacher Questionnaires, compared with subjects receiving placebo ($P = .0001$). The patterns of improvement were similar in adolescents and children. There was no significant relationship between serum DMI levels and clinical response, making the designation of an optimal level inappropriate. Some subjects who improved had serum levels below 100 ng/mL. About one-fourth of the patients had high levels, between 300 and 900 ng/mL; of this group, 80% (12 of 15) improved (Biederman et al., 1989b).

Untoward effects were usually mild and were more frequent in subjects receiving DMI than in the placebo group ($P < .05$); overall, there was no discernible relationship between serum level and untoward effects. Symptoms included dry mouth (32%), decreased appetite (29%), headache (29%), abdominal discomfort (26%), tiredness (25%), dizziness (23%), and insomnia (23%). Although no subjects developed any clinically apparent cardiovascular signs or symptoms, cardiovascular and ECG untoward effects, such as increased diastolic blood pressure, tachycardia, and conduction abnormalities, were statistically more frequent in subjects receiving DMI. There was a suggestion that ECG changes occurred more frequently at higher serum DMI levels. Although side effects were rated as mild, the authors noted that in 71% of patients (22 of 31) receiving DMI and 52% of patients (16 of 31) receiving placebo, untoward effects prevented the medication from being raised to the target dose of 5 mg/kg/day (Biederman et al., 1989b). Of special interest is the fact that in contrast to reports of rapid improvement of subjects with ADD in response to IMI, subjects in this study required 3 to 4 weeks to show significant clinical improvement with DMI as compared with placebo (Biederman et al., 1989b).

Biederman et al. (1989b) suggested that a steady-state serum DMI level between 100 ng/mL and a maximum of 300 ng/mL is probably efficacious and safe for most children and adolescents but that some patients will require daily doses >3.5 mg/kg/day to reach these serum levels. They estimated that optimal doses range between 2.5 and 5 mg/kg/day. The authors (Biederman et al., 1989b) recommended the following parameters as being more clinically relevant in the titration of DMI than accepting an arbitrary maximum limit in dose (e.g., 5 mg/kg):

1. The DMI serum level should be kept under 300 ng/mL.
2. The PR interval on the ECG should be <200 msec.
3. The QRS interval on the ECG should be <120 msec.

Desipramine shows some promise as an alternative medication for children and adolescents diagnosed with ADHD who have unsatisfactory responses to stimulant medication. Gualtieri et al. (1991) reported that DMI improved long-term memory performance, analogous to that reported with stimulants, when used in treating children diagnosed with ADHD. Its use requires strict clinical monitoring, including ECG and serum levels, because of its pharmacokinetics and cardiotoxicity.

Coadministration of Desipramine Hydrochloride and Methylphenidate in the Treatment of Attention-Deficit/Hyperactivity Disorder with Symptoms of Major Depressive Disorder or Comorbid MDD

Rapport et al. (1993) studied the separate and combined effects of methylphenidate and DMI on cognitive functions in 16 hospitalized children (aged 7 years, 9 months to 12 years, 10 months) diagnosed with ADHD and MDD, ADHD with symptoms of MDD, or MDD with symptoms of ADHD. Following a 2-week baseline period, subjects received placebo, DMI, three dose levels of methylphenidate (10, 15, and 20 mg), and combined methylphenidate and DMI at each of the methylphenidate levels. Desipramine was begun at 50 mg/day and increased by 25 mg every 2 days, unless untoward effects prevented the increase and until plasma levels between 125 and 225 mg/mL were reached, because earlier studies had suggested this to be the range of maximum therapeutic efficacy in prepubertal children. Methylphenidate alone improved vigilance, both drugs had positive effects on short-term memory and visual problem solving, and the combination of both drugs affected learning of higher-order relationships. The effects of these drug conditions on mood and behavior were not reported.

In a separate report concerning the same subjects, Pataki et al. (1993) detailed the untoward effects of methylphenidate and DMI alone and in combination in a subset of 13 patients. The mean final dose of DMI during combined administration with methylphenidate was 148 mg/day (range, 75 to 300 mg/day) or 4.4 mg/kg/day (range, 2.5 to 6.6 mg/kg/day). The mean plasma DMI level during combined administration with methylphenidate was 170 ng/mL (range, <50 to 228 ng/mL for the 11 subjects for whom it was available). As methylphenidate is reported to inhibit hepatic enzymes that metabolize tricyclics, DMI plasma levels alone and when coadministered with methylphenidate were compared. The mean final plasma level of DMI when administered alone was 159 ng/mL, compared with a level of 170 ng/mL when administered in combination with methylphenidate, and the difference in plasma levels was not significant. On individual bases, however, the most extreme variations were found in a subject who received 75 mg of DMI daily (2.9 mg/kg/day) in combination with methylphenidate and had a plasma level of 158 ng/mL and another subject who received 300 mg of DMI daily (6.6 mg/kg/day) that resulted in a plasma level of 146 ng/day.

Untoward effects were more frequent in the combined DMI and methylphenidate treatment than in any of the other conditions: nausea (17% vs. 8% in the 40 mg/day methylphenidate group), dry mouth (42% vs. 8% in the 40 mg/day methylphenidate and the DMI-alone groups), and tremor (8% vs. none in any other group). The combination of DMI and methylphenidate resulted in an increase in ventricular heart rate that was significantly greater than that in the other conditions; however, this increase was not in a range that would place the children at clinical risk according to the pediatric cardiologist. Three children had sinus tachycardia on ECG: all three occurred during the combined drug treatment but were not thought to be of clinical significance by the pediatric cardiologist.

The authors concluded that, clinically, the untoward effects of combined DMI and methylphenidate treatment were not significantly greater than those for DMI alone; untoward effects were similar to those during administration of DMI alone, and there was no evidence that the addition of methylphenidate increased DMI levels significantly (Pataki et al., 1993). This study was conducted on a very small number of patients, and much larger samples are needed before definitive conclusions may be reached.

Desipramine Hydrochloride in Comorbid Attention-Deficit/Hyperactivity Disorder and Chronic Motor Tic Disorder or Tourette Syndrome

Although stimulants are the treatment of choice in ADHD, they may exacerbate tics or precipitate them *de novo*. Hence problems arise when children have preexisting tic disorders or when they develop tics while being treated with stimulants. Indeed, some authorities recommend not giving stimulants to children with a family history of tics or Tourette disorder.

Riddle et al. (1988) noted that Tourette disorder and ADHD coexist in approximately 50% of children who are referred for evaluation of Tourette disorder and that between 20% and 50% of such patients develop worsening of their tics if treated with stimulants. The authors treated seven children with DMI, aged 7 to 11 years, all of whom had diagnoses of ADHD and various tic disorders (one with Tourette disorder, three with chronic multiple tics, and two with family histories of Tourette disorder, four of whom had developed chronic tic symptoms when previously treated with methylphenidate). Five of the children had an additional diagnosis of oppositional disorder. Desipramine was begun at 25 mg daily and increased by 25 mg every 2 to 3 days to a maximum of 100 mg, or a lower level when clinical improvement was satisfactory or untoward effects prevented further increase. Four children improved "remarkably," and one child "moderately" when rated on the Clinical Global Impressions–Improvement Scale. Two children were considered nonresponders. Six children showed no change in the status or severity of their tics. One child's intermittent eyeblinking became persistent after 3 weeks of DMI; this had also occurred in this patient during a previous trial of methylphenidate (Riddle et al., 1988).

In a retrospective study of 33 children and adolescents (age range, 5 to 17 years; mean, 12.0 ± 0.6 years) diagnosed with chronic motor tic disorder or Tourette syndrome, 30 of whom had comorbid ADHD, Spencer et al. (1993a) reported

that 27 (82%) of the 33 had significant improvement (P = .0001) in their movement disorders and 24 (80%) of the 30 with ADHD had significant improvements
(P = .0001) in their ADHD symptoms when treated with DMI. The average dose
of DMI was 127 ± 9.8 mg/day or 3.5 ± 0.3 mg/kg/day. Mean serum DMI level was
132 ± 16 ng/mg for the 22 patients for whom such values had been determined.
Untoward effects, rash (one) and abdominal pain (one), caused two patients to
withdraw prematurely from the study, precluding their inclusion in the analysis
of data. The study was discontinued in four patients because of untoward effects:
nausea and vomiting (one), irritability and agitation (two), and worsening of a tic
(one). Eight subjects (24%) had asymptomatic cardiac abnormalities including
new onset of incomplete right bundle branch block (four), junctional rhythms
(two), benign ectopic atrial contractions on Holter monitor (one), and an increase
in the QTc interval (one).

It is unclear why none of the subjects in the study of Riddle et al. (1988)
had improvement in their tic disorders, whereas subjects in the 1993 study of
Spencer et al. showed very significant improvement. Although further experience is
necessary to establish that DMI is both safe and efficacious in treating children and
adolescents with coexisting ADHD and tic disorder, it appears to be a potentially
useful alternative treatment for children whose ADHD is of sufficient severity to
necessitate pharmacological intervention and for those diagnosed with ADHD
who develop tics after the initiation of stimulant therapy.

Clomipramine Hydrochloride (Anafranil)

Clomipramine is an antiobsessional drug that belongs to the class of tricyclic
antidepressants. Clomipramine itself has potent inhibitory effects on the neuronal
reuptake of serotonin as compared with neuronal reuptake of norepinephrine;
however, its primary metabolite, desmethylclomipramine, effectively inhibits norepinephrine uptake.

Flament et al. (1987) studied the actions of clomipramine on peripheral measures of serotonergic and noradrenergic function in children and adolescents diagnosed with obsessive-compulsive disorder. They compared 29 such children and
adolescents (mean age, 13.9 ± 2.5 years; range, 8 to 18 years) with controls and
found that a high pretreatment level of platelet serotonin was a strong predictor
of a favorable clinical response and that clomipramine treatment produced a very
marked decrease in platelet serotonin concentration in all patients (P < .0001).
Clomipramine treatment also produced a trend toward reduction in platelet monoamine oxidase (MAO) activity (P = .11) and increased peripheral noradrenergic
function. The plasma level of norepinephrine in standing subjects increased significantly (P < .008). These data suggest that clomipramine's inhibition of serotonin
uptake may be essential to its antiobsessional effect (Flament et al., 1987).

Pharmacokinetics of Clomipramine Hydrochloride

Clomipramine has a long half-life. The mean half-life of a single 150-mg dose is
32 hours, and the mean half-life of its major metabolite, desmethylclomipramine,
is 69 hours. Steady-state serum levels usually occur within 1 to 2 weeks at a given
daily dosage. Children and adolescents <15 years of age had significantly lower
plasma concentrations for a given dose compared with adults (package insert).
Dugas et al. (1980) reported that peak plasma clomipramine levels were achieved
3 to 4 hours after ingestion in the three children they studied and reported an
apparent plasma terminal half-life of 11.9 to 17.3 hours. The bioavailability of
clomipramine is not significantly affected by ingestion with food, and administering it during initial titration in divided doses with meals helps to reduce gastrointestinal side effects. Clomipramine is metabolized largely into its major bioactive
metabolite, desmethylclomipramine; both compounds are ultimately metabolized

into their glucuronide conjugates by the liver. The metabolites are excreted through the bile duct and the kidneys.

Contraindications for the Administration of Clomipramine Hydrochloride

Known hypersensitivity to clomipramine hydrochloride is a contraindication.

Untoward Effects of Clomipramine Hydrochloride

The most significant risk of clomipramine appears to be the development of seizures. Risk for seizures is cumulative and, for doses up to 300 mg/day, increased from 0.64% at 90 days to 1.45% at 1 year. Other untoward effects that occur in children and adolescents include somnolence, tremor, dizziness, headache, sleep disorders, increased sweating, dry mouth, gastrointestinal effects (constipation and dyspepsia), anorexia, fatigue, cardiovascular effects (postural hypotension, palpitations, tachycardia, and syncope), abnormalities of vision, urinary retention, dysmenorrhea in females, and ejaculation failure in males (package insert). Because of reports of blood dyscrasias, a complete blood cell count should be determined in patients who develop fever and sore throat during the course of treatment.

Dugas et al. (1980) reported in their study of 8 children and 28 adolescents who were administered clomipramine for enuresis or depressive symptomatology that the incidence of untoward effects was clearly related to the clomipramine plasma concentration. Untoward effects occurred in about 15% to 20% of patients with plasma clomipramine levels below 60 ng/mL and were present in more than 90% of cases with serum levels above 90 ng/mL. Hypotension occurred only in cases with serum levels above 80 ng/mL. No discernible relationship was found between untoward effects and plasma levels of desmethylclomipramine.

Indications for Clomipramine Hydrochloride

NOTE: Review the Black Box Warning at the beginning of the chapter or in the package insert before prescribing.

Clomipramine has been approved by the FDA for the treatment of obsessions and compulsions in patients at least 10 years of age who have been diagnosed with obsessive-compulsive disorder.

Clomipramine Dosage Schedule for Children and Adolescents

- *Children ≤9 years of age:* Not recommended.
- *Children and adolescents 10 to 17 years of age:* Initial dose of 25 mg/day, titrated upward to a daily maximum of 100 mg or 3 mg/kg/day, whichever is less, over the first 2 weeks. Subsequently, dosage may be increased gradually to a maximum of 200 mg/day or 3 mg/kg/day, whichever is less. After the optimal dose has been determined, clomipramine may be given in a single bedtime dose to minimize daytime sedation.
- *Adolescents at least 18 years of age and adults:* As above, but the maximum dose can be increased to 250 mg/day.

Clomipramine Withdrawal Syndrome

Abrupt withdrawal of clomipramine may result in withdrawal symptoms similar to those that occur when the tricyclics used in treating depression are suddenly discontinued. Symptoms may include dizziness, nausea, vomiting, headache, malaise, sleep disturbances, hyperthermia, irritability, and worsening of psychiatric status. Hence, a gradual tapering of the dose over a period of 10 days to 2 weeks is recommended.

Clomipramine Hydrochloride Dose Forms Available

- *Capsules:* 25, 50, and 75 mg

Clomipramine Hydrochloride in the Treatment of Obsessive-
Compulsive Disorder in Children and Adolescents

There are few published studies on the use of clomipramine in children and adolescents diagnosed with obsessive-compulsive disorder. Those of Flament et al. (1985, 1987) and of Leonard et al. (1989) include some children below the age of 10 years and are summarized below.

Clomipramine was found to be significantly superior to placebo in a placebo-controlled, double-blind, crossover study of 19 subjects whose ages ranged from 10 to 18 years (mean, 14.5 ± 2.3 years) who were diagnosed with severe primary obsessive-compulsive disorder (Flament et al., 1985). The dose range was 100 to 200 mg/day (mean, 141 ± 30 mg/day). The experimental data suggested that clomipramine has a direct antiobsessional action that is independent of any antidepressant effect. In fact, 10 of the subjects had been previously treated with other tricyclics without significant benefit. Flament et al. (1987) increased the number of their subjects to 29 (mean age, 13.9 ± 2.5 years; range, 8 to 18 years) and reported the continued efficacy of clomipramine; the mean daily dose of clomipramine was 134 ± 33 mg/day.

Leonard et al. (1989) compared the efficacy of clomipramine and DMI in the treatment of severe primary obsessive-compulsive disorder in 49 child and adolescent subjects (31 males and 18 females) (mean age, 13.86 ± 2.87 years; range, 7 to 19 years) in a 10-week crossover-design study. Administration of clomipramine was begun at 25 mg/day for children weighing 25 kg or less and at 50 mg/day for subjects weighing more than 25 kg. Dosage was increased weekly by an amount equal to each subject's initial dose. Maximum dosage did not exceed 250 mg/day or 5 mg/kg/day. The mean dose of clomipramine at week 5 was 150 ± 53 mg/day, with a range of 50 to 250 mg/day. Clomipramine was markedly superior to desipramine DMI in decreasing obsessive-compulsive symptoms on several rating scales. In addition, 64% of patients who improved significantly when initially on clomipramine experienced relapse following the crossover to DMI; this was a relapse rate similar to that for placebo in the preceding Flament et al. (1985) study. The most common side effects reported were dry mouth, tremor, tiredness, dizziness, difficulty sleeping, sweating, constipation, poor appetite, and weakness.

Leonard et al. (1991) reported that, of the 48 children completing the preceding 1989 study, 28 (58%) were still receiving maintenance clomipramine 4 to 32 months later. Twenty-six of these patients agreed to participate in an 8-month double-blind study in which DMI was substituted for clomipramine. At the time of entry to the protocol, subjects' daily doses of clomipramine ranged from 50 to 250 mg (mean dose, 134.7 ± 58.2 mg/day or 2.4 ± 0.6 mg/kg/day). Subjects continued to receive clomipramine at their maintenance level for 3 months, at which time DMI was substituted for clomipramine for the next 2 months. For the final 3-month period, all subjects received clomipramine. Twenty subjects completed the study. Eight of nine patients (89%) randomly assigned to DMI relapsed during the 2-month period, whereas only 2 (18%) of 11 patients remaining on clomipramine relapsed. The authors noted that the eight patients who relapsed on DMI experienced symptom improvement to previous levels within 1 month after clomipramine was reinstituted. This is clinically important because it suggests that a significant percentage of children and adolescents need long-term drug treatment to prevent recurrence of obsessive-compulsive symptoms; however, if relapse occurs when an attempt to discontinue clomipramine is made, comparable clinical control can usually be regained upon reinstating clomipramine.

DeVeaugh-Geiss et al. (1992) reported a multicenter trial in which 60 children and adolescents, aged 10 to 17 years, diagnosed with obsessive-compulsive disorder were administered clomipramine in a 10-week, double-blind, fully randomized, parallel-groups, placebo-controlled study. Thirty-one patients were assigned to the clomipramine group and 29 to the placebo group; except for an excess of males in the clomipramine group, they were comparable. Placebo was administered to all patients under single-blind conditions for the first 2 weeks. During the active drug stage, the initial daily dose was 25 mg of active drug or placebo; over the next 2 weeks, this dose was titrated to either 75 or 100 mg daily based on weight. Subsequent increases to a maximum of 3 mg/kg/day or 200 mg were permitted at the discretion of the investigator. Twenty-seven subjects in each group completed the study. Untoward effects were typical of the tricyclic antidepressants. The patients receiving clomipramine improved significantly compared with those in the placebo group. On the Yale–Brown Obsessive-Compulsive Scale (Y-BOCS), the clomipramine group had a mean reduction in score of 37% and the placebo group a reduction of 8% ($P < .05$), and on the National Institute of Mental Health (NIMH) Global Scale the groups had reductions of 34% and 6%, respectively ($P < .05$).

Evidence suggests that clomipramine is effective for children and adolescents with severe obsessive-compulsive disorder; however, the FDA has not approved for advertising it as effective and safe in treating children <10 years of age.

Clomipramine Hydrochloride in the Treatment of Attention-Deficit/Hyperactivity Disorder

Garfinkel et al. (1983) compared the clinical efficacy of methylphenidate, DMI, and clomipramine in a double-blind, placebo-controlled, crossover study of 12 males (mean age, 7.3 years; range, 5.9 to 11.6 years) diagnosed with ADD who required day hospital or inpatient treatment for severe impulsiveness, attention deficit, and aggression. The mean dose of clomipramine was 85 mg/day and did not exceed 100 mg or 3.5 mg/kg/day for any subject. Methylphenidate was significantly better than the other three conditions in improving overall classroom functioning as rated on the Conners Scale by teachers ($P < .005$) and program child care workers ($P < .001$). Clomipramine, however, was significantly better than DMI in reducing scores reflecting aggressivity, impulsivity, and depressive/affective symptoms. Based on these data, clomipramine would merit further study in treating children and adolescents with ADHD who do not respond satisfactorily to stimulant medication.

Clomipramine Hydrochloride in the Treatment of Autistic Disorder

Gordon et al. (1993) conducted a double-blind comparison of clomipramine, DMI, and placebo in 30 subjects (20 males and 10 females; age range, 6 to 23 years; mean, 10.4 ± 4.11 years) diagnosed with autistic disorder to assess the efficacy of clomipramine in treating obsessive-compulsive and stereotyped motor behaviors. During the initial 2-week, single-blind, placebo washout period, two patients were dropped, one because of positive response and the other because of a refusal to take pills. Fourteen subjects were randomly assigned to a 10-week, double-blind, crossover comparison of clomipramine and placebo, and the other 14 subjects were randomly assigned to a similar comparison of clomipramine and DMI. Two patients were dropped from each group—a 23-year-old man on placebo because of violent outbursts, a 7-year-old girl on clomipramine secondary to a grand mal seizure, and two others for extraneous reasons. The 12 patients in the clomipramine/placebo comparison group showed significantly reduced autistic behaviors ($P = .0001$), anger/uncooperativeness ($P = .0001$), hyperactivity ($P = .001$), but not speech deviance ($P = .27$) in week-5 ratings on the 14-item Autism Relevant Subscale of the Children's Psychiatric Rating Scale (CPRS) while receiving clomipramine. These subjects also had a significant improvement in obsessive-compulsive symptoms ($P = .001$) and overall improvement on the Efficacy Index of the Clinical Global Impressions Scale ($P = .0001$) during the period on the active drug.

The 12 patients in the clomipramine/DMI comparison group improved significantly more during the period on clomipramine than during the period on DMI on week-5 ratings on the Autism Relevant Subscale of the CPRS ($P = .0003$) and anger/uncooperativeness ($P = .008$). The two drugs were not significantly different on the hyperactivity factor, but both were better than placebo; clomipramine showed a trend toward improvement on the speech factor compared with DMI ($P = .08$). Obsessive-compulsive symptoms improved significantly more with clomipramine ($P = .001$), and clomipramine was superior to DMI on the Efficacy Index of the Clinical Global Impressions Scale ($P = .005$). The authors noted that self-injurious behaviors (SIB) such as hitting, kicking, biting, and pinching, which were present in four patients who had not responded to intensive behavioral and drug interventions in two cases, improved significantly in all four subjects when they were receiving clomipramine. Untoward effects of clomipramine were usually minor, and they were not significantly different from placebo or DMI. However, dosage of clomipramine was reduced in one patient because of prolongation of QTc interval to 450 msec and in another because of severe tachycardia (Gordon et al., 1993).

Five patients who continued to be maintained on clomipramine underwent a double-blind placebo substitution for 8 weeks between months 5 and 12 of maintenance therapy. Four (80%) of the five worsened during the period on placebo but regained former clinical improvement when clomipramine was reinstated (Gordon et al., 1993).

Clomipramine Hydrochloride in the Treatment of Enuresis

Dugas et al. (1980) administered clomipramine to 10 enuretic children. A therapeutic effect was observed at plasma clomipramine concentrations of 20 to 60 ng/mL, whereas lower and higher levels were associated with lack of therapeutic efficacy or untoward effects. In a later report, the sample was increased to 31 enuretic children (Morselli et al., 1983). Of the 21 who had good therapeutic outcomes, 16 (76%) had plasma steady-state clomipramine concentrations >15 ng/mL, whereas only 3 of the 10 nonresponders had such high plasma levels. The plasma level differences between the responders and the nonresponders were significant ($P < .05$).

Clomipramine Hydrochloride in the Treatment of Depressive Symptoms

Dugas et al. (1980) treated 1 boy, 8.5 years old, and 25 adolescents, 13 to 19 years old, who had significant depressive symptomatology with clomipramine. Clomipramine doses ranged from 0.24 to 2.93 mg/kg/day. Sixteen patients received other psychoactive medication simultaneously. Twelve of the 26 patients responded positively. Final diagnoses of these patients were school phobia (3), anorexia nervosa (6), manic-depressive psychosis (1), depression (5), and depressive reactions in behavior disorders or borderline personalities (11). Two patients had no therapeutic response, 1 had a minimal response, 11 had moderate improvement, 3 had "good" results, and 9 had excellent results. The patients diagnosed with anorexia responded least favorably; only two had a good response, whereas four of the five diagnosed with depression had excellent responses. Similar plasma levels of clomipramine were present in both responders and nonresponders; however, nonresponders had proportionally higher levels of desmethylclomipramine.

Clomipramine Hydrochloride in the Treatment of School Phobia (Separation Anxiety)

Berney et al. (1981) treated 52 children diagnosed with school refusal, which consisted of a neurotic disorder with a marked reluctance to attend school for at least 4 weeks' duration and was frequently associated with depressive features. The study was double blind and placebo controlled and lasted for 12 weeks. Forty-six patients, aged 9 to 14 years, completed the study; 19 were on placebo and 27 were on clomipramine. The total daily dosage of clomipramine was titrated slowly to 40 mg/day for 9- and 10-year-olds; 50 mg/day for 11- and 12-year-olds; and 75 mg/day for 13- and 14-year-olds. There was no evidence that clomipramine was superior to placebo in reducing separation anxiety and neurotic behavior or being specific for depression. The authors, however, noted that they used proportionally lower doses of clomipramine than the doses used in studies reporting its efficacy in treating school phobia/separation anxiety.

References

Abilify [package insert]. Tokyo, Japan: Otsuka Pharmaceutical Co, Ltd; 2012.

Adler L, Angrist B, Peselow E, et al. A controlled assessment of propranolol in the treatment of neuroleptic-induced akathisia. *Br J Psychiatry*. 1986;149: 42–45.

Adler LA, Rotrosen J, Edson R, et al. Vitamin E treatment of tardive dyskinesia. *Arch Gen Psychiatry*. 1999;56:836–841.

Alaghband-Rad J, Hakimshooshtary M. A randomized controlled clinical trial of Citalopram versus Fluoxetine in children and adolescents with obsessive-compulsive disorder (OCD). *Eur Child Adolesc Psychiatry*. 2009;18(3):131–135.

Alderman J, Wolkow R, Chung M, et al. Sertraline treatment of children and adolescents with obsessive-compulsive disorder or depression: pharmacokinetics, tolerability, and efficacy. *J Am Acad Child Adolesc Psychiatry*. 1998;37:386–394.

Alderman J, Wolkow R, Fogel I. Drug concentration monitoring with tolerability and efficacy assessments during open-label sertraline treatment of children and adolescents. *J Child Adolesc Psychopharmacol*. 2006;16(1–2):117–129.

Alfaro CL, Wudarsky M, Nicolson R, et al. Correlation of antipsychotic and prolactin concentration in children and adolescents acutely treated with haloperidol, clozapine, or olanzapine. *J Child Adolesc Psychopharmacol*. 2002;12:83–91.

Allen RP, Safer D, Covi L. Effects of psychostimulants on aggression. *J Nerv Ment Dis*. 1975;160:138–145.

Altamura AC, Montgomery SA, Wernicke JF. The evidence for 20 mg a day of fluoxetine as the optimal dose in the treatment of depression. *Br J Psychiatry*. 1988;153(suppl 3):109–112.

Althaus M, Vink HJF, Minderaa RB, et al. Lack of effect of clonidine on stuttering in children. *Am J Psychiatry*. 1995;152:1087–1089.

Alvir JMJ, Lieberman JA, Safferman AZ, et al. Clozapine-induced agranulocytosis: incidence and risk factors in the United States. *N Engl J Med*. 1993;329:162–167.

AMA. Informed consent. The American Medical Association; 2012. http://www.ama-assn.org/ama/pub/physician-resources/legal-topics/patient-physician-relationship-topics/informed-consent.page? Accessed March 2, 2013.

Aman MG, Arnold LE, McDougle CJ, et al. Acute and long-term safety and tolerability of risperidone in children with autism. *J Child Adolesc Psychopharmacol.* 2005;15:869–884.

Aman MG, Findling RL, Derivan A, et al. Risperidone versus placebo for severe conduct disorder in children with mental retardation. (Abstract, 40th Annual NCDEU meeting). *J Child Adolesc Psychopharmacol.* 2000;10:253.

Aman MG, Singh NN. Preface. In: Aman MG, Singh NN, eds. *Psychopharmacology of the Developmental Disabilities.* New York, NY: Springer-Verlag; 1988:v–ix.

Ambrosini PJ, Bianchi MD, Rabinovich H, et al. Antidepressant treatments in children and adolescents: I, affective disorders. *J Am Acad Child Adolesc Psychiatry.* 1993;32:1–6.

Ambrosini PJ, Sheikh RM. Increased plasma valproate concentrations when coadministered with guanfacine. *J Child Adolesc Psychopharmacol.* 1998;8:143–147.

Ambrosini PJ, Wagner KD, Biederman J, et al. Multicenter open-label sertraline study in adolescent outpatients with major depression. *J Am Acad Child Adolesc Psychiatry.* 1999;38:566–572.

American Academy of Child and Adolescent Psychiatry. Desipramine and sudden death. Ad hoc committee on DMI [desipramine] and sudden death (J. Biederman, chair). Washington, DC; 1992 Member Forum, 1992 AACAP Program, p. 8.

American Academy of Child and Adolescent Psychiatry. Rating scales. The American Academy of Child and Adolescent Psychiatry website; 2010. http://www.aacap.org/cs/clinical_care_quality_improvement/rating_scales. Accessed March 2, 2013.

American Diabetes Association and American Psychiatric Association. Consensus development conference on antipsychotic drugs and obesity and diabetes. *Diabetes Care.* 2004;27:596–601.

American Medical Association. *Drug Evaluations.* 6th ed. Chicago, IL: American Medical Association; 1986.

American Medical Association. *Drug Evaluations Annual 1994.* Chicago, IL: American Medical Association; 1993.

American Psychiatric Association. *Diagnostic and Statistical Manual of Mental Disorders.* 2nd ed. (DSM-II). Washington, DC: American Psychiatric Association; 1968.

American Psychiatric Association. *Diagnostic and Statistical Manual of Mental Disorders.* 3rd ed. (DSM-III). Washington, DC: American Psychiatric Association; 1980a.

American Psychiatric Association. *Diagnostic and Statistical Manual of Mental Disorders.* 3rd ed. rev. (DSM-III-R). Washington, DC: American Psychiatric Association; 1987.

American Psychiatric Association. *Diagnostic and Statistical Manual of Mental Disorders.* 4th ed. (DSM-IV). Washington, DC: American Psychiatric Association; 1994.

American Psychiatric Association. *Diagnostic and Statistical Manual of Mental Disorders.* 4th ed. Text Revision (DSM-IV-TR). Washington, DC: American Psychiatric Association; 2000.

American Psychiatric Association. *Tardive Dyskinesia: Task Force Report 18.* Washington, DC: American Psychiatric Association; 1980b.

American Psychiatric Association. Task Force on Tardive Dyskinesia. *Tardive Dyskinesia: A Task Force Report of the American Psychiatric Association.* Washington, DC: American Psychiatric Association; 1992.

Amery B, Minichiello MD, Brown GL. Aggression in hyperactive boys: response to d-amphetamine. *J Am Acad Child Psychiatry.* 1984;23:291–294.

Amitai Y, Frischer H. Excess fatality from desipramine in children and adolescents. *J Am Acad Child Adolesc Psychiatry.* 2006;45:54–60.

Anderson LT, Campbell M, Grega DM, et al. Haloperidol in the treatment of infantile autism: effects on learning and behavioral symptoms. *Am J Psychiatry*. 1984;141:1195–1202.

Apter A, Lipschitz A, Fong R, et al. Evaluation of suicidal thoughts and behaviors in children and adolescents taking paroxetine. *J Child Adolesc Psychopharmacol*. 2006;16(1–2):77–90.

Apter A, Ratzone G, King RA, et al. Fluvoxamine open-label treatment of adolescent inpatients with obsessive-compulsive disorder or depression. *J Am Acad Child Adolesc Psychiatry*. 1994;33:342–348.

Armenteros JL, Whitaker AH, Welilson M, et al. Risperidone in adolescents with schizophrenia: an open pilot study. *J Am Acad Child Adolesc Psychiatry*. 1997;36:694–700.

Arnold LE, Huestis RD, Smeltzer DJ, et al. Levoamphetamine vs dextroamphetamine in minimal brain dysfunction. *Arch Gen Psychiatry*. 1976;33:292–301.

Arnold LE, Lindsay RL, Conners K, et al. A double-blind, placebo-controlled withdrawal trial of dexmethylphenidate hydrochloride in children with attention deficit hyperactivity disorder. *J Child Adolesc Psychopharmacol*. 2004;14:542–554.

Arnsten AF, Scahill L, Findling RL. Alpha-2 adrenoreceptors agonists for the treatment of attention-deficit/hyperactivity disorder: emerging concepts from new data. *J Child Adolesc Psychopharmacol*. 2007;17(4):393–406.

Atomoxetine [package insert]. Indianapolis, IN: Eli Lilly and Company; 2012.

Axelson DA, Perel JM, Birmaher B, et al. Sertraline pharmacokinetics and dynamics in adolescents. *J Am Acad Child Adolesc Psychiatry*. 2002;41:1037–1044.

Ayd FJ Jr. *Lexicon of Psychiatry, Neurology and the Neurosciences*. Baltimore, MD: Lippincott Williams & Wilkins; 1995.

Ayd FJ Jr. *Lexicon of Psychiatry, Neurology, and the Neurosciences*. 2nd ed. Baltimore, MD: Lippincott Williams & Wilkins; 2000.

Ayd FJ Jr. Social issues: misuse and abuse. In: Benzodiazepines 1980: current update. *Psychosomatics*. 1980;21(suppl):21–25.

Baldessarini RJ. Drugs and the treatment of psychiatric disorders. In: Gilman AG, Rall TW, Nies AS, et al, eds. *Goodman and Gilman's The Pharmacological Basis of Therapeutics*. 8th ed. New York, NY: Pergamon Press; 1990:383–435.

Baldessarini RJ, Stephens JH. Clinical pharmacology and toxicology of lithium salts. *Arch Gen Psychiatry*. 1970;22:72–77.

Ballenger JC, Carek DJ, Steele JJ, et al. Three cases of panic disorder with agoraphobia in children. *Am J Psychiatry*. 1989;146:922–924.

Balogh S, Hendricks SE, Kang J. Treatment of fluoxetine-induced anorgasmia with amantadine. *J Clin Psych*. 1992;53(6):212–213.

Ban TA, ed. *An Oral History of Neuropsychopharmacology: The First Fifty Years, Peer Interviews*. Brentwood, CA: ACNP; 2011.

Bangs ME, Petti TA, Janus M-D. Fluoxetine-induced memory impairment in an adolescent. *J Am Acad Child Adolesc Psychiatry*. 1994;33:1303–1306.

Bangs ME, Tauscher-Wisniewski S, Polzer J, et al. Meta-analysis of suicide-related behavior events in patients treated with atomoxetine. *J Am Acad Child Adolesc Psychiatry*. 2008;47(2):209–218.

Barrickman L, Noyes R, Kuperman S, et al. Treatment of ADHD with fluoxetine: a preliminary trial. *J Am Acad Child Adolesc Psychiatry*. 1991;30:762–767.

Barrickman LL, Perry PJ, Allen AJ, et al. Bupropion versus methylphenidate in the treatment of attention-deficit hyperactivity disorder. *J Am Acad Child Adolesc Psychiatry*. 1995;34:649–657.

Barzman DH, DelBello MP, Adler CM, et al. The efficacy and tolerability of quetiapine versus divalproex for the treatment of impulsivity and reactive aggression in adolescents with co-occurring bipolar disorder and disruptive behavior disorder. *J Child Adolesc Psychopharmacol*. 2006;16(6):665–670.

Barzman DH, DelBello MP, Kowatch RA, et al. Adjunctive topiramate in hospitalized children and adolescents with bipolar disorders. *J Child Adolesc Psychopharmacol.* 2005;15(6):931–937.

Belsito KM. Lamotrigine therapy for autistic disorder: a randomized, double-blind, placebo-controlled trial. *J Autism Dev Disord.* 2001;31(2):175–181.

Benedek EP, Ash P, Scott CL, eds. *Principles and Practice of Child and Adolescent Forensic Mental Health.* Washington, DC: American Psychiatric Press incorporated; 2010.

Benfield P, Heel RC, Lewis SP. Fluoxetine: a review of its pharmacodynamic and pharmacokinetic properties, and therapeutic efficacy in depressive illness. *Drugs.* 1986;32:481–508.

Berard R, Fong R, Carpenter DJ, et al. An international, multicenter, placebo-controlled trial of paroxetine in adolescents with major depressive disorder. *J Child Adolesc Psychopharmacol.* 2006;16:59–75.

Berg I, Hullin R, Allsopp M, et al. Bipolar manic-depressive psychosis in early adolescence, a case report. *Br J Psychiatry.* 1974;125:416–417.

Bergstrom RF, Lemberger L, Farid NA, et al. Clinical pharmacology and pharmacokinetics of fluoxetine: a review. *Br J Psychiatry.* 1988;153(suppl 3):47–50.

Berney T, Kolvin I, Bhate SR, et al. School phobia: a therapeutic trial with clomipramine and short-term outcome. *Br J Psychiatry.* 1981;138:110–118.

Bernstein GA, Borchardt CM, Perwien AR. Imipramine plus cognitive-behavioral therapy in the treatment of school refusal. *J Am Acad Child Adolesc Psychiatry.* 2000;39:276–283.

Bernstein GA, Carroll ME, Crosby RD, et al. Caffeine effects on learning, performance, and anxiety in normal school-age children. *J Am Acad Child Adolesc Psychiatry.* 1994;33:407–415.

Bernstein GA, Garfinkel BD, Borchardt CM. Comparative studies of pharmacotherapy for school refusal. *J Am Acad Child Adolesc Psychiatry.* 1990;29(5):773–778.

Bevan P, Cools AR, Archer T. *Behavioural Pharmacology of 5-HT.* Hillsdale, NJ: Lawrence Erlbaum; 1989.

Bezchlibnyk-Butler KZ, Virani AS, eds. *Clinical Handbook of Psychotropic Drugs for Children and Adolescents.* Cambridge, MA: Hogrefe & Huber Publishers; 2004.

Biederman J, Baldessarini RJ, Goldblatt A, et al. A naturalistic study of 24-hour electrocardiographic recordings and echocardiographic findings in children and adolescents treated with desipramine. *J Am Acad Child Adolesc Psychiatry.* 1993;32:805–813.

Biederman J, Gastfriend DR, Jellinek MS. Desipramine in the treatment of children with attention deficit disorder. *J Clin Psychopharmacol.* 1986;6:359–363.

Biederman J, Baldessarini RJ, Wright V. A double-blind placebo controlled study of desipramine in the treatment of ADD: I, efficacy. *J Am Acad Child Adolesc Psychiatry.* 1989a;28:777–784.

Biederman J, Baldessarini RJ, Wright V, et al. A double-blind placebo controlled study of desipramine in the treatment of ADD: II, serum drug levels and cardiovascular findings. *J Am Acad Child Adolesc Psychiatry.* 1989b;28:903–911.

Biederman J, Joshi G, Mick E, et al. A prospective open-label trial of lamotrigine monotherapy in children and adolescents with bipolar disorder. *CNS Neurosci Ther.* 2010;16(2):91–102.

Biederman J, Lopez FA, Boellner SW, et al. A randomized, double-blind, placebo-controlled, parallel-group study of SLI381 (Adderall XR) in children with attention-deficit/hyperactivity disorder. *Pediatrics.* 2002;110:258–266.

Biederman J, Mick E, Hammerness P, et al. Open-label, 8 week trial of olanzapine and risperidone for the treatment of bipolar disorder in preschool-age children. *Biol Psychiatry.* 2005a;58(7):589–594.

Biederman J, Mick E, Wozniak J, et al. An open-label trial of risperidone in children and adolescents with bipolar disorder. *J Child Adolesc Psychopharmacol.* 2005b;15:311–317.

Biederman J, Monuteaux M, Spencer T, et al. Stimulant therapy and risk for subsequent substance use disorders in male adults with ADHD: a naturalistic controlled 10-year follow-up study. *Am J Psychiatry.* 2008;165:597–603.

Birmaher B, Axelson DA, Monk K, et al. Fluoxetine for the treatment of childhood anxiety disorders. *J Am Acad Child Adolesc Psychiatry.* 2003;42:415–423.

Birmaher B, Baker R, Kapur S, et al. Clozapine for the treatment of adolescents with schizophrenia. *J Am Acad Child Adolesc Psychiatry.* 1992;31:160–164.

Birmaher B, Greenhill LL, Cooper TB, et al. Sustained release methylphenidate: pharmacokinetic studies in ADDH males. *J Am Acad Child Adolesc Psychiatry.* 1989;28:768–772.

Birmaher B, Quintana H, Greenhill LL. Methylphenidate treatment of hyperactive autistic children. *J Am Acad Child Adolesc Psychiatry.* 1988;27:248–251.

Birmaher B, Waterman GS, Ryan N, et al. Fluoxetine for childhood anxiety disorders. *J Am Acad Child Adolesc Psychiatry.* 1994;33:993–999.

Birmaher B, Waterman GS, Ryan ND, et al. Randomized, controlled trial of amitriptyline versus placebo for adolescents with "treatment resistant" major depression. *J Am Acad Child Adolesc Psychiatry.* 1998;37:527–535.

Black B, Uhde TW. Treatment of elective mutism with fluoxetine: a double-blind, placebo-controlled study. *J Am Acad Child Adolesc Psychiatry.* 1994;33: 1000–1006.

Blader JC, Schooler NR, Jensen PS, et al. Adjunctive divalproex versus placebo for children with ADHD and aggression refractory to stimulant monotherapy. *Am J Psychiatry.* 2009;166(12):1392–1401.

Blanz B, Schmidt MH. Clozapine for schizophrenia [letter]. *J Am Acad Child Adolesc Psychiatry.* 1993;32:223–224.

Bonate PL, Howard DR. *Pharmacokinetics in Drug Development: Clinical Study Design and Analysis.* Vol 1. (Google eBook) Springer; December 5, 2005.

Borison RL, Pathiraja AP, Diamond BI, et al. Risperidone: clinical safety and efficacy in schizophrenia. *Psychopharmacol Bull.* 1992;28:213–218.

Boulos C, Kutcher S, Gardner D, et al. An open naturalistic trial of fluoxetine in adolescents and young adults with treatment-resistant major depression. *J Child Adolesc Psychopharmacol.* 1992;2:103–111.

Boulos C, Kutcher S, Marton P, et al. Response to desipramine treatment in adolescent major depression. *Psychopharmacol Bull.* 1991;27:59–65.

Bowers R, Weston C, Jackson J. Child and adolescent affective disorders and their treatment. In: Klykylo WM, Kay J, eds. *Clinical Child Psychiatry.* 3rd ed. Pennsylvania, PA: John Wiley & Sons Inc; 2012.

Bradley C. The behavior of children receiving Benzedrine. *Am J Psychiatry.* 1937;94:577–585.

Braña-Berríos M, Lam K. In discussion of: Coffey B. Dysphoria associated with neuroleptic withdrawal in an adolescent with Tourette's disorder. *J Child Adolesc Psychopharm.* 2011;21(4):371–374.

Breitner C. An approach to the treatment of juvenile delinquency. *Ariz Med.* 1962;19:82–87.

Brent D, Emslie G, Clarke G, et al. Switching to another SSRI or to venlafaxine with or without cognitive behavioral therapy for adolescents with SSRI-resistant depression: the TORDIA randomized controlled trial. *JAMA.* 2008;299(8):901–913.

Brown S-LB, van Praag HM, eds. *The Role of Serotonin in Psychiatric Disorders.* New York, NY: Brunner/Mazel; 1991.

Bruun R. TSA medical update: treatment with clonidine. *Tourette Syndrome Association Newsletter.* Spring 1983.

Buitelaar JK, van der Gaag RJ, Swaab-Barneveld H, et al. A placebo-controlled comparison of methylphenidate and pindol_ol in ADHD. In: American Academy of Child and Adolescent Psychiatry: Scientific Proceedings of the 41st Annual Meeting; October 25–30, 1994; New York, NY. New Research NR-6. 1994a;X:43.

Buitelaar JK, van der Gaag RJ, Swaab-Barneveld H, et al. Side effects of pindolol, a beta-blocker, in ADHD. In: American Academy of Child and Adolescent Psychiatry: Scientific Proceedings of the 41st Annual Meeting; October 25–30, 1994; New York, NY. New Research NR-7. 1994b;X:43.

Buitelaar JK, van der Gaag RJ, van der Hoeven J. Buspirone in the management of anxiety and irritability in children with pervasive developmental disorders: results of an open-label study. *J Clin Psychiatry*. 1998;59:56–59.

Burke P, Puig-Antich J. Psychobiology of childhood depression. In: Lewis M, Miller SM, eds. *Handbook of Developmental Psychopathology*. New York, NY: Plenum Press; 1990:327–339.

Burke RE, Fahn S, Jankovic J, et al. Tardive dystonia: late-onset and persistent dystonia caused by antipsychotic drugs. *Neurology*. 1982;32:1335–1346.

Cameron OG, Thyer BA. Treatment of pavor nocturnus with alprazolam. *J Clin Psychiatry*. 1985;46:504.

Campbell M, Adams PB, Small AM, et al. Lithium in hospitalized aggressive children with conduct disorder: a double-blind and placebo-controlled study. *J Am Acad Child Adolesc Psychiatry*. 1995;34:445–453.

Campbell M, Anderson LT, Small AM, et al. Naltrexone in autistic children: a double-blind and placebo-controlled study. *Psychopharmacol Bull*. 1990; 26:130–135.

Campbell M, Anderson LT, Small AM, et al. Naltrexone in autistic children: behavioral symptoms and attentional learning. *J Am Acad Child Adolesc Psychiatry*. 1993; 32:1283–1291.

Campbell M, Green WH, Deutsch SI. *Child and Adolescent Psychopharmacology*. Beverly Hills, CA: SAGE; 1985.

Campbell M, Overall JE, Small AM, et al. Naltrexone in autistic children: an acute open dose range tolerance trial. *J Am Acad Child Adolesc Psychiatry*. 1989;28:200–206.

Campbell M, Perry R, Green WH. The use of lithium in children and adolescents. *Psychosomatics*. 1984a;25:95–106.

Campbell M, Silva RR, Kafantars V, et al. Predictors of side effects associated with lithium administration in children. *Psychopharmacol Bull*. 1991;27(3):373–380.

Campbell M, Small AM, Green WH, et al. Behavioral efficacy of haloperidol and lithium carbonate: a comparison in hospitalized aggressive children with conduct disorder. *Arch Gen Psychiatry*. 1984b;41:650–656.

Cantwell DP, Swanson J, Connor DF. Case study: adverse response to clonidine. *J Am Acad Child Adolesc Psychiatry*. 1997;36:539–544.

Carandang CG, Maxwell DJ, Robbins D. Lamotrigine in adolescent mood disorders. *J Am Acad Child Adolesc Psychiatry*. 2003;42(7):750–751.

Carlson JS, Kratochwill TR, Johnston HF. Sertraline treatment of 5 children diagnosed with selective mutism: a single-case research trial. *J Child Adolesc Psychopharmacol*. 1999;9:293–306.

Casat CD, Pleasants DZ, Schroeder DH, et al. Bupropion in children with attention deficit disorder. *Psychopharmacol Bull*. 1989;25:198–201.

Castellanos FX, Giedd JN, Elia J, et al. Controlled stimulant treatment of ADHD and comorbid Tourette's syndrome: efficacy of stimulant and dose. *J Am Acad Child Adolesc Psychiatry*. 1997;36:589–596.

Chakos MH, Lieberman JA, Alvil J, et al. Caudate nuclei volumes in schizophrenic patients treated with typical antipsychotics or clozapine. *Lancet*. 1995;345(8947): 456–457.

Chang K, Saxena K, Howe M. An open-label study of lamotrigine adjunct or monotherapy for the treatment of adolescents with bipolar depression. *J Am Acad Child Adolesc Psychiatry*. 2006;45(3):298–304.

Chappell PB, Riddle MA, Scahill L, et al. Guanfacine treatment of comorbid attention deficit hyperactivity disorder and Tourette's syndrome: preliminary clinical experience. *J Am Acad Child Adolesc Psychiatry*. 1995;34:1140–1146.

Charach A, Figueroa M, Chen S, et al. Stimulant treatment over 5 years: effects on growth. *J Am Acad Child Adolesc Psychiatry*. 2006;45:415–421.

Chatoor I, Wells KC, Conners CK, et al. The effects of nocturnally administered stimulant medication on EEG sleep and behavior in hyperactive children. *J Am Acad Child Psychiatry*. 1983;22:337–342.

Chouinard G, Jones B, Remington G, et al. A Canadian multicenter placebo-controlled study of fixed doses of risperidone and haloperidol in the treatment of chronic schizophrenic patients. *J Clin Psychopharmacol*. 1993;13:25–40.

Cioli V, Corradino C, Piccinelli D, et al. A comparative pharmacological study of trazodone, etoperidone, and 1-(m-chlorophenyl)piperazine. *Pharmacol Res Commun*. 1984;16:85–100.

Ciraulo DA, Shader RI, Greenblatt DJ, et al, eds. *Drug Interactions in Psychiatry*. Baltimore, MD: Williams & Wilkins; 1989.

Clark DB, Birmaher B, Axelson D, et al. Fluoxetine for the treatment of childhood anxiety disorders: open-label, long-term extension to a controlled trial. *J Am Acad Child Adolesc Psychiatry*. 2005;44:1263–1270.

Clarke G, Dickerson J, Gullion CM, et al. Trends in youth antidepressant dispensing and refill limits, 2000 through 2009. *J Child Adolesc Psychopharmacol*. 2012;22(1):11–20.

Clay TH, Gualtieri CT, Evans RW, et al. Clinical and neuropsychological effects of the novel antidepressant bupropion. *Psychopharmacol Bull*. 1988;24:143–148.

Coccaro EF, Murphy DL, eds. *Serotonin in Psychiatric Disorders*. Washington, DC: American Psychiatric Press; 1990.

Coffey B, Shader RI, Greenblatt DJ. Pharmacokinetics of benzodiazepines and psychostimulants in children. *J Clin Psychopharmacol*. 1983;3:217–225.

Coffey BJ. Anxiolytics for children and adolescents: traditional and new drugs. *J Child Adolesc Psychopharmacol*. 1990;1:57–83.

Cohen DJ, Detlor J, Young JG, et al. Clonidine ameliorates Gilles de la Tourette syndrome. *Arch Gen Psychiatry*. 1980;37:1350–1357.

Cohen JA, Mannarino AP, Perel JM, et al. A pilot randomized controlled trial of combined trauma-focused CBT and sertraline for childhood PTSD symptoms. *J Am Acad Child Adolesc Psychiatry*. 2007;46(7):811–819.

Comings DE. *Tourette Syndrome and Human Behavior*. Duarte, CA: Hope Press; 1990.

Comings DE, Comings BG. Tourette's syndrome and attention deficit disorder with hyperactivity: are they genetically related? *J Am Acad Child Psychiatry*. 1984;23:138–146.

Conners CK. Recent drug studies with hyperkinetic children. *J Learn Disabil*. 1971;4:476–483.

Conners CK, Casat CD, Gualtieri CT, et al. Bupropion hydrochloride in attention deficit disorder with hyperactivity. *J Am Acad Child Adolesc Psychiatry*. 1996;34:1314–1321.

Conners CK, Kramer R, Rothschild GH, et al. Treatment of young delinquent boys with diphenylhydantoin sodium and methylphenidate. *Arch Gen Psychiatry*. 1971;24:156–160.

Connor DF, Fletcher KE, Swanson JM. A meta-analysis of clonidine for symptoms of attention-deficit hyperactivity disorder. *J Am Acad Child Adolesc Psychiatry*. 1999;38:1551–1559.

Cooper GL. The safety of fluoxetine: an update. *Br J Psychiatry*. 1988;153(suppl 3):77–86.

Cooper TB, Bergner PE, Simpson GM. The 24-hour lithium level as a prognosticator of dosage requirements. *Am J Psychiatry*. 1973;130:601–603.

Correll CU. Effect of hyperprolactinemia during development in children and adolescents. *J Clin Psychiatry*. 2008;69(8):e24.

Correll CU, Carlson HE. Endocrine and metabolic adverse effects of psychotropic medications in children and adolescents. *J Am Acad Child Adolesc Psychiatry*. 2006;45:771–791.

Correll CU, Manu P, Olshanskiy V, et al. Cardiometabolic risk of second-generation antipsychotic medications during first-time use in children and adolescents. *JAMA*. 2009;302(16):1765–1773.

Corson P, Nopoulos P, Miller D, et al. Change in basal ganglia volume over 2 years in patients with schizophrenia: typical versus atypical neuroleptics. *Am J Psychiatry*. 1999;156:1200–1204.

Craven C, Margaret M. Carbamazepine treatment of bipolar disorder in an adolescent with cerebral palsy. *J Am Acad Child Adolesc Psychiatry*. 2000;39(6):680–681.

Craven C, Murphy M. Carbamazepine treatment of bipolar disorder in an adolescent with cerebral palsy. *J Am Acad Child Adolesc Psychiatry*. 2000;39(6):680–681.

Crismon ML, Trivedi MJ, Pigott TA, et al. The Texas Medication Algorithm Project: report of the Texas consensus conference panel on medication treatment of major depressive disorder. *J Clin Psychiatry*. 1999;60:142–156.

Croarkin PE, Emslie GJ, Mayes TL. Neuroleptic malignant syndrome associated with atypical antipsychotics in pediatric patients: a review of published cases. *J Clin Psychiatry*. 2008;69(7):1157–1165.

Croonenberghs J, Fegert JM, Findling RL, et al; and the Risperidone Disruptive Behavior Study Group. Risperidone in children with disruptive behavior disorders and subaverage intelligence: a 1-year, open-label study of 504 patients. *J Am Acad Child Adolesc Psychiatry*. 2005;44:64–72.

Cross-Disorder Group of the Psychiatric Genomics Consortium. Identification of risk loci with shared effects on five major psychiatric disorders: a genome-wide analysis. *Lancet*. 2013;381(9875):1371–1379. doi:10.1016/S0140-6736(12)62129-1.

Crumrine PK, Feldman HM, Teodori J, et al. The use of methylphenidate in children with seizures and attention deficit disorder. *Ann Neurol*. 1987;22:441–442.

Cueva JE, Overall JE, Small AM, et al. Carbamazepine in aggressive children with conduct disorder: a double-blind and placebo-controlled study. *J Am Acad Child Adolesc Psychiatry*. 1996;35:480–490.

Cutts KK, Jasper HH. Effect of benzedrine sulfate and phenobarbital on behavior problem children with abnormal electroencephalograms. *Arch Neurol Psychiatry*. 1939;411:1138–1145.

D'Amato G. Chlordiazepoxide in management of school phobia. *Dis Nerv Sys*. 1962;23:292–295.

Davanzo P. Mood stabilizers in hospitalized children with bipolar disorder: a retrospective review. *Psychiatry Clin Neurosci*. 2003;57(3):504–510.

Davari-Ashtiani R, Shahrbabaki ME, Razjouyan K, et al. Buspirone versus methylphenidate in the treatment of attention deficit hyperactivity disorder: a double-blind and randomized trial. *Child Psychiatry Hum Dev*. 2010;41(6):641–648.

Davis KL, Charney D, Coyle JT, et al. eds. *Neuropsychopharmacology: The Fifth Generation of Progress*. Philadelphia, PA: Lippincott Williams & Wilkins; 2002.

Daviss WB, Perel JM, Rudolph GR, et al. Steady-state pharmacokinetics of bupropion SR in juvenile patients. *J Am Acad Child Adolesc Psychiatry*. 2005;44:349–357.

De Jong J, Wauben P, Oolders H. Doxazosine, an alpha1-adrenergic antagonist, has positive effects on posttraumatic stress disorder. Poster presented at: The 25th Annual Meeting of The International Society for Traumatic Stress Studies; November 2008; Chicago, IL. Poster # T-208.

De Sousa A. An open-label pilot study of naltrexone in childhood-onset trichotillomania. *J Child Adolesc Psychopharmacol*. 2008;1:30–33.

Dean AJ, Hendy A, McGuire T. Antidepressants in children and adolescents—changes in utilisation after safety warnings. *Pharmacoepidemiol Drug Saf.* 2007;16(9):1048–1053.

DeGatta MF, Garcia MJ, Acosta A, et al. Monitoring of serum levels of imipramine and desipramine and individuation of dose in enuretic children. *Ther Drug Monit.* 1984;6:438–443.

DelBello MP, Findling RL, Kushner S, et al. A pilot controlled study of topiramate for mania in children and adolescents with bipolar disorder. *J Am Acad Child Adolesc Psychiatry.* 2005;44:539–547.

DelBello MP, Kowatch RA, Adler CM, et al. A double-blind randomized pilot study comparing quetiapine and divalproex for adolescent mania. *J Am Acad Child Adolesc Psychiatry.* 2006;45(3):305–313.

DelBello MP, Kowatch RA, Warner J, et al. Adjunctive topiramate treatment for pediatric bipolar disorder: a retrospective chart review. *J Child Adolesc Psychopharmacol.* 2002;12(4):323–330.

DeLong GR, Aldershof AL. Long-term experience with lithium treatment in childhood: correlation with clinical diagnosis. *J Am Acad Child Adolesc Psychiatry.* 1987;26:389–394.

Denckla MB, Bemporad JR, MacKay MC. Tics following methylphenidate administration: a report of 20 cases. *JAMA.* 1976;235:1349–1351.

Deutsch SI. Rationale for the administration of opiate antagonists in treating infantile autism. *Am J Ment Defic.* 1986;90:631–635.

Devane CL, Nemeroff CB. Clinical pharmacokinetics of quetiapine: an atypical antipsychotic. *Clin Pharmacokinet.* 2001;40:509–522.

DeVeaugh-Geiss MD, Moroz G, Biederman J, et al. Clomipramine hydrochloride in childhood and adolescent obsessive-compulsive disorder—a multicenter trial. *J Am Acad Child Adolesc Psychiatry.* 1992;31:45–49.

Dickstein DP, Towbin KE, Van Der Veen JW J, et al. Randomized double-blind placebo-controlled trial of lithium in youths with severe mood dysregulation. *J Child Adolesc Psychopharmacol.* 2009;19(1):61–73.

Diler RS, Avci A. Selective serotonin reuptake inhibitor discontinuation syndrome in children: six case reports. *Curr Ther Res.* 2002;63(3):188–197.

Dockett S, Perry B. Researching with young children: seeking assent. *Child Indicators Res.* 2011;4(2):231–247.

Donnelly M, Zametkin AJ, Rapoport JL, et al. Treatment of childhood hyperactivity with desipramine: plasma drug concentration, cardiovascular effects, plasma and urinary catecholamine levels, and clinical response. *Clin Pharmacol Ther.* 1986;39:72–81.

Donovan SJ, Stewart JW, Nunes EV, et al. Divalproex treatment for youth with explosive temper and mood lability: a double-blind, placebo-controlled crossover design (Published errata appear in *Am J Psychiatry* 157:1038 and *Am J Psychiatry* 157:1192). *Am J Psychiatry.* 2000;157:818–820.

Donovan SJ, Susser ES, Nunes Stewart JW, et al. Divalproex treatment of disruptive adolescents: a report of 10 cases. *J Clin Psychiatry.* 1997;58:12–15.

Dostal T. Antiaggressive effect of lithium salts in mentally retarded adolescents. In: Annell A-L, ed. *Depressive States in Childhood and Adolescence.* Stockholm, Sweden: Almqvist & Wiksell; 1972:491–498.

Drug Facts and Comparisons. 49th ed. St Louis, MO: Facts and Comparisons; 1995.

Dubovsky SL. Severe nortriptyline intoxication due to change from a generic to a trade preparation. *J Nerv Ment Dis.* 1987;175:115–117.

Duff G. Safety of Seroxat (paroxetine) in children and adolescents under 18 years–contraindication in the treatment of depressive illness. Epinet message from Professor G. Duff, Chairman of Committee on Safety of Medicines. 2003. http://www.mhra.gov.uk/Safetyinformation/Safetywarningsalertsandrecalls/Safetywarningsandmessagesformedicines/CON2015704.

Dugas M, Zarifian E, Leheuzey M-F, et al. Preliminary observations of the significance of monitoring tricyclic antidepressant plasma levels in the pediatric patient. *Ther Drug Monit*. 1980;2:307–314.

Dummit ES III, Klein RG, Tancer NK, et al. Fluoxetine treatment of children with selective mutism: an open trial. *J Am Acad Child Adolesc Psychiatry*. 1996;35:615–621.

Duncan MK. Using psychostimulants to treat behavioral disorders of children and adolescents. *J Child Adolesc Psychopharmacol*. 1990;1:7–20.

DuPaul GJ, Barkley RA, McMurray MB. Response of children with ADHD to methylphenidate: interaction with internalizing symptoms. *J Am Acad Child Adolesc Psychiatry*. 1994;33:894–903.

Effron AS, Freedman AM. The treatment of behavioral disorders in children with benadryl. *J Pediatr*. 1953;42:261–266.

Elia J, Borcherding BG, Rapoport JL, et al. Methylphenidate and dextroamphetamine treatments of hyperactivity: are there true nonresponders? *Psychiatry Res*. 1991;36:141–155.

Elliott GR, Popper CW. Tricyclic antidepressants: the QT interval and other cardiovascular parameters [editorial]. *J Child Adolesc Psychopharmacol*. 1990/1991;1:187–189.

Emslie GJ, Findling RL, Yeung PP, et al. Venlafaxine ER for the treatment of pediatric subjects with depression: results of two placebo-controlled trials. *J Am Acad Child Adolesc Psychiatry*. 2007;46(4):479–488.

Emslie GJ, Heiligenstein JH, Wagner KD, et al. Fluoxetine for acute treatment of depression in children and adolescents: a placebo-controlled, randomized clinical trial. *J Am Acad Child Adolesc Psychiatry*. 2002;41(10):1205–1215.

Emslie GJ, Mayes T, Porta G, et al. Treatment of resistant depression in adolescents (TORDIA): week 24 outcomes. *Am J Psychiatry*. 2010;167(7):782–791.

Emslie GJ, Rush AJ, Weinberg WA, et al. A double-blind, randomized, placebo-controlled trial of fluoxetine in children and adolescents with depression. *Arch Gen Psychiatry*. 1997;54:1031–1037.

Emslie GJ, Ventura D, Korotzer A, et al. Escitalopram in the treatment of adolescent depression: a randomized placebo-controlled multisite trial. *J Am Acad Child Adolesc Psychiatry*. 2009;48:721–729.

Emslie GJ, Wagner KD, Kutcher S, et al. Paroxetine treatment in children and adolescents with major depressive disorder: a randomized, multicenter, double-blind, placebo-controlled trial. *J Am Acad Child Adolesc Psychiatry*. 2006;45(6):709–719.

Esposito S, Prange AJ Jr, Golden RN. The thyroid axis and mood disorders: overview and future prospects. *Psychopharmacol Bull*. 1997;33:205–217.

Evans RW, Clay TH, Gualtieri CT. Carbamazepine in pediatric psychiatry. *J Am Acad Child Adolesc Psychiatry*. 1987;26:2–8.

Fairbanks JM, Pine DS, Tancer NK, et al. Open fluoxetine treatment of mixed anxiety disorders in children and adolescents. *J Child Adolesc Psychopharmacol*. 1997;7:17–29.

Famularo R, Kinscherff R, Fenton T. Propranolol treatment for childhood post-traumatic stress disorder, acute type. *Am J Dis Child*. 1988;142:1244–1247.

Fanapt [package insert]. East Hanover, NJ: Novartis Pharmaceuticals Co; 2012.

Faraone SV, Biederman J, Monuteaux M, et al. Long-term effects of extended-release mixed amphetamine salts treatment of attention-deficit/hyperactivity disorder. *J Child Adolesc Psychopharmacol*. 2005;15:191–202.

Faulkner G, Cohn T, Remington G. Interventions to reduce weight gain in schizophrenia. *Cochrane Database Syst Rev*. 2007;(1):CD005148.

Feeney DJ, Klykylo W. TD from Risperidone? *J Am Acad Child Adolesc Psychiatry*. 1997;(7):867.

Feighner JP, Cohen JB. Analysis of individual symptoms in generalized anxiety: a pooled, multi-study double-blind evaluation of buspirone. *Neuropsychobiology*. 1989;21:124–130.

Feldman HM, Kolman BK, Gonzaga AM. Naltrexone and communication skills in young children with autism. *J Am Acad Child Adolesc Psychiatry*. 1999;38:587–593.

Fenichel RR. Combining methylphenidate and clonidine: the role of post-marketing surveillance. *J Child Adolesc Psychopharmacol*. 1995;5:155–156.

Ferguson HB, Simeon JG. Evaluating drug effects on children's cognitive functioning. *Prog Neuropsychopharmacol Biol Psychiatry*. 1984;8:683–686.

Fernández-Jaén A, Fernández-Mayoralas DM, Calleja Pérez B, et al. Atomoxetine for attention deficit hyperactivity disorder in mental retardation. *Pediatr Neurol*. 2010;43(5):341–347.

Findling R, McNamara N, Stansbrey R, et al. Combination lithium and divalproex sodium in pediatric bipolar symptom restabilization. *J Am Acad Child Adolesc Psychiatry*. 2006a;45(2):142–148.

Findling RL, et al. Venlafaxine in the treatment of children and adolescents with attention-deficit/hyperactivity disorder. Presented at: 160th Annual Meeting of the American Psychiatric Association; May 19–24, 2007a; San Diego, CA.

Findling RL, Frazier TW, Youngstrom EA, et al. Double-blind placebo-controlled trial of divalproex monotherapy in the treatment of symptomatic youth at high risk for developing bipolar disorder. *J Clin Psychiatry*. 2007b;68(5): 781–788.

Findling RL, Greenhill LL, McNamara NK, et al. Venlafaxine in the treatment of children and adolescents with attention-deficit/hyperactivity disorder. *J Child Adolesc Psychopharmacol*. 2007c;17(4):433–445.

Findling RL, Kafantaris V, Pavuluri M, et al. Dosing strategies for lithium monotherapy in children and adolescents with bipolar I disorder. *J Child Adolesc Psychopharmacol*. 2011;21(3):195–205.

Findling RL, Kauffman R, Sallee FR, et al. An open-label study of aripiprazole: pharmacokinetics, tolerability, and effectiveness in children and adolescents with conduct disorder. *J Child Adolesc Psychopharmacol*. 2009;19:431–439.

Findling RL, McNamara NK, Branicky LA. A double-blind pilot study of risperidone in the treatment of conduct disorder. *J Am Acad Child Adolesc Psychiatry*. 2000;39:509–516.

Findling RL, McNamara NK, Gracious BL, et al. Quetiapine in nine youths with autistic disorder. *J Child Adolesc Psychopharmacol*. 2004;14:287–294.

Findling RL, McNamara NK, Youngstrom EA, et al. Double-blind 18-month trial of lithium versus divalproex maintenance treatment in pediatric bipolar disorder. *J Am Acad Child Adolesc Psychiatry*. 2005;44:409–417.

Findling RL, Reed MD, Myers C, et al. Paroxetine pharmacokinetics in depressed children and adolescents. *J Am Acad Child Adolesc Psychiatry*. 1999;38:952–959.

Findling RL, Reed MD, O'Riordan MA, et al. Effectiveness, safety, and pharmacokinetics of quetiapine in aggressive children with conduct disorder. *J Am Acad Child Adolesc Psychiatry*. 2006b;45:792–798.

Finniss DG, Kaptchuk TJ, Miller F, et al. Biological, clinical, and ethical advances of placebo effects. *Lancet*. 2010;375(9715):686–695.

Fish B. Drug therapy in child psychiatry: pharmacological aspects. *Compr Psychiatry*. 1960;1:212–227.

Fish B. The "one child, one drug" myth of stimulants in hyperkinesis. *Arch Gen Psychiatry*. 1971;25:193–203.

Fisher S. *Child Research in Psychopharmacology*. Springfield, IL: Charles C Thomas; 1959.

Fitzpatrick PA, Klorman R, Brumaghim JT, et al. Effects of sustained-release and standard preparations of methylphenidate on attention deficit disorder. *J Am Acad Child Adolesc Psychiatry*. 1992;31:226–234.

Flament MF, Rapoport JL, Berg CJ, et al. Clomipramine treatment of childhood obsessive-compulsive disorder: a double blind controlled study. *Arch Gen Psychiatry*. 1985;42:977–983.

Flament MF, Rapoport JL, Murphy DL, et al. Biochemical changes during clomipramine treatment of childhood obsessive-compulsive disorder. *Arch Gen Psychiatry*. 1987;44:219–225.

Fleischhacker WW, Bergmann KJ, Perovich R, et al. The Hillside Akathisia Scale: a new rating instrument for neuroleptic-induced akathisia. *Psychopharmacol Bull*. 1989;25:222–226.

Ford K, Sankey J, Crisp J. Development of children's assent documents using a child-centered approach. *J Child Health Care*. 2007;11(1):19–28.

Franowicz JS, Arnsten AF. Action of α-2 noradrenergic agonists on spatial working memory and blood pressure in rhesus monkeys appear to be mediated by the same receptor subtype. *Psychopharmacology*. 2002;162:304–312.

Fras I. Trazodone and violence [letter]. *J Am Acad Child Adolesc Psychiatry*. 1987;26:453.

Frazier JA, Biederman J, Jacobs TG, et al. Olanzapine in the treatment of bipolar disorder in juveniles. (Abstract 40th Annual NCDEU meeting). *J Child Adolesc Psychopharmacol*. 2000;10:237–238.

Frazier JA, Gordon CT, McKenna K, et al. An open trial of clozapine in 11 adolescents with child-onset schizophrenia. *J Am Acad Child Adolesc Psychiatry*. 1994;33:658–663.

Frazier JA, Meyer MC, Biederman J, et al. Risperidone treatment for juvenile bipolar disorder: a retrospective chart review. *J Am Acad Child Adolesc Psychiatry*. 1999;38:960–965.

Friedman JM, Polifka JE. *The Effects of Neurologic and Psychiatric Drugs on the Fetus and Nursing Infant*. Baltimore, MD: Johns Hopkins University Press; 1998.

Fritz GK, Rockney RM, Yeung AS. Plasma levels and efficacy of imipramine treatment for enuresis. *J Am Acad Child Adolesc Psychiatry*. 1994;33:60–64.

Gadow KD. *Children on Medication: Vol I, Hyperactivity, Learning Disabilities, and Mental Retardation*. San Diego, CA: College-Hill Press; 1986a.

Gadow KD. *Children on Medication: Vol II, Epilepsy, Emotional Disturbance, and Adolescent Disorders*. San Diego, CA: College-Hill Press; 1986b.

Gadow KD, Nolan EE, Sverd J. Methylphenidate in hyperactive boys with comorbid tic disorder: II, short-term behavioral effects in school settings. *J Am Acad Child Adolesc Psychiatry*. 1992;31:462–471.

Gadow KD, Poling AG. *Pharmacotherapy and Mental Retardation*. Boston, MA: College-Hill Press; 1988.

Gadow KD, Sverd J, Sprafkin J, et al. Efficacy of methylphenidate for attention-deficit hyperactivity disorder in children with tic disorder. *Arch Gen Psychiatry*. 1995;52:444–455.

Gadow KD, Sverd J, Sprafkin J, et al. Long-term methylphenidate therapy in children with comorbid attention-deficit hyperactivity disorder and chronic multiple tic disorder. *Arch Gen Psychiatry*. 1999;56:330–336.

Gammon GD, Brown TE. Fluoxetine and methylphenidate in combination for treatment of attention deficit disorder and comorbid depressive disorder. *J Child Adolesc Psychopharmacol*. 1993;3:1–10.

Garfinkel BD, Wender PH, Sloman L, et al. Tricyclic antidepressant and methylphenidate treatment of attention deficit disorder in children. *J Am Acad Child Psychiatry*. 1983;22:343–348.

Gastfriend DR, Biederman J, Jellinek MS. Desipramine in the treatment of adolescents with attention deficit disorder. *Am J Psychiatry*. 1984;141:906–908.

Geller B. Commentary on unexplained deaths of children on Norpramin. *J Am Acad Child Adolesc Psychiatry*. 1991;30:682–684.

Geller B, Carr LG. Similarities and differences between adult and pediatric major depressive disorders. In: Georgotas A, Cancro R, eds. *Depression and Mania*. New York, NY: Elsevier; 1988:565–580.

Geller B, Cooper TB, Carr LG, et al. Prospective study of scheduled withdrawal from nortriptyline in children and adolescents. *J Clin Psychopharmacol*. 1987a;7:252–254.

Geller B, Cooper TB, Chestnut EC, et al. Child and adolescent nortriptyline single dose kinetics predict steady state plasma levels and suggested dose: preliminary data. *J Clin Psychopharmacol*. 1985;5:154–158.

Geller B, Cooper TB, Chestnut EC, et al. Preliminary data on the relationship between nortriptyline plasma level and response in depressed children. *Am J Psychiatry*. 1986;143:1283–1286.

Geller B, Cooper TB, Graham DL, et al. Double-blind placebo-controlled study of nortriptyline in depressed adolescents using a "fixed plasma level" design. *Psychopharmacol Bull*. 1990;26:85–90.

Geller B, Cooper TB, Graham DL, et al. Pharmacokinetically designed double-blind placebo-controlled study of nortriptyline in 6- to 12-year-olds with major depressive disorder. *J Am Acad Child Adolesc Psychiatry*. 1992;31:34–44.

Geller B, Cooper TB, McCombs HG, et al. Double-blind placebo-controlled study of nortriptyline in depressed children using a "fixed plasma level" design. *Psychopharmacol Bull*. 1989;25:101–108.

Geller B, Cooper TB, Schluchter MD, et al. Child and adolescent nortriptyline single dose pharmacokinetic parameters: final report. *J Clin Psychopharmacol*. 1987b;7:321–323.

Geller B, Cooper TB, Sun K, et al. Double-blind and placebo-controlled study of lithium for adolescent bipolar disorders with secondary substance dependency. *J Am Acad Child Adolesc Psychiatry*. 1998;37:171–178.

Geller B, Fox LW, Fletcher M. Effect of tricyclic antidepressants on switching to mania and on the onset of bipolarity in depressed 6- to 12-year-olds. *J Am Acad Child Adolesc Psychiatry*. 1993;32:43–50.

Geller B, Guttmacher LB, Bleeg M. Coexistence of childhood onset pervasive developmental disorder and attention deficit disorder with hyperactivity. *Am J Psychiatry*. 1981;138:388–389.

Geller B, Luby JL, Joshi P, et al. A randomized controlled trial of risperidone, lithium, or divalproex sodium for initial treatment of bipolar I disorder, manic or mixed phase, in children and adolescents. *Arch Gen Psychiatry*. 2012;69(5):515–528.

Geller D, Donnelly C, Lopez F, et al. Atomoxetine treatment for pediatric patients with attention-deficit/hyperactivity disorder with comorbid anxiety disorder. *J Am Acad Child Adolesc Psychiatry*. 2007;46(9):1119–1127.

Geller DA, Hoog SL, Heiligenstein JH, et al. Fluoxetine treatment for obsessive-compulsive disorder in children and adolescents: a placebo-controlled clinical trial. *J Am Acad Child Adolesc Psychiatry*. 2001;40(7):773–779.

Geller DA, Wagner KD, Emslie G, et al. Paroxetine treatment in children and adolescents with obsessive-compulsive disorder: a randomized, multicenter, double-blind, placebo-controlled trial. *J Am Acad Child Adolesc Psychiatry*. 2004;43:1387–1396.

Geodon [package insert]. New York, NY: Pfizer Inc; 2012.

Gerbino-Rosen G, Roofeh D, Tompkins DA, et al. Hematological adverse events in clozapine-treated children and adolescents. *J Am Acad Child Adolesc Psychiatry*. 2005;44:1024–1031.

Gharabawi GM, Bossie CA, Lasser RA, et al. Abnormal Involuntary Movement Scale (AIMS) and Extrapyramidal Symptom Rating Scale (ESRS): cross-scale comparison in assessing tardive dyskinesia. *Schizophr Res*. 2005;77(2–3):119–128.

Ghaziuddin N, Alessi NE. An open clinical trial of trazodone in aggressive children. *J Child Adolesc Psychopharmacol*. 1992;2:291–297.

Giacino JT, Whyte J, Bagiella E, et al. Placebo-controlled trial of amantadine for severe traumatic brain injury. *N Engl J Med*. 2012;366:819–826.

Gibbons RD, Brown CH, Hur K, et al. Early evidence on the effects of regulators' suicidality warnings on SSRI prescriptions and suicide in children and adolescents. *Am J Psychiatry*. 2007;164:1356–1363.

Gilbert AR, Moore GJ, Keshavan MS, et al. Decrease in thalamic volumes of pediatric patients with obsessive-compulsive disorder who are taking paroxetine. *Arch Gen Psychiatry*. 2000;57:449–456.

Gilbert DL, Batterson JR, Sethuraman G, et al. Tic reduction with risperidone versus pimozide in a randomized, double-blind, crossover trial. *J Am Acad Child Adolesc Psychiatry*. 2004;43:206–214.

Gillberg C, Melander H, von Knorring A-L, et al. Long-term stimulant treatment of children with attention-deficit hyperactivity disorder symptoms. *Arch Gen Psychiatry*. 1997;54:857–864.

Ginsburg GS, Kendall PC, Sakolsky D, et al. Remission after acute treatment in children and adolescents with anxiety disorders: findings from the CAMS. *J Consult Clin Psychol*. 2011;79(6):806–813.

Gittelman-Klein R, Klein D. Controlled imipramine treatment of school phobia. *Arch Gen Psychiatry*. 1971;25:204–207.

Gittelman-Klein R, Klein DF, Katz S, et al. Comparative effects of methylphenidate and thioridazine in hyperkinetic children: I, clinical results. *Arch Gen Psychiatry*. 1976;33:1217–1231.

GlaxoSmithKline [prescribing information]. EL:L50.2003.

Glick BS, Schulman D, Turecki S. Diazepam (Valium) treatment in childhood sleep disorder. *Dis Nerv Sys*. 1971;32:565–566.

Good CR, Feaster CS, Krecko VF. Tolerability of oral loading of divalproex sodium in child psychiatry inpatients. *J Child Adolesc Psychopharmacol*. 2001;11:53–56.

Goodyer I, Dubicka B, Wilkinson P, et al. Selective serotonin reuptake inhibitors (SSRIs) and routine specialist care with and without cognitive behavior therapy in adolescents with major depression: randomised controlled trial. *BMJ*. 2007;335:142–146.

Gordon CT, State RC, Nelson JE, et al. A double-blind comparison of clomipramine, desipramine, and placebo in the treatment of autistic disorder. *Arch Gen Psychiatry*. 1993;50:441–447.

Graae F, Milner J, Rizzotto L, et al. Clonazepam in childhood anxiety disorders. *J Am Acad Child Adolesc Psychiatry*. 1994;33:372–376.

Gray KM, Carpenter MJ, Baker NL, et al. Bupropion SR and contingency management for adolescent smoking cessation. *J Subst Abuse Treat*. 2011;40(1):77–86.

Green WH. Pervasive developmental disorders. In: Kestenbaum CJ, Williams DT, eds. *Handbook of Clinical Assessment of Children and Adolescents*. Vol 1. New York, NY: New York University Press; 1988:469–498.

Green WH. Psychosocial dwarfism: psychological and etiological considerations. In: Lahey BB, Kazdin AE, eds. *Advances in Clinical Child Psychology*. Vol 9. New York, NY: Plenum Press; 1986:245–278.

Green WH. Schizophrenia with childhood onset. In: Kaplan HI, Sadock BJ, eds. *Comprehensive Textbook of Psychiatry*. 5th ed. Baltimore, MD: Williams & Wilkins; 1989:1975–1981.

Green WH. The treatment of attention-deficit hyperactivity disorder with nonstimulant medications. *Child Adolesc Psychiatr Clin N Am*. 1995;4:169–195.

Green WH, Campbell M, Hardesty AS, et al. A comparison of schizophrenic and autistic children. *J Am Acad Child Psychiatry*. 1984;23:399–409.

Green WH, Deutsch SI. Biological studies of schizophrenia with childhood onset. In: Deutsch SI, Weizman A, Weizman R, eds. *Application of Basic Neuroscience to Child Psychiatry*. New York, NY: Plenum Medical Book; 1990:217–229.

Green WH, Deutsch SI, Campbell M, et al. Neuropsychopharmacology of the childhood psychoses: a critical review. In: Morgan DW, ed. *Psychopharmacology:*

Impact on Clinical Psychiatry. St Louis, MO: Ishiyaku EuroAmerica; 1985:139–173.

Green WH, Padron-Gayol M, Hardesty AS, et al. Schizophrenia with childhood onset: a phenomenological study of 38 cases. *J Am Acad Child Adolesc Psychiatry*. 1992;31:968–976.

Greenblatt DJ, Shader RI, Abernethy DR. Current status of benzodiazepines (first of two parts). *N Engl J Med*. 1983;309:354–358.

Greenblatt DJ, Shader RI. *Benzodiazepines in Clinical Practice*. New York, NY: Raven Press; 1974.

Greenhill LL. Attention-deficit hyperactivity disorder in children. In: Garfinkel BD, Carlson GA, Weller EB, eds. *Psychiatric Disorders in Children and Adolescents*. Philadelphia, PA: WB Saunders; 1990:149–182.

Greenhill LL, Pliszka S, Dulcan MK; and the Work Group on Quality Issues. Practice parameters for the use of stimulant medications in the treatment of children, adolescents, and adults. *J Am Acad Child Adolesc Psychiatry*. 2002;41(suppl):26S–49S.

Greenhill LL, Solomon M, Pleak R, et al. Molindone hydrochloride treatment of hospitalized children with conduct disorder. *J Clin Psychiatry*. 1985;46:20–25.

Grizenko N, Vida S. Propranolol treatment of episodic dyscontrol and aggressive behavior in children [letter]. *Can J Psychiatry*. 1988;33:776–778.

Groh C. The psychotropic effect of Tegretol in non-epileptic children, with particular reference to the drug's indications. In: Birkmayer W, ed. *Epileptic Seizures-Behaviour-Pain*. Bern, Germany: Hans Huber Publishers; 1976:259–263.

Gross MD. Imipramine in the treatment of minimal brain dysfunction in children. *Psychosomatics*. 1973;14:283–285.

Gross MD, Wilson WC. *Minimal Brain Dysfunction*. New York, NY: Brunner/Mazel; 1974.

Grothe DR, Calis KA, Jacobsen L, et al. Olanzapine pharmacokinetics in pediatric and adolescent inpatients with childhood-onset schizophrenia. *J Clin Psychopharmacol*. 2000;20:220–225.

Gualtieri CT. *Brain Injury and Mental Retardation: Psychopharmacology and Neuropsychiatry*. Philadelphia, PA: Lippincott Williams and Wilkins; 2002:294.

Gualtieri CT, Golden R, Evans RW, et al. Blood level measurement of psychoactive drugs in pediatric psychiatry. *Ther Drug Monit*. 1984a;6:127–141.

Gualtieri CT, Golden RN, Fahs JJ. New developments in pediatric psychopharmacology. *J Dev Behav Pediatr*. 1983;4:202–209.

Gualtieri CT, Johnson LG. Antidepressant side effects in children and adolescents. *J Child Adolesc Psychopharmacol*. 2006;16(1–2):147–157.

Gualtieri CT, Keenan PA, Chandler M. Clinical and neuropsychological effect on desipramine in children with attention deficit hyperactivity disorder. *J Clin Psychopharmacol*. 1991;11:155–159.

Gualtieri CT, Quade D, Hicks RE, et al. Tardive dyskinesia and other clinical consequences of neuroleptic treatment in children and adolescents. *Am J Psychiatry*. 1984b;141:20–23.

Gualtieri CT, Wafgin W, Kanoy R, et al. Clinical studies of methylphenidate serum levels in children and adults. *J Am Acad Child Psychiatry*. 1982;21:19–26.

Gutgesell H, Atkins D, Barst R, et al; Members, Taubert KA, AHA staff. AHA scientific statement: cardiovascular monitoring of children and adolescents receiving psychotropic drugs. *J Am Acad Child Adolesc Psychiatry*. 1999;38:1047–1050. (Reprinted from *Circulation* 1999;99:979–982.)

Guy W. Dosage Record and Treatment Emergent Symptoms Scale (DOTES). In: *ECDEU Assessment Manual for Psychopharmacology—Revised* [DHEW Publ No ADM 76–338]. Rockville, MD: US Department of Health, Education, and Welfare, Public Health Service, Alcohol, Drug Abuse, and Mental Health

Administration, NIMH Psychopharmacology Research Branch, Division of Extramural Research Programs; 1976a:223–244.

Guy W. *ECDEU assessment manual for psychopharmacology* (NIMH Publ No 76–338). Washington, DC: DHEW, NIMH; 1976b.

Hallowell EM, Ratey JJ. *Delivered from Distraction: Getting the Most Out of Life with Attention Deficit Disorder*. New York, NY: Random House Publishing Group; 2005:253–255.

Hamill PVV, Drizd TA, Johnson CL, et al. NCHS growth charts, 1976. *Monthly Vital Statistics Reports*. 1976;25(suppl 3):1–22. (Health Examination Survey Data, National Center for Health Statistics Publication [HRA] 76–1120.)

Handen BJ, Feldman HM, Lurier A, et al. Efficacy of methylphenidate among preschool children with developmental disabilities and ADHD. *J Am Acad Child Adolesc Psychiatry*. 1999;38:805–812.

Handen BJ, Johnson CR, Lubetsky M. Efficacy of methylphenidate among children with autism and symptoms of attention-deficit hyperactivity disorder. *J Autism Dev Disord*. 2000;30:245–255.

Hanwella R, Senanayake M, de Silva V. Comparative efficacy and acceptability of methylphenidate and atomoxetine in treatment of attention deficit hyperactivity disorder in children and adolescents: a meta-analysis. *BMC Psychiatry*. 2011;11:176.

Harfterkamp M, van de Loo-Neus G, Minderaa RB, et al. A randomized double-blind study of atomoxetine versus placebo for attention-deficit/hyperactivity disorder symptoms in children with autism spectrum disorder. *J Am Acad Child Adolesc Psychiatry*. 2012;51(7):733–741.

Hayes PE, Schulz SC. Beta-blockers in anxiety disorders. *J Affect Disord*. 1987;13:119–130.

Hayes TA, Logan Panitch M, Marker E. Imipramine dosage in children: a comment on "imipramine and electrocardiographic abnormalities in hyperactive children." *Am J Psychiatry*. 1975;132:546–547.

Hellings JA, Weckbaugh M, Nickel EJ, et al. A double-blind, placebo-controlled study of valproate for aggression in youth with pervasive developmental disorders. *J Child Adolesc Psychopharmacol*. 2005;15:682–692.

Hersh CB, Sokol MS, Pfeffer CR. Transient psychosis with fluoxetine [letter]. *J Am Acad Child Adolesc Psychiatry*. 1991;31:851.

Herskowitz J. Developmental neurotoxicology. In: Popper C, ed. *Psychiatric Pharmacosciences of Children and Adolescents*. Washington, DC: American Psychiatric Press; 1987:81–123.

Hollander E, Chaplin W, Soorya L, et al. Divalproex sodium vs. placebo for the treatment of irritability in children and adolescents with autism spectrum disorders. *Neuropsychopharmacology*. 2010;35:990–998.

Hollander E, Phillips A, Chaplin W, et al. A placebo controlled crossover trial of liquid fluoxetine on repetitive behaviors in childhood and adolescent autism. *Neuropsychopharmacology*. 2005;30:582–589.

Hollander E, Soorya L, Wasserman S, et al. Divalproex sodium vs. placebo in the treatment of repetitive behaviours in autism spectrum disorder. *Int J Neuropsychopharmacol*. 2006;9(2):209–213.

Holzer JF. The process of informed consent. *Bull Am Coll Surg*. 1989;74:10–14.

Horrigan JP, Barnhill LJ. Does guanfacine trigger mania in children? [letter]. *J Child Adolesc Psychopharmacol*. 1998;8:149–150.

Horrigan JP, Barnhill LJ. Guanfacine for treatment of attention-deficit hyperactivity disorder in boys. *J Child Adolesc Psychopharmacol*. 1995;5:215–223.

Horrigan JP, Barnhill LJ. Risperidone and explosive aggressive autism. *J Autism Dev Disord*. 1997;27:313–323.

Hosenbocus S, Chahal R. SSRIs and SNRIs: a review of the discontinuation syndrome in children and adolescents. *J Can Acad Child Adolesc Psychiatry*. 2011;20(1):60–67.

Howell C, Larson J, Coffey B. Treatment of bipolar disorder in an adolescent with autistic disorder: a diagnostic and treatment dilemma. *J Child Adolesc Psychopharmacol*. 2011;21(3):283–286.

Huessy HR, Wright AL. The use of imipramine in children's behavior disorders. *Acta Paedopsychiatr*. 1970;37:194–199.

Hughes CW, Emslie GJ, Crismon ML, et al. The Texas Children's Medication Algorithm Project: report of the Texas Consensus Conference Panel on Medication Treatment of Childhood Major Depressive Disorder. *J Am Acad Child Adolesc Psychiatry*. 1999;38:1442–1454.

Hughes CW, Emslie GJ, Crismon ML, et al. Texas Children's Medication Algorithm Project: Update from Texas Consensus Conference Panel on Medication Treatment of Childhood Major Depressive Disorder. *J Am Acad Child Adolesc Psychiatry*. 2007;46(6):667–686.

Hunt RD. Treatment effects of oral and transdermal clonidine in relation to methylphenidate: an open pilot study in ADD-H. *Psychopharmacol Bull*. 1987;23:111–114.

Hunt RD, Arnsten AFT, Asbell MD. An open trial of guanfacine in the treatment of attention-deficit hyperactivity disorder. *J Am Acad Child Adolesc Psychiatry*. 1995;34:50–54.

Hunt RD, Capper L, O'Connell P. Clonidine in child and adolescent psychiatry. *J Child Adolesc Psychopharmacol*. 1990;1:87–102.

Hunt RD, Cohen DJ, Shaywitz SE, et al. Strategies for study of the neurochemistry of attention deficit disorder in children. *Schizophr Bull*. 1982;8:236–252.

Hunt RD, Lau S, Ryu J. Alternative therapies for ADHD. In: Greenhill LL, Osman BB, eds. *Ritalin: Theory and Patient Management*. New York, NY: Mary Ann Liebert; 1991:75–95.

Hunt RD, Minderaa RB, Cohen DJ. Clonidine benefits children with attention deficit disorder and hyperactivity: report of a double-blind placebo-crossover therapeutic trial. *J Am Acad Child Psychiatry*. 1985;24:617–629.

Invega Sustenna [package insert]. Titusville, NJ: Janssen Pharmaceuticals Inc; 2012.

Isojarvi JIT, Laatikainen TJ, Pakarinen AJ, et al. Polycystic ovaries and hyperandrogenism in women taking valproate for epilepsy. *N Engl J Med*. 1993;329:1383–1388.

Jafri AB. Fluoxetine side effects [letter]. *J Am Acad Child Adolesc Psychiatry*. 1991;31:852.

Jankovic J, Jimenez-Shahed J, Brown LW. A randomized, double-blind, placebo-controlled study of topiramate in the treatment of Tourette syndrome. *J Neurol Neurosurg Psychiatry*. 2010;81(1):70–73.

Jann MW. Clozapine. *Pharmacotherapy*. 1991;11:179–195.

Jaselskis CA, Cook EH, Fletcher KE, et al. Clonidine treatment of hyperactive and impulsive children with autistic disorder. *J Clin Psychopharmacol*. 1992;12:322–327.

Jasinski DR, Krishnan S. Abuse liability and safety of oral lisdexamfetamine dimesylate in individuals with a history of stimulant abuse. *J Psychopharmacol*. 2009a;23(4):419–427.

Jasinski DR, Krishnan S. Human pharmacology of intravenous lisdexamfetamine dimesylate: abuse liability in adult stimulant abusers. *J Psychopharmacol*. 2009b;23(4):410–418.

Jatlow PI. Psychotropic drug disposition during development. In: Popper C, ed. *Psychiatric Pharmacosciences of Children and Adolescents*. Washington, DC: American Psychiatric Press; 1987:27–44.

Jefferson JW, Greist JH, Ackerman DL, et al. *Lithium Encyclopedia for Clinical Practice*. 2nd ed. Washington, DC: American Psychiatric Press; 1987.

Jefferson JW, Greist JH, Clagnaz PJ, et al. Effect of strenuous exercise on serum lithium level in man. *Am J Psychiatry*. 1982;139:1593–1595.

Jerome L. Hypomania with fluoxetine [letter]. *J Am Acad Child Adolesc Psychiatry.* 1991;30:850–851.

Jeste DV, Wyatt RJ. *Understanding and Treating Tardive Dyskinesia.* New York, NY: Guilford Press; 1982.

Johnston C, Pelham WE, Hoza J, et al. Psychostimulant rebound in attention deficit disordered boys. *J Am Acad Child Adolesc Psychiatry.* 1988;27:806–810.

Johnston HF. More on valproate and polycystic ovaries [letter]. *J Am Acad Child Adolesc Psychiatry.* 1999;38:354.

Joshi G, Wozniak J, Mick E, et al. A prospective open-label trial of extended-release carbamazepine monotherapy in children with bipolar disorder. *J Child Adolesc Psychopharmacol.* 2010;20(1):7–14.

Joshi PT, Capozzoli JA, Coyle JT. Low-dose neuroleptic therapy for children with childhood-onset pervasive developmental disorder. *Am J Psychiatry.* 1988;145:335–338.

Joshi PT, Walkup JT, Capozzoli JA, et al. The use of fluoxetine in the treatment of major depressive disorder in children and adolescents. Paper presented at: the 36th Annual Meeting of the American Academy of Child and Adolescent Psychiatry; October 11–15, 1989; New York, NY.

Kafantaris V, Campbell M, Padron-Gayol MV, et al. Carbamazepine in hospitalized aggressive conduct disorder children: an open pilot study. *Psychopharmacol Bull.* 1992;28:193–199.

Kafantaris V, Coletti D, Dicker R, et al. Lithium treatment of acute mania in adolescents: a large open trial. *J Am Acad Child Adolesc Psychiatry.* 2003;42:1038–1045.

Kafantaris V, Coletti DJ, Dicker R, et al. Lithium treatment of acute mania in adolescents: a placebo-controlled discontinuation study. *J Am Acad Child Adolesc Psychiatry.* 2004;43(8):984–993.

Kallen B, Tandberg A. Lithium and pregnancy. *Acta Psychiatr Scand.* 1983;68:134–139.

Kandemir H, Yumru M, Kul M, et al. Behavioral disinhibition, suicidal ideation, and self-mutilation related to clonazepam. *J Child Adolesc Psychopharmacol.* 2008;18(4):409–410.

Kane JM, Lieberman JA. *Adverse Effects of Psychotropic Drugs.* New York, NY: Guilford Press; 1992.

Kapetanovic S. Oxcarbazepine in youths with autistic disorder and significant disruptive behaviors. *Am J Psychiatry.* 2007;164(5):832–833.

Kaplan SL, Simms RM, Busner J. Prescribing practices of outpatient child psychiatrists. *J Am Acad Child Adolesc Psychiatry.* 1994;33:35–44.

Kashani JH, Shekim WO, Reid JC. Amitriptyline in children with major depressive disorder: a double-blind crossover pilot study. *J Am Acad Child Psychiatry.* 1984;23:348–351.

Kastner T, Finesmith R, Walsh K. Long-term administration of valproic acid in the treatment of affective symptoms in people with mental retardation. *J Clin Psychopharmacol.* 1993;13:448–451.

Kastner T, Friedman DL, Plummer AT, et al. Valproic acid for the treatment of children with mental retardation and mood symptomatology. *Pediatrics.* 1990;86:467–472.

Kaufmann CA, Wyatt RJ. Neuroleptic malignant syndrome. In: Meltzer HY, ed. *Psychopharmacology: The Third Generation of Progress.* New York, NY: Raven Press; 1987:1421–1430.

Kemner JE, Starr HL, Ciccone PE, et al. Outcomes of OROS methylphenidate compared with atomoxetine in children with ADHD: a multicenter, randomized prospective study. *Adv Ther.* 2005;22:498–512.

Kemph JP, DeVane CL, Levin GM, et al. Treatment of aggressive children with clonidine: results of an open pilot study. *J Am Acad Child Adolesc Psychiatry.* 1993;32:577–581.

Kennard B, Silva SG, Tonev S, et al. Remission and recovery in the treatment for adolescents with depression study (TADS): acute and long-term outcomes. *J Am Acad Child Adolesc Psychiatry*. 2009;48(2):186–195.

Kennard B, Silva S, Vitiello B, et al. Remission and residual symptoms after short-term treatment in the treatment of adolescents with depression study (TADS). *J Am Acad Child Adolesc Psychiatry*. 2006;45(12):1404–1411.

King BH, Hollander E, Sikich L, et al. Lack of efficacy of citalopram in children with autism spectrum disorders and high levels of repetitive behavior; citalopram ineffective in children with autism. *Arch Gen Psychiatry*. 2009;66(6):583–590.

King RA, Riddle MA, Chappell PB, et al. Emergence of self-destructive phenomena in children and adolescents during fluoxetine treatment. *J Am Acad Child Adolesc Psychiatry*. 1991;30:179–186.

Klein DF, Gittelman R, Quitkin F, et al. *Diagnosis and Drug Treatment of Psychiatric Disorders: Adults and Children*. Baltimore, MD: Williams & Wilkins; 1980.

Klein DJ, Cottingham EM, Sorter M, et al. A randomized, double-blind, placebo-controlled trial of metformin treatment of weight gain associated with initiation of atypical antipsychotic therapy in children and adolescents. *Am J Psychiatry*. 2006;163:2072–2079.

Klein RG. Pharmacotherapy of childhood hyperactivity: an update. In: Meltzer HY, ed. *Psychopharmacology: The Third Generation of Progress*. New York, NY: Raven Press; 1987:1215–1224.

Klein RG. Thioridazine effects on the cognitive performance of children with attention-deficit hyperactivity disorder. *J Child Adolesc Psychopharmacol*. 1990/1991;1:263–270.

Klein RG, Abikoff H, Klass E, et al. Clinical efficacy of methylphenidate in conduct disorder with and without attention deficit hyperactivity disorder. *Arch Gen Psychiatry*. 1997;54:1073–1080.

Klein RG, Koplewicz HS, Kanner A. Imipramine treatment of children with separation anxiety disorder. *J Am Acad Child Adolesc Psychiatry*. 1992;31:21–28.

Klein RG, Landa B, Mattes JA, et al. Methylphenidate and growth in hyperactive children: a controlled withdrawal study. *Arch Gen Psychiatry*. 1988;45:1127–1130.

Klein RG, Last CG. *Anxiety Disorders in Children*. Newbury Park, CA: SAGE; 1989.

Klein RG, Mannuzza S. Hyperactive boys almost grown up: III, methylphenidate effects on ultimate height. *Arch Gen Psychiatry*. 1988;45:1131–1134.

Klorman R, Brumaghim JT, Salzman LF, et al. Effects of methylphenidate on attention-deficit hyperactivity disorder with and without aggressive/noncompliant features. *J Abnorm Psychol*. 1988a;97:413–422.

Klorman R, Coons HW, Brumaghim JT, et al. Stimulant treatment for adolescents with attention deficit disorder. *Psychopharmacol Bull*. 1988b;24:88–92.

Koelch M, Pfalzer A, Kliegl K, et al. Therapeutic drug monitoring of children and adolescents treated with fluoxetine. *Pharmacopsychiatry*. 2012;45(2):72–76.

Kofoed L, Tadepalli G, Oesterheld JR, et al. Case series: clonidine has no systematic effects on PR or QTc intervals in children. *J Am Acad Child Adolesc Psychiatry*. 1999;38:1193–1196.

Kolman BK, Feldman HM, Handen BL, et al. Naltrexone in young autistic children: a double-blind, placebo-controlled crossover study. *J Am Acad Child Adolesc Psychiatry*. 1995;34:223–231.

Kolman BK, Feldman HM, Handen BJ, et al. Naltrexone in young autistic children: replication study and learning measures. *J Am Acad Child Adolesc Psychiatry*. 1997;36:1570–1578.

Korein J, Fish B, Shapiro T, et al. EEG and behavioral effects of drug therapy in children: chlorpromazine and diphenhydramine. *Arch Gen Psychiatry*. 1971;24:552–563.

Kotler LA, Devlin MJ, Davies M, et al. An open trial of fluoxetine for adolescents with bulimia nervosa. *J Child Adolesc Psychopharmacol*. 2003;13(3):329–335.

Kowatch RA, DelBello MP. The use of mood stabilizers and atypical antipsychotics in children and adolescents with bipolar disorders. *CNS Spectr*. 2003;8(4):273–280.

Kowatch RA, Suppes T, Carmody TJ, et al. Effect size of lithium, divalproex sodium, and carbamezapine in children and adolescents with bipolar disorder. *J Am Acad Child Adolesc Psychiatry*. 2000;39(6):713–720.

Kraft IA, Ardall C, Duffy JH, et al. A clinical study of chlordiazepoxide used in psychiatric disorders of children. *Int J Neuropsychiatry*. 1965;1:433–437.

Krakowski AJ. Amitriptyline in treatment of hyperkinetic children. *Psychosomatics*. 1965;6:355–360.

Krakowski AJ. Chlordiazepoxide in treatment of children with emotional disturbances. *N Y State J Med*. 1963;63:3388–3392.

Kramer AD, Feiguine RJ. Clinical effects of amitriptyline in adolescent depression: a pilot study. *J Am Acad Child Psychiatry*. 1981;20:636–644.

Kranzler H, Roofeh D, Gerbino-Rosen G, et al. Clozapine: its impact on aggressive behavior among children and adolescents with schizophrenia. *J Am Acad child Adolesc Psychiatry*. 2005;44:55–63.

Kranzler HR. Use of buspirone in an adolescent with overanxious disorder. *J Am Acad Child Adolesc Psychiatry*. 1988;27:789–790.

Krener PK, Mancina RA. Informed consent or informed coercion? Decision-making in pediatric psychopharmacology. *J Child Adolesc Psychopharmacol*. 1994;4(3):183–200.

Kuhn-Gebhart V. Behavioural disorders in non-epileptic children and their treatment with carbamazepine. In: Birkmayer W, ed. *Epileptic Seizures-Behaviour-Pain*. Bern, Germany: Hans Huber Publishers; 1976:264–267.

Kumra S, Frazier JA, Jacobson LK, et al. Childhood-onset schizophrenia: a double-blind clozapine-haloperidol comparison. *Arch Gen Psychiatry*. 1996;53:1090–1097.

Kumra S, Herion D, Jacobsen LK, et al. Case study: risperidone-induced hepatotoxicity in pediatric patients. *J Am Acad Child Adolesc Psychiatry*. 1997;36:701–705.

Kumra S, Jacobson LK, Lenane M, et al. Childhood-onset schizophrenia: an open-label study of olanzapine in adolescents. *J Am Acad Child Adolesc Psychiatry*. 1998;37:377–385.

Kuperman S, Stewart MA. Use of propranolol to decrease aggressive outbursts in younger patients. *Psychosomatics*. 1987;28:315–319.

Kurdyak PA, Juurlink DN, Mamdani MM. The effect of antidepressant warnings on prescribing trends in Ontario, Canada. *Am J Public Health*. 2007;97(4):750–754.

Kurian BT, Ray WA, Arbogast PG, et al. Effect of regulatory warnings on antidepressant prescribing for children and adolescents. *Arch Pediatr Adolesc Med*. 2007;161(7):690–696.

Kutcher S, ed. *Practical Child and Adolescent Psychopharmacology*. Cambridge, UK: Cambridge University Press; 2002.

Kutcher S, Boulos C, Ward B, et al. Response to desipramine treatment in adolescent depression: a fixed-dose, placebo-controlled trial. *J Am Acad Child Adolesc Psychiatry*. 1994;33:686–694.

Kutcher SP. *Child and Adolescent Psychopharmacology*. Philadelphia, PA: WB Saunders; 1997.

Kutcher SP, MacKenzie S. Successful clonazepam treatment of adolescents with panic disorder [letter]. *J Clin Psychopharmacol*. 1988;8:299–301.

Kutcher SP, MacKenzie S, Galarraga W, et al. Clonazepam treatment of adolescents with neuroleptic-induced akathisia. *Am J Psychiatry*. 1987;144:823–824.

Kutz G. Foster children: HHS guidance could help states improve oversight of psychotropic prescriptions. GAO-12-270T. Washington, DC: The Government

Accountability Office; 2011. www.gao.gov/assets/590/586570.pdf. Accessed March 2, 2013.

Labellarte M, Biederman J, Emslie G, et al. Multiple-dose pharmacokinetics of fluvoxamine in children and adolescents. *J Am Acad Child Adolesc Psychiatry*. 2004;43:1497–1505.

Lader M. Fluoxetine efficacy vs comparative drugs: an overview. *Br J Psychiatry*. 1988:153(suppl 3):51–58.

Latuda [package insert]. Marlborough, MA: Sunovion Pharmaceuticals, Inc; 2012.

Latz SR, McCracken JT. Neuroleptic malignant syndrome in children and adolescents: two case reports and a warning. *J Child Adolesc Psychopharmacol*. 1992;2:123–129.

Law SF, Schachar RJ. Do typical clinical doses of methylphenidate cause tics in children treated for attention-deficit hyperactivity disorder? *J Am Acad Child Adolesc Psychiatry*. 1999;38:944–951.

Leckman JF, Cohen DJ, Detlor J, et al. Clonidine in the treatment of Tourette syndrome: a review of data. In: Friedhoff AJ, Chase TN, eds. *Gilles de la Tourette Syndrome*. New York, NY: Raven Press; 1982:391–401.

Leckman JF, Detlor J, Harcherik DF, et al. Short- and long-term treatment of Tourette's syndrome with clonidine: a clinical perspective. *Neurology*. 1985;35:343–351.

Leckman JF, Hardin MT, Riddle MA, et al. Clonidine treatment of Gilles de la Tourette's syndrome. *Arch Gen Psychiatry*. 1991;48:324–328.

Lefkowitz MM. Effects of diphenylhydantoin on disruptive behavior. *Arch Gen Psychiatry*. 1969;20:643–651.

Lena B, Surtees SJ, Maggs R. The efficacy of lithium in the treatment of emotional disturbance in children and adolescents. In: Johnson FN, Johnson S, eds. *Lithium in Medical Practice*. Baltimore, MD: University Park Press; 1978:79–83.

Leonard HL, Swedo SE, Lenane MC, et al. A double-blind desipramine substitution during long-term clomipramine treatment in children and adolescents with obsessive-compulsive disorder. *Arch Gen Psychiatry*. 1991;48:922–927.

Leonard HL, Swedo SE, Rapoport JL, et al. Treatment of obsessive-compulsive disorder with clomipramine and desipramine in children and adolescents: a double-blind crossover comparison. *Arch Gen Psychiatry*. 1989;46:1088–1092.

Leonard HL, Topol D, Bukstein O, et al. Clonazepam as an augmenting agent in the treatment of childhood-onset obsessive-compulsive disorder. *J Am Acad Child Adolesc Psychiatry*. 1994;33:692–694.

Levin GM, Burton-Teston K, Murphy T. Development of precocious puberty in two children treated with clonidine for aggressive behavior. *J Child Adolesc Psychopharmacol*. 1993;3:127–131.

Levkovitch Y, Kaysar N, Kronnenberg Y, et al. Clozapine for schizophrenia [letter]. *J Am Acad Child Adolesc Psychiatry*. 1994;33:431.

Levy RH. Psychopharmacological interventions. In: Katz SE, Nardacci D, Sabatini A, eds. *Intensive Treatment of the Homeless Mentally Ill*. Washington, DC: American Psychiatric Press; 1993:129–165.

Liebenluft E, Charney DS, Towbin KE, et al. Defining clinical phenotypes of juvenile mania. *Am J Psychiatry*. 2003;160:430–437.

Lingjaerde O, Ahlfors UG, Bech P, et al. The UKU side effect rating scale: a new comprehensive rating scale for psychotropic drugs, and a cross sectional study of side effects in neuroleptic-treated patients. *Acta Psychiatr Scand Suppl*. 1987;76:1–100.

Linnoila M, Dejong J, Virkkunen M. Monoamines, glucose metabolism, and impulse control. *Psychopharmacol Bull*. 1989;25:404–406.

Linnoila M, Gualtieri CT, Jobson K, et al. Characteristics of the therapeutic response to imipramine in hyperactive children. *Am J Psychiatry*. 1979;136:1201–1203.

Looker A, Conners CK. Diphenylhydantoin in children with severe temper tantrums. *Arch Gen Psychiatry*. 1970;23:80–89.

Lowe TL, Cohen DJ, Detlor J, et al. Stimulant medications precipitate Tourette's syndrome. *JAMA*. 1982;247:1729–1931.

Lucas AR, Pasley FC. Psychoactive drugs in the treatment of emotionally disturbed children: haloperidol and diazepam. *Compr Psychiatry*. 1969;10:376–386.

MacLeod CM, Dekaban AS, Hunt E. Memory impairment in epileptic patients: selective effects of phenobarbital concentration. *Science*. 1978;202:1102–1104.

Malhotra S, Santosh PR. An open clinical trial of buspirone in children with attention-deficit/hyperactivity disorder. *J Am Acad Child Adolesc Psychiatry*. 1998;37:364–371.

Malhotra S, Subodh BN. Informed consent & ethical issues in paediatric psychopharmacology. *Indian J Med Res*. 2009;129(1):19–32.

Malone RP, Delaney MA, Luebbert JF, et al. A double-blind placebo-controlled study of lithium in hospitalized aggressive children and adolescents with conduct disorder. *Arch Gen Psychiatry*. 2000;57:649–654.

Malone RP, Delaney MA, Luebbert JF, et al. The lithium test dose prediction method in aggressive children. *Psychopharmacol Bull*. 1995;31(2):379–382.

Mandoki M. Clozapine for adolescents with psychosis: literature review and two case reports. *J Child Adolesc Psychopharmacol*. 1993;3:213–221.

Mann JJ, Marzuk PM, Arango V, et al. Neurochemical studies of violent and nonviolent suicide. *Psychopharmacol Bull*. 1989;25:407–413.

Manos MJ, Short EJ, Findling RL. Differential effectiveness of methylphenidate and Adderall in school-age youth with attention-deficit/hyperactivity disorder. *J Am Acad Child Adolesc Psychiatry*. 1999;38:813–819.

March J, Franklin ME, Leonard H, et al. Tics moderate treatment outcome with sertraline but not cognitive-behavior therapy in pediatric obsessive-compulsive disorder. *Biol Psychiatry*. 2007a;61(3):344–347.

March J, Silva S, Curry J, et al; TADS Team. The treatment for adolescents with depression study (TADS): outcomes over 1 year of naturalistic follow-up. *Am J Psychiatry*. 2009;166(10):1141–1149.

March JS, Biederman J, Wolkow R, et al. Sertraline in children and adolescents with obsessive-compulsive disorder: a multicenter randomized controlled trial. *JAMA*. 1998;280:1752–1756.

March JS, Entusah AR, Rynn M, et al. A randomized controlled trial of venlafaxine ER versus placebo in pediatric social anxiety disorder. *Biol Psychiatry*. 2007b;62(10):1149–1154.

March JS, Foa E, Gammon P, et al; The Pediatric OCD Treatment Study (POTS) Team. Cognitive-behavioral therapy, sertraline, and their combination for children and adolescents with obsessive-compulsive disorder. *JAMA*. 2004;292:1969–1976.

Martin A, Koenign K, Scahill L, et al. Open-label quetiapine in the treatment of children and adolescents with autistic disorder. *J Child Adolesc Psychopharmacol*. 1999;9:99–107.

Martin A, Landau J, Leebens P, et al. Risperidone-associated with gain in children and adolescents: a retrospective chart review. *J Child Adolesc Psychopharmacol*. 2000;10:259–268.

Martin A, Scahill L, Charney DS, et al, eds. *Pediatric Psychopharmacology: Principles and Practice*. New York, NY: Oxford University Press; 2003.

Mattai A, Fung L, Bakalar J, et al. Adjunctive use of lithium carbonate for the management of neutropenia in clozapine-treated children. *Hum Psychopharmacol*. 2009;24(7):584–589.

Mattes JA, Gittelman R. Growth of hyperactive children on maintenance regimen of methylphenidate. *Arch Gen Psychiatry*. 1983;40:317–321.

Mazzone L, Reale L, Mannino V, et al. Lower IQ is associated with decreased clinical response to atomoxetine in children and adolescents with attention-deficit hyperactivity disorder. *CNS Drugs*. 2011;25(6):503–509.

Mazzone L, Reale L. Topiramate in children with autistic spectrum disorders. *Brain Dev*. 2006;28(10):668.

McBride MC, Wang DD, Torres C. Methylphenidate in therapeutic doses does not lower seizure threshold. *Ann Neurol.* 1986;20:428.

McConville BJ, Arvanitis LA, Thyrum PT. Pharmacokinetics, tolerability, and clinical effectiveness of quetiapine fumarate: an open-label trial in adolescents with psychotic disorders. *J Clin Psychiatry.* 2000;61:252–260.

McConville BJ, Minnery KL, Sorter MT, et al. An open study of the effects of sertraline on adolescent major depression. *J Child Adolesc Psychopharmacol.* 1996;6:41–51.

McCormick LH. Treatment with buspirone in a patient with autism. *Arch Fam Med.* 1997;6(4):368–370.

McCormick LH, Rizzuto GT, Knuckles HB. A pilot study of buspirone in attention-deficit hyperactivity disorder. *Arch Fam Med.* 1994;3:68–70.

McCracken JT, Biederman J, Greenhill LL, et al. Analog classroom assessment of a once-daily mixed amphetamine formulations, SLI381 (Adderall XR) in children with ADHD. *J Am Acad Child Adolesc Psychiatry.* 2003;42:673–683.

McCracken JT, Martin W. Clonidine side effect [letter]. *J Am Acad Child Adolesc Psychiatry.* 1997;36:160–161.

McCracken JT, McGough J, Shah B, et al; Research Units on Pediatric Psychopharmacology Autism Network. Risperidone in children with autism and serious behavioral problems. *N Engl J Med.* 2002;347:314–321.

McDonagh M, Peterson K, Carson S, et al. *Drug Class Review: Atypical Antipsychotic Drugs: Final Update 3 Report.* Portland, OR: Oregon Health & Science University; 2010.

McDougle CJ, Kem DL, Posey DJ. Case series: use of ziprasidone for maladaptive symptoms in youths with autism. *J Am Acad Child Adolesc Psychiatry.* 2002;41:921–927.

McGough JJ, Biederman J, Wigal SB, et al. Long-term tolerability and effectiveness of once-daily mixed amphetamine salts (Adderall XR) in children with ADHD. *J Am Acad Child Adolesc Psychiatry.* 2005;44:539–547.

McVoy M, eds. *Clinical Manual of Child and Adolescent Psychopharmacology.* 2nd ed. Washington, DC: American Psychiatric Press Inc; 2012.

Meyers B, Tune LE, Coyle JT. Clinical response and serum neuroleptic levels in childhood schizophrenia. *Am J Psychiatry.* 1980;137:1459–1460.

Michelson D, Allen AJ, Busner J, et al. Once-daily atomoxetine treatment for children and adolescents with attention deficit hyperactivity disorder: a randomized, placebo-controlled study. *Am J Psychiatry.* 2002;159(11):1896–1901.

Michelson D, Faries D, Wernicke J, et al. Atomoxetine in the treatment of children and adolescents with attention-deficit/hyperactivity disorder: a randomized, placebo-controlled, dose-response study. *Pediatrics.* 2001;108(5):E83.

Michelson D, Read HA, Ruff DD, et al. CYP2D6 and clinical response to atomoxetine in children and adolescents with ADHD. *J Am Acad Child Adolesc Psychiatry.* 2007;46(2):242–251.

Mitsunaga MM, Garrett A, Howe M, et al. Increased subgenual cingulate cortex volume in pediatric bipolar disorder associated with mood stabilizer exposure. *J Child Adolesc Psychopharmacol.* 2011;21(2):149–155.

MMDLN. Newsletter update: Antipsychotic medication use in medicaid children and adolescents: a study of 16 state programs. *The Medicaid Medical Directors' Learning Network Newsletter.* Spring 2011. http://chsr.rutgers.edu/MMDLNAPKIDS/mmdlnnews1.pdf. Accessed March 2, 2013.

Molitch M, Eccles AK. The effect of benzedrine sulfate on the intelligence scores of children. *Am J Psychiatry.* 1937;94:587–590.

Molitch M, Poliakoff S. The effect of benzedrine sulfate on enuresis. *Arch Pediatr.* 1937;54:499–501.

Molitch M, Sullivan JP. The effect of benzedrine sulfate on children taking the New Stanford Achievement Test. *Am J Orthopsychiatry.* 1937;7:519–522.

Morselli PL, Bianchetti G, Dugas M. Therapeutic drug monitoring of psychotropic drugs in children. *Pediatr Pharmacol.* 1983;3:149–156.

Mozes T, Toren P, Chernauzan N, et al. Clozapine treatment in very early onset schizophrenia. *J Am Acad Child Adolesc Psychiatry.* 1994;33:65–70.

Mrakotsky C, Masek B, Biederman J, et al. Prospective open-label pilot trial of mirtazapine in children and adolescents with social phobia. *J Anxiety Disord.* 2008;22(1):88–97.

MTA Cooperative Group. A 14-month randomized clinical trial of treatment strategies for attention-deficit/hyperactivity disorder. *Arch Gen Psychiatry.* 1999a;56:1073–1086.

MTA Cooperative Group. Moderators and mediators of treatment response for children with attention-deficit/hyperactivity disorder. *Arch Gen Psychiatry.* 1999b;56:1088–1096.

Musten LM, Firestone P, Pisterman S, et al. Effects of methylphenidate on pre-school children with ADHD: cognitive and behavioral functions. *J Am Acad Child Adolesc Psychiatry.* 1997;36:1407–1415.

Myers WC, Carrera F III. Carbamazepine-induced mania with hypersexuality in a 9-year-old boy. *Am J Psychiatry.* 1989;146:400.

Nasrallah HA, White T, Nasrallah AT. Lower mortality in geriatric patients receiving risperidone and olanzapine versus haloperidol: a preliminary analysis of retrospective data. *Am J Geriatr Psychiatry.* 2004;12(4):437–439.

National Institute of Mental Health/National Institutes of Health Consensus Development Panel. Mood disorders: pharmacologic prevention of recurrences. *Am J Psychiatry.* 1985;142:469–476.

Neppe VM, Ward NG. The evaluation and management of neuroleptic-induced acute extrapyramidal syndromes. In: Neppe VM, ed. *Innovative Psychopharmacology.* New York, NY: Raven Press; 1989:152–176.

New York State Department of Health. *Safe, Effective and Therapeutically Equivalent Prescription Drugs.* 7th ed. Albany, NY: New York State Department of Health Office of Health Systems Management; 1988.

Newcomer JW. Metabolic considerations in the use of antipsychotic medications: a review of recent evidence. *J Clin Psychiatry.* 2007;68(suppl 1):20–27.

Newcorn JH, Spencer TJ, Biederman J, et al. Atomoxetine treatment in children and adolescents with attention-deficit/hyperactivity disorder and comorbid oppositional defiant disorder. *J Am Acad Child Adolesc Psychiatry.* 2005;44(3):240–248.

Newcorn JH, Sutton VK, Weiss MD, et al. Clinical responses to atomoxetine in attention-deficit/hyperactivity disorder: the Integrated Data Exploratory Analysis (IDEA) study. *J Am Acad Child Adolesc Psychiatry.* 2009;48(5):511–518.

Newton JEO, Cannon DJ, Couch L, et al. Effects of repeated drug holidays on serum haloperidol concentration, psychiatric symptoms, and movement disorders in schizophrenic patients. *J Clin Psychiatry.* 1989;50:132–135.

Nobile M, Bellotti B, Marino C, et al. An open trial of paroxetine in the treatment of children and adolescents diagnosed with dysthymia. *J Child Adolesc Psychopharmacol.* 2000;10:103–109.

Noyes R. Beta-adrenergic blockers. In: Last CG, Hersen M, eds. *Handbook of Anxiety Disorders.* New York, NY: Pergamon Press; 1988:445–459.

Nurcombe B. Malpractice. In: Lewis M, ed. *Child and Adolescent Psychiatry: A Comprehensive Textbook.* Baltimore, MD: Williams & Wilkins; 1991:1127–1139.

Nurcombe B, Partlett DF. *Child Mental Health and the Law.* New York, NY: Free Press; 1994:220–272.

Olfson M, Marcus SC, Druss BG. Effects of Food and Drug Administration warnings on antidepressant use in a national sample. *Arch Gen Psychiatry.* 2008;65(1):94–101.

Olvera RL, Pliszka SR, Luh J, et al. An open trial of venlafaxine in the treatment of attention-deficit/hyperactivity disorder in children and adolescents. *J Child Adolesc Psychopharmacol.* 1996;6:241–250.

Orsagh-Yentis DK, Wink LK, Stigler KA, et al. Buspirone for bruxism in a child with pervasive developmental disorder-not otherwise specified. *J Child Adolesc Psychopharmacol.* 2011;21(6):643–645.

Owens JA, Rosen CL, Mindell JA, et al. Use of pharmacotherapy for insomnia in child psychiatry practice: a national survey. *Sleep Med.* 2010;11(7):692–700.

Owley T, Walton L, Salt J, et al. An open-label trial of escitalopram in pervasive developmental disorders. *J Am Acad Child Adolesc Psychiatry.* 2005;44(4):343–348.

Oxford English Dictionary. 2nd ed. Oxford, England: Oxford University Press; 1989.

Pandina G, Bossie C, Youssef E, et al. Risperidone improves behavioral symptoms in children with autism in a randomized, double-blind, placebo-controlled trial. *J Autism Dev Disord.* 2007;37:367–373.

Papatheodorou G, Kutcher SP, Katic M, et al. The efficacy and safety of divalproex sodium in the treatment of acute mania in adolescents and young adults: an open clinical trial. *J Clin Psychopharmacol.* 1995;15:110–116.

Pappagallo M, Silva R. The effect of atypical antipsychotic agents on prolactin levels in children and adolescents. *J Child Adolesc Psychopharmacol.* 2004;14:359–371.

Pare CMB, Kline N, Hallstrom C, et al. Will amitriptyline prevent the "cheese" reaction of monoamine oxidase inhibitors? *Lancet.* 1982;2:183–186.

Pataki CS, Carlson GA, Kelly KL, et al. Side effects of methylphenidate and desipramine alone and in combination in children. *J Am Acad Child Adolesc Psychiatry.* 1993;32:1065–1072.

Patel N, Delbello M, Bryan H, et al. Open-label lithium for the treatment of adolescents with bipolar depression. *J Am Acad Child Adolesc Psychiatry.* 2006;45(3):289–297.

Patrick KS, Mueller RA, Gualtieri CT, et al. Pharmacokinetics and actions of methylphenidate. In: Meltzer HY, ed. *Psychopharmacology: The Third Generation of Progress.* New York, NY: Raven Press; 1987:1387–1395.

Pavuluri MN, Henry DB, Carbray JA, et al. A one-year open-label trial of risperidone augmentation in lithium nonresponder youth with preschool-onset bipolar disorder. *J Child Adolesc Psychopharmacol.* 2006;16(3):336–350.

Pavuluri MN, Henry DB, Carbray JA, et al. Divalproex sodium for pediatric mixed mania: a 6-month prospective trial. *Bipolar Disord.* 2005;7(3):266–273.

Pavuluri MN, Henry DB, Findling RL, et al. Double-blind randomized trial of risperidone versus divalproex in pediatric bipolar disorder. *Bipolar Disord.* 2010a;12(6):593–605.

Pavuluri MN, Henry DB, Moss M, et al. Effectiveness of lamotrigine in maintaining symptom control in pediatric bipolar disorder. *J Child Adolesc Psychopharm.* 2009;19(1):75–82.

Pavuluri MN, Passarotti AM, Mohammed T, et al. Enhanced working and verbal memory after lamotrigine treatment in pediatric bipolar disorder. *Bipolar Disord.* 2010b;12(2):213–220.

PDR.net. *FDA Drug Safety Communication Information for Healthcare Professionals: Suicidal Behavior and Ideation and Antiepileptic Drugs.* PDR.net; 2008.

PDR.net. *Drug Information: Drug Summary.* PDR.net; 2012.

Pearson DA, Lane DM, Santos CW, et al. Effects of methylphenidate treatment in children with mental retardation and ADHD: individual variation in medication response. *J Am Acad Child Adolesc Psychiatry.* 2004a;43:686–698.

Pearson DA, Santos CW, Casat CD, et al. Treatment effects of methylphenidate on cognitive functioning in children with mental retardation and ADHD. *J Am Acad Child Adolesc Psychiatry.* 2004b;43:677–685.

Pearson DA, Santos CW, Roache JD, et al. Treatment effects of methylphenidate on behavioral adjustment in children with mental retardation and ADHD. *J Am Acad Child Adolesc Psychiatry.* 2003;42:209–216.

Pelham WE, Bender ME, Caddell J, et al. Methylphenidate and children with attention deficit disorder. *Arch Gen Psychiatry*. 1985;42:948–952.

Pelham WE, Greenslade KE, Vodde-Hamilton M, et al. Relative efficacy of long-acting stimulants on children with attention deficit-hyperactivity disorder: a comparison of standard methylphenidate, sustained-release methylphenidate, sustained-release dextroamphetamine, and pemoline. *Pediatrics*. 1990;86: 226–237.

Pelham WE, Sturges J, Hoza JA, et al. Sustained release and standard methylphenidate effects on cognitive and social behavior in children with attention deficit disorder. *Pediatrics*. 1987;80:491–501.

Perry R, Campbell M, Adams P, et al. Long-term efficacy of haloperidol in autistic children: continuous versus discontinuous drug administration. *J Am Acad Child Adolesc Psychiatry*. 1989;28:87–92.

Perry R, Campbell M, Green WH, et al. Neuroleptic-related dyskinesias in autistic children: a prospective study. *Psychopharmacol Bull*. 1985;21:140–143.

Pesikoff RB, Davis PC. Treatment of pavor nocturnus and somnambulism in children. *Am J Psychiatry*. 1971;128:778–781.

Peterson CE, Amaral S, Frosch E. Lithium-induced nephrotic syndrome in a prepubertal boy. *J Child Adolesc Psychopharmacol*. 2008;18(2):210–213.

Petti TA, Fish B, Shapiro T, et al. Effects of chlordiazepoxide in disturbed children: a pilot study. *J Clin Psychopharmacol*. 1982;2:270–273.

Pfeffer CR, Jiang H, Domeshek LJ. Buspirone treatment of psychiatrically hospitalized children with symptoms of anxiety and moderately severe aggression. *J Child Adolesc Psychopharmacol*. 1997;7:145–155.

Pfefferbaum G, Overall JE, Boren HA, et al. Alprazolam in the treatment of anticipatory and acute situational anxiety in children with cancer. *J Am Acad Child Adolesc Psychiatry*. 1987;26:532–535.

Phan H, Casavant M, Crockett S, et al. Serotonin syndrome following a single 50 mg dose of sertraline in a child. *Clin Toxicol*. 2008;46(9):845–849.

Physicians' Desk Reference (PDR). 44th ed. Oradell, NJ: Medical Economics; 1990.

Physicians' Desk Reference (PDR). 49th ed. Oradell, NJ: Medical Economics; 1995.

Physicians' Desk Reference (PDR). 54th ed. Oradell, NJ: Medical Economics; 2000.

Physician's Desk Reference (PDR). 58th ed. Montvale, NJ: Thomson PDR; 2005.

Physicians' Desk Reference (PDR). 59th ed. Montvale, NJ: Thomson PDR; 2006.

Piontek CM, Wisner KL. Appropriate clinical management of women taking valproate. *J Clin Psychiatry*. 2000;61:161–163.

Platt JE, Campbell M, Green WH, et al. Cognitive effect of lithium carbonate and haloperidol in treatment resistant aggressive children. *Arch Gen Psychiatry*. 1984;41:657–662.

Pleak RR, Birmaher B, Gavrilescu A, et al. Mania and neuropsychiatric excitation following carbamazepine. *J Am Acad Child Adolesc Psychiatry*. 1988;27:500–503.

Pliszka S, Bernet W, Bukstein O, et al. Practice parameter for the assessment and treatment of children and adolescents with attention-deficit/hyperactivity disorder. *J Am Acad Child Adolesc Psychiatry*. 2007;46(7):894–921.

Pliszka SR. Tricyclic antidepressants in the treatment of children with attention deficit disorder. *J Am Acad Child Adolesc Psychiatry*. 1987;26:127–132.

Pliszka SR, Browne RG, Olvera RL, et al. A double-blind, placebo-controlled study of Adderall and methylphenidate in the treatment of attention-deficit/hyperactivity disorder. *J Am Acad Child Adolesc Psychiatry*. 2000;39:619–626.

Pliszka SR, Crismon ML, Hughes CW, et al. The Texas children's medication algorithm project: revision of the algorithm for pharmacotherapy of attention-deficit/hyperactivity disorder. *J Am Acad Child Adolesc Psychiatry*. 2006;45(6):642–657.

Pliszka SR, Greenhill LL, Crismon ML, et al. The Texas Children's Medication Algorithm Project: report of the Texas Consensus Conference Panel on

Medication Treatment of Childhood Attention-Deficit/Hyperactivity Disorder: part I, attention-deficit/hyperactivity disorder. *J Am Acad Child Adolesc Psychiatry*. 2000a;39:908–919.

Pliszka SR, Greenhill LL, Crismon ML, et al. The Texas Children's Medication Algorithm Project: report of the Texas Consensus Conference Panel on Medication Treatment of Childhood Attention-Deficit/Hyperactivity Disorder: part II, tactics. *J Am Acad Child Adolesc Psychiatry*. 2000b;39:920–927.

Pool D, Bloom W, Mielke DH, et al. A controlled evaluation of loxitane in seventy-five adolescent schizophrenic patients. *Curr Ther Res Clin Exp*. 1976;19:99–104.

Popper C. Medical unknown and ethical consent: prescribing psychotropic medications for children in the face of uncertainty. In: Popper C, ed. *Psychiatric Pharmacosciences of Children and Adolescents*. Washington, DC: American Psychiatric Press; 1987a.

Popper C, ed. *Psychiatric Pharmacosciences of Children and Adolescents*. Washington, DC: American Psychiatric Press; 1987b.

Popper CW. Combining methylphenidate and clonidine: pharmacologic questions and news reports about sudden death. *J Child Adolesc Psychopharmacol*. 1995;5:157–166.

Popper CW, Zimnitzky B. Sudden death putatively related to desipramine treatment in youth: a fifth case and a review of speculative mechanisms. *J Child Adolesc Psychopharmacol*. 1995;5:283–300.

Potenza MN, Holmes JP, Kanes SJ, et al. Olanzapine treatment of children, adolescents, and adults with pervasive developmental disorders: an open-label pilot study. *J Clin Psychopharmacol*. 1999;19:37–44.

Potter WZ, Calil HM, Sutfin TA, et al. Active metabolites of imipramine and desipramine in man. *Clin Pharmacol Ther*. 1982;31:393–401.

Poussaint AF, Ditman KS. A controlled study of imipramine (Tofranil) in the treatment of childhood enuresis. *J Pediatr*. 1965;67:283–290.

Prakash A, Lobo E, Kratochvil CJ, et al. An open-label safety and pharmacokinetics study of duloxetine in pediatric patients with major depression. *J Child Adolesc Psychopharmacol*. 2012;22:48–55.

Preskorn SH, Bupp SJ, Weller EB, et al. Plasma levels of imipramine and metabolites in 68 hospitalized children. *J Am Acad Child Adolesc Psychiatry*. 1989a;28:373–375.

Preskorn SH, Jerkovich GS, Beber JH, et al. Therapeutic drug monitoring of tricyclic antidepressants: a standard of care issue. *Psychopharmacol Bull*. 1989b;25:281–284.

Preskorn SH, Weller E, Jerkovich G, et al. Depression in children: concentration dependent CNS toxicity of tricyclic antidepressants. *Psychopharmacol Bull*. 1988;24:275–279.

Preskorn SH, Weller EB, Hughes CW, et al. Depression in prepubertal children: dexamethasone nonsuppression predicts differential response to imipramine vs. placebo. *Psychopharmacol Bull*. 1987;23:128–133.

Prien RF. Methods and models for placebo use in pharmacotherapeutic trials. *Psychopharmacol Bull*. 1988;24:4–8.

Prince JB, Wilens TE, Biederman J, et al. A controlled study of nortriptyline in children and adolescents with attention deficit hyperactivity disorder. *J Child Adolesc Psychopharmacol*. 2000;10:193–204.

Psychopharmacology Bulletin. Special issue: *Pharmacotherapy of Children*. Rockville, MD: US Department of Health, Education, and Welfare; 1973. Publication No (HSM) 73–9002.

Puente RM. The use of carbamazepine in the treatment of behavioural disorders in children. In: Birkmayer W, ed. *Epileptic Seizures-Behaviour-Pain*. Bern, Germany: Hans Huber Publishers; 1976:243–252.

Puig-Antich J. Affective disorders in children and adolescents: diagnostic validity and psychobiology. In: Meltzer HY, ed. *Psychopharmacology: The Third Generation of Progress.* New York, NY: Raven Press; 1987:843–859.

Puig-Antich J. Major depression and conduct disorder in prepuberty. *J Am Acad Child Adolesc Psychiatry.* 1982;21:118–128.

Puig-Antich J, Perel JM, Lupatkin W, et al. Imipramine in prepubertal major depressive disorders. *Arch Gen Psychiatry.* 1987;44:81–89.

Quiason H, Ward D, Kitchen T. Buspirone for aggression [letter]. *J Am Acad Child Adolesc Psychiatry.* 1991;30:1026.

Quinn PO, Rapoport JL. One-year follow-up of hyperactive boys treated with imipramine or methylphenidate. *Am J Psychiatry.* 1975;132:241–245.

Quintana H, Birmaher B, Stedge D, et al. Use of methylphenidate in the treatment of children with autistic disorder. *J Autism Dev Disord.* 1995;25:283–294.

Rall TW. Hypnotics and sedatives; ethanol. In: Gilman AG, Rall TW, Nies AS, et al, eds. *Goodman and Gilman's The Pharmacological Basis of Therapeutics.* 8th ed. New York, NY: Pergamon Press; 1990:345–382.

Rapoport JL, Buchsbaum MS, Weingartner H, et al. Dextroamphetamine: its cognitive and behavioral effects in normal and hyperactive boys and normal men. *Arch Gen Psychiatry.* 1980a;37:933–943.

Rapoport JL, Buchsbaum MS, Zahn TP, et al. Dextroamphetamine: cognitive and behavioral effects in normal prepubertal boys. *Science.* 1978a;199:560–563.

Rapoport JL, Mikkelsen EJ. Antidepressants. In: Werry JS, ed. *Pediatric Psychopharmacology: The Use of Behavior Modifying Drugs in Children.* New York, NY: Brunner/Mazel; 1978b:208–233.

Rapoport JL, Mikkelsen EJ, Werry JS. Antimanic, antianxiety, hallucinogenic and miscellaneous drugs. In: Werry JS, ed. *Pediatric Psychopharmacology: The Use of Behavior Modifying Drugs in Children.* New York, NY: Brunner/Mazel; 1978c:316–355.

Rapoport JL, Mikkelsen EJ, Zavadil A, et al. Childhood enuresis: psychopathology, plasma tricyclic concentration and antienuretic effect. *Arch Gen Psychiatry.* 1980b;37:1146–1152.

Rapoport JL, Quinn PO, Bradbard G, et al. Imipramine and methylphenidate treatment of hyperactive boys. *Arch Gen Psychiatry.* 1974;30:789–798.

Rapport MD, Carlson GA, Kelly KL, et al. Methylphenidate and desipramine in hospitalized children: I, separate and combined effects on cognitive function. *J Am Acad Child Adolesc Psychiatry.* 1993;32:333–342.

Rapport MD, Denney C, DuPaul GJ, et al. Attention deficit disorder and methylphenidate: normalization rates, clinical effectiveness, and response prediction in 76 children. *J Am Acad Child Adolesc Psychiatry.* 1994;33:882–893.

Raskind MA, Peskind ER, Hoff DJ, et al. A parallel group placebo controlled study of prazosin for trauma nightmares and sleep disturbance in combat veterans with post-traumatic stress disorder. *Biol Psychiatry.* 2007;61:928–934.

Rating scales and assessment instruments for use in pediatric psychopharmacology research. *Psychopharmacol Bull.* 1985;21:713–1124.

Realmuto G. Neurobiological assessment. In: Klykylo W, Kay J, eds. *Clinical Child Psychiatry.* 3rd ed. Chichester, UK: John Wiley and Sons; 2012.

Realmuto GM, August GJ, Garfinkel BD. Clinical effect of buspirone in autistic children. *J Clin Psychopharmacol.* 1989;9:122–125.

Realmuto GM, Erickson WD, Yellin AM, et al. Clinical comparison of thiothixene and thioridazine in schizophrenic adolescents. *Am J Psychiatry.* 1984;141:440–442.

Redden L, DelBello M, Wagner KD, et al. Long-term safety of divalproex sodium extended-release in children and adolescents with bipolar I disorder. *J Child Adolesc Psychopharmacol.* 2009;19(1):83–89.

Reisberg B, Gershon S. Side effects associated with lithium therapy. *Arch Gen Psychiatry.* 1979;36:879–887.

Reiss AL, O'Donnell DJ. Carbamazepine-induced mania in two children: case report. *J Clin Psychiatry*. 1984;45:272–274.

Reite ML, Nagel KE, Ruddy JR. *Concise Guide to Evaluation and Management of Sleep Disorders*. Washington, DC: American Psychiatric Press; 1990.

Remschmidt H. The psychotropic effect of carbamazepine in non-epileptic patients, with particular reference to problems posed by clinical studies in children with behavioural disorders. In: Birkmayer W, ed. *Epileptic Seizures-Behaviour-Pain*. Bern, Germany: Hans Huber Publishers; 1976:253–258.

Remschmidt H, Schulz E, Martin PDM. An open trial of clozapine in thirty-six adolescents with schizophrenia. *J Child Adolesc Psychopharmacol*. 1994;4:31–41.

Richardson MA, Haugland G, Craig TJ. Neuroleptic use, parkinsonian symptoms, tardive dyskinesia and associated factors in child and adolescent psychiatric patients. *Am J Psychiatry*. 1991;148:1322–1328.

Riddle MA, ed. Pediatric psychopharmacology I. *Child Adolesc Psychiatr Clin N Am*. 1995a;4:1–260. (Entire issue.)

Riddle MA, ed. Pediatric psychopharmacology II. *Child Adolesc Psychiatr Clin N Am*. 1995b;4:261–520. (Entire issue.)

Riddle MA, Geller B, Ryan N. Another sudden death in a child treated with desipramine. *J Am Acad Child Adolesc Psychiatry*. 1993;32:792–797.

Riddle MA, Geller B, Ryan ND. The safety of desipramine: reply [letter]. *J Am Acad Child Adolesc Psychiatry*. 1994;33:589–590.

Riddle MA, Hardin MT, Cho SC, et al. Desipramine treatment of boys with attention-deficit hyperactivity disorder and tics: preliminary clinical experiences. *J Am Acad Child Adolesc Psychiatry*. 1988;27:811–814.

Riddle MA, Hardin MT, King R, et al. Fluoxetine treatment of children and adolescents with Tourette's and obsessive compulsive disorders: preliminary clinical experience. *J Am Acad Child Adolesc Psychiatry*. 1990;29:45–48.

Riddle MA, King RA, Hardin MT, et al. Behavioral side effects of fluoxetine in children and adolescents. *J Child Adolesc Psychopharmacol*. 1990/1991;1:193–198.

Riddle MA, Nelson JC, Kleinman CS, et al. Sudden death in children receiving norpramin: a review of three reported cases and commentary. *J Am Acad Child Adolesc Psychiatry*. 1991;30:104–108.

Riddle MA, Scahill L, King RA, et al. Double-blind, crossover trial of fluoxetine and placebo in children and adolescents with obsessive-compulsive disorder. *J Am Acad Child Adolesc Psychiatry*. 1992;31:1062–1069.

Rifkin A, Quitkin F, Klein DF. Akinesia: a poorly recognized drug-induced extrapyramidal behavior disorder. *Arch Gen Psychiatry*. 1975;32:672–674.

Riggs PD, Leon SL, Mikulich SK, et al. An open trial of bupropion for ADHD in adolescents with substance use disorders and conduct disorder. *J Am Acad Child Adolesc Psychiatry*. 1998;37:1271–1278.

Risperdal [prescribing information]. Titusville, NJ: Janssen L.P.; 2007.

Risperdal [package insert]. Titusville, NJ: Janssen Pharmaceuticals, Inc; 2010.

Rivera-Calimlim L, Griesbach PH, Perlmutter R. Plasma chlorpromazine concentrations in children with behavioral disorders and mental illness. *Clin Pharmacol Ther*. 1979;26:114–121.

Rivera-Calimlim L, Nasrallah H, Strauss J, et al. Clinical response and plasma levels: effect of dose, dosage schedules, and drug interactions on plasma chlorpromazine levels. *Am J Psychiatry*. 1976;133:646–652.

Robb AS, Cueva JE, Sporn J, et al. Sertraline treatment of children and adolescents with posttraumatic stress disorder: a double-blind placebo-controlled trial. *J Child Adolesc Psychopharmacol*. 2010;20(6):463–471.

Roessner V, Schoenefeld K, Buse J, et al. Pharmacological treatment of tic disorders and Tourette syndrome. *Neuropharmacology*. 2012;68:143–149.

Rosenberg DR, Davanzo PA, Gershon S. *Pharmacotherapy for Child and Adolescent Psychiatric Disorders*. 2nd ed. New York, NY: Marcel Dekker, Inc; 2002.

Rosenberg DR, Holttum J, Gershon S. *Textbook of Pharmacotherapy for Child and Adolescent Psychiatric Disorders*. New York, NY: Brunner/Mazel; 1994.

Rosenberg DR, Johnson K, Sahl R. Evolving mania in an adolescent treated with low-dose fluoxetine. *J Child Adolesc Psychopharmacol*. 1992;2:299–306.

Rosenberg DR, Stewart CM, Fitzgerald KD, et al. Paroxetine open-label treatment of pediatric outpatients with obsessive-compulsive disorder. *J Am Acad Child Adolesc Psychiatry*. 1999;38:1180–1185.

Rosenbaum JF, Fava M, Hoog SL, et al. Selective serotonin reuptake inhibitor discontinuation syndrome: a randomized clinical trial. *Biol Psychiatry*. 1998;44:77–87.

Ross DC, Piggott LR. Clonazepam for OCD [letter]. *J Am Acad Child Adolesc Psychiatry*. 1993;32:470–471.

Rosse RB, Giese AA, Deutsch SI, et al. *Laboratory Diagnostic Testing in Psychiatry*. Washington, DC: American Psychiatric Press; 1989.

Rossenu S, Cleton A, Talluri K, et al. Evaluation of the pharmacokinetics of an extended-release formulation of paliperidone with an immediate-release formulation of risperidone. *Clin Pharm Ther*. 2007;81(suppl 1):S62.

Rossenu SAC, Rusch S, Janssens S, et al. Extended-release formulation of paliperidone shows dose proportional pharmacokinetics. Presented at: the American Association of Pharmaceutical Sciences Annual Meeting and Exposition; October 29–November 2, 2006; San Antonio, TX; 2006. Poster number: T3123.

Rudorfer MV, Potter WZ. Pharmacokinetics of antidepressants. In: Meltzer HY, ed. *Psychopharmacology: The Third Generation of Progress*. New York, NY: Raven Press; 1987:1353–1363.

Russo RM, Gururaj VJ, Allen JE. The effectiveness of diphenhydramine HCl in pediatric sleep disorders. *J Clin Pharmacol*. 1976;4:284–288.

Ryan ND. Heterocyclic antidepressants in children and adolescents. *J Child Adolesc Psychopharmacol*. 1990;1:21–31.

Ryan ND, Meyer V, Dachille S, et al. Lithium antidepressant augmentation in TCA-refractory depression in adolescents. *J Am Acad Child Adolesc Psychiatry*. 1988a;27:371–376.

Ryan ND, Puig-Antich J, Cooper T, et al. Imipramine in adolescent major depression: plasma level and clinical response. *Acta Psychiatr Scand*. 1986;73:275–288.

Ryan ND, Puig-Antich J, Rabinovich H, et al. MAOIs in adolescent major depression unresponsive to tricyclic antidepressants. *J Am Acad Child Adolesc Psychiatry*. 1988b;27:755–758.

Rynn M, Siqueland L, Rickels K. Placebo-controlled trial of sertraline in the treatment of children with generalized anxiety disorder. *Am J Psychiatry*. 2001;158:2008–2014.

Rynn M, Wagner KD, Donnelly C, et al. Long-term sertraline treatment of children and adolescents with major depressive disorder. *J Child Adolesc Psychopharmacol*. 2006;16(1–2):103–116.

Sabuncuoglu O, Ekinci O, Berkem M. Fluoxetine-induced sleep bruxism in an adolescent treated with buspirone: a case report. *Spec Care Dentist*. 2009;29(5): 215–217.

Safer D, Allen RP, Barr E. Depression of growth in hyperactive children on stimulant drugs. *N Engl J Med*. 1972;287:217–220.

Safer DJ, Krager M. A survey of medication treatment for hyperactive/inattentive students. *JAMA*. 1988;260:2256–2258.

Safer DJ, Zito JM. Treatment-emergent adverse events from selective serotonin reuptake inhibitors by age group: children versus adolescents. *J Child Adolesc Psychopharmacol*. 2006;16(1–2):159–169.

Saito E, Correll CU, Gallelli K, et al. A prospective study of hyperprolactinemia in children and adolescents treated with atypical antipsychotic agents. *J Child Adolesc Psychopharmacol*. 2004;14:350–358.

Sakarcan A, Thomas DB, O'Reilly KP, et al. Lithium-induced nephrotic syndrome in a young pediatric patient. *Pediatr Nephrol*. 2002;17(4):290–292.

Sakkas P, Davis JM, Han J, et al. Pharmacotherapy of NMS. *Psychiatr Ann*. 1991;21:157–164.

Salazar DE, Frackiewicz EJ, Dockens R. Pharmacokinetics and tolerability of buspirone during oral administration to children and adolescents with anxiety disorder and normal healthy adults. *J Clin Pharmacol*. 2001;41:1351–1358.

Sallee FR, DeVane CL, Ferrell RE. Fluoxetine-related death in a child with cytochrome P-450 2D6 genetic deficiency. *J Child Adolesc Psychopharmacol*. 2000a;10:27–34.

Sallee FR, Kurlan R, Goetz CG, et al. Ziprasidone treatment of children and adolescents with Tourette's syndrome: a pilot study. *J Am Acad Child Adolesc Psychiatry*. 2000b;39(3):292–299.

Sallee FR, Nesbitt L, Jackson C, et al. Relative efficacy of haloperidol and pimozide in children and adolescents with Tourette's disorder. *Am J Psychiatry*. 1997;154:1057–1062.

Sallee FR, Sethuraman G, Rock CM. Effects of pimozide on cognition in children with Tourette syndrome: interaction with comorbid attention deficit hyperactivity disorder. *Acta Psychiatr Scand*. 1994;90(1):4–9.

Salzman C. Benzodiazepine dependency: summary of the APA task force on benzodiazepines. *Psychopharmacol Bull*. 1990;26:61–62.

Saphris [package insert]. Whitehouse Station, NJ: Merck & Co, Inc; 2009.

Saraf KR, Klein DF, Gittelman-Klein R, et al. Imipramine side effects in children. *Psychopharmacologia (Berlin)*. 1974;37:265–274.

Saul RC. Nortriptyline in attention deficit disorder. *Clin Neuropharmacol*. 1985;8:382–384.

Scahill L, Chappell PB, Kim YS, et al. Guanfacine in the treatment of children with tic disorders and ADHD: a placebo-controlled study [Abstract, 40th Annual NCDEU meeting]. *J Child Adolesc Psychopharmacol*. 2000;10:250.

Scahill L, McCracken J, Mcdougle CJ, et al. Methodological issues in designing a multisite trial of risperidone in children and adolescents with autism. *J Child Adolesc Psychopharmacol*. 2001;11:377–388.

Scharko AM, Schumacher J. Prolonged QTc interval in a 14-year-old girl with escitalopram overdose. *J Child Adolesc Psychopharmacol*. 2008;18(3):297–298.

Schmidt MH, Trott G-E, Blanz B, et al. Clozapine medication in adolescents. In: Stefania CN, Rabavilas AD, Soldatos CR, eds. *Psychiatry: A World Perspective*. Vol 1. Proceedings of the Eighth World Congress of Psychiatry. Amsterdam, The Netherlands: Excerpta Medica; 1990:1100–1104.

Schooler N, Gharabawi G, Bossie C, et al. A virtual comparison of Paliperidone ER and oral Risperidone in patients with schizophrenia. Presented at: the 45th Annual Meeting of the American College of Neuropharmacology; December 3–7, 2006; Hollywood, FL; 2006.

Schooler NR, Kane JM. Research diagnoses for tardive dyskinesia. *Arch Gen Psychiatry*. 1982;38:486–487.

Schou M. Lithium: elimination rate, dosage, control, poisoning, goiter, mode of action. *Acta Psychiatr Scand*. 1969;207(suppl):49–59.

Schroeder JS, Mullin AV, Elliott GR, et al. Cardiovascular effects of desipramine in children. *J Am Acad Child Adolesc Psychiatry*. 1989;28:376–379.

Schumann A, Ewigman B. Can metformin undo weight gain induced by antipsychotics? *J Fam Pract*. 2008;57(8):526–530.

Scott LL. Iloperidone: in schizophrenia. *CNS Drugs*. 2009;23(10):867–880.

Shamseddeen W, Clarke G, Keller MB, et al. Adjunctive sleep medications and depression outcome in the treatment of serotonin-selective reuptake inhibitor resistant depression in adolescents study. *J Child Adolesc Psychopharmacol*. 2012;22(1):29–36.

Shapiro AK, Shapiro E. Controlled study of pimozide vs. placebo in Tourette's syndrome. *J Am Acad Child Psychiatry*. 1984;23:161–173.

Shapiro AK, Shapiro E. Do stimulants provoke, cause, or exacerbate tics and Tourette syndrome? *Compr Psychiatry*. 1981;22:265–273.

Shapiro AK, Shapiro E. Tic disorders. In: Kaplan HI, Sadock BJ, eds. *Comprehensive Textbook of Psychiatry*. 5th ed. Baltimore, MD: Williams & Wilkins; 1989:1865–1878.

Shapiro AK, Shapiro E, Eisenkraft GJ. Treatment of Gilles de la Tourette syndrome with pimozide. *Am J Psychiatry*. 1983;140:1183–1186.

Sharko AM. Selective serotonin reuptake inhibitor-induced sexual dysfunction in adolescents: a review. *J Am Acad Child Adolesc Psychiatry*. 2004;43:1071–1079.

Shea S, Turgay A, Carroll A, et al. Risperidone in the treatment of disruptive behavioral symptoms in children with autistic and other pervasive developmental disorders. *Pediatrics*. 2004;114(5):634–641.

Sheitman BB, Bird PM, Binz W, et al. Olanzapine-induced elevation of plasma triglyceride levels. *Am J Psychiatry*. 1999;156:1471–1472.

Shin L, Bregman H, Breeze J, et al. Metformin for weight control in pediatric patients on atypical antipsychotic medication. *J Child Adolesc Psychopharmacol*. 2009;3:275–279.

Shirazi E, Alaghband-Rad J. An open trial of citalopram in children and adolescents with depression. *J Child Adolesc Psychopharmacol*. 2005;15:233–239.

Shojaei AH, Rong-Kun C, Pennick M. Guanfacine extended release tablets as treatment for attention-deficit/hyperactivity disorder: formulation characteristics. Poster presented at: USPMH Congress; November 16, 2006; New Orleans, LA.

Sholevar EH, Baron DA, Hardie TL. Treatment of childhood-onset schizophrenia with olanzapine. *J Child Adolesc Psychopharmacol*. 2000;10:69–78.

Siefen G, Remschmidt H. Behandlungsergebnisse mit clozapin bei schizophrenen jugendlichen [Clozapine in the treatment of adolescents with schizophrenia: treatment outcome]. *Zeitschrift fur Kinder-und-Jugendpsychiatrie*. 1986;14:245–257. (English translation by the Ralph McElroy Co, provided by the manufacturer.)

Sikich L, Frazier JA, McClellan J, et al. Double-blind comparison of first- and second-generation antipsychotics in early-onset schizophrenia and schizoaffective disorder: findings from the Treatment of Early-Onset Schizophrenia Spectrum Disorders (TEOSS) study. *Am J Psychiatry*. 2008;165(11):1420–1431.

Silva RR. May-June 2012 update: psychopharmacology news and views. *J Child Adolesc Psychopharmacol*. 2012;22(3):249.

Silva RR, Muniz R, Pestreich L, et al. Efficacy and duration of effect of extended-release dexmethylphenidate versus placebo in schoolchildren with attention-deficit/hyperactivity disorder. *J Child Adolesc Psychopharmacol*. 2006;16:239–251.

Silva RR, Munoz DM, Alpert M. Carbamazepine use in children and adolescents with features of attention-deficit hyperactivity disorder: a meta-analysis. *J Am Acad Child Adolesc Psychiatry*. 1996;35:352–358.

Simeon JG, Carrey NJ, Wiggins DM, et al. Risperidone effects in treatment-resistant adolescents: preliminary case reports. *J Child Adolesc Psychopharmacol*. 1995;5:69–79.

Simeon JG, Dinicola VF, Ferguson HB, et al. Adolescent depression: a placebo-controlled fluoxetine treatment study and follow-up. *Prog Neuropsychopharmacol Biol Psychiatry*. 1990;14:791–795.

Simeon JG, Ferguson HB. Alprazolam effects in children with anxiety disorders. *Can J Psychiatry*. 1987;32:570–574.

Simeon JG, Ferguson HB. Recent developments in the use of antidepressant and anxiolytic medications. *Psychiatr Clin North Am*. 1985;8:893–907.

Simeon JG, Ferguson HB, Fleet JVW. Bupropion effects in attention deficit and conduct disorder. *Can J Psychiatry*. 1986;31:581–585.

Simeon JG, Ferguson HB, Knott V, et al. Clinical, cognitive, and neurophysiological effects of alprazolam in children and adolescents with overanxious and avoidant disorders. *J Am Acad Child Adolesc Psychiatry*. 1992;31:29–33.

Simeon JG, Knott VJ, DuBois C, et al. Buspirone therapy of mixed anxiety disorders in childhood and adolescence: a pilot study. *J Child Adolesc Psychopharmacol.* 1994;4:159–170.

Simon GE, Savarino J, Operskalski B, et al. Suicidal risk during antidepressant treatment. *Am J Psychiatry.* 2006;163:41–47.

Singer HS. Treatment of tics and Tourette syndrome. *Curr Treat Options Neurol.* 2010;12(6):539–561.

Sleator EK. Diagnosis. In: Sleator EK, Pelham WE Jr, eds. *Attention Deficit Disorder: Dialogues in Pediatric Management.* Vol 1, No 3. Norwalk, CT: Appleton-Century-Crofts; 1986:11–42.

Sleator EK, von Neumann A, Sprague RL. Hyperactive children: a continuous long-term placebo-controlled follow-up. *JAMA.* 1974;229:316–317.

Small JG, Milstein V, Marhenke JD, et al. Treatment outcome with clozapine in tardive dyskinesis, neuroleptic sensitivity, and treatment resistant psychosis. *J Clin Psychiatry.* 1987;48:263–267.

Smathers SA, Wilson JG, Nigro MA. Topiramate effectiveness in Prader-Willi syndrome. *Pediatr Neurol.* 2003;28(2):130–133.

Smith TC, Wollman H. History and principles of anaesthesiology. In: Gilman AF, Goodman LS, Rall TW, et al, eds. *Goodman and Gilman's The Pharmacological Basis of Therapeutics.* 7th ed. New York, NY: Macmillan; 1985:260–275.

Snyder R, Turgay A, Aman M, et al; and the Risperidone Conduct Study Group. Effects of risperidone on conduct and disruptive behavior disorders in children with subaverage IQs. *J Am Acad Child Adolesc Psychiatry.* 2002;41:1026–1036.

Sokol MS, Campbell M. Novel psychoactive agents in the treatment of developmental disorders. In: Aman MG, Singh NN, eds. *Psychopharmacology of the Developmental Disabilities.* New York, NY: Springer-Verlag; 1988:147–167.

Sondheimer AN, Klykylo WM. The Ethics Committees of the American Academy of Child and Adolescent Psychiatry and the American Psychiatric Association: history, process, education, and advocacy. *Child Adolesc Psychiatr Clin N Am.* 2008;17(1):225–236.

Soutullo CA, Casuto LS, Keck PE Jr. Gabapentin in the treatment of adolescent mania: a case report. *J Child Adolesc Psychopharmacol.* 1998;8(1):81–85.

Soutullo CA, Diez-Suarez A, Figueroa-Quintana A. Adjunctive lamotrigine treatment for adolescents with bipolar disorder: retrospective report of five cases. *J Child Adolesc Psychopharmacol.* 2006;16(3):357–364.

Spencer EK, Kafantaris V, Padron-Gayol MV, et al. Haloperidol in schizophrenic children: early findings from a study in progress. *Psychopharmacol Bull.* 1992;28:183–186.

Spencer T, Biederman J, Kerman K, et al. Desipramine treatment of children with attention-deficit hyperactivity disorder and tic disorder or Tourette's syndrome. *J Am Acad Child Adolesc Psychiatry.* 1993a;32:354–360.

Spencer T, Biederman J, Steingard R, et al. Bupropion exacerbates tics in children with attention-deficit hyperactivity disorder and Tourette's syndrome. *J Am Acad Child Adolesc Psychiatry.* 1993b;32:211–214.

Spencer T, Biederman J, Wilens T, et al. Nortriptyline treatment of children with attention-deficit hyperactivity disorder and tic disorder or Tourette's syndrome. *J Am Acad Child Adolesc Psychiatry.* 1993c;32:201–210.

Spitzer RL, Endicott J, Robins E. Research diagnostic criteria. *Arch Gen Psychiatry.* 1978;35:773–782.

Sprague RL, Sleator EK. Methylphenidate in hyperkinetic children: differences in dose effects on learning and social behavior. *Science.* 1977;198:1274–1276.

Stahl SM. *Essential Psychopharmacology: Neuroscientific Basis and Practical Applications.* 2nd ed. Cambridge, England: Cambridge; 2000.

Staller JA. Intramuscular ziprasidone in youth: a retrospective chart review. *J Child Adolesc Psychopharmacol.* 2004;14:590–592.

Staller JA, Kunwar A, Simionescu M. Oxcarbazepine in the treatment of child psychiatric disorders: a retrospective review. *J Child Adolesc Psychopharmacol.* 2005;15:964–969.

Stanley B. An integration of ethical and clinical considerations in the use of placebos. *Psychopharmacol Bull.* 1988;24:18–20.

Starr HL, Kemner J. Multicenter, randomized, open-label study of OROS methylphenidate versus atomoxetine: treatment outcomes in African-American children with ADHD. *J Natl Med Assoc.* 2005;97(10 suppl):11S–16S.

Steingard R, Biederman J, Spencer T, et al. Comparison of clonidine response in the treatment of attention-deficit hyperactivity disorder with and without comorbid tic disorders. *J Am Acad Child Adolesc Psychiatry.* 1993;32:350–353.

Steingard R, Khan A, Gonzales A, et al. Neuroleptic malignant syndrome: review of experience with children and adolescents. *J Child Adolesc Psychopharmacol.* 1992;2:183–198.

Stigler K, Erickson C, Mullet J, et al. Paliperidone for irritability in autistic disorder [letters to the editor]. *J Child Adolesc Psychopharmacol.* 2010;20(1):75–78.

Stoddard FJ, Luthra R, Sorrentina EA, et al. A randomized controlled trial of sertraline to prevent posttraumatic stress disorder in burned children. *J Child Adolesc Psychopharmacol.* 2011;21(5):469–477.

Strayhorn JM, Rapp N, Donina W, et al. Randomized trial of methylphenidate for an autistic child. *J Am Acad Child Adolesc Psychiatry.* 1988;27:244–247.

Strober M, Freeman R, Rigali J. The pharmacotherapy of depressive illness in adolescents: I, an open label trial of imipramine. *Psychopharmacol Bull.* 1990;26:80–84.

Strober M, Freeman R, Rigali J, et al. The pharmacotherapy of depressive illness in adolescents: II, effects of lithium augmentation in nonresponders to imipramine. *J Am Acad Child Adolesc Psychiatry.* 1992;31:16–20.

Sudden death in children treated with a tricyclic antidepressant. *Med Lett.* 1990;32:53.

Sussman N. The potential benefits of serotonin receptor-specific agents. *J Clin Psychiatry.* 1994a;55(suppl 1):45–51.

Sussman N. The uses of buspirone in psychiatry. *J Clin Psychiatry Monograph.* 1994b;12:3–19.

Sussman N, Ginsberg D. Valproate and risk of polycystic ovary syndrome. *Prim Psychiatry.* 1998;5:42–48.

Sverd J. Methylphenidate treatment for children with attention deficit hyperactivity disorder and tic disorder: inadvisable or indispensable? In: Greenhill LL, Osman BB, eds. *Ritalin: Theory and Practice.* 2nd ed. Larchmont, NY: Mary Ann Liebert, Inc; 2000:301–319.

Swanson J, Greenhill L, Pelham W, et al. Initiating Concerta (OROS methylphenidate HCl) qd in children with attention-deficit hyperactivity disorder. *J Clin Res.* 2000;3:59–76.

Swanson JM, Connor DF, Cantwell D. Combining methylphenidate and clonidine: ill-advised/and negative rebuttal (debate forum). *J Am Acad Child Adolesc Psychiatry.* 1999;38:614–622.

Swanson JM, Flockhart D, Udrea D, et al. Clonidine in the treatment of ADHD: questions about safety and efficacy [letter]. *J Child Adolesc Psychopharmacol.* 1995;5:301–304.

Swanson JM, Lerner M, Cantwell D. Blood levels and tolerance to stimulants in ADDH children. *Clin Neuropharmacol.* 1986;9(suppl 4):523–525.

Swanson JM, Lerner MA, Gupta S, et al. Development of a new once-a-day formulation of methylphenidate for the treatment of ADHD. *Arch Gen Psychiatry.* 2003;60:204–211.

Swanson JM, Wigal S, Greenhill LL, et al. Analog classroom assessment of Adderall in children with ADHD. *J Am Acad Child Adolesc Psychiatry.* 1998;37:519–526.

Szigethy E, Wiznitzer M, Branicky LA, et al. Risperidone-induced hepatotoxicity in children and adolescents? A chart review study. *J Child Adolesc Psychopharmacol.* 1999;9:93–98.

Tauscher-Wisniewski S, Nilsson M, Caldwell C, et al. Meta-analysis of aggression and/or hostility-related events in children and adolescents treated with fluoxetine compared with placebo. *J Child Adolesc Psychopharmacol.* 2007;17(5):713–718.

Taylor E, Schachar R, Thorley G, et al. Which boys respond to stimulant medication? A controlled trial of methylphenidate in boys with disruptive behavior. *Psychol Med.* 1987;17:121–143.

Teicher MH, Baldessarini RJ. Developmental pharmacodynamics. In: Popper C, ed. *Psychiatric Pharmacosciences of Children and Adolescents.* Washington, DC: American Psychiatric Press; 1987:45–80.

Teitelbaum M. Oxcarbazepine in bipolar disorder [letter]. *J Am Acad Child Adolesc Psychiatry.* 2001;40:993–994.

Thase ME, Kupfer DJ, Frank E, et al. Treatment of imipramine-resistant recurrent depression: II, an open clinical trial of lithium augmentation. *J Clin Psychiatry.* 1989;50:413–417.

Thompson PM, Vidal C, Giedd JN, et al. Mapping adolescent brain change reveals a dynamic wave of accelerated gray matter loss in very early-onset schizophrenia. *Proc Natl Acad Sci U S A.* 2001;98(20):11650–11655.

Thomsen PH. Child and adolescent obsessive-compulsive disorder treated with citalopram: findings from an open trial of 23 cases. *J Child Adolesc Psychopharmacol.* 1997;7:157–166.

Tierney E, Joshi PT, Llinas JF, et al. Sertraline for major depression in children and adolescents: preliminary clinical experience. *J Child Adolesc Psychopharmacol.* 1995;5:13–27.

Treatment for Adolescents with Depression Study (TADS) Team [March JS, Silva S, Petrycki S, et al]. Fluoxetine, cognitive-behavioral therapy, and their combination for adolescents with depression: treatment for adolescents with depression study (TADS) randomized controlled trial. *JAMA.* 2004;292:807–820.

Trivedi H, Chang K. *Psychopharmacology, an Issue of Child and Adolescent Psychiatric Clinics of North America.* Vol 21-4. Philadelphia, PA: WB Saunders; 2012.

Tsapakis EM, Soldani F, Tondo L, et al. Efficacy of antidepressants in juvenile depression: meta-analysis. *Br J Psychiatry.* 2008;193:10–17.

United States Pharmacopeial Dispensing Information (USPDI). *Drug Information for the Health Care Professional.* Rockville, MD: United States Pharmacopeial Convention; 1990.

United States Pharmacopeial Dispensing Information (USPDI). Thompson Healthcare, eds. *Drug Information for the Health Care Professional.* 25th ed, Vol 1. Greenwood Village, CO: Thomson MICROMEDEX; 2005.

Upadhyaya HP, Brady KT, Wang W. Bupropion SR in adolescents with comorbid ADHD and nicotine dependence: a pilot study. *J Am Acad Child Adolesc Psychiatry.* 2004;43:199–205.

US Food and Drug Administration. FDA statement regarding the anti-depressant paxil for pediatric population. *FDA Talk Paper.* 2003.

Usala T, Clavenna A, Zuddas A, et al. Randomised controlled trials of selective serotonin reuptake inhibitors in treating depression in children and adolescents: a systematic review and meta-analysis. *Eur Neuropsychopharmacol.* 2008;18(1):62–73.

Van Putten T, Marder SR. Behavioral toxicity of antipsychotic drugs. *J Clin Psychiatry.* 1987;48(suppl 9):13–19.

Van Putten T, May PRA, Marder SR. Akathisia with haloperidol and thiothixene. *Arch Gen Psychiatry.* 1984;41:1036–1039.

Varley CK, McClellan J. Case study: two additional sudden deaths with tricyclic antidepressants. *J Am Acad Child Adolesc Psychiatry.* 1997;36:390–394.

Veatch RM. *The Patient-Physician Relation: The Patient As Partner, Part 2*. Bloomington, IN: Indiana University Press; 1991.

Venkataraman S, Naylor MW, King CA. Mania associated with fluoxetine treatment in adolescents. *J Am Acad Child Adolesc Psychiatry*. 1992;31:276–281.

Vermeir M, Boom S, Naessens I, et al. Absorption, metabolism and excretion of a single oral dose of 14C-paliperidone 1 mg in healthy subjects. *Eur Neuropsychopharmacol*. 2005;30:S191–S192.

Vetro A, Szentistvanyi I, Pallag L, et al. Therapeutic experience with lithium in childhood aggressivity. *Pharmacopsychiatry*. 1985;14:121–127.

Villeneuve A. The rabbit syndrome: a peculiar extrapyramidal reaction. *Can Psychiatr Assoc J*. 1972;17:69–72.

Vincent J, Varley CK, Leger P. Effects of methylphenidate on early adolescent growth. *Am J Psychiatry*. 1990;147:501–502.

Vitiello B, Behar D, Malone R, et al. Pharmacokinetics of lithium carbonate in children. *J Clin Psychopharmacol*. 1988;8:355–359.

Vitiello B, Emslie G, Clarke G, et al. Long-term outcome of adolescent depression initially resistant to selective serotonin reuptake inhibitor treatment: a follow-up study of the TORDIA sample. *J Clin Psychiatry*. 2011;72(3):388–396.

Volavka J. The effects of clozapine on aggression and substance abuse in schizophrenic patients. *J Clin Psychiatry*. 1999;60(suppl 12):43–46.

Volkers AC, Heerdink ER, van Dijk L. Antidepressant use and off-label prescribing in children and adolescents in Dutch general practice (2001–2005). *Pharmacoepidemiol Drug Saf*. 2007;16(9):1054–1062.

Vyvanse [package insert]. Wayne, PA: Shire US Inc; 2007.

Wagner KD, Ambrosinie P, Rynn M, et al. Efficacy of sertraline in the treatment of children and adolescents with major depressive disorder two randomized controlled trials. *JAMA*. 2003;290:1033–1041.

Wagner KD, Arsarnow JR, Vitiello B, et al. Out of the black box: treatment of resistant depression in adolescents and the antidepressant controversy. *J Child Adolesc Psychopharmacol*. 2012;22(1):5–10.

Wagner KD, Berard R, Stein MB, et al. A multicenter, randomized, double-blind, placebo-controlled trial of paroxetine in children and adolescents with social anxiety disorder. *Arch Gen Psychiatry*. 2004a;61:1153–1162.

Wagner KD, Kowatch RA, Emslie GJ, et al. A double-blind, randomized, placebo-controlled trial of oxcarbazepine in the treatment of bipolar disorder in children and adolescents. *Am J Psychiatry*. 2006;163(7):1179–1186.

Wagner KD, Redden L, Kowatch R, et al. A double-blind, randomized, placebo-controlled trial of divalproex extended-release in the treatment of bipolar disorder in children and adolescents. *J Am Acad Child Adolesc Psychiatry*. 2009;48(5):519–532.

Wagner KD, Robb AS, Findling RL, et al. A randomized placebo-controlled trial of citalopram for the treatment of major depression in children and adolescents. *Am J Psychiatry*. 2004b;161(6):1079–1083.

Wagner KD, Weller E, Carlson G, et al. An open-label trial of divalproex in children and adolescents with bipolar disorder. *J Am Acad Child Adolesc Psychiatry*. 2002;41(10):1224–1230.

Waizer J, Hoffman SP, Polizos P, et al. Outpatient treatment of hyperactive school children with imipramine. *Am J Psychiatry*. 1974;131:587–591.

Walkup JT, Albano AM, Piacentini J, et al. Cognitive behavioral therapy, sertraline, or a combination in childhood anxiety. *N Engl J Med*. 2008;359:2753–2766.

Walkup JT, Labellarte MJ, Riddle MA, et al. Fluvoxamine for the treatment of anxiety disorders in children and adolescents. *N Engl J Med*. 2001;344:1279–1285.

Walsh BT, ed. *Child Psychopharmacology*. Washington, DC: American Psychiatric Press; 1998.

Walsh BT, Giardina E-GV, Sloan RP, et al. Effects of desipramine on autonomic control of the heart. *J Am Acad Child Adolesc Psychiatry*. 1994;33:191–197.

Walsh BT, Greenhill LL, Giardina E-GV, et al. Effects of desipramine on autonomic input to the heart. *J Am Acad Child Adolesc Psychiatry*. 1999;38:1186–1192.

Wang HD, Dunnavant FD, Jarman T, et al. Effects of antipsychotic drugs on neurogenesis in the forebrain of adult rat. *Neuropsychopharmacology*. 2004;29(7):1230–1238.

Ware JC, Pittard JT. Increased deep sleep after trazodone use: a double-blind placebo-controlled study in healthy young adults. *J Clin Psychiatry*. 1990;51:18–22.

Wechsler D. *Manual for the Wechsler Intelligence Scale for Children—Revised*. San Antonio, TX: The Psychological Corporation; 1974.

Wehmeier PM, Schacht A, Dittmann RW, et al. Effect of atomoxetine on quality of life and family burden: results from a randomized, placebo-controlled, double-blind study in children and adolescents with ADHD and comorbid oppositional defiant or conduct disorder. *Qual Life Res*. 2011;20(5):691–702.

Wehmeier PM, Schacht A, Dittmann RW, et al. Minor differences in ADHD-related difficulties between boys and girls treated with atomoxetine for attention-deficit/hyperactivity disorder. *Atten Defic Hyperact Disord*. 2010;2(2):73–85.

Wehmeier PM, Schacht A, Escobar R, et al. Differences between children and adolescents in treatment response to atomoxetine and the correlation between health-related quality of life and attention deficit/hyperactivity disorder core symptoms: meta-analysis of five atomoxetine trials. *Child Adolesc Psychiatry Ment Health*. 2010;4:30.

Weiden PJ. Switching antipsychotics as a treatment strategy for antipsychotic-induced weight gain and dyslipidemia. *J Clin Psychiatry*. 2007;68(suppl 4):34–39.

Weiner JM, Jaffe SL. Historical overview of childhood and adolescent psychopharmacology. In: Weiner JM, ed. *Diagnosis and Psychopharmacology of Childhood and Adolescent Disorders*. New York, NY: John Wiley; 1985:3–50.

Weiner N. Norepinephrine, epinephrine, and the sympathomimetic amines. In: Gilman AG, Goodman LS, Gilman A, eds. *Goodman and Gilman's The pharmacological Basis of Therapeutics*. 6th ed. New York, NY: Macmillan; 1980:138–175.

Weiss G, Hechtman LT. *Hyperactive Children Grown Up: Empirical Findings and Theoretical Considerations*. New York, NY: Guilford Press; 1986.

Weiss G, Kruger E, Danielson U, et al. Effect of long-term treatment of hyperactive children with methylphenidate. *Can Med Assoc J*. 1975;112:159–165.

Weiss M, Tannock R, Kratochvil C, et al. A randomized, placebo-controlled study of once-daily atomoxetine in the school setting in children with ADHD. *J Am Acad Child Adolesc Psychiatry*. 2005;44(7):647–655.

Weizman A, Weitz R, Szekely GA, et al. Combination of neuroleptic and stimulant treatment in attention deficit disorder with hyperactivity. *J Am Acad Child Psychiatry*. 1984;23:295–298.

Weller EB, Weller RA, Fristad MA. Lithium dosage guide for prepubertal children: a preliminary report. *J Am Acad Child Psychiatry*. 1986;25:92–95.

Weller EB, Weller RA, Preskorn SH, et al. Steady-state plasma imipramine levels in prepubertal depressed children. *Am J Psychiatry*. 1982;139:506–508.

Wender PH. Attention deficit hyperactivity disorder. In: Howells JG, ed. *Modern Perspectives in Clinical Psychiatry*. New York, NY: Brunner/Mazel; 1988:149–169.

Wernicke JF. The side effect profile and safety of fluoxetine. *J Clin Psychiatry*. 1985;46:59–67.

Werry J, Aman M. Methylphenidate and haloperidol in children: effects on attention, memory, and activity. *Arch Gen Psychiatry*. 1975;32:790–795.

Werry J, Aman MG, Diamond E. Imipramine and methylphenidate in hyperactive children. *J Child Psychol Psychiatry*. 1980;21:27–35.

Werry J, Weiss G, Douglas V, et al. Studies on the hyperactive child III: the effects of chlorpromazine upon behavior and learning ability. *J Am Acad Child Psychiatry*. 1966;5:292–312.

Werry JS. The safety of desipramine [letter]. *J Am Acad Child Adolesc Psychiatry*. 1994;33:588–589.

Werry JS, ed. *Pediatric Psychopharmacology: The Use of Behavior Modifying Drugs in Children*. New York, NY: Brunner/Mazel; 1978.

Werry JS, Aman MG, eds. *Practitioner's Guide to Psychoactive Drugs for Children and Adolescents*. 2nd ed. New York, NY: Plenum Medical Book; 1999.

West L, Brunssen S, Waldrop J. Review of the evidence for treatment of children with autism with selective serotonin reuptake inhibitors. *J Spec Pediatr Nurs*. 2009;14:183–191.

Whalen CK, Henker B, Swanson JM, et al. Natural social behaviors in hyperactive children: dose effects of methylphenidate. *J Consult Clin Psychol*. 1987;55:187–193.

White L, Tursky B, Schwartz GE, eds. *Placebo: Theory, Research, and Mechanisms*. New York, NY: Guilford Press; 1985.

Wigal S, Swanson JM, Feifel D, et al. A double-blind, placebo-controlled trial of dexmethylphenidate hydrochloride and *d, l-threo*-methylphenidate hydrochloride in children with attention-deficit/hyperactivity disorder. *J Am Acad Child Adolesc Psychiatry*. 2004;43:1406–1414.

Wigal SB, McGough JJ, McCracken JT, et al. A laboratory school comparison of mixed amphetamine salts extended release (Adderall XR) and atomoxetine (Strattera) in school-aged children with attention deficit/hyperactivity disorder. *J Atten Disord*. 2005;9(1):275–289.

Wilens T, McBurnett K, Stein M, et al. ADHD treatment with once-daily OROS methylphenidate: final results from a long-term open-label study. *J Am Acad Child Adolesc Psychiatry*. 2005;44:1015–1023.

Wilens TE, Biederman J, Baldessarini RJ, et al. Developmental changes in serum concentrations of desipramine and 2-hydroxydesipramine during treatment with desipramine. *J Am Acad Child Adolesc Psychiatry*. 1992;31:691–698.

Wilens TE, Biederman J, Baldessarini RJ, et al. Electrocardiographic effects of desipramine and 2-hydroxydesipramine in children, adolescents, and adults treated with desipramine. *J Am Acad Child Adolesc Psychiatry*. 1993a;32:798–804.

Wilens TE, Biederman J, Geist DE, et al. Nortriptyline in the treatment of ADHD: a chart review of 58 cases. *J Am Acad Child Adolesc Psychiatry*. 1993b;32:343–349.

Wilens TE, Biederman J, March JS, et al. Absence of cardiovascular adverse effects of sertraline in children and adolescents. *J Am Acad Child Adolesc Psychiatry*. 1999;38:573–577.

Wilens TE, Biederman J, Spencer T. Clonidine for sleep disturbances associated with attention-deficit hyperactivity disorder. *J Am Acad Child Adolesc Psychiatry*. 1994;33:424–426.

Wilens TE, Spencer TJ. Combining methylphenidate and clonidine: a clinically sound medication option/and affirmative rebuttal [Debate Forum]. *J Am Acad Child Adolesc Psychiatry*. 1999;38:614–622.

Wilens TE, Spencer TJ. The stimulants revisited. *Child Adolesc Psychiatr Clin N Am*. 2000;9:573–603.

Williams DT, Mehl R, Yudofsky S, et al. The effect of propranolol on uncontrolled rage outbursts in children and adolescents with organic brain dysfunction. *J Am Acad Child Psychiatry*. 1982;21:129–135.

Winsberg BG, Kupietz SS, Sverd J, et al. Methylphenidate oral dose plasma concentrations and behavioral response in children. *Psychopharmacology*. 1982;76:329–332.

Wolf DV, Wagner KD. Tardive dyskinesia, tardive dystonia, and tardive Tourette's syndrome in children and adolescents. *J Child Adolesc Psychopharmacol*. 1993;3:175–198.

Woolston J. Case study: carbamazepine treatment of juvenile-onset bipolar disorder. *J Am Acad Child Adolesc Psychiatry*. 1999;38:335–338.

Wozniak J, Mick E, Waxmonsky J, et al. Comparison of open-label 8-week trials of olanzapine monotherapy and topiramate augmentation of olanzapine for the treatment of pediatric bipolar disorder. *J Child Adolesc Psychopharmacol.* 2009;19(5):539–545.

Wu R-R, Zhao J-P, Jin H, et al. Lifestyle intervention and metformin for treatment of antipsychotic-induced weight gain: a randomized controlled trial. *JAMA.* 2008;299:185–193.

Wudarsky M, Nicolson R, Hamburger SD, et al. Elevated prolactin in pediatric patients on typical and atypical antipsychotics. *J Child Adolesc Psychopharmacol.* 1999;9:239–245.

Wysowski DK, Barash D. Adverse behavioral reactions attributed to triazolam in the Food and Drug Administration's spontaneous reporting system. *Arch Intern Med.* 1991;151:2003–2008.

Yepes LE, Balka EB, Winsberg BG, et al. Amitriptyline and methylphenidate treatment of behaviorally disordered children. *J Child Psychol Psychiatry.* 1977;18:39–52.

Zametkin A, Rapoport JL, Murphy DL, et al. Treatment of hyperactive children with monoamine oxidase inhibitors: I, clinical efficacy. *Arch Gen Psychiatry.* 1985;42:962–966.

Zametkin AJ, Rapoport JL. Noradrenergic hypothesis of attention deficit disorder with hyperactivity: a critical review. In: Meltzer HY, ed. *Psychopharmacology: The Third Generation of Progress.* New York, NY: Raven Press; 1987:837–842.

Zrull JP, Westman JC, Arthur B, et al. A comparison of chlordiazepoxide, d-amphetamine, and placebo in the treatment of the hyperkinetic syndrome in children. *Am J Psychiatry.* 1963;120:590–591.

Zrull JP, Westman JC, Arthur B, et al. A comparison of diazepam, d-amphetamine, and placebo in the treatment of the hyperkinetic syndrome in children. *Am J Psychiatry.* 1964;121:388–389.

Zubieta JK, Alessi NE. Acute and chronic administration of trazodone in the treatment of disruptive behavior disorders in children. *J Clin Psychopharmacol.* 1992;12:346–351.

Zubieta JK, Bueller JA, Jackson LR, et al. Placebo effects mediated by endogenous opioid activity on μ-opioid receptors. *J Neurosci.* 2005;25(34):7754–7762.

Zuckerman ML, Vaughan BL, Whitney J, et al. Tolerability of selective serotonin reuptake inhibitors in thirty-nine children under age seven: a retrospective chart review. *J Child Adolesc Psychopharmacol.* 2007;17(2):165–174.

Zwier KJ, Rao U. Buspirone use in an adolescent with social phobia and mixed personality disorder (cluster A type). *J Am Acad Child Adolesc Psychiatry.* 1994;33:1007–1011.

Zyprexa [package insert]. Indianapolis, IN: Lilly USA, LLC; 2011.

Index

Note: Page numbers followed by *t* indicate tables.